DEPRESSION

Primers On Psychiatry

Stephen M. Strakowski, MD, Series Editor

DEPRESSION

Edited by
Madhukar H. Trivedi, MD
University of Texas Southwestern Medical Center

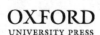
OXFORD
UNIVERSITY PRESS

Oxford University Press is a department of the University of Oxford. It furthers
the University's objective of excellence in research, scholarship, and education
by publishing worldwide. Oxford is a registered trade mark of Oxford University
Press in the UK and certain other countries.

Published in the United States of America by Oxford University Press
198 Madison Avenue, New York, NY 10016, United States of America.

Library of Congress Control Number: 2019949817
ISBN 978–0–19–092956–5

This material is not intended to be, and should not be considered, a substitute for medical or other professional
advice. Treatment for the conditions described in this material is highly dependent on the individual
circumstances. And, while this material is designed to offer accurate information with respect to the subject
matter covered and to be current as of the time it was written, research and knowledge about medical and
health issues is constantly evolving and dose schedules for medications are being revised continually, with
new side effects recognized and accounted for regularly. Readers must therefore always check the product
information and clinical procedures with the most up-to-date published product information and data sheets
provided by the manufacturers and the most recent codes of conduct and safety regulation. The publisher
and the authors make no representations or warranties to readers, express or implied, as to the accuracy
or completeness of this material. Without limiting the foregoing, the publisher and the authors make no
representations or warranties as to the accuracy or efficacy of the drug dosages mentioned in the material.
The authors and the publisher do not accept, and expressly disclaim, any responsibility for any liability,
loss or risk that may be claimed or incurred as a consequence of the use and/or application of any of the
contents of this material.

9 8 7 6 5 4 3 2 1

Printed by Marquis, Canada

CONTENTS

FOREWORD

Dear Reader,

Thank you for purchasing this primer on depression. For this volume, Dr. Madhukar H. Trivedi, as editor, recruited leading experts in depressive disorders from around the world to provide early stage practitioners with current evidence about the etiology and pathophysiology of these conditions, common comorbidities and differential diagnoses, pharmacotherapy strategies, psychotherapeutic and neuromodulation interventions, novel and nontraditional treatment strategies, and considerations in special populations. Major depression is one of the most common causes of disability worldwide, so we hope the information provided here will guide practitioners as they manage this common problem. We believe you will find this book exceptionally informative and helpful to you in your work.

This volume is part of the Oxford University Press "Primer On" series; I have been honored to lead this series since 2016 and was particularly pleased to join an already successful venture. The "Primer On" series has been designed specifically to support psychiatry residents, early stage practicing psychiatrists, psychology graduate students, and other interested medical trainees and practitioners. Specifically, in this series we have asked international experts to create books that focus on a specific set of conditions to provide the basic science and clinical tools to diagnose, treat, and manage these major psychiatric disorders. We have expanded the scope of the series to provide information and guidance about major aspects of mental health care practices. With these considerations in mind, each volume is written with an eye toward early stage practitioners to present current evidence and recommendations in a format that is user-friendly and informative. These texts complement other resources, such as the Oxford American Psychiatry Library, by offering more comprehensive basic and clinical knowledge so that psychiatric and other trainees can better understand these disorders in ways that will prepare them for clinical practice and fellowships (and to take board exams). As they are released, each volume will be available in print, e-book, and Oxford Medicine Online (http://oxfordmedicine. com/). We have aimed to make these affordable books that bridge handbooks and more lengthy and expensive highly specialized textbooks. I hope you enjoy this text!

Best wishes,

Steve Strakowski, MD
Associate Vice President, Regional Mental Health
Dell Medical School, University of Texas at Austin
Series Editor

CONTRIBUTORS

David Benrimoh, MD
McGill Group for Suicide Studies
Department of Psychiatry
McGill University
Montreal, Quebec, Canada

John P. Coetzee, PhD
Postdoctoral Scholar
Department of Psychiatry and
    Behavioral Sciences
Stanford University School of Medicine
Health Fellow
Division of Polytrauma
Veteran's Health Administration
Palo Alto, CA, USA

Callan M. Coghlan, BA
Research Specialist
Department of Psychiatry and
    Behavioral Sciences
Emory University School of Medicine
Atlanta, GA, USA

Evan Collins, MD, FRCPC
Assistant Professor
Department of Psychiatry
University of Toronto
Toronto, Canada

C. Munro Cullum, PhD, ABPP
Professor of Psychiatry, Neurology, and
    Neurosurgery
Department of Psychiatry
University of Texas Southwestern
    Medical Center
Dallas, TX, USA

Andrew H. Czysz, MD, PhD
Center for Depression Research and
    Clinical Care
Department of Psychiatry
University of Texas Southwestern
    Medical Center
Dallas, TX, USA

Sabrina C. da Costa, MD
Department of Psychiatry
Yale University School of Medicine
Addiction Psychiatry Program
New Haven, CT, USA
Department of Psychiatry and
    Behavioral Sciences
McGovern Medical School
University of Texas Health Science
    Center at Houston
Houston, TX, USA

Sylvanne Daniels, PhD
McGill Group for Suicide Studies
Department of Psychiatry
McGill University
Montreal, Quebec, Canada

Brett Davis, BA
Semel Institute for Neuroscience
    and Behavior
David Geffen School of Medicine
University of California
    Los Angeles
Los Angeles, California

Lori L. Davis, MD
Department of Psychiatry and
    Behavioral Neurobiology
University of Alabama
    at Birmingham
Birmingham, AL
Research and Development Service
Tuscaloosa VA Medical Center
Tuscaloosa, AL

Zhi-De Deng, PhD
Director, Computational
    Neurostimulation Research
    Program Noninvasive
    Neuromodulation Unit
Experimental Therapeutics and
    Pathophysiology Branch
National Institute of Mental
    Health
Bethesda, MD, USA

Andrew Diederich, MD
Assistant Professor
Child and Adolescent Division
University of Texas Southwestern
    Department of Psychiatry
University of Texas Southwestern
    Medical Center
Dallas, TX, USA

Steven C. Dufour, BA
Department of Psychiatry
Massachusetts General Hospital
Boston, MA, USA

Graham J. Emslie, MD
Professor
Department of Psychiatry
University of Texas Southwestern
    Medical Center
Dallas, TX, USA

Maurizio Fava, MD
Director
Division of Clinical Research/MGH
    Research Institute
Massachusetts General Hospital
Boston, MA, USA

Bharathi S. Gadad, PhD
Assistant Professor
Department of Psychiatry
Texas Tech University Health
    Science Center
El Paso, TX, USA
Center for Depression Research
    and Clinical Care, Department of
    Psychiatry, University of Texas
    Southwestern Medical Center
Dallas, TX, USA

Tracy L. Greer, PhD, MSCS
Center for Depression Research and
    Clinical Care
Department of Psychiatry
University of Texas Southwestern
    Medical Center
Dallas, TX, USA

Thorhildur Halldorsdottir, PhD
Centre of Public Health Sciences
Faculty of Medicine
University of Iceland
Reykjavik, Iceland
Department of Translational Research
   in Psychiatry
Max Planck Institute of Psychiatry
Munich, Germany

David J. Hellerstein, MD
Professor of Clinical Psychiatry
Department of Psychiatry
Columbia University Irving
   Medical Center
New York, NY, USA

Ioline D. Henter, MA
Technical Publications Writer
Section on the Neurobiology and
   Treatment of Mood Disorders
Intramural Research Program, National
   Institute of Mental Health
Bethesda, MD, USA

Steven D. Hollon, PhD
Gertrude Conway Vanderbilt Professor
Department of Psychology
Vanderbilt University
Nashville, TN, USA

Jennifer L. Hughes, PhD, MPH
Center for Depression Research and
   Clinical Care
Department of Psychiatry
University of Texas Southwestern
   Medical Center
Dallas, TX, USA

Sonia Israel
McGill Group for Suicide Studies
Department of Psychiatry
McGill University Douglas Mental
   Health University Institute
Montreal, Quebec, Canada

Jessica A. Janos, BA
Department of Psychology and
   Neuroscience
University of North Carolina
Chapel Hill, NC

Manish K. Jha, MBBS
Department of Psychiatry
Icahn School of Medicine at
   Mount Sinai
New York, NY, USA

Jessica M. Jones, MA
Research Scientist
Department of Psychiatry
University of Texas Southwestern
   Medical Center
Dallas, TX, USA

Bashkim Kadriu, MD
Clinical Fellow
National Institute of Mental Health
National Institutes of Health
Bethesda, MD, USA

Farra Kahalnik, MSSW, MPH
Department of Psychiatry
Center for Depression Research and
   Clinical Care
University of Texas Southwestern
   Medical Center
Dallas, TX, USA

Alexander Kane, MD
Assistant Professor of Clinical
   Psychiatry
Weill Cornell Medical College
Assistant Inpatient Attending
NewYork-Presbyterian Hospital
New York, NY, USA

Jordan F. Karp, MD
Department of Psychiatry
University of Pittsburgh School of
   Medicine
Pittsburgh, PA, USA

Robert S. Kinney, BSc
McGill Group for Suicide Studies
Department of Psychiatry
McGill University
Montreal, Quebec, Canada

Emily B. Kroska
Department of Psychiatry
University of Wisconsin Madison
Madison, WI

Raymond W. Lam, MD, FRCPC
Professor and BC Leadership Chair in
    Depression Research
Department of Psychiatry
University of British Columbia
Vancouver, BC, Canada

Eric J. Lenze, MD
Wallace and Lucille K. Renard
    Professor of Psychiatry
Department of Psychiatry
Washington University School of
    Medicine
St. Louis, MO, USA

Julio Licinio, MD, PhD, MBA
Professor of Psychiatry, Pharmacology,
    Medicine, and Neuroscience &
    Physiology, College of Medicine
SUNY Upstate Medical University
Syracuse, NY, USA

Rajnish Mago, MD
Editor-in-Chief
Simple and Practical Mental Health
Clinical Assistant Professor of
    Psychiatry, Perelman School of
    Medicine, University of Pennsylvania
Philadelphia, PA, USA

Brittany L. Mason, PhD
Assistant Professor
Department of Psychiatry
University of Texas Southwestern
    Medical Center
Dallas, TX, USA

Taryn L. Mayes, MS
University of Texas Southwestern
    Medical Center
Dallas, TX, USA

Catherine Munro, PhD
Professor of Psychiatry, Neurology, and
    Neurosurgery
Department of Psychiatry
University of Texas Southwestern
    Medical Center
Dallas, TX, USA

Hanadi Ajam Oughli, MD
Healthy Mind Lab
Department of Psychiatry
Washington University in Saint Louis
    School of Medicine
St. Louis, MO, USA

George I. Papakostas, MD
Clinical Trials Network and Institute
Massachusetts General Hospital
Harvard Medical School
Boston, MA, USA

Lawrence T. Park, MD
Director
Experimental Therapeutics and
    Pathophysiology Branch
National Institute of Mental Health
Bethesda, MD, USA

Nikita Patel, BS, Psych
Department of Psychiatry
University of Wisconsin Madison
Madison, WI

Seth W. Perry, PhD
Associate Professor of Psychiatry, and
 Neuroscience & Physiology
Department of Psychiatry
SUNY Upstate Medical University
Syracuse, NY, USA

Patricia Pilkinton, MD
Department of Psychiatry and
 Behavioral Medicine
University Medical Center, University
 of Alabama
Tuscaloosa, AL
Research and Development Service
Tuscaloosa VA Medical Center
Tuscaloosa, AL

Radu Pop, PhD
Department of Psychiatry, Center
 for Depression Research and
 Clinical Care
University of Texas Southwestern
 Medical Center
Dallas, TX, USA

Chad D. Rethorst, PhD
Center for Depression Research and
 Clinical Care
Department of Psychiatry
University of Texas Southwestern
 Medical Center
Dallas, TX, USA

Barbara O. Rothbaum, PhD, ABPP
Professor in Psychiatry
Department of Psychiatry and
 Behavioral Sciences
Emory University School of Medicine
Atlanta, GA, USA

Naji C. Salloum, MD
Clinical Trials Network and Institute
Massachusetts General Hospital,
 Harvard Medical School
Boston, MA, USA

Marsal Sanches, MD, PhD
Associate Professor
Department of Psychiatry and
 Behavioral Sciences
McGovern Medical School
Houston, TX, USA

Eduardo J. Sanchez, MD, MPH
Chief Medical Officer for Prevention
Chief, Center for Health Metrics and
 Evaluation
American Heart Association
Dallas, TX, USA

Katherine Sanchez, PhD, LCSW
Associate Professor
School of Social Work
The University of Texas at Arlington
Arlington, TX, USA

Zindel Segal, PhD, CPsych
Departments of Psychological Clinical
 Science and Psychiatry
University of Toronto
Toronto, Ontario, Canada

Bonnie Seifert, BS
Project Coordinator and Data
 Information Specialist
Department of Psychiatry and
 Behavioral Sciences
Emory University School of Medicine
Atlanta, GA, USA

Jair C. Soares, MD, PhD
Professor and Chairman Pat
 R. Rutherford Chair in Psychiatry
Department of Psychiatry and
 Behavioral Sciences
Executive Director, UT Harris County
 Psychiatric Center Director, UT
 Center of Excellence on Mood
 Disorders UTHealth School of
 Medicine
Houston, TX, USA

Zachary N. Stowe
Department of Psychiatry
University of Wisconsin Madison
Madison, WI

Subha Subramanian, MD
Section on the Neurobiology and
    Treatment of Mood Disorders
Intramural Research Program, National
    Institute of Mental Health
Bethesda, MD, USA

Louisa G. Sylvia, PhD
Department of Psychiatry
Massachusetts General Hospital
Department of Psychiatry
Harvard Medical School
Boston, MA, USA

Madhukar H. Trivedi, MD
Professor of Psychiatry; Director,
    Center for Depression Research
    and Clinical Care; Betty Jo Hay
    Distinguished Chair in Mental
    Health; Julie K. Hersh Chair
    for Depression Research and
    Clinical Care
Department of Psychiatry
University of Texas Southwestern
    Medical Center
Dallas, TX, USA

Gustavo Turecki, MD, PhD
Professor
Department of Psychiatry
McGill University
Montreal, Quebec, Canada

Nolan Williams, MD
Assistant Professor
Director, Interventional Psychiatry
    Clinical Research
Director, Brain Stimulation Laboratory
Department of Psychiatry and
    Behavioral Sciences
Stanford University Medical Center
Palo Alto, CA, USA

Ma-Li Wong, MD, PhD
Professor of Psychiatry, and
    Neuroscience & Physiology
College of Medicine, SUNY Upstate
    Medical University
Syracuse, NY, USA

Carly Yasinski, PhD
Assistant Professor
Department of Psychiatry and
    Behavioral Sciences
Emory University School of Medicine
Atlanta, GA, USA

Hildur Ýr Hilmarsdottir, BS
Centre of Public Health Sciences
Faculty of Medicine
University of Iceland
Reykjavik, Iceland

Carlos A. Zarate Jr., MD
Chief Experimental Therapeutics &
    Pathophysiology Branch & Section
    Neurobiology and Treatment of Mood
    Disorders
Division of Intramural Research
    Program
National Institute of Mental Health
Bethesda, MD, USA

DEPRESSION

/// 1 /// PRIMER ON DEPRESSION

Introduction and Overview

MADHUKAR H. TRIVEDI, TRACY L. GREER, AND TARYN L. MAYES

1.1. HISTORY AND CHARACTERISTICS OF DEPRESSION

Depression has been discussed in philosophy, literature, and medicine for hundreds of years, including early descriptions in Greek culture of "melancholia" with associated symptoms resulting from an overproduction of "black bile." Early conceptualizations of mental illness were thought of as separate from medical science, corresponding to early views on dualism and the distinction of the mind–body connection. The compilation of symptoms associated with depression began to take the form of diagnostic categories in the late 19th century (Kendler and Engstrom 2017), stemming largely from the concepts of "manic depressive insanity," and its evolution to "depressive states" proposed by Emil Kraepelin (Kraepelin 1921; Trede, Salvatore et al. 2005; Zivanovic and Nedic 2012; Kendler and Engstrom 2017). Categorical and diagnostic definitions have evolved over the years, but there has been significant stability in the core symptoms that have been used (Kendler and Engstrom 2017).

1.1.1. Defining Depression

The *Diagnostic and Statistical Manual of Mental Disorders*, fifth edition (DSM-5) (American Psychiatric Association 2013) characterizes a major depressive episode (MDE) by the presence of five or more symptoms. One of these must include diminished interest or pleasure in activities, or sad or depressed mood, and the rest must include changes in weight/appetite, sleep, arousal, and/or fatigue/energy; feelings of worthlessness/guilt; diminished ability to think, concentrate, or make decisions; and suicidal thoughts or actions (Table 1.1). Of note, symptom presentations may vary

TABLE 1.1. Symptoms of an MDE

- Depressed mood most of the day (**Note**: In children and adolescents, can be irritable mood)
- Diminished interest or pleasure in activities most of the day
- Significant changes in appetite or weight **(Note:** In children, consider failure to make expected weight gains)
- Insomnia or hypersomnia
- Psychomotor agitation or retardation
- Fatigue or loss of energy
- Feelings of worthlessness or guilt
- Diminished ability to concentrate, or indecisiveness
- Recurrent thoughts of death, suicidal ideation or without a specific plan, or a suicide attempt

Symptoms are present most days.

Patient A Symptom Presentation	Patient B Symptom Presentation
Depressed mood	Decreased interest in most activities
Reduced appetite	Increased appetite
Psychomotor agitation	Psychomotor retardation
Insomnia	Hypersomnia
Difficulty concentrating	Fatigue
Feelings of worthlessness	Thoughts of suicide

dramatically from one individual to the next, as evidenced by two common symptom presentations outlined in Table 1.1. In addition, DSM-5 has several diagnoses related to depression, including major depressive disorder (MDD), persistent depressive disorder (previously dysthymia), premenstrual dysphoric disorder, depressive disorder due to another medical condition, and other specified depressive disorder (previously depression not otherwise specified [NOS]) (Box 1.1). For an MDE, symptoms must be present most of the time over at least a two-week period, be associated with impairments in daily life and functioning, and not be attributed better to another medical condition or substance use. Of particular importance, depression is quite heterogeneous—it is possible for individuals with completely non-overlapping symptoms to both have a diagnosis of depression. This heterogeneity is a significant contributor to the variability in treatment response, and a major focus of recent research endeavors to identify biologically based subtypes.

Symptom-based subtypes have been used to identify more homogenous groups of depressed patients for some time and include melancholic, atypical, psychotic, and catatonic subtypes. These subtypes are included as specifiers in the DSM-5, along with newer specifiers: anxious distress, mixed features, seasonal pattern, and peripartum onset (see Lam, McIntosh et al. 2016 for a nice synthesis of this information). Additional proposed subtypes have been developed throughout the years,

BOX 1.1.

DEPRESSIVE ILLNESS DIAGNOSTIC CATEGORIES

MAJOR DEPRESSIVE DISORDER (MDD)

A. Five (or more) symptoms of an MDE (see Table 1.1); symptoms last for a minimum of two weeks, and represent a change from previous functioning; at least one of the symptoms must be either depressed mood or loss of interest or pleasure.

B. Symptoms cause significant distress or impairment in functioning.

C. The episode is not attributable to substances or a medical condition.

D. The MDE is not better explained by a psychotic disorder.

E. There has never been a manic episode or a hypomanic episode.

Specifiers:

With anxious distress
With mixed features
With melancholic features
With atypical features
With mood-congruent psychotic features
With mood-incongruent psychotic features
With peripartum onset
With seasonal pattern

PERSISTENT DEPRESSIVE DISORDER

A. Depressed mood for most of the day, for more days than not, for at least 2 years. (Note: In children and adolescents, duration must be at least 1 year, and mood can be irritable)

B. While depressed, also has two (or more) of the following:
   1) Changes in appetite
   2) Insomnia or hypersomnia
   3) Fatigue or loss of energy
   4) Low self-esteem
   5) Poor concentration or indecisiveness
   6) Feelings of hopelessness

C. During the 2-year period (1 year for children or adolescents), the person has never been without the symptoms in Criteria A and B for more than 2 months at a time.

D. Criteria for a major depressive disorder may be continuously present for 2 years.

E. There has never been a manic episode or a hypomanic episode, and criteria have never been met for cyclothymic disorder.

F. The disturbance is not better explained by a psychotic disorder.

G. The symptoms are not attributed to the physiological effects of a substance or medical condition.

H. The symptoms cause significant distress or impairment in functioning.

PREMENSTRUAL DYSPHORIC DISORDER (PMDD)

A. At least five symptoms (from below categories B and C) are present in the final week before the onset of menses in the majority of menstrual cycles; in addition, these symptoms start to improve within a few days after the onset of menses, becoming minimal or absent following menses.

B. One (or more) of the following symptoms must be present:

1) Affective lability (e.g. mood swings; sudden sadness or tearfulness; sensitivity to rejection)

2) Marked irritability, anger, or increased interpersonal conflicts

3) Marked depressed mood; feelings of hopelessness; self-deprecating thoughts

4) Marked anxiety, tension, or feeling keyed up or on edge

C. One (or more) of the following symptoms must also be present, totaling at least five symptoms, when combined with symptoms from criterion B above.

1) Decreased interest in usual activities (e.g. work, school, friends and hobbies)

2) Difficulty in concentration

3) Lack of energy

4) Changes in appetite or specific food cravings

5) Insomnia or hypersomnia

6) A sense of being overwhelmed or out of control.

7) Physical symptoms (e.g. breast tenderness or swelling, joint or muscle pain, feeling bloated or having weight gain)

The symptoms in criteria A–C must be present for most menstrual cycles in the preceding year.

D. The symptoms cause significant distress or impairment in functioning.

E. The disturbance is not an exacerbation of another disorder, such as MDD, persistent depressive disorder, panic disorder, or personality disorder; however, PMDD may co-occur with any of these disorders.

F. Criterion A should be confirmed by daily ratings for at least two symptomatic cycles. (Note: The diagnosis may be made provisionally prior to this confirmation).

G. The symptoms are not attributed to the physiological effects of a substance, medical condition, or treatment for another medical condition.

DEPRESSIVE DISORDER DUE TO ANOTHER MEDICAL CONDITION

A. Persistent depressed mood or markedly diminished interest or pleasure in activities

B. There is evidence that the disturbance is a direct pathophysiological consequence of another medical condition.

C. The disturbance is not better explained by another mental disorder (e.g. adjustment disorder, with depressed mood, where the medical condition is the stressor).

D. The disturbance does not occur exclusively during delirium.

E. The symptoms cause significant distress or impairment in functioning.

OTHER SPECIFIED DEPRESSIVE DISORDER

This category applies to depressive disorder symptoms that cause significant distress or impairment functioning, but that do not meet the full criteria for any specific depressive disorders. The following categories may be used to define "Other Specified Depressive Disorder":

1. **Recurrent brief depression:** Presence of depressed mood and at least four other symptoms of a MDE, lasting only 2–13 days at least once per month (and not associated with the menstrual cycle) for at least 12 consecutive months; the symptoms have never met criteria for any other depressive or bipolar disorder, or active or residual criteria for any psychotic disorder.

2. **Short-duration depressive disorder (4–13 days):** Depressed mood and at least four other symptoms of a MDE, and symptoms persists for more than 4 days, but less than 14 days; symptoms cause significant distress or impairment; the symptoms have never met criteria for any other depressive or bipolar disorder, active or residual criteria for any psychotic disorder, or recurrent brief depression.

3. **Depressive episode with insufficient symptoms:** Depressed mood and at least one other symptom of a MDE, with significant distress or impairment; symptoms persist for at least two weeks; symptoms have never met criteria for any other depressive or bipolar disorder, active or residual criteria for any psychotic disorder, or mixed anxiety and depressive disorders.

with vascular depression being perhaps one of the most important. The concept of vascular depression developed in recognition of vascular alterations in brain circuits known to regulate affect (Krishnan and McDonald 1995; Alexopoulos, Meyers et al. 1997) and speaks to the comorbidity between vascular disease and depression. The definition and utility of this subtype has been variably supported, but the vascular depression concept illustrates the complexity and bidirectional nature of the relationship between vascular disease and depression, and it also highlights the need to examine potential underlying factors, such as inflammation, that are associated with both disease processes (Baldwin 2005).

In addition, depression often presents concurrently with other conditions. In a large study of 1,500 adults with MDD, 52.8% reported a concurrent medical condition (Yates, Mitchell et al. 2004). Chapters 9 and 10 provide additional details about the interplay of depression and comorbid medical conditions. Depression also commonly presents with comorbid psychiatric conditions. In 2012–2013, the National Epidemiological Survey on Alcohol and Related Conditions III study was conducted, with over 36,000 adults participating in the survey. MDD was associated with psychiatric conditions ranging from an adjusted odds ratio (aOR) of 2.1 (95% confidence interval [CI], 1.84–2.35) for specific phobia to an aOR of 5.7 (95% CI, 4.98–6.50) for generalized anxiety disorder. Substance use disorders were also common, ranging from an aOR of 1.8 (95% CI, 1.63–2.01) for alcohol use disorder to an aOR of 3.0 (95% CI, 2.57–3.55) for any drug (Hasin, Sarvet et al. 2018).

1.1.2. Course of Depression

Depression often begins early in life and is often chronic, both of which significantly increase burden. Definitions for terminology related to depression course were initially defined by Frank (Frank, Prien et al. 1991; Kupfer 1991). In clinical trials, *response* is usually defined as a specified level of improvement in symptoms, typically using a measure of clinical global improvement or change in depressive severity. *Remission* is defined as minimal or no remaining depressive symptomatology, often defined using a cutoff on a clinical depression rating scale. *Recovery* refers to a more extended period of time (i.e., at least two months) of remitted symptoms. *Relapse* is referred to as a return of symptoms within a treated episode, while *recurrence* is a return of symptoms after someone is identified as having recovered from his or her index episode.

There is quite a bit of variability in illness course, but most studies show that the mean length of episode duration is 12 to 22 weeks (Solomon, Keller et al. 1997; Kessler, Berglund et al. 2003; Eaton, Shao et al. 2008; Hasin, Sarvet et al. 2018). In a 13-year follow-up study, about 15% of individuals with depression never recovered (Eaton et al., 2008). Unfortunately, after symptom remission or recovery, recurrence is common, with over half experiencing a relapse or recurrence of symptoms, and most recurrences occur within 6 to 12 months after recovery (Solomon, Keller et al. 2000).

1.1.3. Prevalence and Burden

Data from the National Epidemiologic Survey on Alcoholism and Related Conditions III, which are based on over 36,000 in-person interviews within US households, estimate the 12-month and lifetime prevalence of MDD as 10.4% and 20.6%, respectively, with 12-month and lifetime prevalence of 13.4% and 26.1% among women and 7.2% and 14.7% among men (Hasin, Sarvet et al. 2018). In addition to gender differences, being of African American or Asian/Pacific Islander race or of Hispanic ethnicity (compared to white adults) was associated with lower odds of MDD within a 12-month period, whereas younger age (18–29 years) or lower income ($19,999 or less) was associated with higher odds (Hasin, Sarvet et al. 2018). Depression is often comorbid with other chronic health conditions, including anxiety and substance disorders, diabetes, cardiovascular disease, and cancer.

Depression has detrimental effects on all aspects of social functioning (e.g., self-care, social role, and family life, including household, marital, kinship, and parental roles). Furthermore, depression is one of the leading chronic illnesses contributing to disability (GBD 2015 DALYs and HALE Collaborators 2016; World Health Organization 2018), costing the United States over $200 billion per year in direct and indirect costs (Greenberg, Fournier et al. 2015). Specifically, the annual cost of depression (approximately $210.5 billion in 2010) includes 45% in direct medical costs (e.g., diagnosis, treatments, and overall cost to the community), 5% in suicide-related mortality costs, and 50% in workplace costs (Greenberg, Fournier et al. 2015). Depression substantially impairs work productivity, increasing work absence and reducing work performance. Depressed workers report significantly more total health-related lost productive time than nondepressed workers (mean 5.6 hours/week vs. expected 1.5 hours/week) (Stewart, Ricci et al. 2003). In a study examining the impact of many medical and psychiatric conditions on work productivity, depression had the largest effect on work performance of any individual condition examined (Kessler, White et al. 2008). However, recovery from depression is associated with reduced lost time from work and improved productivity (Simon, Chisholm et al. 2002; Jha, Minhajuddin et al. 2016).

1.1.4. Functional Impairments

Much of the burden associated with depression relates to impaired functioning. Impairments are seen across a broad range of life domains, including family, occupational, and social life. Importantly, aspects of depression, such as cognitive impairments that are not sufficiently captured in current diagnostic criteria, are increasingly being recognized as having a significant impact on disease course and quality of life. While assessment of symptom changes over time is critical during treatment, it is equally important to assess functional outcomes. In fact, patients report that functional improvements are as important or even more important than the reduction of symptoms (Zimmerman, McGlinchey et al. 2006). Furthermore, even when remission of symptoms is achieved, there are frequently residual symptoms, which may be depressive symptoms or associated symptoms that affect functioning. In a study of duloxetine, Sheehan, Harnett-Sheehan et al. (2011) reported that 38%

of participants reached remission of depressive symptoms and 32% achieved functional remission, but only 23% achieved both.

1.2. MEASUREMENT OF DEPRESSIVE SYMPTOMS

For many years, clinical evaluation of depression relied predominantly on an interview and discussion with the patient, sometimes including input from a significant other or family member. Symptom severity scales were developed to assist with quantification of symptoms and to facilitate a common metric for evaluation of symptom types and severity, as well as to monitor changes in symptoms over time. Hamilton (1960) developed the commonly used Hamilton Rating Scale for Depression (HRSD) to incorporate the type, frequency, and intensity of individual symptoms, with an intended use of quantifying the results of clinical interview in individuals already diagnosed with depression. Measurements evolved to be more sensitive to treatment change (e.g., the Montgomery–Åsberg Depression Rating Scale [MADRS]; Montgomery 1979), and later evolutions of symptom severity scales began to focus on the need to use measurements to screen for depression (e.g., the Patient Health Questionnaire–9; Kroenke, Spitzer et al. 2001), as well as to encompass a broader array of related symptoms (e.g., the Inventory for Depressive Symptomatology [IDS]; Rush et al., 1986, 1996). Clinical research endeavors began to use scales as a metric of treatment success, with the common metric of treatment response being a reduction in symptom severity of 50% or more.

Beyond the initial assessment, it is crucial to continue measuring changes in symptoms. Measurement-based care is defined as basing clinical decisions on patient symptoms and functioning throughout treatment (Trivedi and Daly 2007). As a result, measurement-based care is increasingly employed in clinical settings, and symptom severity scales are useful tools in evaluating treatment response. A list of commonly used symptom severity scales is presented in Table 1.2.

1.3. TREATMENT OF DEPRESSION

Currently, there are a wide variety of treatment approaches employed for depression, including antidepressants and psychotherapeutic interventions. Yet many people do not receive any treatment, and more are inadequately treated, with clinicians changing medications too quickly or not quickly enough (Rush, Crismon et al. 2003). In acute (six- to eight-week) treatment studies, typically with relatively uncomplicated, non-chronic forms of MDD, response rates (e.g., 50% or greater reduction in depressive symptoms) range between 45% and 55%. However, remission rates are low (around 30–35%) with first-line interventions (Trivedi, Rush et al. 2006). Furthermore, almost one-third show minimal or no improvement (Sackeim 2001; Corey-Lisle, Nash et al. 2004). Unfortunately, non-remission leads to poorer outcomes, with increased psychosocial impairment and risk of relapse (Paykel, Ramana et al. 1995; Judd, Paulus et al. 2000). Similarly, the efficacy of psychotherapy for the treatment of

TABLE 1.2. Common Symptom Rating Scales

Rating Scale	Rater	Source	Scoring Cutoff
Hamilton Rating Scale for Depression (HRSD)	Clinician-rated	Hamilton, M. (1960). "A rating scale for depression." J Neurol Neurosurg Psychiatry **23**: 56–62.	0–7: normal 8–16: mild depression 17–23: moderate depression ≥23: severe depression (based on 17-item HRSD)
Beck Depression Inventory (BDI-II)	Self-report	Beck, A. T., C. H. Ward, M. Mendelson, J. Mock and J. Erbaugh (1961). "An inventory for measuring depression." Arch Gen Psychiatry **4**: 561–571.	0–13: minimal depression 14–19: mild depression 20–28: moderate depression 29–63: severe depression
Montgomery–Åsberg Depression Rating Scale (MADRS)	Clinician-rated	Montgomery, S. A., and M. Åsberg (1979). "A new depression scale designed to be sensitive to change." Br J Psychiatry **134**(4): 382–389.	0–6: normal 7–19: mild depression 20–34: moderate depression >34: severe depression
Patient Health Questionnaire (PHQ-9)	Self-report	Kroenke, K., and R. Spitzer (2002). "The PHQ-9: a new depression diagnostic and severity measure." Psychiatric Annals **32**(9): 509–515.	1–4: none 5–9: mild depression 10–14: moderate depression 15–19: moderately severe depression 20–27: severe depression
Inventory of Depressive Symptomatology (IDS)	Self-report and clinician rating	Rush, A. J., D. E. Giles, M. A. Schlesser, C. L. Fulton, J. Weissenburger, and C. Burns (1986). "The Inventory for Depressive Symptomatology (IDS): preliminary findings." Psychiatry Res **18**: 65–87.	28 items scored on a 0–3 scale; higher scores indicate worse depressive symptoms

(continued)

TABLE 1.2. Continued

Rating Scale	Rater	Source	Scoring Cutoff
Quick Inventory of Depressive Symptomatology (QIDS)	Self-report and clinician rating	Rush, A. J., M. H. Trivedi, H. M. Ibrahim, T. J. Carmody, B. Arnow, D. N. Klein, J. C. Markowitz, P. T. Ninan, S. Kornstein, R. Manber, M. E. Thase, J. H. Kocsis and M. B. Keller (2003). "The 16-Item Quick Inventory of Depressive Symptomatology (QIDS), clinician rating (QIDS-C), and self-report (QIDS-SR): a psychometric evaluation in patients with chronic major depression." Biol Psychiatry **54**: 573–583.	1–5: no depression 6–10: mild depression 11–15: moderate depression 16–20: severe depression 21–27: very severe depression
Mood and Feelings Questionnaire	Self-report	Angold, A., E. J. Costello, S. C. Messer, A. Pickles, F. Winder and D. Silver (1995). "The development of a short questionnaire for use in epidemiological studies of depression in children and adolescents." Int J Methods Psychiatr Res **5**: 237–249.	Short version: Range 0–26 Scores ≥12 indicate the presence of depression. Long version: Range 0–66 Scores ≥27 indicate the presence of depression.

depression has been found to be modest, with small effect sizes comparable to those of standard antidepressants (Cuijpers, van Straten et al. 2010). Although the combination of antidepressants and psychotherapy appears to be somewhat more efficacious than either one approach alone, the efficacy of this combination treatment remains limited (Cuijpers, Dekker et al. 2009; Cuijpers, van Straten et al. 2010). Clearly, more research is sorely needed to help improve outcomes for millions of patients with depression worldwide.

1.4. MOVING TOWARD A PRECISION MEDICINE APPROACH FOR UNDERSTANDING AND TREATING DEPRESSION

It has become increasingly recognized that a multifaceted approach to understanding and treating depression is needed. With the development and expansion of technological tools to allow us to better understand biomarkers of depression, we have gained a wealth of knowledge in recent years regarding fluid-based, brain-based, and cognitive changes associated with disease development, course, and treatment response. However, this field is still in its early stages, with current efforts focused on how such data may be integrated to better characterize depressive subtypes and predictors of treatment response. This book provides an introduction to the etiology and pathophysiology of depression, common comorbidities and differential diagnoses, pharmacotherapy strategies, psychotherapeutic and neuromodulation interventions, novel and nontraditional treatment strategies, and considerations in special populations.

REFERENCES

Alexopoulos, G. S., B. S. Meyers, R. C. Young, S. Campbell, D. Silbersweig, and M. Charlson (1997). "'Vascular depression' hypothesis." Arch Gen Psychiatry **54**: 915–922.

American Psychiatric Association (2013). *Diagnostic and statistical manual of mental disorders*, 5th ed. Washington, D.C.: American Psychiatric Association.

Baldwin, R. C. (2005). "Is vascular depression a distinct sub-type of depressive disorder? A review of causal evidence." Int J Geriatr Psychiatry **20**(1): 1–11.

Corey-Lisle, P. K., R. Nash, P. Stang and R. Swindle (2004). "Response, partial response, and nonresponse in primary care treatment of depression." Arch Intern Med **164**(11): 1197–1204.

Cuijpers, P., A. van Straten, E. Bohlmeijer, S. D. Hollon and G. Andersson (2010). "The effects of psychotherapy for adult depression are overestimated: a meta-analysis of study quality and effect size." Psychol Med **40**(2): 211–223.

Cuijpers, P., A. van Straten, S. D. Hollon and G. Andersson (2010). "The contribution of active medication to combined treatments of psychotherapy and pharmacotherapy for adult depression: a meta-analysis." Acta Psychiatr Scand **121**(6): 415–423.

Cuijpers, P., J. Dekker, S. D. Hollon and G. Andersson (2009). "Adding psychotherapy to pharmacotherapy in the treatment of depressive disorders in adults: a meta-analysis." J Clin Psychiatry **70**(9): 1219–1229.

Eaton, W. W., H. Shao, G. Nestadt, H. B. Lee, O. J. Bienvenu and P. Zandi (2008). "Population-based study of first onset and chronicity in major depressive disorder." Arch Gen Psychiatry **65**(5): 513–520.

Frank, E., R. F. Prien, R. B. Jarrett, M. B. Keller, D. J. Kupfer, P. W. Lavori, A. J. Rush and M. M. Weissman (1991). "Conceptualization and rationale for consensus definitions of terms in major depressive disorder. Remission, recovery, relapse, and recurrence." Arch Gen Psychiatry 48(9): 851–855.

GBD 2015 DALYs and HALE Collaborators (2016). "Global, regional, and national disability-adjusted life-years (DALYs) for 315 diseases and injuries and healthy life expectancy (HALE), 1990-2015: a systematic analysis for the Global Burden of Disease Study 2015." Lancet 388(10053): 1603–1658.

Greenberg, P. E., A. A. Fournier, T. Sisitsky, C. T. Pike and R. C. Kessler (2015). "The economic burden of adults with major depressive disorder in the United States (2005 and 2010)." J Clin Psychiatry 76(2): 155–162.

Hamilton, M. (1960). "A rating scale for depression." J Neurol Neurosurg Psychiatry 23: 56–62.

Hasin, D. S., A. L. Sarvet, J. L. Meyers, T. D. Saha, W. J. Ruan, M. Stohl and B. F. Grant (2018). "Epidemiology of adult DSM-5 major depressive disorder and its specifiers in the United States." JAMA Psychiatry 75(4): 336–346.

Jha, M. K., A. Minhajuddin, T. L. Greer, T. Carmody, A. J. Rush and M. H. Trivedi (2016). "Early improvement in work productivity predicts future clinical course in depressed outpatients: findings from the CO-MED trial." Am J Psychiatry 173(12): 1196–1204.

Judd, L. L., M. J. Paulus, P. J. Schettler, H. S. Akiskal, J. Endicott, A. C. Leon, J. D. Maser, T. Mueller, D. A. Solomon and M. B. Keller (2000). "Does incomplete recovery from first lifetime major depressive episode herald a chronic course of illness?" Am J Psychiatry 157(9): 1501–1504.

Kendler, K. S. and E. J. Engstrom (2017). "Kahlbaum, Hecker, and Kraepelin and the transition from psychiatric symptom complexes to empirical disease forms." Am J Psychiatry 174(2): 102–109.

Kessler, R. C., P. Berglund, O. Demler, R. Jin, D. Koretz, K. R. Merikangas, A. J. Rush, E. E. Walters, P. S. Wang and National Comorbidity Survey Replication (2003). "The epidemiology of major depressive disorder: results from the National Comorbidity Survey Replication (NCS-R)." JAMA 289(23): 3095–3105.

Kessler, R., L. A. White, H. Birnbaum, Y. Qiu, Y. Kidolezi, D. Mallett and R. Swindle (2008). "Comparative and interactive effects of depression relative to other health problems on work performance in the workforce of a large employer." J Occup Environ Med 50(7): 809–816.

Kraepelin, E. (1921). Manic-Depressive Insanity and Paranoia. Edinburgh: E&S, Livingstone.

Krishnan, K. R. and W. M. McDonald (1995). "Arteriosclerotic depression." Med Hypotheses 44(2): 111–115.

Kroenke, K., R. L. Spitzer and J. B. Williams (2001). "The PHQ-9: validity of a brief depression severity measure." J Gen Intern Med 16(9): 606–613.

Kupfer, D. J. (1991). "Long-term treatment of depression." J Clin Psychiatry 52 (Suppl): 28–34.

Lam, R. W., D. McIntosh, J. Wang, M. W. Enns, T. Kolivakis, E. E. Michalak, J. Sareen, W. Y. Song, S. H. Kennedy, G. M. MacQueen, R. V. Milev, S. V. Parikh, and A. V. Ravindran; CANMAT Depression Work Group. (2016). "Canadian Network for Mood and Anxiety Treatments (CANMAT) 2016 clinical guidelines for the management of adults with major depressive disorder: section 1: disease burden and principles of care." Can J Psychiatry 61(9): 510–523.

Montgomery, S. M. (1979). "Depressive symptoms in acute schizophrenia." Prog Neuropsychopharmacol 3(4): 429–433.

Paykel, E. S., R. Ramana, Z. Cooper, H. Hayhurst, J. Kerr and A. Barocka (1995). "Residual symptoms after partial remission: an important outcome in depression." Psychol Med 25(6): 1171–1180.

Rush, A. J., M. L. Crismon, T. M. Kashner, M. G. Toprac, T. J. Carmody, M. H. Trivedi, T. Suppes, A. L. Miller, M. M. Biggs, K. Shores-Wilson, B. P. Witte, S. P. Shon, W. V. Rago,

K. Z. Altshuler and T. R. Group (2003). "Texas Medication Algorithm Project, phase 3 (TMAP-3): rationale and study design." J Clin Psychiatry **64**(4): 357–369.

Rush, A. J., D. E. Giles, M. A. Schlesser, et al. (1986). "The Inventory for Depressive Symptomatology (IDS): preliminary findings." Psychiatry Res **18**: 65–87.

Rush, A. J., C. M. Gullion, M. R. Basco, et al. (1996). "The Inventory of Depressive Symptomatology (IDS): psychometric properties." Psychol Med **26**: 477–486.

Sackeim, H. A. (2001). "The definition and meaning of treatment-resistant depression." J Clin Psychiatry **62** (Suppl 16): 10–17.

Sheehan, D. V., K. Harnett-Sheehan, M. E. Spann, H. F. Thompson and A. Prakash (2011). "Assessing remission in major depressive disorder and generalized anxiety disorder clinical trials with the Discan metric of the Sheehan Disability Scale." Int Clin Psychopharmacol **26**(2): 75–83.

Simon, G. E., D. Chisholm, M. Treglia, D. Bushnell and LIDO Group (2002). "Course of depression, health services costs, and work productivity in an international primary care study." Gen Hosp Psychiatry **24**(5): 328–335.

Solomon, D. A., M. B. Keller, A. C. Leon, T. I. Mueller, P. W. Lavori, M. T. Shea, W. Coryell, M. Warshaw, C. Turvey, J. D. Maser and J. Endicott (2000). "Multiple recurrences of major depressive disorder." Am J Psychiatry **157**(2): 229–233.

Solomon, D. A., M. B. Keller, A. C. Leon, T. I. Mueller, M. T. Shea, M. Warshaw, J. D. Maser, W. Coryell and J. Endicott (1997). "Recovery from major depression: A 10-year prospective follow-up across multiple episodes." Arch Gen Psychiatry **54**(11): 1001–1006.

Stewart, W. F., J. A. Ricci, E. Chee, S. R. Hahn and D. Morganstein (2003). "Cost of lost productive work time among US workers with depression." JAMA **289**(23): 3135–3144.

Trede, K., P. Salvatore, C. Baethge, A. Gerhard, C. Maggini and R. J. Baldessarini (2005). "Manic-depressive illness: evolution in Kraepelin's textbook, 1883–1926." Harv Rev Psychiatry **13**(3): 155–178.

Trivedi, M. H., and E. J. Daly (2007). "Measurement-based care for refractory depression: a clinical decision support model for clinical research and practice." Drug Alcohol Depend **88** (Suppl 2): S61–S71.

Trivedi, M. H., A. J. Rush, S. R. Wisniewski, A. A. Nierenberg, D. Warden, L. Ritz, G. Norquist, R. H. Howland, B. Lebowitz, P. J. McGrath, K. Shores-Wilson, M. M. Biggs, G. K. Balasubramani, M. Fava and STAR*D Study Team (2006). "Evaluation of outcomes with citalopram for depression using measurement-based care in STAR*D: implications for clinical practice." Am J Psychiatry **163**(1): 28–40.

World Health Organization (2018). "Depression." http://www.who.int/news-room/fact-sheets/detail/depression.

Yates, W. R., J. Mitchell, A. J. Rush, M. H. Trivedi, S. R. Wisniewski, D. Warden, R. B. Hauger, M. Fava, B. N. Gaynes, M. M. Husain and C. Bryan (2004). "Clinical features of depressed outpatients with and without co-occurring general medical conditions in STAR*D." Gen Hosp Psychiatry **26**(6): 421–429.

Zimmerman, M., J. B. McGlinchey, M. A. Posternak, M. Friedman, N. Attiullah and D. Boerescu (2006). "How should remission from depression be defined? The depressed patient's perspective." Am J Psychiatry **163**(1): 148–150.

Zivanovic, O., and A. Nedic. (2012). "Kraepelin's concept of manic-depressive insanity: one hundred years later." J Affect Disord **137**(1-3):15–24.

Etiology/Pathophysiology of Depression

/// 2 /// NEUROBIOLOGY

SONIA ISRAEL, DAVID BENRIMOH,
SYLVANNE DANIELS, AND GUSTAVO TURECKI

2.1. HISTORICAL NOTE: THE MONOAMINE HYPOTHESIS

For many years, depression was thought to be caused exclusively by chemical imbalances of monoamine neurotransmitters, particularly serotonin and catecholamines (i.e., norepinephrine, dopamine). Much of this hypothesis was based initially on work from the 1950s investigating reserpine,[1] an antihypertensive agent that depletes presynaptic storage of monoamines and was found to cause depression in a proportion of hypertensive patients. Around the same time, iproniazid, a monoamine oxidase inhibitor (MAOI) used to treat tuberculosis,[1] was found to have antidepressant properties. Since then, a large number of studies have focused on monoamines in depression, and many effective antidepressant drugs have been developed, most of which act at monoaminergic neurons and their synapses. Despite their utility, monoaminergic antidepressants do not always work.[2,3] Increasing monoamine release and/or activity is not directly associated with antidepressant effects, as indicated by the fact that monoamine antidepressants typically have a delayed therapeutic onset of several weeks.[4] Newer findings suggest that the monoaminergic system may be only one of multiple interacting contributors to depression (see Figure 2.1).

2.2. NEUROTRANSMITTERS IN DEPRESSION

2.2.1. Serotonin

Serotonin (also known as 5-hydroxytryptophan [5-HT]) is a monoamine neurotransmitter produced in the raphe nuclei of the brainstem.[5] These serotonergic neurons

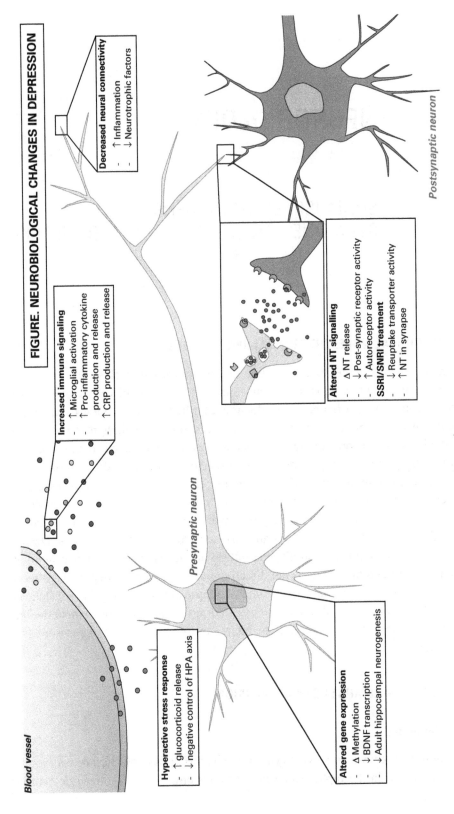

FIGURE 2.1. The diverse neurobiological changes that occur in depression.

send projections to many brain areas involved in depression, including the limbic areas,[6] frontal cortex, amygdala, and hippocampus.[5] Serotonin is implicated in many brain functions that can be impaired in depression, including mood, sleep, pain, and memory.[5] Due to multiple distinct serotonin receptor subtypes, the effects of serotonin can differ depending on the receptor stimulated.[3,5] Many monoaminergic antidepressants, however, act primarily or exclusively on serotonin reuptake, such as selective serotonin reuptake inhibitors (SSRIs).

Much evidence suggests serotonergic changes in depression. In addition to the fact that most antidepressants act on serotonergic receptors, neuroimaging studies demonstrate reduced global serotonin binding to 5-HT1A receptors in depressed patients[7] (which can persist even after patients are medicated[8]), and postmortem brain studies reveal abnormalities of the serotonergic system in depressed individuals.[9] In addition, studies on cerebrospinal fluid (CSF) of depressed suicidal patients and on brainstem tissue of individuals who died by suicide found decreased levels of 5-hydroxyindoleacetic acid (5-HIAA), a serotonin metabolite.[10,11]

But what is the significance of these serotonergic abnormalities? One possible answer is that some people may have a "serotonergic vulnerability" to developing depression when stressed.[11–13] This notion is supported by a meta-analysis showing that tryptophan depletion can trigger depressive symptoms in individuals with a history of depression.[14] Such a vulnerability could partially explain the high relapse rates seen in depression. Interestingly, a much-investigated polymorphism in the serotonin transporter gene—linked to anxiety and greater amygdalar response to fearful stimuli—is associated with increased vulnerability to stress during development.[13,15] Normal serotonin functioning therefore seems important for resilience to stress in addition to healthy cognitive and emotional processing.

2.2.2. Norepinephrine

Norepinephrine is produced in the locus coeruleus, which innervates brain areas that are believed to be important in depression, including the amygdala, hippocampus, and frontal cortex.[16] Decreased norepinephrine levels have been related to low energy, reduced attention and arousal, and depressed mood.[16,17] Noradrenergic agents may be more effective in patients with severe fatigue and lack of arousal.[17,18]

Findings from both animal and human studies posit a role for norepinephrine in the pathogenesis and treatment of depression. In animal models, decreased norepinephrine is associated with depression-like symptoms, including learned helplessness,[17] and mice lacking the norepinephrine reuptake transporter are more resilient toward stress.[19] Depleting norepinephrine causes relapse in patients recently recovered from depression, but not in healthy controls.[16] Postmortem brain studies of unmedicated depressed individuals who died by suicide showed increased expression of α2 and β1 adrenoceptors compared to controls, indicating a possible role of norepinephrine deficiency in depression.[20]

Several established antidepressants target norepinephrine in part, such as sero-tonin and norepinephrine reuptake inhibitors (SNRIs) and tricyclic antidepressants (TCAs). Blockade of norepinephrine reuptake using these agents allows for increased binding to α and β adrenoceptors, which may mediate antidepressant effects.[16] Evidence also suggests that α1 and α2 receptor agonists improve working memory and attention,[21] both of which can be impaired in depression. Despite this, specifically targeting the norepinephrine pathway has not been a promising avenue, since reboxetine, an SNRI, has been shown to be overall ineffective in relieving the symptoms of depression.[22]

2.2.3. Dopamine

Changes in dopamine levels are associated with anhedonia, psychomotor re-tardation, and loss of motivation, as seen in depression.[23–25] Dopaminergic neurons project from the ventral tegmental area and substantia nigra to areas associated with depression, such as the limbic system and frontal cortex.[25,26] Animal studies have supported the role of dopamine in the pathophysiology of depression, with reports of altered mesolimbic dopaminergic function in an-imal models of depression,[27] and decreased motor function and motivation in animals following inhibition of dopamine release.[28] In some cases, pretreatment with dopaminergic agents protects animals against the development of learned helplessness.[25] In humans, depression is often present in Parkinson's disease, where dopamine is significantly decreased,[25,29] and patients with depression who have attempted suicide have reduced levels of dopamine metabolites in their CSF.[25,30] Unmedicated depressed patients have decreased binding at stri-atal D1 dopamine receptors, as seen by positron emission tomography (PET) imaging.[31]

Dopamine receptor antagonists can cause relapse in patients previously treated for depression, whereas dopamine receptor agonists and reuptake inhibitors can alleviate depression.[30] For example, the antidepressant bupropion, which works at least partially by blocking the dopamine transporter (DAT) in the basal gan-glia, is effective,[32,33] though it also inhibits norepinephrine reuptake. Similarly, MAOIs (e.g., selegiline, phenelzine) increase catecholamine activity in the syn-aptic cleft.[25]

It remains unclear which dopamine receptors are most important in the path-ogenesis and treatment of depression. Anhedonia may be linked to altered dopa-mine function, potentially through reduced D2 and D3 receptor sensitivity in limbic areas.[27,34,35] Conversely, electroconvulsive therapy and antidepressant treatment upregulate the expression of D3 messenger RNA in the nucleus accumbens.[36] These results imply that several members of the dopamine receptor family may be impor-tant in the pathophysiology and treatment of depression.

2.2.4. Other Neurotransmitters

Additional neurotransmitters may also be involved in the pathophysiology of depression. Glutamate is the major excitatory neurotransmitter in the brain and is thought to mediate many of the cognitive and emotional functions that are also affected by the monoamines described earlier in the chapter.[37] In mood-disordered patients, glutamatergic alterations have been reported in CSF, brain tissue, and plasma and on imaging studies; however, no clear pattern has yet emerged regarding glutamate dysregulation.[37] The "glutamate theory" of depression has been bolstered by recent evidence of rapid relief of depression by N-methyl-D-aspartate (NMDA) receptor antagonists like ketamine.[38] Glutamate has a role in neurogenesis and plasticity,[37] as it stimulates neurogenesis through AMPA receptors[39] and mediates synaptic plasticity through NMDA receptors.[40] Evidence from human and animal studies points to altered activity of gamma-aminobutyric acid (GABA), glutamate's inhibitory counterpart.[41] Alterations are specific to brain regions, and no clear pathophysiological mechanism has yet been proposed.[41–43]

The role of neurotransmitters in pathophysiology and treatment may also be influenced by their interactions.[17,25] For example, interactions between serotonin and dopamine release in the nucleus accumbens contribute to pathogenesis in mouse models of depression.[30] Such interactions make it difficult to assign depression vulnerability to defects in any one neurotransmitter pathway.

2.3. NEUROGENESIS

During adulthood, newly differentiated neurons are sparse.[44] The hippocampus is one of the few regions with—albeit slow—neurogenesis in the adult brain.[45] The neurogenic theory of depression[46] suggests that depression is associated with impaired adult hippocampal neurogenesis (AHN), whereas recovery results from restoring AHN. Hippocampal neurons generated in adulthood are required for cognitive functions that are reduced in patients with depression.[47,48] The neurobiological underpinnings of depression might therefore be partly explained by deficiencies in AHN, which is demonstrably altered in animal models of depression.[49]

Most neurobiological accounts of depression recognize stress as a major risk factor.[50] The hypothalamic–pituitary–adrenal (HPA) axis is a critical regulator of stress response and adaptation.[51] Cortisol produced in the adrenal cortex provides a negative stimulus to other structures of the axis to maintain hormone homeostasis.[51] The hippocampus is a key structure in mediating this negative feedback loop.[52] Though a causal link has yet to be established, some studies examining the effects of stress have reported reductions in hippocampal volume (suggested as a marker of impaired AHN[53]) and depressive behavior.[54]

In animals, sustained activation of the HPA axis by stress, and subsequent glucocorticoid elevation, impairs AHN,[54,55] while treatment with SSRIs boosts AHN.[56] In the brains of depressed individuals, the HPA axis may be hyperactive due to impaired negative feedback signaling by cortisol in the hippocampus, resulting in increased glucocorticoid release.[52,57,58] In addition, hippocampal neurogenesis is particularly active during adolescence in rodents, and it has been hypothesized that stress in adolescence can have a negative impact on hippocampal development. This effect may be potentiated by altered HPA axis and neuroinflammatory response to stress in adolescence and might contribute to the development of depression and sustained cognitive changes.[59] Neuroimaging experiments in animals and humans with depressed phenotypes reveal reduced hippocampal activity and smaller hippocampal volume.[60,61] In humans, longitudinal magnetic resonance imaging (MRI) studies show that depressed patients treated with SSRIs have larger hippocampi in comparison to nonmedicated patients with depression.[62] Evidence from rodent studies suggests that AHN is necessary for treatment response to the antidepressant fluoxetine,[63,64] as well as for normalization of the HPA axis by fluoxetine.[65]

Increasing AHN is a potential treatment avenue for depression. In rodents, administering compounds to boost AHN has antidepressant effects that are blocked by AHN ablation.[66] Antidepressants,[67] exercise,[67–69] and electroconvulsive therapy[70] are all thought to upregulate activity of brain-derived neurotrophic factor (BDNF), a key modulator of neuronal cell growth, neuroplasticity, and antidepressant effects.[71] In depressed patients, BDNF levels are significantly higher following effective antidepressant treatment,[72] suggesting that the efficacy of depression treatments might be partially explained by their ability to increase neurogenesis and/or plasticity.

While evidence for the neurogenic theory of depression in animal models is promising, current limitations in methodology prevent more precise investigation in humans. Whether AHN leads to depression or vice versa remains debatable. These findings should be interpreted cautiously, as more recent, methodologically robust evidence disputes the occurrence of AHN in humans and suggests that neurogenic findings may be species-specific.[45]

2.4. INFLAMMATION

Multiple lines of evidence involve inflammation in the pathophysiology of depression. Roughly one-third of patients with depression who are not otherwise ill have increased markers of inflammation in the brain or the periphery.[73] Inflammatory molecules, such as interleukin (IL)-6, tumor necrosis factor-α, and C-reactive protein, have been implicated in depression,[73–75] and inflammatory markers are elevated in postmortem brain studies of patients with depression who have died by suicide.[75] The glucocorticoid receptor (GR), which is involved in stress response, is specifically targeted by certain cytokines. Evidence shows that IL-1α reduces GR-mediated gene transcription, and both IL-1α and IL-1β block dexamethasone-induced translocation of GR from the cytoplasm to the cell nucleus.[76] These results may help explain the lack of dexamethasone suppression seen in depressed patients.[76–79]

The elevated cytokine levels observed in depression could be a result, rather than a cause, of the disease. Nevertheless, the risk for depression is increased in individuals taking pro-inflammatory treatments for conditions like hepatitis C infection—up to 40% of these patients develop depression.[73,74] Furthermore, certain cytokines decrease levels of norepinephrine, serotonin, and dopamine by several mechanisms (including monoamine reuptake),[74,75] suggesting that elevated cytokine levels might precipitate a depressed state.

In addition, abnormalities in microglia—the immune cells of the central nervous system—have been demonstrated by PET imaging in humans, and despite varied study outcomes linked to the methodology employed, recent studies seem to support abnormal microglia activation.[80] Evidence from animal models indicates a mediating role of microglia in stress-induced depression.[80,81] Antidepressants may also reduce inflammatory markers,[82] suggesting that normalizing abnormal inflammatory signals is part of their mechanism of action.

Additionally, many risk factors for depression are associated with increased inflammation (e.g., obesity, childhood trauma or adversity).[75] Inflammation in brain regions and circuits relevant to depression may influence their function: Elevated inflammatory markers have been shown to modulate the functional connectivity between the subgenual anterior cingulate cortex and the amygdala during response to threatening or fearful stimuli.[75,83] Finally, a large prospective study of 3,000 subjects found that while levels of C- reactive protein and IL-6 at baseline predicted cognitive symptoms of depression (i.e., thoughts of worthlessness and hopelessness, belief that life is not worth living, and impairment in activity because of "nerves") 12 years later, baseline depressive symptoms did not predict inflammation at follow-up, suggesting that inflammation preceded the cognitive symptoms of depression.[84]

Of clinical relevance, the presence of inflammatory markers is correlated with impaired response to antidepressants.[73] Anti-inflammatory drugs, such as nonsteroidal anti-inflammatory drugs (NSAIDs), are currently under investigation for adjunct or monotherapy treatment of depression.[85] The balance of evidence in the literature indicates that inflammation may be an important pathophysiological factor in certain depressed patients, and this may lead to clinically relevant developments, such as new treatments or reliable biomarkers of treatment response.[75,82]

2.5. FUNCTIONAL GENOMICS

2.5.1. Epigenetics

As in many other psychopathologies, genetic and environmental risk factors contribute to the onset of depression.[86,87] Exposure to stress or adverse life events,[88] especially in early life,[89,90] is one of the strongest risk factors for developing depression and other mood disorders. In response to stress, resilient individuals are able to maintain normal psychological functioning, whereas vulnerable individuals may develop psychopathology.[91,92] The epigenetic theory of depression suggests that severe environmental stress contributes to vulnerability to depression by triggering sustained changes in gene expression through epigenetic modifications.[91,92]

Epigenetics has been proposed as a mechanism to explain the phenomenon of biological embedding, which is the translation of experiences into differential regulation of biological systems and development.[59,93] Epigenetics refers to the processes that alter gene expression—and subsequently protein function—without making any changes to the underlying DNA sequence;[92] of these epigenetic mechanisms, DNA methylation and histone modification have received particular attention in studies of depression.[94] Methylation of cytosine bases in DNA is a posttranscriptional modification that usually represses gene expression.[92] Histone modifications include methylation and acetylation, which promote changes in chromatin conformation, allowing for increased or decreased gene expression, depending on the type and location of histone modification.[92]

Epigenetic modifications can be studied on a gene-specific or genome-wide level.[92] Although overall methylation changes may be indicative of widespread changes, the relationship between global levels and pathology has not been well described, and most informative studies have focused on depression-related genes.

As described earlier in the chapter, the HPA axis is a critical regulator of physiological and behavioral responses to stressful stimuli,[95] and a wealth of evidence indicates that epigenetic changes resulting from environmental stressors regulate HPA axis genes.[87,96,97] Pioneering epigenetic studies in animal models have linked variables in early life environment (i.e., maternal care, environmental enrichment, social support) to HPA axis function in adulthood.[98–100] For instance, the NR3C1 gene encodes GR, a critical component of the HPA axis. Abundance of GR dictates glucocorticoid sensitivity via a negative feedback loop of the HPA axis. Early life environment and early life adversity (including childhood maltreatment, parental stress, and social stress) affect the HPA axis and lead to differential methylation of the GR gene and altered receptor expression in the hippocampus.[98,100–102] Childhood maltreatment is also associated with altered methylation of FKBP5, a gene involved in the feedback regulation of GR signaling.[103–105]

Animal models of early life adversity provide evidence for stress-induced epigenetic changes in neurotrophic gene expression. For example, BDNF is repressed through increased methylation of both DNA and histones,[106,107] while glial cell line–derived neurotrophic factor is repressed through increased DNA methylation, decreased histone acetylation, and increased repressive histone methylation.[108] Additionally, studies using brain tissue from individuals who died by suicide reported altered methylation patterns in the gene encoding the BDNF receptor tropomyosin receptor kinase B (TrkB), which could potentially explain their relationship with depression.[109,110] Effective antidepressant treatment may also depend on epigenetic regulation of key genes that confer risk for depression.[111,112] For instance, in animal models of depression, antidepressant response is mediated by chromatin modification of critical genes, such as BDNF.[107]

2.5.2 Noncoding RNA

Contrary to messenger RNAs that encode proteins (and make up less than 2% of the human genome), noncoding RNAs (ncRNAs) are important regulators of gene expression.[113,114] Dysregulation of ncRNA is implicated in disease etiology;[115] investigations on their relation to depression has been growing rapidly.[116] Advances in genomics reveal several associations of various ncRNAs with depression, but their specific mechanisms often remain poorly characterized. A commonly studied class of ncRNAs is micro-RNAs (miRNA), since expression levels of over a dozen different miRNAs are demonstrably altered in both animal models and depressed individuals.[116] Manipulating expression levels of particular miRNAs in the brains of animal models can alter depressive behavior.[117,118]

Numerous miRNAs targeting the genetic regulation of various neural systems are under investigation as biomarkers of depression susceptibility[119] and of antidepressant treatment response.[117,118,120–123] For instance, landmark studies identified miR-16 as a mediator of fluoxetine antidepressant action in the raphe and locus coeruleus of mice[120] with specific effects on AHN.[124] Expression of miR-135a, thought to target the serotonin transporter, is upregulated in the raphe nuclei of mice, and in depressed patients, peripheral blood levels of miR-135a are lower than in healthy controls.[118] Strikingly, blood miR-135a levels significantly increased after three months of cognitive-behavioral therapy, but not after SSRI treatment.[118]

Other studies also identified several miRNAs in humans that may mediate antidepressant response, via different pathways. For example, expression levels of the miRNAs146a-5p, 146b-5p, 425-3p, and 24-3p change with depression symptom improvement, and all act on the MAPK/Wnt pathway.[122] Another interesting finding relates to the primate-specific and brain-enriched miR-1202, which is downregulated both in the prefrontal cortex of depressed individuals who died by suicide and in blood samples from unmedicated depressed patients who go on to achieve remission.[121] The same study showed that, specifically in patients who achieved remission with citalopram treatment, miR-1202 levels increased significantly following treatment, indicating its potential for use as a peripheral biomarker and predictor of antidepressant response. This finding is of particular interest since miR-1202 may be implicated in regulating the glutamatergic network, as demonstrated by its effects on levels of a glutamatergic metabotropic receptor (GRM4) and by imaging studies.[121,125] Overall, increasing evidence highlights the importance of miRNAs in the pathophysiology and treatment of depression, as potentially powerful biomarkers of susceptibility and treatment response.

2.6. CONCLUSION

While no single biological cause is likely to explain depression, the complex interplay between the different systems described herein—as well as their interactions with the social environment of the individual and with personal history—reflects the complexity in clinical presentation of depression. Existing evidence for neurobiological pathways of depressive pathophysiology and symptomatology has prompted future research directions. The overall state of knowledge in this field emphasizes the importance of considering alterations in and interactions between multiple pathways, in multiple regions, to fully grasp the changes occurring in the depressed brain. Further investigation of neural circuitry and genomics will undoubtedly facilitate such understanding, as will the continued study of genetic, environmental, social, and psychological factors associated with depression.

AUTHOR NOTE

G.T. holds a Canada Research Chair (Tier 1) and a NARSAD Distinguished Investigator Award. He is supported by grants from the Canadian Institute of Health Research (CIHR) (FDN148374 and EGM141899), by the FRQS through the Quebec Network on Suicide, Mood Disorders and Related Disorders. S.I. and D.B. contributed equally to this work.

REFERENCES

1. Coppen A. The biochemistry of affective disorders. *Br J Psychiatry*. 1967;113(504):1237–1264.
2. Rush AJ, Trivedi MH, Wisniewski SR, et al. Acute and longer-term outcomes in depressed outpatients requiring one or several treatment steps: a STAR*D report. *Am J Psychiatry*. 2006;163(11):1905–1917.
3. Fakhoury M. Revisiting the serotonin hypothesis: implications for major depressive disorders. *Mol Neurobiol*. 2016;53(5):2778–2786.
4. Tylee A, Walters P. Onset of action of antidepressants. *BMJ*. 2007;334(7600):911–912.
5. Charnay Y, Leger L. Brain serotonergic circuitries. *Dialogues Clin Neurosci*. 2010;12(4):471–487.
6. Zhang TY, Labonte B, Wen XL, et al. Epigenetic mechanisms for the early environmental regulation of hippocampal glucocorticoid receptor gene expression in rodents and humans. *Neuropsychopharmacology*. 2013;38(1):111–123.
7. Cowen PJ. Serotonin and depression: pathophysiological mechanism or marketing myth? *Trends Pharmacol Sci*. 2008;29(9):433–436.
8. Sargent PA, Kjaer KH, Bench CJ, et al. Brain serotonin 1A receptor binding measured by positron emission tomography with [11C]WAY-100635: effects of depression and antidepressant treatment. *Arch Gen Psychiatry*. 2000;57(2):174–180.
9. Stockmeier CA. Involvement of serotonin in depression: evidence from postmortem and imaging studies of serotonin receptors and the serotonin transporter. *J Psychiatr Res*. 2003;37(5):357373.
10. Bach H, Arango V. Neuroanatomy of serotonergic abnormalities in suicide. In: Dwivedi Y, ed. *The Neurobiological Basis of Suicide*. Boca Raton, FL: CRC Press/Taylor & Francis; 2012.
11. Asberg M, Traskman L, Thoren P. 5-HIAA in the cerebrospinal fluid. A biochemical suicide predictor? *Arch Gen Psychiatry*. 1976;33(10):1193–1197.
12. Jans LA, Riedel WJ, Markus CR, Blokland A. Serotonergic vulnerability and depression: assumptions, experimental evidence and implications. *Mol Psychiatry*. 2007;12(6):522543.

13. Mann JJ. The serotonergic system in mood disorders and suicidal behaviour. *Philos Trans Royal Soc London B Biol Sciences*. 2013;368(1615):20120537.

14. Ruhe HG, Mason NS, Schene AH. Mood is indirectly related to serotonin, norepinephrine and dopamine levels in humans: a meta-analysis of monoamine depletion studies. *Mol Psychiatry*. 2007;12(4):331–359.

15. Hariri AR, Mattay VS, Tessitore A, et al. Serotonin transporter genetic variation and the response of the human amygdala. *Science*. 2002;297(5580):400–403.

16. Maletic V, Eramo A, Gwin K, et al. The role of norepinephrine and its alpha-adrenergic receptors in the pathophysiology and treatment of major depressive disorder and schizophrenia: a systematic review. *Front Psychiatry*. 2017;8:42.

17. Nutt DJ. The role of dopamine and norepinephrine in depression and antidepressant treatment. *J Clin Psychiatry*. 2006;67(suppl 6):3–8.

18. Werner FM, Covenas R. Classical neurotransmitters and neuropeptides involved in major depression: a review. *Int J Neurosci*. 2010;120(7):455–470.

19. Haenisch B, Bilkei-Gorzo A, Caron MG, Bönisch H. Knockout of the norepinephrine transporter and pharmacologically diverse antidepressants prevent behavioral and brain neurotrophin alterations in two chronic stress models of depression. *J Neurochem*. 2009;111(2):403–416.

20. Rivero G, Gabilondo AM, Garcia-Sevilla JA, et al. Increased alpha2- and beta1-adrenoceptor densities in postmortem brain of subjects with depression: differential effect of antidepressant treatment. *J Affect Disord*. 2014;167:343–350.

21. Berridge CW, Spencer RC. Differential cognitive actions of norepinephrine a2 and a1 receptor signaling in the prefrontal cortex. *Brain Res*. 2016;1641:189–196.

22. Eyding D, Lelgemann M, Grouven U, et al. Reboxetine for acute treatment of major depression: systematic review and meta-analysis of published and unpublished placebo and selective serotonin reuptake inhibitor controlled trials. *BMJ*. 2010;341:c4737.

23. Nutt DJ. Relationship of neurotransmitters to the symptoms of major depressive disorder. *J Clin Psychiatry*. 2008;69(suppl E1):4–7.

24. Belujon P, Grace AA. Dopamine system dysregulation in major depressive disorders. *Int J Neuropsychopharmacol*. 2017;20(12):1036–1046.

25. Dunlop BW, Nemeroff CB. The role of dopamine in the pathophysiology of depression. *Arch Gen Psychiatry*. 2007;64(3):327–337.

26. Arias-Carrion O, Stamelou M, Murillo-Rodriguez E, et al. Dopaminergic reward system: a short integrative review. *Int Arch Med*. 2010;3:24.

27. Willner P, Lappas S, Cheeta S, Muscat R. Reversal of stress-induced anhedonia by the dopamine receptor agonist, pramipexole. *Psychopharmacology*. 1994;115(4):454–462.

28. Salamone JD, Aberman JE, Sokolowski JD, Cousins MS. Nucleus accumbens dopamine and rate of responding: neurochemical and behavioral studies. *Psychobiology*. 1999;27(2):236–247.

29. Schrag A, Jahanshahi M, Quinn NP. What contributes to depression in Parkinson's disease? *Psychol Med*. 2001;31(1):65–73.

30. Yadid G, Friedman A. Dynamics of the dopaminergic system as a key component to the understanding of depression. *Progress Brain Res*. 2008;172:265–286.

31. Cannon DM, Klaver JM, Peck SA, et al. Dopamine type-1 receptor binding in major depressive disorder assessed using positron emission tomography and [11C]NNC-112. *Neuropsychopharmacology*. 2009;34(5):1277–1287.

32. Learned-Coughlin SM, Bergström M, Savitcheva I, et al. In vivo activity of bupropion at the human dopamine transporter as measured by positron emission tomography. *Biol Psychiatry*. 2003;54(8):800–805.

33. Patel K, Allen S, Haque MN, et al. Bupropion: a systematic review and meta-analysis of effectiveness as an antidepressant. *Ther Adv Psychopharmacol*. 2016;6(2):99–144.

34. Beaulieu JM, Gainetdinov RR. The physiology, signaling, and pharmacology of dopamine receptors. *Pharmacol Rev*. 2011;63(1):182–217.
35. Der-Avakian A, Markou A. The neurobiology of anhedonia and other reward-related deficits. *Trends Neurosci*. 2012;35(1):68–77.
36. Lammers CH, Diaz J, Schwartz JC, Sokoloff P. Selective increase of dopamine D3 receptor gene expression as a common effect of chronic antidepressant treatments. *Mol Psychiatry*. 2000;5:378.
37. Sanacora G, Treccani G, Popoli M. Towards a glutamate hypothesis of depression: an emerging frontier of neuropsychopharmacology for mood disorders. *Neuropharmacology*. 2012;62(1):6377.
38. Mathews DC, Henter ID, Zarate CA. Targeting the glutamatergic system to treat major depressive disorder: rationale and progress to date. *Drugs*. 2012;72(10):1313–1333.
39. Lauterborn JC, Lynch G, Vanderklish P, et al. Positive modulation of AMPA receptors increases neurotrophin expression by hippocampal and cortical neurons. *J Neurosci*. 2000;20(1):8.
40. Citri A, Malenka RC. Synaptic plasticity: multiple forms, functions, and mechanisms. *Neuropsychopharmacology*. 2008;33(1):18–41.
41. Lener MS, Niciu MJ, Ballard ED, et al. Glutamate and gamma-aminobutyric acid systems in the pathophysiology of major depression and antidepressant response to ketamine. *Biol Psychiatry*. 2017;81(10):886–897.
42. Ghose S, Winter MK, McCarson KE, et al. The GABA(B) receptor as a target for antidepressant drug action. *Br J Pharmacol*. 2011;162(1):1–17.
43. Cryan JF, Slattery DA. GABA(B) receptors and depression: current status. *Adv Pharmacology*. 2010;58:427–451.
44. Spalding KL, Bergmann O, Alkass K, et al. Dynamics of hippocampal neurogenesis in adult humans. *Cell*. 2013;153(6):1219–1227.
45. Sorrells SF, Paredes MF, Cebrian-Silla A, et al. Human hippocampal neurogenesis drops sharply in children to undetectable levels in adults. *Nature*. 2018;555(7696):377–381.
46. Jacobs BL, van Praag H, Gage FH. Adult brain neurogenesis and psychiatry: a novel theory of depression. *Mol Psychiatry*. 2000;5(3):262–269.
47. Sahay A, Scobie KN, Hill AS, et al. Increasing adult hippocampal neurogenesis is sufficient to improve pattern separation. *Nature*. 2011;472:466.
48. Burghardt NS, Park EH, Hen R, Fenton AA. Adult-born hippocampal neurons promote cognitive flexibility in mice. *Hippocampus*. 2012;22(9):1795–1808.
49. Miller BR, Hen R. The current state of the neurogenic theory of depression and anxiety. *Curr Opin Neurobiol*. 2015;30:51–58.
50. Mahar I, Bambico FR, Mechawar N, Nobrega JN. Stress, serotonin, and hippocampal neurogenesis in relation to depression and antidepressant effects. *Neurosci Biobehav Rev*. 2014;38:173–192.
51. Herman JP, McKlveen JM, Ghosal S, et al. Regulation of the hypothalamic-pituitary-adrenocortical stress response. *Compr Physiol*. 2016;6(2):603–621.
52. Jacobson L, Sapolsky R. The role of the hippocampus in feedback regulation of the hypothalamic-pituitary-adrenocortical axis. *Endocr Rev*. 1991;12(2):118–134.
53. Schoenfeld TJ, McCausland HC, Morris HD, et al. Stress and loss of adult neurogenesis differentially reduce hippocampal volume. *Biol Psychiatry*. 2017;82(12):914–923.
54. Campbell S, Macqueen G. The role of the hippocampus in the pathophysiology of major depression. *J Psychiatry Neurosci*. 2004;29(6):417–426.
55. Wong EY, Herbert J. Raised circulating corticosterone inhibits neuronal differentiation of progenitor cells in the adult hippocampus. *Neuroscience*. 2006;137(1):83–92.
56. Levone BR, Cryan JF, O'Leary OF. Role of adult hippocampal neurogenesis in stress resilience. *Neurobiol Stress*. 2015;1:147–155.

57. Anacker C, Zunszain PA, Carvalho LA, Pariante CM. The glucocorticoid receptor: pivot of depression and of antidepressant treatment? *Psychoneuroendocrinology*. 2011;36(3):415–425.
58. Turecki G. The molecular bases of the suicidal brain. *Nat Rev Neurosci*. 2014;15(12):802–816.
59. Hueston CM, Cryan JF, Nolan YM. Stress and adolescent hippocampal neurogenesis: diet and exercise as cognitive modulators. *Transl Psychiatry*. 2017;7(4):e1081.
60. MacQueen GM, Campbell S, McEwen BS, et al. Course of illness, hippocampal function, and hippocampal volume in major depression. *Proc Nat Acad Sci USA*. 2003;100(3):1387–1392.
61. Sapolsky RM. Depression, antidepressants, and the shrinking hippocampus. *Proc Nat Acad Sci USA*. 2001;98(22):12320–12322.
62. Huang Y, Coupland NJ, Lebel RM, et al. Structural changes in hippocampal subfields in major depressive disorder: a high-field magnetic resonance imaging study. *Biol Psychiatry*. 2013;74(1):62–68.
63. Santarelli L, Saxe M, Gross C, et al. Requirement of hippocampal neurogenesis for the behavioral effects of antidepressants. *Science*. 2003;301(5634):805–809.
64. David DJ, Samuels BA, Rainer Q, et al. Neurogenesis-dependent and -independent effects of fluoxetine in an animal model of anxiety/depression. *Neuron*. 2009;62(4):479–493.
65. Surget A, Tanti A, Leonardo ED, et al. Antidepressants recruit new neurons to improve stress response regulation. *Mol Psychiatry*. 2011;16(12):1177–1188.
66. Walker AK, Rivera PD, Wang Q, et al. The P7C3 class of neuroprotective compounds exerts antidepressant efficacy in mice by increasing hippocampal neurogenesis. *Mol Psychiatry*. 2015;20(4):500–508.
67. Baj G, D'Alessandro V, Musazzi L, et al. Physical exercise and antidepressants enhance BDNF targeting in hippocampal CA3 dendrites: further evidence of a spatial code for BDNF splice variants. *Neuropsychopharmacology*. 2012;37:1600.
68. Phillips C. Brain-derived neurotrophic factor, depression, and physical activity: making the neuroplastic connection. *Neural Plast*. 2017;2017:7260130.
69. Oliff HS, Berchtold NC, Isackson P, Cotman CW. Exercise-induced regulation of brain-derived neurotrophic factor (BDNF) transcripts in the rat hippocampus. *Brain Res Mol Brain Res*. 1998;61(1-2):147–153.
70. Tendolkar I, van Beek M, van Oostrom I, et al. Electroconvulsive therapy increases hippocampal and amygdala volume in therapy refractory depression: a longitudinal pilot study. *Psychiatry Res*. 2013;214(3):197–203.
71. Bjorkholm C, Monteggia LM. BDNF—a key transducer of antidepressant effects. *Neuropharmacology*. 2016;102:72–79.
72. Sen S, Duman R, Sanacora G. Serum brain-derived neurotrophic factor, depression, and antidepressant medications: meta-analyses and implications. *Biol Psychiatry*. 2008;64(6):527–532.
73. Leighton SP, Nerurkar L, Krishnadas R, et al. Chemokines in depression in health and in inflammatory illness: a systematic review and meta-analysis. *Mol Psychiatry*. 2018;23(1):48–58.
74. Mechawar N, Savitz J. Neuropathology of mood disorders: do we see the stigmata of inflammation? *Transl Psychiatry*. 2016;6(11):e946.
75. Miller AH, Raison CL. The role of inflammation in depression: from evolutionary imperative to modern treatment target. *Nature Rev Immunol*. 2016;16(1):22–34.
76. Pace TW, Miller AH. Cytokines and glucocorticoid receptor signaling: relevance to major depression. *Ann NY Acad Sci*. 2009;1179:86–105.
77. Pariante CM, Pearce BD, Pisell TL, et al. The proinflammatory cytokine, interleukin-1-alpha, reduces glucocorticoid receptor translocation and function. *Endocrinology*. 1999;140(9):43594366.
78. Wang X, Wu H, Miller AH. Interleukin 1α (IL-1α) induced activation of p38 mitogen-activated protein kinase inhibits glucocorticoid receptor function. *Mol Psychiatry*. 2003;9:65.

79. Raddatz D, Toth S, Schwörer H, Ramadori G. Glucocorticoid receptor signaling in the intestinal epithelial cell lines IEC-6 and Caco-2: evidence of inhibition by interleukin-1beta. *Int J Colorectal Dis.* 2001;16(6):377–383.

80. Yirmiya R, Rimmerman N, Reshef R. Depression as a microglial disease. *Trends Neurosci.* 2015;38(10):637–658.

81. Hinwood M, Morandini J, Day TA, Walker FR. Evidence that microglia mediate the neurobiological effects of chronic psychological stress on the medial prefrontal cortex. *Cereb Cortex.* 2012;22(6):1442–1454.

82. Martin C, Tansey KE, Schalkwyk LC, Powell TR. The inflammatory cytokines: molecular biomarkers for major depressive disorder? *Biomarkers Med.* 2015;9(2):169–180.

83. Harrison NA, Brydon L, Walker C, et al. Inflammation causes mood changes through alterations in subgenual cingulate activity and mesolimbic connectivity. *Biol Psychiatry.* 2009;66(5):407–414.

84. Gimeno D, Kivimaki M, Brunner EJ, et al. Associations of C-reactive protein and interleukin-6 with cognitive symptoms of depression: 12-year follow-up of the Whitehall II study. *Psychol Med.* 2009;39(3):413–423.

85. Kohler O, Krogh J, Mors O, Benros ME. Inflammation in depression and the potential for anti-inflammatory treatment. *Curr Neuropharmacol.* 2016;14(7):732–742.

86. Sullivan PF, Neale MC, Kendler KS. Genetic epidemiology of major depression: review and metaanalysis. *Am J Psychiatry.* 2000;157(10):1552–1562.

87. Nagy C, Vaillancourt K, Turecki G. A role for activity-dependent epigenetics in the development and treatment of major depressive disorder. *Genes Brain Behavior.* 2018;17(3):e12446.

88. Mazure CM. Life stressors as risk factors in depression. *Clin Psychol Sci Practice.* 1998;5(3):291–313.

89. Saleh A, Potter GG, McQuoid DR, et al. Effects of early life stress on depression, cognitive performance and brain morphology. *Psychol Med.* 2017;47(1):171–181.

90. Juruena MF. Early-life stress and HPA axis trigger recurrent adulthood depression. *Epilepsy Behav.* 2014;38:148–159.

91. Zannas AS, West AE. Epigenetics and the regulation of stress vulnerability and resilience. *Neuroscience.* 2014;264:157–170.

92. Nestler EJ. Epigenetic mechanisms of depression. *JAMA Psychiatry.* 2014;71(4):454–456.

93. Hertzman C. Putting the concept of biological embedding in historical perspective. *Proc Nat Acad Sci USA.* 2012;109(Suppl 2):1716017167.

94. Turecki G, Ota VK, Belangero SI, et al. Early life adversity, genomic plasticity, and psychopathology. *Lancet Psychiatry.* 2014;1(6):461–466.

95. Burns SB, Szyszkowicz JK, Luheshi GN, et al. Plasticity of the epigenome during early-life stress. *Semin Cell Devel Biol.* 2017.

96. Skinner MK. Environmental stress and epigenetic transgenerational inheritance. *BMC Med.* 2014;12:153.

97. Anacker C, O'Donnell KJ, Meaney MJ. Early life adversity and the epigenetic programming of hypothalamic-pituitary-adrenal function. *Dialogues Clin Neurosci.* 2014;16(3):321–333.

98. Weaver IC, Cervoni N, Champagne FA, et al. Epigenetic programming by maternal behavior. *Nature Neurosci.* 2004;7(8):847–854.

99. Meaney MJ. Maternal care, gene expression, and the transmission of individual differences in stress reactivity across generations. *Annu Rev Neurosci.* 2001;24(1):1161–1192.

100. Meaney MJ, Szyf M. Environmental programming of stress responses through DNA methylation: life at the interface between a dynamic environment and a fixed genome. *Dialogues Clin Neurosci.* 2005;7(2):103–123.

101. McGowan PO, Sasaki A, D'Alessio AC, et al. Epigenetic regulation of the glucocorticoid receptor in human brain associates with childhood abuse. *Nature Neurosci*. 2009;12(3):342–348.
102. Turecki G, Meaney MJ. Effects of the social environment and stress on glucocorticoid receptor gene methylation: a systematic review. *Biol Psychiatry*. 2016;79(2):87–96.
103. Klengel T, Binder EB. FKBP5 allele-specific epigenetic modification in gene by environment interaction. *Neuropsychopharmacology*. 2015;40(1):244–246.
104. Klengel T, Mehta D, Anacker C, et al. Allele-specific FKBP5 DNA demethylation mediates gene–childhood trauma interactions. *Nature Neurosci*. 2013;16(1):33–41.
105. Lutz PE, Almeida D, Fiori LM, Turecki G. Childhood maltreatment and stress-related psychopathology: the epigenetic memory hypothesis. *Curr Pharmaceut Design*. 2015;21(11):1413–1417.
106. Roth TL, Lubin FD, Funk AJ, Sweatt JD. Lasting epigenetic influence of early-life adversity on the BDNF gene. *Biol Psychiatry*. 2009;65(9):760–769.
107. Tsankova NM, Berton O, Renthal W, et al. Sustained hippocampal chromatin regulation in a mouse model of depression and antidepressant action. *Nature Neurosci*. 2006;9(4):519–525.
108. Uchida S, Hara K, Kobayashi A, et al. Epigenetic status of GDNF in the ventral striatum determines susceptibility and adaptation to daily stressful events. *Neuron*. 2011;69(2):359–372.
109. Ernst C, Chen ES, Turecki G. Histone methylation and decreased expression of TrkB.T1 in orbital frontal cortex of suicide completers. *Mol Psychiatry*. 2009;14(9):830–832.
110. Maussion G, Yang J, Suderman M, et al. Functional DNA methylation in a transcript specific 3′UTR region of TrkB associates with suicide. *Epigenetics*. 2014;9(8):1061–1070.
111. Lopez JP, Mamdani F, Labonte B, et al. Epigenetic regulation of BDNF expression according to antidepressant response. *Mol Psychiatry*. 2013;18(4):398–399.
112. Menke A, Binder EB. Epigenetic alterations in depression and antidepressant treatment. *Dialogues Clin Neurosci*. 2014;16(3):395–404.
113. Mattick JS. RNA regulation: a new genetics? *Nat Rev Genet*. 2004;5(4):316–323.
114. Qureshi IA, Mehler MF. Emerging roles of non-coding RNAs in brain evolution, development, plasticity and disease. *Nat Rev Neurosci*. 2012;13(8):528–541.
115. Taft RJ, Pang KC, Mercer TR, et al. Non-coding RNAs: regulators of disease. *J Pathol*. 2010;220(2):126–139.
116. Lin R, Turecki G. Noncoding RNAs in depression. *Adv Exp Med Biol*. 2017;978:197–210.
117. Issler O, Chen A. Determining the role of microRNAs in psychiatric disorders. *Nat Rev Neurosci*. 2015;16(4):201–212.
118. Issler O, Haramati S, Paul ED, et al. MicroRNA 135 is essential for chronic stress resiliency, antidepressant efficacy, and intact serotonergic activity. *Neuron*. 2014;83(2):344–360.
119. Torres-Berrio A, Lopez JP, Bagot RC, et al. DCC confers susceptibility to depression-like behaviors in humans and mice and is regulated by miR-218. *Biol Psychiatry*. 2017;81(4):306–315.
120. Baudry A, Mouillet-Richard S, Schneider B, et al. miR-16 targets the serotonin transporter: a new facet for adaptive responses to antidepressants. *Science*. 2010;329(5998):1537–1541.
121. Lopez JP, Lim R, Cruceanu C, et al. miR-1202 is a primate-specific and brain-enriched microRNA involved in major depression and antidepressant treatment. *Nat Med*. 2014;20(7):764–768.
122. Lopez JP, Fiori LM, Cruceanu C, et al. MicroRNAs 146a/b-5 and 425-3p and 24-3p are markers of antidepressant response and regulate MAPK/Wnt-system genes. *Nat Commun*. 2017;8:15497.

123. Lopez JP, Kos A, Turecki G. Major depression and its treatment: microRNAs as peripheral biomarkers of diagnosis and treatment response. *Curr Opin Psychiatry*. 2018;31(1):7–16.

124. Launay JM, Mouillet-Richard S, Baudry A, et al. Raphe-mediated signals control the hippocampal response to SRI antidepressants via miR-16. *Trans Psychiatry*. 2011;1:e56.

125. Lopez JP, Pereira F, Richard-Devantoy S, et al. Co-variation of peripheral levels of miR-1202 and brain activity and connectivity during antidepressant treatment. *Neuropsychopharmacology*. 2017;42(10):20432051.

/// 3 /// GENETIC RISK FACTORS OF DEPRESSION

THORHILDUR HALLDORSDOTTIR
AND HILDUR ÝR HILMARSDOTTIR

3.1. INTRODUCTION

The goal of understanding the genetic underpinnings of depression is to create more homogeneous neurobiological diagnostic criteria than are available in our current diagnostic framework. Such fine-tuning of our diagnostic criteria will in turn improve an individual's prognosis through personalized medicine and targeted therapeutic interventions. With the combination of technological advances allowing a deeper understanding of human genomic variation, cost-effective genotyping techniques, and large-scale international consortia, there have been extraordinary advances in molecular genetic studies on depression in the past decade. In this chapter, we provide an overview of these advances in the genetics of depression. We will start with a brief summary of genetic epidemiology findings, in particular family and twin studies, and then move on to more recent molecular genetic studies. Figure 3.1 provides an overview of common genetic epidemiological and molecular study designs used to determine the genetic basis for depression. Within the molecular studies, genome-wide association studies (GWAS) on depression outcomes will be introduced and summarized. Given the ongoing debate within the field, we discuss findings from GWAS on individuals with a clinical diagnosis of major depressive disorder (MDD) and GWAS on a broader definition of depression separately. Then, main findings from studies focused on specific genes believed to play a role in the neurobiology of depression, or so-called candidate gene studies, will be detailed. Findings from prominent gene-by-environment interaction (GxE) studies on depression will also

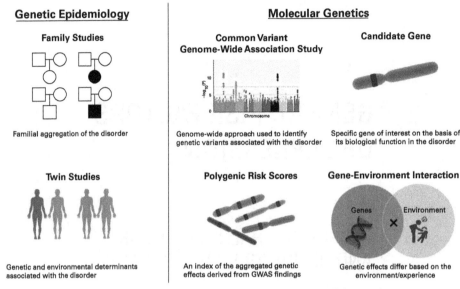

FIGURE 3.1. Methodological approaches used to study the genetics of depression.

be summarized. Lastly, the clinical implications of the collective findings will be discussed.

3.2. FAMILY AND TWIN STUDIES

It has long been recognized that depression runs in families. However, the first empirical studies conducted to establish the familial risk for depression relied on family- and twin-based designs. Family studies are designed to answer whether a disorder aggregates in families. In these studies, the occurrence of a disorder among first-degree relatives of affected individuals (referred to as probands) is compared to the occurrence of the disorder in either first-degree relatives of unaffected controls or to the population prevalence. The family studies using modern methodology show substantial familial aggregation for depression. A meta-analysis of high-quality family studies reported the odds ratio of 2.84 (95% confidence interval [CI]: 2.31–3.49) among first-degree relatives of subjects with MDD compared to controls.[1,2] In other words, individuals with MDD are almost three times more likely to have a first-degree relative who also has MDD than those without the disorder. Similar risk ratio estimates has been reported in more recent family studies.[3]

Twin studies are used to distinguish between genetic and environmental influences associated with disease status by comparing disorder concordance rates between monozygotic twins, who share 100% of their DNA, and dizygotic twin pairs, who share on average 50% of their DNA like other sibling pairs. Higher occurrence of depression among monozygotic twins than dizygotic twins suggests at least a partial genetic basis. Twin studies have shown that up to 40% of the liability toward depression can be attributed to genetic factors.[1] It is, however, believed that this is on the lower bound of the heritability range[4,5] and that the level of heritability would be much higher for reliably diagnosed MDD or certain depression subtypes (e.g., recurrent and earlier-onset depression).

3.3. GWAS

Coinciding with technological advancements and related cost reductions, GWAS are now a widely used, hypothesis-free approach to examine specific loci associated with disease risk.[6] More specifically, GWAS involves a systematic examination of whether genotype frequencies for variants across the genome differ between individuals affected with a specific disorder and those who are unaffected. GWAS typically involve one million or more common genetic variants (defined as alleles that are carried by >5% of the population) known as *single nucleotide polymorphisms* (SNPs). To correct for the large number of tests conducted in GWAS, the threshold for a genetic variant to be considered a genome-wide significant is a *p*-value of less than 5×10^{-8}. Given that the effects of common genetic variants are typically modest, GWAS require large sample sizes (>10,000 cases and controls) to have sufficient power to detect such effects at this statistical threshold.

As described earlier in the chapter, epidemiological studies on depression show that it is a modestly heritable disorder. With such relatively high heritability estimates, it has been surprising that large-scale consortia using a GWAS design have historically been unsuccessful in identifying genetic loci associated with depression. Given these difficulties, GWAS have been conducted on a number of depression phenotypes, including clinician-diagnosed MDD, depressive symptoms, self-declared depression, and depression ascertained via hospital records. The general trend in these studies has favored greater sample size over clinical precision, with a steady increase over time in the number of genome-wide significant variants for ever more diverse depression-related phenotypes. Here, we will discuss findings from GWAS using a clinician-diagnosed MDD first, followed by GWAS findings on more broadly defined depression phenotypes to provide a full picture of the current GWAS literature. When this is written, just under 20 GWAS on depression phenotypes have been published in peer-reviewed journals. Table 3.1 provides an overview of these studies.

3.3.1. GWAS on Clinician-Diagnosed MDD

The first GWAS on MDD was conducted in 2009 and yielded no genetic variants directly associated with disease status.[7] Although this study yielded no genome-wide significant hits, the researchers' investigation of the top 200 SNPs in the study implicated *PCLO* SNPs in depression. *PCLO* encodes a presynaptic protein involved in monoaminergic neurotransmitter release named piccolo. Since these initial findings, *PCLO* SNPs have been implicated in candidate gene studies on

TABLE 3.1. Published GWAS on MDD, Recurrent MDD, and/or Depressive Symptoms

Study	Cohort(s)	Definition of Depression	Participants	Cases	Controls	Mean Age (SD)	Female:Male Ratio	Ethnicity	Loci
Clinical Diagnosis of MDD									
Sullivan et al., 2009[7]	NESDA; NTR; NEMESIS; ARIADNE	Clinical diagnosis	3540	1738	1802	Cases: 42.6 (12.6) Controls: 45.1 (14.1)	2.3:1 1.6:1	Western European	0
Rietschel et al., 2010[10]	Bonn; PopGen; KORA	Clinical diagnosis	1968	604	1364	Cases: 47.5 (13.9) Controls: *	1.8:1 1:1.05	European	0
Muglia et al., 2010[16]	GSK	Clinical diagnosis of recurrent MDD	1792	926	866	Cases: 50.7 (13.7) Controls: 52.4 (13.2)	2:1 2.1:1	European	0
	Colaus Study		1544	492	1052	Cases: 50.9 (8.6) Controls: 51.9 (8.7)	2.7:1 1:1.5		
Lewis et al., 2010[17]	DeCC; DeNT; GENDEP	Clinical diagnosis of recurrent MDD	3230	1636	1594	Cases: * Controls: *	2.4:1 *	European	0

Study	Cohort	Diagnosis	N total	N cases	N controls	Age, mean (SD)	Sex ratio	Ancestry	
Shi et al., 2011[18]	GenRED	Clinical diagnosis of recurrent early onset MDD	2656	1020	1636	Cases: 40.5 (11.9) Controls: 52.5 (17.2)	2.4:1 1:1.3	European	0
Aragam et al., 2011[11]	NESDA; NTR	Clinical diagnosis of MDD	3356	1726	1630	Cases: 42.4 (12.6) Controls: 45.2 (14.1)	2.3:1 1.6:1	Western European	0
Kohli et al., 2011[15]	MARS	Clinical diagnosis of MDD	719	353	366	Cases: 49.5 (14.3) Controls: +	1.3:1 +	European	1
			1939	917	1022	Cases: 51.0 (13.8) Controls: +	2:1 +		
Shyn et al., 2011[12]	STAR*D; GenRED; GAIN-MDD	Clinical diagnosis of MDD	7385	3957	3428	Cases: * Controls: *	2:1 1.1:1	European	0
Wray et al., 2012[13]	MDD2000+ (QIMR; NESDA; NTR; UoE, MGS)	Clinical diagnosis of MDD	6104	2431	3673	Cases: 41.1 (11.4) Controls: 48.0 (15.8)	1.8:1 1.1:1	European	0
			12664	5763	6901	Cases: * Controls: *	* *		

(continued)

TABLE 3.1. Continued

Study	Cohort(s)	Definition of Depression	Participants	Cases	Controls	Mean Age (SD)	Female:Male Ratio	Ethnicity	Loci
Power et al., 2012[19]	RADIANT	Clinical diagnosis of recurrent depression	3064	1480	1584	Cases: * Controls: 43.7 (14.3)	2.5:1 1.3:1	European	0
Ripke et al., 2013[14]	MDD Working Group of the PGC	Clinical diagnosis of MDD	18759	9240	9519	Cases: * Controls: *	2:1 1.3:1	European	0
			57478	6783	50695	Cases: * Controls: *	* *		
Cai et al., 2015[20]	CONVERGE	Clinical diagnosis	10640	5303	5337	Cases: * Controls: *	1:0 1:0	Asian	2
Broader Depression Phenotype									
Terracciano et al., 2010[28]	SardiNIa BLSA	Depressive symptoms	3972 839	– –	– –	42.8 (17.0) 58.5 (17.0)	1.3:1 1:1.2	European	0
Luciano et al., 2012[29]	LBC1921; LBC1936; Manchester; Nijmegen	Depressive symptoms	4525	–	–	*	*	European	0
Hek et al., 2013[27]	CHARGE	Depressive symptoms	34549	–	–	66.5 (np)	*	European	0

Study	Cohort	Phenotype	Total N	Cases	Controls			Ancestry	Ref
Okbay et al., 2016[30]	PGC; UK Biobank; GERA	Depressive symptoms	162107	-	-	*	*	European	2
	23andMe		368890	-	-	*	*	European	5
Hyde et al., 2016[26]	23andMe	Self-reported clinical diagnosis	307354	75607	231747	Cases: * Controls: *	1.6:1 1:1.3	European	15
			152127	45773	106354	Cases: * Controls: *	2:1 1:1.1		
Howard et al., 2018[23]	UK Biobank	Depression phenotypes (self-reported past help-seeking for problems with "nerves, anxiety, tension or depression," self-reported depressive symptoms associated with impairment, and MDD according to hospital admission records)	322580	113769	208811	Cases: * Controls: *	* *	European	17

(continued)

TABLE 3.1. Continued

Study	Cohort(s)	Definition of Depression	Participants	Cases	Controls	Mean Age (SD)	Female:Male Ratio	Ethnicity	Loci
Wray et al., 2018[25]	MDD Working Group of the PGC	Clinical diagnosis, registry records, self-reported diagnosis/ treatment	480359	135458	344901	Cases: * Controls: *	* *	European	44
Howard et al., 2018+[24]	23andMe, UK Biobank, MDD Working Group of the PGC	Clinical diagnosis, registry records, self-reported diag- nosis/treatment	807553	246363	561190	Cases: * Controls: *	* *	European	102

* Not reported or not reported for the whole sample.

+ Participants matched on age, gender, and ethnicity.

++ Caution is advised in interpreting results from the Howard et al. (2018) study as it has not been peer-reviewed when this manuscript is written. Although listed here, the study is not featured in the text since it has not been peer-reviewed.

Note: The publication by the MDD Working Group of the PGC in 2013 includes samples from Bonn/Mannheim, Genetic Association Information Network (GAIN)-MDD, GenRED, Glaxo-Smith-Kline (GSK), MDD2000, MARS, RADIANT, STAR*D, deCODE, GenPod/NEWMEDS, Harvard i2b3, PsyCoLaus, SHIP-LEGEND, TwinGene, GenRED Phase II, Depression Genes and Networks.[14] The publication by the MDD Working Group of the PGC included the aforementioned cohorts, in addition to cohorts from deCODE, GenScotland, GERA, iPSYCH, UK Biobank, 23andMe.

Abbreviations: ARIADNE = Adolescents at Risk for Anxiety and Depression; BLSA = Baltimore Longitudinal Study of Aging; Bonn = Department of Psychiatry of the University of Bonn = Germany; CHARGE = Cohorts for Heart and Age Research in Genomic Epidemiology Consortium; Colaus Study = Caucasian population of Lausanne; CONVERGE = China, Oxford and Virginia Commonwealth University Experimental Research on Genetic Epidemiology; DeCC = Depression Case Control Study; DeNT = Depression Network; GAIN-MDD = Genetic Association Information Network MDD; GENDEP = Genome-Based Therapeutic Drugs for Depression; GenRED = Genetics of Recurrent Early-Onset Depression; GERA = Genetic Epidemiology Research on Adult Health and Aging; GSK = GlaxoSmithKline cohort; KORA = Cooperative Health Research in the Region of Augsburg; LBC1921 and LBC1936 = Lothian Birth Cohorts 1921 and 1936; Manchester = University of Manchester Longitudinal Study of Cognition; MARS = Munich Antidepressant Response Study; MGS = Molecular Genetics of Schizophrenia study; NEMESIS = Netherlands Mental Health Survey and Incidence Study; NESDA = Netherlands Study of Depression and Anxiety; Nijmegen = Nijmegen Biomedical Study; NTR = Netherlands Twin Registry; PGC = Psychiatric Genomics Consortium; PopGen = Population-based recruitment of patients and controls for the analysis of complex genotype-phenotype relationships; QIMR = Queensland Institute of Medical Research; STAR*D = Sequenced Treatment Alternatives to Relieve Depression; UoE = University of Edinburgh.

depression.[8,9] After this initial study, a surge of GWAS on MDD ensued, but these studies were also unable to detect any genome-wide hits.[10–14]

In 2011, Kohli and colleagues were the first to report a genome-wide significant hit, rs1545843, associated with a clinician diagnosis of MDD.[15] This SNP is in *SLC6A15*, a gene that plays a role in transporting neutral amino acids. However, the mega-analysis of the Psychiatric Genomics Consortium—Major Depressive Disorder Working Group (PGC-MDD) published in 2013 with over 60,000 individuals did not replicate the finding; in fact, the study yielded no genome-wide significant SNPs.

Given the higher heritability among certain subtypes of depression, GWAS with a narrower definition of the type of clinician-diagnosed MDD have been conducted.[16–19] Among these studies, the most successful to date was reported by the CONVERGE Consortium in 2015.[20] They reported two genome-wide significant loci associated with recurrent MDD in a sample of 5,303 Han Chinese women diagnosed with recurrent MDD compared to 5,337 controls. One of the SNPs, rs12415800, is on chromosome 10 near *SIRT1*, which has previously been implicated in reward-related neural and behavioral phenotypes in animal models and anxiety in humans.[21,22] The second SNP, rs35936514, is in an intron of *LHPP*, which encodes the enzyme phospholysine phosphohistidine inorganic pyrophosphate phosphatase. In their replication sample of the more severe melancholic subtype, the findings for *SIRT1* association were even stronger despite the smaller sample size. Of note, the association between these loci and MDD may be specific to Han Chinese samples since the risk alleles are relatively rare in European ancestry samples and have not been associated with MDD in the larger PGC-MDD mega-analysis.

In total, 12 GWAS comparing individuals with clinician-diagnosed MDD with controls have been conducted to date. Overall, their success has been limited. Difficulties with identifying genetic variants associated with MDD have been in part attributed to the heterogeneity of the disorder and absence of a biological gold standard diagnosis. These early GWAS, however, do suggest that substantially larger sample sizes are needed to identify genetic variants associated with depression in order to detect the small effect sizes of most SNPs.

3.3.2. GWAS on Broader Depression Phenotypes

Research has shown strong correlations between clinician-diagnosed MDD (measured on a dichotomous scale) and self-reported depressive symptoms,[23,24] and both phenotypes are associated with similar patterns of risk factors, suggesting shared etiology with varying severity. Moreover, the genetic correlation between clinician-diagnosed MDD and depressive symptoms has been found to exceed 0.90.[25] These collective findings suggest that MDD and depressive symptoms likely have similar underlying genetic architecture. Building on these findings, recent GWAS have focused on a broader phenotype of depression[23,25,26] or even as a quantitative phenotype.[27–30]

These recent efforts using a broader phenotype of depression have proven more successful in identifying genome-wide significant variants. In 2016, leveraging the large population-based 23andMe cohort, Hyde and colleagues detected 15 genetic variants associated with a self-reported diagnosis of MDD.[26] More recently, with more than 460,000 participants, the recent meta-analysis from the PGC-MDD successfully identified 44 genome-wide significant loci associated with the broad phenotype depression, including participants with clinician-diagnosed MDD or a self-reported depression diagnosis.[25] Of these 44 identified loci, 14 loci had been identified in prior studies of MDD (12 loci in the Hyde et al. study) or depressive symptoms (1 locus from the meta-analysis by the CHARGE Consortium and 1 locus from the SSGAC). The remaining 30 loci had not previously been associated with depression.

Again, although successful, this pragmatic approach of including cohorts with broader definitions of depression has been criticized by some researchers given that self-reported diagnosis or the treatment of MDD does not necessarily correspond to the gold standard of a diagnosis of MDD derived from a standardized clinical interview. However, the findings do suggest that brief methods of assessing major depression, such as relying on treatment registers or self-report of an MDD, may be informative for the genetics of depression.[25]

3.4. POLYGENIC RISK SCORES

These GWAS findings have shown that depression is a complex, polygenic disorder influenced by many genetic variants each of small effect. One of the methods used to study such complex disorders are polygenic risk scores (PRSs).[31] PRSs are typically created by taking genetic variants up to varying thresholds of significance from a GWAS discovery sample and applying a score from these variants, weighted by the associations in the discovery sample to predict a trait in an independent target sample. As such, PRS represents the additive effect of multiple SNPs, with a higher PRS suggesting a greater genetic predisposition toward the psychiatric disorder. These scores give a much better representation of the genetic risk profile than a single candidate gene. PRSs hold great promise for supporting the identification of disease risk within different contexts, including identifying individuals at high risk for early age at onset.[31]

Analyses using PRS are relatively new and their utility is completely dependent on the success of the GWAS they are derived from. PRSs derived from the most successful published GWAS on depression to date have been found to predict 1.9% of the variance in liability toward MDD in adults[25] and 5% of the variance in liability towards MDD in children and adolescents.[32] Here, PRSs derived from larger, and consequently better-powered, discovery GWAS are likely to explain more variance in depression in the future.[33] It should also be noted that PRSs derived from other psychiatric disorders have also been found to predict depression outcomes.[33]

3.5. CANDIDATE GENE STUDIES

Prior to the availability of GWAS, the examination of genetic factors associated with depression was limited to candidate genes. In these studies, researchers choose a specific gene of interest on the basis of its biological function in a psychiatric disorder and test its association with the disorder. In spite of the hundreds of candidate genes that have been investigated, few findings are generally accepted by the genetics community. This is because results across these studies have not been consistent, likely due to the studies being underpowered when it comes to detecting the modest effect expected for common variants.[34] Larger meta-analyses of candidate gene studies have found nominal support for the association between depression and specific variants—specifically, several serotonergic genes (*SLC6A4, HTR1A, HTR2A, TPH2*), dopaminergic genes (*DRD4, SLC6A3*). and genes associated with neurodegeneration (*APOE*). Other genes associated with depression include *GNB3* and *MTHFR*, which have also been associated with other psychiatric and physical conditions. Leveraging findings from previous candidate gene studies, Lee and colleagues in 2012 examined 188 MDD candidate genes and 178 biological gene sets related to these genes in pathway analyses in previous GWAS data sets. Their findings supported the role of genes involved in the glutamatergic synaptic neurotransmission in MDD.[35]Importantly, none of these candidate gene variants have been replicated in GWAS, suggesting that their effect may be dependent on environmental factors.

3.6. GxE INTERACTION

Numerous environmental factors have been implicated in depression, including poverty, child maltreatment, and other stressful life events more generally.[36–38] However, there is marked variability in the outcomes of individuals exposed to such, raising questions about individual differences in genetic vulnerability to adverse environments. Accordingly, researchers have been interested in examining the interaction between genetic factors with established environmental risk factors for depression in GxE studies. Such studies have been conducted with candidate genes, and more recently genome-wide GxE studies have begun to emerge. Here, we will first feature prominent GxE findings for candidate genes and then provide a summary of the depression PRSxE findings.

In their landmark 2003 study, Caspi and colleagues reported that stressful life events interact with a polymorphism in the promoter of the serotonin transporter gene (*5-HTTLPR*) to increase the risk of depression.[39] This study has been highly influential as it was the first to demonstrate genetically driven individual differences in the response to environmental influences and susceptibility to psychopathology. However, these findings remain highly controversial because replication studies have yielded incongruent results.[40]

Multiple other candidate gene GxE studies of depression have been reported. Of these studies, the strongest empirical support has been found for genes involved in the regulation of the hypothalamic–pituitary–adrenal (HPA) axis, in particular FK506 binding protein-5 (*FKBP5*) and corticotropin-releasing hormone receptor 1 (*CRHR1*).[34] *FKBP5* plays an important role in the HPA axis through its regulation of the glucocorticoid receptor. *FKBP5* has found to robustly interact with childhood adversity to predict risk for depression outcomes, as well as other psychiatric disorders.[41] Interestingly, this interaction with *FKBP5* appears to be confined to the environmental stressor occurring during childhood, but not adulthood. *CRHR1* is a guanine nucleotide-binding protein receptor and is a major regulator of the HPA axis as it binds corticotropin-releasing hormone. *CRHR1* polymorphisms have also been found to interact with childhood adversity to predict risk for depression. In addition to the GxE effect at the gene association level, both *FKBP5* and *CRHR1* have extensive multilevel validation for their interaction with environmental factors, including corroborating molecular, endocrine, and neuroimaging findings.[34] Recently, in the largest systemic GxE analysis in MDD to date, the interaction between candidate genes implicated with depression—including those featured in this chapter—and early trauma yielded no significant hits.[42]

Similarly, the PRSxE studies have yielded inconclusive findings. Some studies, including a recent meta-analysis, suggest that the interaction between PRS of depression and environmental risk factors does not predict depression.[32] Yet other studies do report a significant interaction, albeit the directionality of the effect has varied across studies.[43–46]

Taken together, these inconclusive findings from GxE likely reflect the methodological challenges (e.g., limited power, heterogeneity across samples and measures of the environmental exposure, GWAS used to create the PRS) within this field. In regard to the depression PRS, future studies in which the PRS is derived from a larger sample may explain a greater proportion of the variance in depression as well as shed light on these discrepant findings.

3.7. CLINICAL IMPLICATIONS

Personalized medicine builds on the assumption that unique characteristics, including clinical presentation, history of environmental influences, and genetic predisposition, influence how (and whether) an individual develops a psychiatric disorder, as well as whether he or she will respond to a certain treatment.[47] The ultimate goal of personalized medicine is then to predict an individual's risk of developing depression, obtain an accurate diagnosis, and determine the most effective and favorable treatment option.

Within the framework of personalized medicine, the findings on genetic factors associated with depression that we have detailed may pave the way toward identifying individuals at risk for the disorder in order to target them in prevention efforts. A number of studies have investigated whether genetic markers predict response to psychotropic medication for depression.[48] Candidate gene studies have focused on genetic variants previously implicated in depression (e.g., *5-HTTLPR*, *CRHR1*) and genes involved in the metabolism of many antidepressants (i.e., genes of the cytochrome p450 system). However, the findings from these studies have been inconsistent. Also, when a genetic variant is associated with treatment response, the effect size tends to be too small to be clinically relevant.

It has become increasingly clear that most psychiatric medications are processed by and interact with multiple biological pathways. GWAS have been conducted to identify markers across the genome associated with response to psychotropic medication. To date, no genome-wide significant genes or gene sets associated with antidepressant treatment or treatment resistance have been identified.[49–51] Studies examining the predictive effect of PRS on pharmacotherapy efficacy are also now emerging. In a recent large-scale multisite study, the PRS derived from the MDD PGC did not predict response to antidepressants (i.e., escitalopram or citalopram).[52] For both the GWAS and PRS studies, larger samples may be more successful in identifying a predictors of antidepressant response.

Another novel approach within pharmacogenetics is the use of pharmacogenetic-guided decision support tools. These tools are designed to assess and interpret multiple genetic markers simultaneously in order to inform what medication is prescribed. A meta-analysis of the five existing randomized controlled trials revealed that the use of pharmacogenetic-guided decision support tools outperformed treatment as usual in relation to remission likelihood, especially among patients with severe depressive symptoms and a history of inadequate response or intolerability to previous psychotropic medication.[53] Although the findings are promising, substantial further investigation of these tools is needed to investigate the generalizability of these findings given that the samples in the extant studies have comprised predominantly 40- to 50-year-old women of European descent.

Taken together, evidence that pharmacogenetics may be successfully applied to guide the selection of psychotropic medication for depression is just emerging. However, there are still many challenges within this field. For instance, when genetic variants are robustly associated with treatment response, the effect size of the findings tends to be small and thus not suitable for clinical prediction.[54] There is also evidence suggesting that other factors influence treatment response, including demographic and clinical characteristics as well as history of trauma. For example, individuals with depression and a history of childhood trauma have been found to respond more favorably to psychotherapy than to pharmacotherapy.[55] The collective findings suggest differences in the etiology and pathogenesis of depressed individuals based on their developmental history. These findings also indicate that treatment response may be determined by a combination of factors, such as G×E effects.

3.8. CONCLUSIONS

Each of the methodological approaches introduced in this chapter has played an important role in uncovering the genetic basis of depression. They have collectively shown that genetic factors account for a substantial portion of risk for depression; however, the genetic architecture of depression is complex and polygenic. Recent large-scale efforts have finally been able to identify specific genetic variants associated with depression. These findings will open new doors in terms of future investigations. Moving forward, identifying the causal variation underlying the GWAS-associated locus with depression will be a challenge. This will require complex fine-mapping followed by functional studies of gene expression in animal and human brain, and high-resolution immunohistochemistry. Mechanistic investigations using powerful new technologies to study systems genomics and neuroscience (e.g., induced pluripotent stem cells, gene-editing methods, and optogenetic interrogation of brain circuits) will provide valuable insight into the functional effects of risk variants and pathways discovered. Pharmacogenetics will without a doubt play an important role toward personalized medicine of depression in the future. However, this field remains in its infancy and more studies with larger sample sizes are required for the promise of pharmacogenetics to materialize.

In sum, the genetics of depression is an exciting and rapidly evolving research field that will ultimately result in a deeper understanding of the underlying pathobiology of depression and, consequently, more targeted prevention and treatment strategies. However, to be successful, several challenges must be overcome and studies comprising larger cohorts or consortia will be necessary.

AUTHOR NOTE

Thorhildur Halldorsdottir and Hildur Ýr Hilmarsdottir are funded by an ERC Consolidator Grant (StressGene, grant no:726413, Prof. Valdimarsdóttir).

REFERENCES

1. Sullivan PF, Neale MC, Kendler KS. Genetic epidemiology of major depression: review and meta-analysis. *Am J Psychiatry*. 2000;157(10):1552–1562.
2. Kendler KS, Gatz M, Gardner CO, Pedersen NL. A Swedish national twin study of lifetime major depression. *Am J Psychiatry*. 2006;163(1):109–114.
3. Merikangas KR, Cui L, Heaton L, et al. Independence of familial transmission of mania and depression: results of the NIMH family study of affective spectrum disorders. *Mol Psychiatry*. 2014;19(2):214.
4. Kendler KS, Heath AC, Neale MC, et al. Alcoholism and major depression in women: a twin study of the causes of comorbidity. *Arch Gen Psychiatry*. 1993;50(9):690–698.
5. McGuffin P, Katz R, Watkins S, Rutherford J. A hospital-based twin register of the heritability of DSM-IV unipolar depression. *Arch Gen Psychiatry*. 1996;53(2):129–136.
6. Sullivan PF, Agrawal A, Bulik CM, et al. Psychiatric genomics: an update and an agenda. *Am J Psychiatry*. 2018;175(1):15–27.
7. Sullivan PF, de Geus EJC, Willemsen G, et al. Genome-wide association for major depressive disorder: a possible role for the presynaptic protein piccolo. *Mol Psychiatry*. 2009;14(4):359.
8. Hek K, Mulder CL, Luijendijk HJ, et al. The PCLO gene and depressive disorders: replication in a population-based study. *Hum Mol Genet*. 2010;19(4):731–734.
9. Minelli A, Scassellati C, Cloninger CR, et al. PCLO gene: its role in vulnerability to major depressive disorder. *J Affect Disord*. 2012;139(3):250–255.

10. Rietschel M, Mattheisen M, Frank J, et al. Genome-wide association-, replication-, and neuroimaging study implicates HOMER1 in the etiology of major depression. *Biol Psychiatry*. 2010;68(6):578–585.

11. Aragam N, Wang K-S, Pan Y. Genome-wide association analysis of gender differences in major depressive disorder in the Netherlands NESDA and NTR population-based samples. *J Affect Disord*. 2011;133(3):516–521.

12. Shyn SI, Shi J, Kraft JB, et al. Novel loci for major depression identified by genome-wide association study of Sequenced Treatment Alternatives to Relieve Depression and meta-analysis of three studies. *Mol Psychiatry*. 2011;16(2):202.

13. Wray NR, Pergadia ML, Blackwood DHR, et al. Genome-wide association study of major depressive disorder: new results, meta-analysis, and lessons learned. *Mol Psychiatry*. 2012;17(1):36.

14. Ripke S, Wray NR, Lewis CM, et al. A mega-analysis of genome-wide association studies for major depressive disorder. *Mol Psychiatry*. 2013;18(4):497–511.

15. Kohli MA, Lucae S, Saemann PG, et al. The neuronal transporter gene SLC6A15 confers risk to major depression. *Neuron*. 2011;70(2):252–265.

16. Muglia P, Tozzi F, Galwey NW, et al. Genome-wide association study of recurrent major depressive disorder in two European case-control cohorts. *Mol Psychiatry*. 2010;15(6):589.

17. Lewis CM, Ng MY, Butler AW, et al. Genome-wide association study of major recurrent depression in the UK population. *Am J Psychiatry*. 2010;167(8):949–957.

18. Shi J, Potash JB, Knowles JA, et al. Genome-wide association study of recurrent early-onset major depressive disorder. *Mol Psychiatry*. 2011;16(2):193.

19. Power RA, Keers R, Ng MY, et al. Dissecting the genetic heterogeneity of depression through age at onset. *Am J Med Genet B Neuropsychiatr Gen*. 2012;159(7):859–868.

20. Cai N, Bigdeli TB, Kretzschmar W, et al. Sparse whole-genome sequencing identifies two loci for major depressive disorder. *Nature*. 2015;523(7562):588.

21. Kishi T, Yoshimura R, Kitajima T, et al. SIRT1 gene is associated with major depressive disorder in the Japanese population. *J Affect Disord*. 2010;126(1-2):167–173.

22. Libert S, Pointer K, Bell EL, et al. SIRT1 activates MAO-A in the brain to mediate anxiety and exploratory drive. *Cell*. 2011;147(7):1459–1472.

23. Howard DM, Adams MJ, Shirali M, et al. Genome-wide association study of depression phenotypes in UK Biobank identifies variants in excitatory synaptic pathways. *Nature Commun*. 2018;9(1):1470.

24. Howard DM, Adams MJ, Clarke T-K, et al. Genome-wide meta-analysis of depression in 807,553 individuals identifies 102 independent variants with replication in a further 1,507,153 individuals. *bioRxiv*. 2018:433367.

25. Wray NR, Ripke S, Mattheisen M, et al. Genome-wide association analyses identify 44 risk variants and refine the genetic architecture of major depression. *Nature Genet*. 2018; 50(5):668.

26. Hyde CL, Nagle MW, Tian C, et al. Identification of 15 genetic loci associated with risk of major depression in individuals of European descent. *Nature Genet*. 2016;48(9):1031–1036.

27. Hek K, Demirkan A, Lahti J, et al. A genome-wide association study of depressive symptoms. *Biol Psychiatry*. 2013;73(7):667–678.

28. Terracciano A, Tanaka T, Sutin AR, et al. Genome-wide association scan of trait depression. *Biol Psychiatry*. 2010;68(9):811–817.

29. Luciano M, Huffman JE, Arias-Vásquez A, et al. Genome-wide association uncovers shared genetic effects among personality traits and mood states. *Am J Med Genet B Neuropsychiatric Genet*. 2012;159(6):684–695.

30. Okbay A, Baselmans BML, De Neve J-E, et al. Genetic variants associated with subjective well-being, depressive symptoms, and neuroticism identified through genome-wide analyses. *Nature Genet*. 2016;48(6):624.

31. Torkamani A, Wineinger NE, Topol EJ. The personal and clinical utility of polygenic risk scores. *Nature Rev Genet.* 2018;19(9):581–590.

32. Halldorsdottir T, Piechaczek C, Matos AP, et al. Polygenic risk: predicting depression outcomes in clinical and epidemiological cohorts of youth. *Am J Psychiatry.* 2019 [Epub ahead of print].

33. Bogdan R, Baranger DAA, Agrawal A. Polygenic risk scores in clinical psychology: bridging genomic risk to individual differences. *Annu Rev Clin Psychology.* 2018;14:119–157.

34. Halldorsdottir T, Binder EB. Gene-by-environment interactions: from molecular mechanisms to behavior. *Annu Rev Psychol.* 2017;68:215–241.

35. Lee PH, Perlis RH, Jung J-Y, et al. Multi-locus genome-wide association analysis supports the role of glutamatergic synaptic transmission in the etiology of major depressive disorder. *Transl Psychiatry.* 2012;2(11):e184.

36. Kessler RC, McLaughlin KA, Green JG, et al. Childhood adversities and adult psychopathology in the WHO World Mental Health Surveys. *Br J Psychiatry.* 2010;197(5):378–385.

37. Chapman DP, Whitfield CL, Felitti VJ, et al. Adverse childhood experiences and the risk of depressive disorders in adulthood. *J Affect Disord.* 2004;82(2):217–225.

38. Widom CS, DuMont K, Czaja SJ. A prospective investigation of major depressive disorder and comorbidity in abused and neglected children grown up. *Arch Gen Psychiatry.* 2007;64(1):49–56.

39. Caspi A, Sugden K, Moffitt TE, et al. Influence of life stress on depression: moderation by a polymorphism in the 5-HTT gene. *Science.* 2003;301(5631):386–389.

40. Culverhouse RC, Saccone NL, Horton AC, et al. Collaborative meta-analysis finds no evidence of a strong interaction between stress and 5-HTTLPR genotype contributing to the development of depression. *Mol Psychiatry.* 2018;23(1):133–142.

41. Matosin N, Halldorsdottir T, Binder EB. Understanding the molecular mechanisms underpinning gene by environment interactions in psychiatric disorders: the FKBP5 model. *Biol Psychiatry.* 2018;83(10):821–830.

42. Van der Auwera S, Peyrot WJ, Milaneschi Y, et al. Genome-wide gene–environment interaction in depression: a systematic evaluation of candidate genes. *Am J Med Genet B Neuropsychiatr Genet.* 2018;177(1):40–49.

43. Coleman JRI, Purves KL, Davis KAS, et al. Genome-wide gene–environment analyses of depression and reported lifetime traumatic experiences in UK Biobank. *bioRxiv.* 2018:247353.

44. Peyrot WJ, Milaneschi Y, Abdellaoui A, et al. Effect of polygenic risk scores on depression in childhood trauma. *Br J Psychiatry.* 2014;205(2):113–119.

45. Mullins N, Power RA, Fisher HL, et al. Polygenic interactions with environmental adversity in the aetiology of major depressive disorder. *Psychol Med.* 2016;46(04):759–770.

46. Musliner KL, Seifuddin F, Judy JA, et al. Polygenic risk, stressful life events and depressive symptoms in older adults: a polygenic score analysis. *Psychol Med.* 2015;45(08):1709–1720.

47. Ozomaro U, Wahlestedt C, Nemeroff CB. Personalized medicine in psychiatry: problems and promises. *BMC Med.* 2013;11(1):132.

48. Crisafulli C, Fabbri C, Porcelli S, et al. Pharmacogenetics of antidepressants. *Frontiers Pharmacol.* 2011;2:6.

49. Wigmore EM, Hafferty JD, Hall LS, et al. Genome-wide association study of antidepressant treatment resistance in a population-based cohort using health service prescription data and meta-analysis with GENDEP. *Pharmacogenomics J.* 2019 [Epub ahead of print].

50. GENDEP Investigators, MARS Investigators, STAR*D Investigators. Common genetic variation and antidepressant efficacy in major depressive disorder: a meta-analysis of three genome-wide pharmacogenetic studies. *Am J Psychiatry.* 2013;170(2):207–217.

51. Tansey KE, Guipponi M, Perroud N, et al. Genetic predictors of response to serotonergic and noradrenergic antidepressants in major depressive disorder: a genome-wide analysis of individual-level data and a meta-analysis. *PLoS Med.* 2012;9(10):e1001326.

52. García-González J, Tansey KE, Hauser J, et al. Pharmacogenetics of antidepressant response: a polygenic approach. *Prog Neuropsychopharmacol Biol Psychiatry*. 2017;75:128–134.
53. Bousman CA, Arandjelovic K, Mancuso SG, et al. Pharmacogenetic tests and depressive symptom remission: a meta-analysis of randomized controlled trials. *Pharmacogenomics*. 2019;20(1):37–47.
54. Keers R, Aitchison KJ. Pharmacogenetics of antidepressant response. *Exp Rev Neurotherapeutics*. 2011;11(1):101–125.
55. Nemeroff CB, Heim CM, Thase ME, et al. Differential responses to psychotherapy versus pharmacotherapy in patients with chronic forms of major depression and childhood trauma. *Proc Nat Acad Sci USA*. 2003;100(24):14293–14296.

/// 4 /// ENVIRONMENTAL AND SOCIAL RISK FACTORS IN DEPRESSION

KATHERINE SANCHEZ
AND EDUARDO J. SANCHEZ

Since 1987, psychiatry and behavioral health have relied on the *Diagnostic and Statistical Manual of Mental Disorders* (DSM) multi-axial system to formulate a diagnostic impression, and Axis IV was used for identifying psychosocial and environmental problems that may affect treatment and prognosis.[1] Despite evidence that Axis IV identification of primary support group problems, occupational problems, and childhood adversity effectively predicted increased risks of depressive episodes and suicidal ideation,[2] the systematic assessment of psychosocial stressors was eliminated in DSM-5.[3]

A nonaxial assessment does not mean that psychosocial and environmental stressors are not important for the manifestation or management of mental disorders. In fact, such stressors are present for many, if not most, patients, and they should be considered as part of a complete diagnostic assessment. Essentially, the social determinants of health are what were previously considered in Axis IV evaluation. Today's clinician should address social and environmental factors that might be etiologically relevant to the current episode or to the future course of the disorder in order to customize treatment and optimize outcomes.

4.1. DEPRESSION AND THE SOCIAL DETERMINANTS

The World Health Organization (WHO) has defined mental health as "a state of well-being in which every individual realizes his or her own potential, can cope with the normal stresses of life, can work productively and fruitfully, and is able to make a contribution to her or his community."[4] A life course perspective considers risk exposure in the formative stages of life, which can affect mental well-being or predispose individuals and populations made vulnerable by deep-rooted poverty, social inequality, and discrimination. Various risk and protective factors at the individual, family, community, policy, and population levels act to improve or perpetuate inequalities in health status.[5]

The social determinants of health include societal conditions and psychosocial factors, such as opportunities for employment, adequate income, hopefulness, and freedom from racism.[6] US adults living in poverty are more than five times as likely to report being in fair or poor health compared to adults with incomes at least four times the federal poverty level.[7] The social determinants are thought to impact health indirectly through mechanisms that may include stress associated with low socioeconomic status, experiences of disempowerment and violence, hopelessness, helplessness, and income insecurity; they impact health more directly through reduced access to health services for physical and mental health problems.[8,9]

WHO has declared depression to be the leading cause of medical disability, health burden, and increased medical cost in the world, and it is associated with the highest rates of unemployment of all disabilities.[10,11] One in five Americans is diagnosed in their lifetime, and a chronic or relapsing course is common.[12] The increase in worldwide disability has been attributed to social and environmental factors such as changes in family structure, substance abuse, and growing socioeconomic inequalities.[4,13]

Efforts to address the double and coexisting burden of economic disadvantage and depression are critical yet tricky to tease out. An understanding of the social and environmental factors that contribute to risk for developing depression is important for illustrating the potential for primary prevention and identification of target groups and social contexts (Figure 4.1).[14] Specifically, understanding how patient characteristics such as socioeconomic status, race, ethnicity, health beliefs and attitudes, and access to medical care influence the underutilization of services is critical.[15–17]

4.1.1. Societal and Individual Burden

The economic burden of depression is significant, with a recent 21.5% increase in cost attributable to direct medical care costs (inpatient, outpatient, and pharmacy), to suicide-related costs, and to workplace costs such as "presenteeism" (reduced productivity while at work) and absenteeism (missed days of work). During the period of 2005 to 2010, treatment rates remained low, which increased the related economic costs—for every dollar spent on treatment, an additional $1.90 was spent on indirect costs (suicide and workplace) and another $4.70 was spent on comorbidity costs for people with depression.[18] Thus, there exists a complex interplay of work status, depression symptoms, and treatment.

Other documented societal burdens for individuals with depression include the greater likelihood of loss of employment and diminished employment prospects compared with their counterparts without depression.[18] Low socioeconomic status is

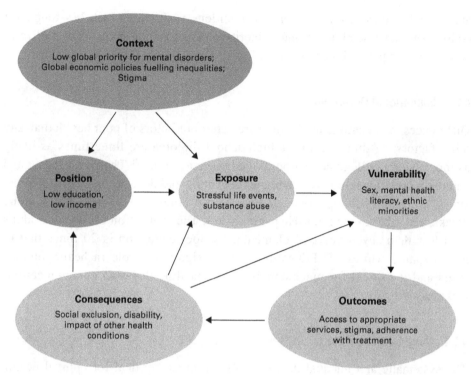

FIGURE 4.1. WHO cycle of social determinants and mental disorders. *Reprinted with permission from WHO,* Equity, Social Determinants and Public Health Programmes *(2010; pp. 115–134). https://www.who. int/sdhconference/resources/EquitySDandPH_eng.pdf ISBN 978 92 4 156397 0 (NLM classification: WA 525).*

associated with greater odds of depression and likelihood of a persistent depression,[8] and women experience social, economic, and environmental factors in ways that put them at even greater risk than men.[14] Additionally, people with depression are disproportionately affected by downturns in the economy and availability of part-time work.[18]

4.1.2. Environmental Determinants

Environmental factors appear to increase risk even before birth, and disadvantage accumulates throughout life.[5] Recent public health efforts, particularly in the past two decades, have identified a select array of conditions in which people are born, grow, live, work, and age that significantly affect health.[19] Simply put, place matters.[20] The inequitable impact of the environmental and social conditions in which people live creates persistent and pervasive health disparities that plague discrete populations. Low education level, racial segregation, low social support, and poverty are all social determinants that are attributable to increased death rates.[21]

Unsafe or unhealthy housing; proximity to highways, factories, or other sources of toxic agents; and other hazards like overcrowding significantly affect the physical and mental health of the residents of a community.[22] Adverse environments are strongly linked with exposure to hazardous toxicants, which has long-term consequences.[23] Racial and ethnic minority populations are more likely to live in conditions that put their health at risk.[5]

4.1.3. Educational Determinants

Differences in education and income are better predictors of poor health than any other factors.[24] Adults without a high school diploma are three times as likely as those with a college education to die before age 65.[25,26] There is a strong and significant relationship between higher education and decreasing rates of depression.[4,8] The high school dropout rate is 18.3% among Hispanics, 9.9% among blacks, and 4.8% among non-Hispanic whites. The proportion of Hispanic adults with less than seven years of elementary school education is 20 times that of non-Hispanic whites.[27,28] Education plays a significant role in health literacy skills and is critical for understanding basic health education communications and messaging.[29]

4.1.4. Neighborhood Determinants

The systematic and unequal distribution of resources critical for optimal health, such as access to affordable healthy food or safe environments in which to exercise, has a significant impact on populations marginalized by low socioeconomic status and geographic location.[19] Furthermore, physical activities such as walking, running, cycling, and gardening outdoors have known mental health benefits, such as reducing stress, anxiety, and depression.[30] Opportunities for residents of some neighborhoods are limited; it is simply unsafe for children to play and adults to exercise outside.[22]

Stores and restaurants selling unhealthy food may outnumber markets with fresh produce or restaurants with nutritious food.[22] Low-income neighborhoods have one-third fewer grocery stores than their higher-income counterparts. Additionally, corner stores and gas stations typically charge one and a half times the price of similar items available in grocery stores.[31] Not having an automobile or adequate public transportation can reduce access to affordable, healthy food. Less expensive, more accessible foods are often high in calories and fat. Limited time and lack of knowledge of food preparation can increase demand for and consumption of prepackaged or processed foods.[31]

Gaps in health across neighborhoods stem from multiple factors. Communities with weak tax bases cannot support high-quality schools, and jobs are often scarce in neighborhoods with struggling economies. Features that isolate communities, such as highways, can lead to residential segregation, which limits social cohesion, stifles economic growth, and perpetuates cycles of poverty.[22] Conversely, people living in less segregated neighborhoods, with better schools and family stability, have a higher probability of socioeconomic upward mobility.[32,33]

4.1.5. Racial and Ethnic Determinants

Poverty and poor health are associated with higher rates of mental disorders.[34] Data from a number of studies suggest that people from racial and ethnic minority groups and underserved populations are particularly unlikely to receive specialty mental health care treatment.[35,36] Hispanics and other ethnic minorities experience a disproportionate burden of disability associated with mental disorders because of these disparities in mental health care.[37,38] And while effective treatments exists, only 20% of people with diagnosed depression receive guideline-concordant, evidence-based treatment.[39,40]

Undertreatment is particularly common in racial and ethnic minority populations; ability to speak English and affordability are the greatest predictors of use of antidepressant medication.[15,41,42] In one study of depression (self-report, diagnosed, and treated) among Hispanics and African Americans in public housing in Los Angeles, a high incidence of depression, both by self-report and physician diagnosed, was not being treated.[15] Access to care is affected by a dearth of, or poorly conducted, outreach campaigns to communities, lack of availability of materials in a variety of languages, and the fear of retribution and reporting to government agencies of their immigration status when applying for public benefits.[43] Other access-to-care barriers include low parental education, transportation problems, and excessive wait times.[44,45]

The seminal Surgeon General report *Mental Health: Culture, Race and Ethnicity* emphasized the importance of history and culture to understanding mental health, mental illness, and disparities in services for racial and ethnic minority populations.[42] In particular, understanding the cultural and historical experiences of different groups and examining how patient characteristics such as socioeconomic status, ethnicity, health beliefs and attitudes, and accessibility to medical care influence the utilization of services, will allow a health care delivery system to respond appropriately and better meet the unique needs of patients whose culture may be different than the larger culture in which they live.[16,17,46,47]

Lastly, there now exits extensive evidence documenting the role of racism and discrimination experienced on a daily basis by Hispanics, African Americans, and other ethnic minorities that leads to poor health outcomes, especially mental health.[15–17,48–50] Though current research cannot adequately explain the exact mechanism of discrimination and its role in poor health outcomes, it suggests that the daily experience of emotional distress leads to a substantially increased risk of disease.[48]

4.2. ADVERSE CHILDHOOD EXPERIENCES

Adverse childhood experiences (ACEs) are stressful or traumatic events that occur in childhood, including suffering abuse and neglect, witnessing domestic violence or family members who have substance use disorders or mental illness, or even having an incarcerated parent.[51] Evidence from neurobiology and epidemiology suggests that early life stress and related adverse experiences cause enduring brain dysfunction and are a significant risk factor for the development and prevalence of a wide range of health problems throughout a person's lifespan, including substance misuse/abuse, depression, and obesity.[52,53] Much of what is known about the long-term impacts of childhood adversity comes from the landmark Centers for Disease Control and Prevention (CDC)-Kaiser Permanente Adverse Childhood Experiences (ACE) Study[51] and subsequent studies using ACE data collected on the Behavioral Risk Factor Surveillance System (BRFSS).[54]

Measurement of ACEs is categorized into three groups: abuse, neglect, and family/household challenges. Each category is further divided into multiple subcategories. All ACE questions refer to the respondent's first 18 years of life.[55]

Abuse:emotional abuse;physical abuse; sexual abuse
Neglect: emotional neglect; physical neglect
Family/Household Challenges: mother treated violently; household substance abuse;mental illness in household;parental separation or divorce; criminal household member

ACE studies use an index, a sum of the different categories of ACEs reported by participants, to assess cumulative childhood stress, and the framework is conceptualized as a pyramid (Figure 4.2). Findings repeatedly indicate a

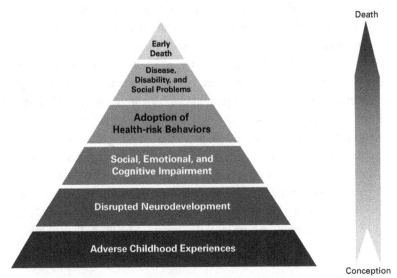

Mechanism by Which Adverse Childhood Experiences
Influence Health and Well-being Throughout the Lifespan

FIGURE 4.2. The ACE pyramid conceptual framework. *Reprinted with permission from Felitti VJ, Anda RF, Nordenberg D, et al., Relationship of childhood abuse and household dysfunction to many of the leading causes of death in adults: the Adverse Childhood Experiences (ACE) Study.* Am J Prev Med. *1998;14(4):245–258. doi: 10.1016/s0749-3797(98)00017-8*

dose–response relationship between ACE scores and the likelihood of moderate to heavy drinking, drug use, depressed affect, and suicide attempts in adulthood.[56,57] The number of ACEs strongly predicts both lifetime and recent depressive disorders, up to decades after their occurrence.[58] There is a startlingly significant association between the number of ACEs related to all forms of abuse, repeated physical abuse, and forced sexual intercourse, and late-life depression and suicidality.[59,60]

4.3. ACHIEVING QUALITY HEALTH CARE OUTCOMES

In 2015, the US Department of Health and Human Services set a goal of tying Medicare payments to value using measurable goals aimed at paying providers based on the quality, rather than the quantity, of care they give patients. A subsequent requisite report to Congress in 2016 examined the effect of individuals' social risk factors on quality measures, resource use, and other measures under the Medicare program, as well as analyses of the impact of Medicare's current value-based payment programs on providers serving socially at-risk beneficiaries. Two significant findings emerged from the report:

1. Beneficiaries with social risk factors had worse outcomes on many quality measures, regardless of the providers they saw, and dual enrollment status (Medicare plus Medicaid) was the most powerful predictor of poor outcomes.
2. Providers who disproportionately served beneficiaries with social risk factors tended to have worse performance on quality measures. As a result, safety net providers were more likely to face financial penalties in most of the value-based purchasing programs.[61]

Amid the growing discussion about whether payment and quality measurement should be adjusted to account for social risk factors, the National Academies of Sciences, Engineering, and Medicine (NAM) convened an ad hoc committee to identify social risk factors that affect the health outcomes of Medicare beneficiaries and methods to account for these factors in Medicare payment programs. The NAM ultimately concluded that it is possible to deliver high-quality care to socially at-risk populations.[62]

For over 50 years, a set of social and demographic characteristics have been collected during routine clinical assessments and recorded in patients' medical records.[63] They generally include race/ethnicity, occupation, marital status, living situation, use of alcohol, use of tobacco, and recent travel. In 2016, the Institute of Medicine (IOM) Committee on the Recommended Social and Behavioral Domains and Measures for Electronic Health Records (EHRs) provided a concrete approach to include social and behavioral determinants of health in the clinical record to increase awareness and provide crucial information about factors that influence health and the effectiveness of diagnosis, treatment choices, policy, health care system design, and innovations to improve health outcomes and reduce health care costs.[64]

IOM recommended that all EHRs should include race/ethnicity, educational attainment, financial resource strain, stress, depression, physical activity, tobacco use and exposure, alcohol use, social connections and isolation, exposure to violence, and neighborhood and community composition. Sincere and comprehensive measurement of the social and behavioral domains will enable more effective treatment of individual patients, more effective population management for health care systems and for public health agencies, and discovery of the pathways that link social and behavioral factors to functioning, disease processes, and mortality that may inform new treatments and interventions.[65]

Standardized collection of social determinants of health is necessary but not sufficient to create meaningful change. Use of the measures in psychiatry can help providers to better act on patients' social determinants of health and identify socioeconomic drivers of poor outcomes and higher costs. Providers can measure and document the increased complexity of their patients, and potentially transform care with integrated services and community partnerships to meet the needs of their patients and advocate for change in their communities.[65]

4.4. CONCLUSION

Castrucci and Auerbach remind us that assessing and addressing social determinants of health at an individual level in the clinical setting by providing or referring for housing vouchers, travel vouchers, and medication assistance is important to address the individual burden at a point in time.[66] This approach complements clinical care and may improve individual health outcomes. However, there is a need to assess and address social determinants of health at a population, policy-driven level. The recently released report titled "How States Can Improve Community Health Working Through Policy Change" identifies many policies that are within social determinants of health areas identified in this chapter.[67]

Taking action to improve the conditions of daily life includes environmental, structural, and local interventions to reduce the risk of mental disorders and to promote mental health in the population.[5] The practicing psychiatrist will be a better clinician by delivering evidence-based clinical care that is informed by individuals' burden of social and environmental factors and by understanding and, in some instances, advocating for policies that can ease the burden of social determinants on populations.

REFERENCES

1. American Psychiatric Association. *Diagnostic and Statistical Manual of Mental Disorders.* 4th ed. Washington, D.C.: American Psychiatric Association; 1994.
2. Gilman SE, Trinh NH, Smoller JW, et al. Psychosocial stressors and the prognosis of major depression: a test of Axis IV. *Psychol Med.* 2013;43(2):303–316.
3. American Psychiatric Association. *Diagnostic and Statistical Manual of Mental Disorders.* 5th ed. Washington, D.C.: American Psychiatric Association; 2013.

4. World Health Organization. Mental health: a state of well-being. 2014; https://www.who.int/features/factfiles/mental_health/en/.
5. World Health Organization and Calouste Gulbenkian Foundation. *Social Determinants of Mental Health*. Geneva: World Health Organization; 2014.
6. Smedley BD. The lived experience of race and its health consequences. *Am J Public Health*. 2012;102(5):933–935.
7. Heron M, Hoyert DL, Murphy SL, et al. *Deaths: Final Data for 2006*. Atlanta: Centers for Disease Control and Prevention; 2009.
8. Lorant V, Deliege D, Eaton W, et al. Socioeconomic inequalities in depression: a meta-analysis. *Am J Epidemiol*. 2003;157(2):98–112.
9. Allen J, Balfour R, Bell R, Marmot M. Social determinants of mental health. *Int Rev Psychiatry*. 2014;26(4):392–407.
10. WHO. *Depression and Other Common Mental Disorders: Global Health Estimates*. Geneva: World Health Organization; 2017.
11. Kessler RC. The costs of depression. *Psychiatr Clin North Am*. 2012;35(1):1–14.
12. Hasin DS, Sarvet AL, Meyers JL, et al. Epidemiology of adult DSM-5 major depressive disorder and its specifiers in the United States. *JAMA Psychiatry*. 2018;75(4):336–346.
13. Cross-National Collaborative Group. The changing rate of major depression. Cross-national comparisons. *JAMA*. 1992;268(21):3098–3105.
14. Patel V, Lund C, Hatheril S, et al. Mental disorders: equity and social determinants. In: E Blas, A Sivasankara Kurup, eds. *Equity, Social Determinants and Public Health Programmes*. Geneva: World Health Organization; 2010:115–134.
15. Bazargan M, Bazargan-Hejazi S, Baker RS. Treatment of self-reported depression among Hispanics and African Americans. *J Health Care Poor Underserved*. 2005;16(2):328–344.
16. Gelberg L, Andersen RM, Leake BD. The behavioral model for vulnerable populations: application to medical care use and outcomes for homeless people. *Health Serv Res*. 2000;34(6):1273–1302.
17. Wu CH, Erickson SR, Kennedy J. Patient characteristics associated with the use of antidepressants among people diagnosed with DSM-IV mood disorders: results from the National Comorbidity Survey Replication. *Curr Med Res Opin*. 2009;25(2):471–482.
18. Greenberg PE, Fournier AA, Sisitsky T, et al. The economic burden of adults with major depressive disorder in the United States (2005 and 2010). *J Clin Psychiatry*. 2015;76(2): 155–162.
19. Ramirez L, Baker E, Metzler M. *Promoting Health Equality: A Resource to Help Communities Address Social Determinates of Health*. Atlanta: Centers for Disease Control and Prevention; 2008.
20. Bell J, Rubin V. *Why Place Matters: Building a Movement for Healthy Communities*. PolicyLink. 2007. https://www.policylink.org/resources-tools/why-place-matters-building-the-movement-for-healthy-communities.
21. Galea S, Tracy M, Hoggatt KJ, et al. Estimated deaths attributable to social factors in the United States. *Am J Public Health*. 2011;101(8):1456–1465.
22. VCU Center on Society and Health. Mapping Life Expectancy. 2016. https://societyhealth.vcu.edu/work/the-projects/mapping-life-expectancy.html.
23. Glass TA, Bilal U. Are neighborhoods causal? Complications arising from the "stickiness" of ZNA. *Soc Sci Med*. 2016;166:244–253.
24. National Academies of Sciences. *Communities in Action: Pathways to Health Equity*. Washington, D.C.: National Academies Press; 2017.
25. Bravemen P, Egerter S. *Overcoming Obstacles to Health*. Princeton, NJ: Robert Wood Johnson Foundation; 2008.
26. Institute of Medicine. *Crossing the Quality Chasm: A New Health System for the 21st Century*. Washington, D.C.: National Academy Press; 2001.

27. DeNavas-Walt C, Proctor BD, Smith JC. *Income, Poverty, and Health Insurance Coverage in the United States: 2009.* Washington, D.C.: US Census Bureau; 2010.

28. Taylor P, Kochhar R, Fry R, et al. *Wealth Gaps Rise to Record Highs Between Whites, Blacks, and Hispanics.* Washington, D.C.: Pew Research Center; 2011.

29. Lopez V, Sanchez K, Killian MO, Eghaneyan BH. Depression screening and education: an examination of mental health literacy and stigma in a sample of Hispanic women. *BMC Public Health.* 2018;18(1):018–5516.

30. Thompson Coon J, Boddy K, Stein K, et al. Does participating in physical activity in outdoor natural environments have a greater effect on physical and mental wellbeing than physical activity indoors? A systematic review. *Environ Sci Technol.* 2011;45(5):1761–1772.

31. International City/County Management Association. *Community Health and Food Access: The Local Government Role.* Washington, D.C.; 2006.

32. Chetty R, Hendren N, Kline P, Saez E. Where is the land of opportunity? The geography of intergenerational mobility in the United States. *Q J Econ.* 2014;129(4):1553–1623.

33. Chetty R, Hendren N. The impacts of neighborhoods on intergenerational mobility I: Childhood exposure effects. *Q J Econ.* 2018;133(3):1107–1162.

34. McGuire T, Miranda J. New evidence regarding racial and ethnic disparities in mental health: policy implications. *Health Aff.* 2008;27(2):393–403.

35. Jackson-Triche ME, Greer Sullivan J, Wells KB, et al. Depression and health-related quality of life in ethnic minorities seeking care in general medical settings. *J Affect Disord.* 2000;58(2):89–97.

36. The President's New Freedom Commission on Mental Health. *Achieving the Promise: Transforming Mental Health Care in America.* Rockville, MD: Department of Health and Human Services; 2003.

37. Cabassa LJ, Zayas LH, Hansen MC. Latino adults' access to mental health care: a review of epidemiological studies. *Admin Policy Mental Health.* 2006;33(3):316–330.

38. Dwight-Johnson M, Lagomasino IT. Addressing depression treatment preferences of ethnic minority patients. *Gen Hosp Psychiatry.* 2007;29(3):179–181.

39. Young AS, Klap R, Sherbourne CD, Wells KB. The quality of care for depressive and anxiety disorders in the United States. *Arch Gen Psychiatry.* 2001;58(1):55–61.

40. Kessler RC, Demler O, Frank RG, et al. Prevalence and treatment of mental disorders, 1990 to 2003. *N Engl J Med.* 2005;352(24):2515–2523.

41. Karasz A, Watkins L. Conceptual models of treatment in depressed Hispanic patients. *Ann Fam Med.* 2006;4(6):527–533.

42. US Department of Health and Human Services. *Mental Health: Culture, Race, and Ethnicity: A Supplement to Mental Health: A Report to the Surgeon General.* Rockville, MD; 2001.

43. Sanchez K, Chapa T, Ybarra R, Martinez ON. Eliminating health disparities through culturally and linguistically centered integrated health care: consensus statements, recommendations, and key strategies from the field. *J. Health Care Poor Underserved.* 2014;25(2): 469–477.

44. Flores G, Fuentes-Afflick E, Barbot O, et al. The health of Latino children: urgent priorities, unanswered questions, and a research agenda. *JAMA.* 2002;288(1):82–90.

45. Sanchez K, Ybarra R, Chapa T, Martinez ON. Eliminating behavioral health disparities and improving outcomes for racial and ethnic minority populations. *Psychiatr Serv.* 2016;67(1):13–15.

46. Bazargan M, Ani CO, Hindman DW, et al. Correlates of complementary and alternative medicine utilization in depressed, underserved African American and Hispanic patients in primary care settings. *J Altern Complement Med.* 2008;14(5):537–544.

47. Office of Minority Health. *National Standards for Culturally and Linguistically Appropriate Services in Health Care, Final Report.* Washington, D.C.: US Department of Health and Human Services; 2001.

48. Williams DR, Neighbors HW, Jackson JS. Racial/ethnic discrimination and health: findings from community studies. *Am J Public Health*. 2003;93(2):200–208.

49. Clark R, Anderson NB, Clark VR, Williams DR. Racism as a stressor for African Americans: a biopsychosocial model. *Am Psychol*. 1999;54(10):805–816.

50. Alderete E, Vega WA, Kolody B, Aguilar-Gaxiola S. Lifetime prevalence of and risk factors for psychiatric disorders among Mexican migrant farmworkers in California. *Am J Public Health*. 2000;90(4):608–614.

51. Felitti VJ, Anda RF, Nordenberg D, et al. Relationship of childhood abuse and household dysfunction to many of the leading causes of death in adults: the Adverse Childhood Experiences (ACE) Study. *Am J Prev Med*. 1998;14(4):245–258.

52. Substance Abuse and Mental Health Services Administration (SAMHSA). Adverse Childhood Experiences. 2018. https://www.samhsa.gov/capt/practicing-effective-prevention/prevention-behavioral-health/adverse-childhood-experiences.

53. Anda RF, Felitti VJ, Bremner JD, et al. The enduring effects of abuse and related adverse experiences in childhood. A convergence of evidence from neurobiology and epidemiology. *Eur Arch Psychiatry Clinical Neurosci*. 2006;256(3):174–186.

54. Behavioral Risk Factor Surveillance System (BRFSS). 2019. https://www.cdc.gov/brfss/index.html.

55. Centers for Disease Control and Prevention. CDC-Kaiser Permanente Adverse Childhood Experiences (ACE) Study. 2016. https://www.cdc.gov/violenceprevention/childabuseandneglect/acestudy/about.html.

56. Merrick MT, Ports KA, Ford DC, et al. Unpacking the impact of adverse childhood experiences on adult mental health. *Child Abuse Neglect*. 2017;69:10–19.

57. Brown DW, Anda RF, Tiemeier H, et al. Adverse childhood experiences and the risk of premature mortality. *Am J Prev Med*. 2009;37(5):389–396.

58. Chapman DP, Whitfield CL, Felitti VJ, et al. Adverse childhood experiences and the risk of depressive disorders in adulthood. *J Affect Disord*. 2004;82(2):217–225.

59. Sachs-Ericsson NJ, Rushing NC, Stanley IH, Sheffler J. In my end is my beginning: developmental trajectories of adverse childhood experiences to late-life suicide. *Aging Ment Health*. 2016;20(2):139–165.

60. Ege MA, Messias E, Thapa PB, Krain LP. Adverse childhood experiences and geriatric depression: results from the 2010 BRFSS. *Am J Geriatric Psychiatry*. 2015;23(1):110–114.

61. US Department of Health and Human Services; Office of the Assistant Secretary for Planning and Evaluation. *Report to Congress: Social Risk Factors and Performance Under Medicare's Value-Based Purchasing Programs*. Washington, D.C.; 2016.

62. National Academies of Sciences Engineering and Medicine. *Accounting for Social Risk Factors in Medicare Payment: Identifying Social Risk Factors*. Washington, D.C.; 2017.

63. Delbanco T, Walker J, Darer JD, et al. Open notes: doctors and patients signing on. *Ann Intern Med*. 2010;153(2):121–125.

64. Committee on the Recommended Social and Behavioral Domains and Measures for Electronic Health Records; Board on Population Health and Public Health Practice. *Capturing Social and Behavioral Domains and Measures in Electronic Health Records: Phase 2*. Washington, D.C.: National Academies Press; 2015.

65. DeVoe JE, Bazemore AW, Cottrell EK, et al. Perspectives in primary care: a conceptual framework and path for integrating social determinants of health into primary care practice. *Ann Fam Med*. 2016;14(2):104–108.

66. Castrucci B, Auerbach J. Meeting individual social needs falls short of addressing social determinants of health. *Health Affairs Blog*. 2019. https://www.healthaffairs.org/do/10.1377/hblog20190115.234942/full//

67. Trust for America's Health. *Promoting Health and Cost Control in States: How States Can Improve Community Health & Well-Being Through Policy Change*. Washington, D.C.; 2019.

BIOMARKERS PREDICTING
ANTIDEPRESSANT
TREATMENT RESPONSE

An Overview

BHARATHI S. GADAD, MANISH K. JHA,
AND MADHUKAR H. TRIVEDI

5.1. INTRODUCTION

Patients with major depressive disorder (MDD) often stay on ineffective treatments for too long or switch/discontinue too early [1–3]. Even when taken for adequate duration, treatment outcomes are suboptimal and the side-effect burden is substantial [4–6]. With the availability of several effective treatments, detailed in other chapters, patients and their clinicians often struggle with selecting the right treatment. However, in the absence of any evidence demonstrating the efficacy of one treatment over another, treatments are often selected based on patient or provider preferences, cost, side effects, tolerability, and/or response during previous episode(s) [7]. Unlike other fields of medicine, like breast cancer [8], asthma [9], macular degeneration [10], and multiple sclerosis [11], there are no available and valid biomarkers to move toward precision medicine for this devastating lifelong illness. Personalized treatments, which maximize the likelihood of treatment response and continuation, are urgently needed to reduce the burden of MDD [12, 13].

Factors that adversely impact the search for biomarkers of treatment response in MDD include the heterogeneity of disease [14] and the limitation of current diagnostic categories [15]. Factors previously studied include demographic features (like gender [16], race [17], employment status [4]), illness characteristics (like baseline severity of depression [18], duration of illness [19], number of previous episodes

[20], age of onset [21], family history of mood disorders [20], presence of anxious features [22], depression subtypes [23], comorbid psychiatric disorders [17], psychosocial functioning [24]), and social factors (like marital status [20], level of social support, social status) [25], with little to no clinical utility [23, 26–30]. Among currently available features that can be easily measured in clinics, body mass index (BMI) has been shown to guide treatment selection in two separate studies [31]. Biological markers, which are objective and can be measured externally [32, 33], have the potential to bridge the knowledge gap needed to personalize MDD treatment. To maximize the chances of success, we may need to go beyond individual biomarkers toward generating biosignatures by systematically evaluating combinations of both clinical and biological markers.

In this chapter, we briefly review the current state of technology available for blood-based biomarker research, as well as the status of biomarker research to date for antidepressant treatment response. Finally, we discuss exciting new innovations that have the potential to galvanize the search for breakthrough biomarker discovery.

5.2. BIOMARKERS FOR ANTIDEPRESSANT RESPONSE

In recent years, researchers have aimed to identify several different types of putative biomarkers, including genomic, endocrine, neuroimaging, neurophysiological, proteomic-immune, and many others that could predict future response to antidepressant treatment; some of these are targeted by antidepressants and may change over the course of treatment. The latest advancement in technologies has enabled providers to screen for these biomarkers that enhance the better understanding of the disease, the treatment, and the response. In this chapter, we discuss in detail the advanced methodologies, protocols, and validation techniques that aim to apply multiple technologies for the screening of blood-based biomarkers.

5.2.1. Current State of Technology

In the field of pharmacogenomics, advanced technologies that have been extensively used in large-scale trials including genome-wide association studies (GWAS) and single nucleotide polymorphism (SNP) genotyping in the Sequenced Treatment Alternatives to Relieve Depression (STAR*D) study [34], the Munich Antidepressant Response Signature (MARS) study [35], the Genome-Based Therapeutic Drugs for Depression (GENDEP) [36] study, and the Mayo Clinic Pharmacogenomics Research Network Antidepressant Medication Pharmacogenomics Study (PGRN-AMPS) [37]; whole exome sequencing; targeted gene sequencing; and epigenetic changes including DNA methylation and post-translational modifications of histones in MDD [37]. Genotype imputation is now an essential tool in the analysis of GWAS. Imputed genotype data increase the power of analysis and provide greater coverage and higher resolutions than did tag SNP genotyping, as evidenced by the "1000" genomes imputed SNPs associated with selective serotonin reuptake inhibitors

(SSRIs) [38]. In addition, epigenetic profiling or modifications serve as an important and promising tool for a better understanding of antidepressant treatment effect and could be a more robust biomarker.

In proteomics, there are several traditional methods, including two-dimensional gel electrophoresis (2DE) for protein separation and mass spectrometry (MS) for protein identification. 2DE has been extensively and successfully used in studies of brain tissue or body fluids of patients with psychiatric disorders such as depression, schizophrenia, and bipolar disorder as well as in studies of neurodegenerative disorders such as Alzheimer's diseasee [39–41]. 2DE–MS-based proteomics presents some limitations such as a difficulty in detecting low-abundance, acidic or basic proteins as well as proteins with extremes of high or low molecular weight. Later, an alternative direct MS-based approach was developed to target proteins. Generally known as shotgun proteomics or liquid chromatography–tandem mass spectrometry (LC-MS), this uses a combination of chromatographic steps prior to MS analyses in a high-throughput way. Shotgun proteomics has been used in MDD, revealing some differentially expressed proteins that have not been found by 2DE methods. Shotgun LC-MS analysis of MDD patients with and without psychosis showed significant differences in proteomic profiles [39, 41]. Xu et al. showed that using the 2D ITRAQ LC-MS approach in MDD led to upregulation and downregulation of proteins such as apolipoprotein D, B-100, ceruloplasmin histidine-rich glycoprotein, semaphorin, and α-2-macroglobulin [42].

The latest introduction of advanced multiplex Luminex-based technologies comprises rules-based medicine (RBM), bioplex, meso-scale discovery (MSD), SomaLogic, and others that allow measurement of multiple analytes in individual small-volume samples, revolutionizing proteomic analyses. These platforms are suitable for the development of convenient, rapid, sensitive, and specific assays for a wide range of diseases [42, 43]. This technology employs multiplexed dye-coded microspheres, coated with specific capture reagents (antibodies in case of enzyme-linked immunosorbent assay [ELISA] or aptamers for microarray-based high-throughput approach for SomaLogic) assaying targeted analytes within biological samples. The format allows multiplexing of up to 25 to 1,100 analytes for a single sample. This approach minimizes sampling errors, the amount of sample required for each analysis, and the need for and costs of assay reagents. Expression levels were significantly different between normal controls and MDD patients. There are several other studies based on the different proteomic approaches that support the findings that protein biomarkers are primarily involved in lipid metabolism and immunoregulation. These studies suggest that early perturbation of lipid metabolism and immunoregulation may be involved in the pathophysiology of MDD. The initiation of high-resolution proton nuclear magnetic resonance spectroscopy (^{1}H-NMR) provided a means of multiplexing analyses of metabolites and provided greater accuracy and higher throughput. Moreover, high-performance liquid chromatography, gas chromatography, and targeted electrochemistry-based metabolomics platforms have also been widely used to quantify significant metabolic biomarkers in serum, plasma, and cerebrospinal fluid of patients with MDD. Biomarkers based on the "omics" category can be analyzed using different biospecimens such as plasma, serum, cerebrospinal fluid, etc., using the right method of approach. The approach or the methodology must be based on the specific targets that a person is screened for. For example, for identifying SNPs, genotyping based on GWAS is performed (Figure 5.1).

2DE, LC-MS, and shotgun or multiplex proteomic approaches are used to reveal the global protein expression of a given tissue or biological sample. They are more useful as discovery-based panels. However, other methods, such as Western blot (WB), ELISA, singleplex, multiple reaction monitoring mass spectrometry, and antibody arrays, are employed commonly to validate differentially expressed proteins observed in the discovery-based panel. Validation is necessary to demonstrate that the differences found in a limited small set of samples are found in a broader universe of samples, considering factors such as age, gender, and different ethnicities. Moreover, there is a necessity to implement and improve high-throughput methods for validation studies such that high sample numbers are not a limiting factor. Since all of the molecular profiling methods described here have their strengths and weaknesses, the combined use of two or more platforms to screen putative biomarkers for depression and antidepressant drug response would be best to maximize coverage of the relevant molecular pathways. Several types of biomarkers, including genomics, transcriptomics, epigenomics, proteomics, and metabolomics, show promise for predicting antidepressant treatment response. The evidence supporting each type of biomarker is considered separately next.

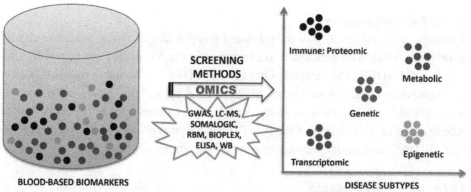

FIGURE 5.1. Characterization of biomarkers from the biological samples into subsets of the markers: proteomics, immune, metabolomics, genetic, transcriptomic, and epigenomic. The biomarkers are screened based on the antidepressant treatment based on the appropriate analyses: GWAS, multiplex, singleplex, ELISA.

5.2.2. Genomics, Epigenomics, and Transcriptomics

Genomics and transcriptomics enable the study of genes and their structure, function, and expression. Large-scale GWAS of the STAR*D (n = 1,953) sample [34], MARS (n = 339) sample [35], GENDEP (n = 706), sample [36], and PGRN-AMPS (n = 529) sample [37] have failed to detect any gene at the level of genome-wide significance in predicting antidepressant response.

5.2.2.1. Multidrug-Resistance Gene

Genetic polymorphisms in the multidrug-resistance gene (MDR1) have been investigated for predicting response to antidepressant medications. P-glycoprotein (P-GP), the gene product of MDR1, is present at the blood–brain barrier and influences absorption of antidepressants that are substrates of P-GP (like citalopram, venlafaxine, or paroxetine). There are multiple positive [44–48] and negative [49–51] studies showing an association of SNPs in MDR1 and differential treatment outcomes with antidepressant medications that are P-GP substrates.

5.2.2.2. Serotonin Transporter

Polymorphisms in the serotonin transporter linked polymorphic region (5-HTTLPR) of the SLC6A4 gene influence serotonin reuptake and have been investigated widely for antidepressant response. Using samples from the STAR*D study, while an initial report suggested no significant association [52], a follow-up study of polymorphisms in 5-HTTLPR showed differential treatment outcomes with citalopram in non-Hispanic white subjects but not in Hispanic white and black subjects [53]. In a systematic meta-analysis, Porcelli et al. found a strong association between a polymorphism in 5-HTTLPR and treatment outcomes with SSRIs in Caucasians but not in Asians [54].

5.2.2.3. Serotonin Receptor

A specific SNP (rs7997012) of the serotonin receptor 2A (HTR2A) gene was significantly associated with antidepressant response in the STAR*D [55,56] and MARS [57] and GENDEP [58] samples. Other studies failed to replicate this association but found an association with other SNPs of HTR2A and antidepressant treatment outcomes [55, 59–61]. Adding to the variability of these findings, several studies failed to find an association of the 5-HTTLPR polymorphism [62–64] and HTR2A SNPs [63, 65] with antidepressant treatment outcomes.

5.2.2.4. Dopamine Metabolism

An SNP at codon 158 of the catechol-O-methyl transferase (COMT) gene (rs4680) results in the substitution of valine by methionine and is commonly referred to as the COMT val158met polymorphism. Met/met genotype is associated with decreased activity [66, 67] of the COMT enzyme, the main catalytic enzyme of dopamine in the brain [68–70] and has been reported to have favorable outcomes with antidepressants in some studies [71–77] but not others [63, 78–80]. In contrast, treatment-resistant patients with the Val/Val genotype had a much higher chance of responding to electroconvulsive therapy [81]. Domschke et al. found that higher rates of improvement after electroconvulsive therapy in treatment-resistant patients with the Val/Val genotype were found only in female patients [82].

5.2.2.5. Glutamate Receptor

Polymorphisms in the glutamate inotropic kainite (GRIK) 4 receptor gene were shown to be associated with treatment response in samples from the STAR*D [83], MARS [60], and other [84] studies. However, Perlis et al. [64] and Serretti et al. [85] failed to replicate these associations.

5.2.2.6. Brain-Derived Neurotrophic Factor

Associations of polymorphisms of the brain-derived neurotrophic factor (BDNF) gene and antidepressant response [7, 86, 87] were not replicated in other studies [88–90]. In samples from the STAR*D [91] MARS [92], and GENDEP [59] studies, BDNF polymorphisms were not associated with antidepressant response [93–95].

5.2.2.7. Cytochrome P450 Enzymes

Tests for common polymorphisms in genes encoding for cytochrome P450 enzymes are included in commercially available kits [96] and may be used to classify individuals as extensive metabolizers, intermediate metabolizers, poor metabolizers, or ultra-rapid metabolizers [97]. While these polymorphisms can be helpful in predicting adverse effects [97–99], their association with response to SSRIs in the STAR*D [49, 51], the GENDEP [100, 101], and other studies [102–104] has been either negative or only weakly positive [105].

5.2.2.8. Multiple SNPs

Taking an innovative approach of developing and testing models using multiple developmental and validation cohorts of MDD outpatients of Asian ethnicity, Lim et al. found that a model incorporating SNPs of GRIK 2 (rs543196) and glutamate decarboxylase 1 (rs3828275 of GAD1) and haplotypes of tryptophan hydroxylase 2 (TPH2) and 5-HTTLPR predicted response to SSRI with 87% accuracy [99, 106, 107]. Interestingly, their model was not accurate for predicting response to non-SSRI medications, raising the possibility of developing genetic profiles to predict differential response to antidepressants.

5.2.2.9. Monoamine Oxidase A

Genetic variations of monoamine oxidase A (MAO-A) are altered by the mechanism of action of SSRIs through interaction with 5-HT transporters. But a recent study in bipolar depression revealed that the link of rs6323 in the MAO-A gene is associated with mirtazapine response in girls and women. Other studies on fluoxetine and bupropion by Tiwari et al. [61] and Peters et al. [107], respectively, have shown no association with the antidepressant response in Mexican ($n = 319$) and Caucasian ($n = 96$) populations.

5.2.2.10. FK506 Binding Protein 5

FK506 binding protein 5 genetic variants like rs1360780, rs4713916, and rs3800373 have shown a stronger link with the various antidepressant treatments in Caucasian subjects ($n = 294$) [35]. However, several other studies, such as Mayo-PGRN-AMPS, have not replicated these findings in different cohorts and Antidepressant Medications (ADMs) [108]. Uher et al. [58] and Perlis et al. [64] have found no association with the SNPs on antidepressants such as escitalopram and duloxetine ($n = 760$ and 250).

5.2.2.11. ALX4

Recently, Gadad et al. (2018) [109] showed the association of novel ALX4 gene polymorphisms with antidepressant treatment response in CO-MED clinical trial subjects ($n = 459$) of Caucasian ethnicity. Haplotype analysis on all the positive ALX4 variants showed that a regulatory haplotype CAAACTG was significantly associated (odds ratio = 3.4, $p = 2.00E-04$) with response to escitalopram monotherapy. ALX4 is most strongly known for its association with bone development, and MDD patients frequently have significant decreases in bone density.

So far, the genes listed in MDD are in the coding region, so it is also important to determine whether any genes related to MDD and antidepressant response are encoded in the noncoding regulatory regions. All the genes and SNPs discussed in this section and their association with different antidepressant treatments are summarized in Table 5.1.

5.2.3. Transcriptomics

In an exploration of transcriptomic biomarkers with whole-genome gene expression study of MDD remitters versus nonresponders, Hennings et al. [110] initially identified messenger ribonucleic acid (mRNA) transcripts of interest and then used a replication sample of 142 patients from the MARS study. They found that lower pretreatment levels of retinoid-related orphan receptor alpha (RORa) mRNA, germinal center expressed transcript 2 (GCET2) mRNA, and chitinase 3-like protein 2 (CHI3L2) mRNA were associated with a greater likelihood of antidepressant response. Using convergent functional genomics analysis with data from human blood gene expression, genetic linkage/association, and postmortem brain studies as well as animal model gene expression data, Le-Niculescu et al. identified candidate blood biomarker genes involved in myelination and growth factor signaling as predictors of high and low mood states [111]. Keri et al. then tested the expression of these genes in MDD patients, before and after cognitive–behavioral therapy, and control subjects and found that clinical improvement with cognitive–behavioral therapy was associated with increased expression of genes associated with high mood state versus genes associated with low mood states [112].

TABLE 5.1. Genes Associated with Antidepressant Treatment Response

	Gene	Author and Year	Ethnicity	Discovered	Antidepressant	Association and Favorable Outcome	n
1	SLC6A4			No association	SSRI, SSNRI, SNRI, TCA		
2	HTR2A	Tiwari et al. (2013)	European African Mexican	44 SNPs within HTR2A	Bupropion	rs277096 GG genotype	319
3	HTR2A	Uher et al. (2009)	Caucasian	36 SNPs within seroto-nergic genes	Escitalopram	rs9316233 G allele rs1923884 A allele	424
4	HTR2A	Peters et al. (2009)	Mainly Caucasian (78%)	15 SNPs within HTR2A	Citalopram	rs787012 A allele rs1923884 CC genotype	1631
5	HTR2A	Perlis et al. (2009)	Caucasian	41 SNPs within HTR2A	Duloxetine	rs9534505, rs1923884, rs2760351	250
6	HTR2A	Hortsmann et al. (2009)	Caucasian	38 SNPs within HTR2A	Various	rs7997012 G allele	300
7	HTR2A	Peters et al. (2004)	Mainly Caucasian (78%)	17 SNPs within HTR2A	Fluoxetine	rs1923882 CC genotype rs6314 GG genotype rs3125 GG genotype	96
8	TPH1/ TPH2	Uher et al. (2009)	Caucasian	36 SNPs within seroto-nergic genes	Escitalopram	No association	424
9	TPH1/ TPH2	Tsai et al. (2009)	Asian	5 SNPs within TPH2	Fluoxetine, Citalopram (SSRI)	Rs2171363 T/C genotype	187
10	TPH1/ TPH2	Peters et al. (2009)	Mainly Caucasian (78%)	6 SNPs within TPH1 and 9 SNPs within TPH2	Citalopram	No association	1631

(continued)

TABLE 5.1. Continued

	Gene	Author and Year	Ethnicity	Discovered	Antidepressant	Association and Favorable Outcome	n
11	TPH1/TPH2	Tzvetkov et al. (2008)	Caucasian	10 SNPs within TPH2	Various	No association	183
12	TPH1/TPH2	Peters et al. (2004)	Mainly Caucasian (78%)	19SNPs within TPH1 and 14SNPs within TPH2	Fluoxetine	T-7180G; T-7065C, T-5806G (TPH1); rs1843809, rs1386492; rs1487276 (TPH2)	96
13	MAO-A	Tiwari et al. (2013)	Mixed (European African Mexican)	7 SNPs within MAO-A	Bupropion	No association	319
14	MAO-A	Peters et al. (2004)	Mainly Caucasian (78%)	8SNPs within MAO-A and MAO-VNTR	Fluoxetine	No association	96
15	COMT	Houston et al. (2011)	Caucasian	24 SNPs within COMT	Duloxetine	Rs165737 CC genotype; 2 SNP diplotype	225
16	COMT	Kocabas et al. (2010)	Caucasian	7 SNPs within COMT	Various	Rs2075507 GG genotype; 3 SNP haplotype	396
17	COMT	Perlis et al. (2009)	Caucasian	19 SNPs within COMT	Duloxetine	Rs165599 GG; rs165774 GG; rs174696 CC	250
18	GRIK4	Pu et al. (2013)	Asian	5 SNPs within GRIK4	Paroxetine, fluoxetine, sertraline, escitalopram (SSRIs) or venlafaxine (SNRI)	Rs1954787 G allele; 3 SNP haplotype with AGG (rs 1954787-rs2230297-rs2298725)	281

#	Gene	Study	Ethnicity	SNPs examined	Drug	Result	N
19	BDNF	Hennings et al. (2013) MARS Study	Caucasian	18 SNPs within BDNF	Various	7 BDNF SNPs and haplotypes	398
		Hennings et al. (2013) 2 replication samples	Caucasian	7 SNPs within BDNF	Various	Rs11602246	496
		Hennings et al. (2013) Combined sample	Caucasian	7 SNPs within BDNF	Various	Rs2049046 T allele	894
20	BDNF	Murphy et al. (2013)	Caucasian	13 SNPs within BDNF	Paroxetine, mirtazapine	Rs11030086 AA genotype; rs6265 GG genotype; rs988712 CC genotype; rs988748 CC genotype	216
21	BDNF	Kocabas et al. (2011)	Caucasian	8 tagging SNPs within BDNF (including 66 val/met)	Various	Rs10501087 C allele; rs6265 A allele; rs 1491850 C allele and various haplotypes	206
22	BDNF	Domschke et al. (2010) STAR*D (replication sample)	Mixed	10 SNPs within BDNF	Various	No association	1953
23	BDNF	Licinio et al. (2009)	Mixed Americans	130 SNPs within BDNF	Fluoxetine, desipramine	Rs61888800 GG genotype	272
24	BDNF	Uher et al. (2009)	Caucasian	57 tagging SNps within BDNF (including 66 val/met)	Escitalopram, nortriptyline	No association	760

(continued)

TABLE 5.1. Continued

	Gene	Author and Year	Ethnicity	Discovered	Antidepressant	Association and Favorable Outcome	n
25	BDNF	Gratacos et al. (2008)	Caucasian	8 tagging SNPs within BDNF (including val/met)	Various	Rs908867 A allele; TAT haplotype	374
26	FKBP5	Ellsworth et al. (2013) Mayo-PGRN-AMPS	White non-Hispanic	481 SNPS; 127 FKBP5 SNPs and 354 FKBP5 eQTL SNPs	Citalopram; escitalopram	24 FKBP5 SNPs; 21 FKBP5 eQTL SNPs	512
27	FKBP5	Ellsworth et al. (2013) Mayo-PGRN-AMPS	White non-Hispanic	6SNPs; 3 FKBP5 SNPs and 3FKBP5 eQTL SNPs	Citalopram	Rs352428 GG genotype	960
28	FKBP5	Uher et al. (2009)	Caucasian	57 SNPs within common pathway genes	Escitalopram, nortriptyline	No association	760
29	FKBP5	Perlis et al. (2009)	Caucasian	4 SNPs within FKBP5	Duloxetine	No association	250
30	FKBP5	Binder et al. (2004)	Caucasian	21 SNPs within FKBP5	Various	Rs1360780 TT genotype; rs4713916 AA genotype; rs 3800373 CC genotype	294
31	ALX4	Gadad et al. (2018)	Caucasian	14 SNPs with ALX4	Escitalopram, venlafaxine, mirtazapine, bupropion	Rs10769025, CAAACTG	450

Listed are the major SNPs from the previous studies from the literature, which are known to be associated with the treatment response.

5.2.4. Epigenomics

DNA methylation has emerged as a target of antidepressant medications, and methylation of the serotonin transporter has been shown to predict treatment outcome. Domschke et al. observed a higher methylation status of the SLC6A4 gene in MDD patients who showed a better response following six weeks of treatment with escitalopram [113].

5.2.5. MicroRNAs

MicroRNAs (miRNAs) play an important role in the fundamental and physiological processes in the central nervous system (CNS). MiRNAs are small regulatory RNAs that could cause post-transcriptional silencing of the gene by base pairing with the target mRNA. MiRNAs are known to play several important functions in the brain, such as synaptic plasticity, regulating neuronal differentiation and development. In recent years, there have been several pieces of evidence that suggest alterations in the levels of miRNAs in MDD patients. In addition, miRNAs are known to be used by antidepressant drugs as downstream signaling effectors.

5.2.6. Proteomics

The major proteomics biomarkers reported in the literature based on the antidepressant response are summarized in Table 5.2. Proteomics, the next step after genomics and transcriptomics, involves profiling the entire set of proteins in a biological system to recognize their structure and functions. Proteomic biomarkers have shown some potential in predicting treatment response. While levels of peripheral blood inflammatory cytokines are reduced with SSRIs [114], they have limited utility in predicting antidepressant response [115, 116]. Low (<1 mg/mL) levels of C-reactive protein (CRP), a marker of inflammation, at baseline successfully identified patients who would respond to escitalopram versus nortriptyline in the GENDEP study [117]. As Compared to escitalopram, the use of nortriptyline in patients with higher CRP levels at baseline was associated with a greater reduction in their depression severity. Raison et al. [118] found that elevated levels of high-sensitivity CRP (>5 mg/mL) at baseline were associated with a significantly greater likelihood of treatment response with infliximab versus placebo. Levels of protein p11 in natural killer (NK) cells and monocytes may be potential biomarker, as Svenningsson et al. found that reduction in p11 after one to two weeks of citalopram treatment was significantly correlated with a subsequent reduction in depression severity [119]. Janssen et al. found that antidepressants modulate cytokine functioning and directly influence treatment outcome in MDD [120]. Further, they showed that antidepressants normalize serum levels of cytokines, including interleukin (IL)-6, IL-1 β, tumor necrosis factor alpha (TNF-α), and interferon gamma (IFN-γ) [120]. Maes et al. examined the effects of clomipramine, sertraline, and trazodone on the stimulated production of IFN-γ and

TABLE 5.2. Proteomic Markers Associated with Antidepressant Response

	Method/Sample	Author and Year	Biomarkers Discovered	Drug/Context	N
1	LC-MS and Multiplex (Serum)	Stelzhammer et al. (2014)	Ferritin, MIF, EN-RAGE, SOD-1, IL-1, IL-16; tenascin-C, BDNF, serotransferrin, growth hormone	Drug-naive vs. controls	Drug-naive MDD N = 23 and 15 and N = 42 and 21 controls
2	LC-MS (Serum)	Lee et al. (2015)	Platelet basic protein, ceruloplasmin, plasma kallikrein, inter-alpha trypsin inhibitor HC4, neutrophil, complement component 1qC, immunoglobulin J chain, apolipoprotein C-III, immunoglobulin HC3, fetuin B	Baseline vs. remission after treatment	N = 5 MDD; N = 8 matched controls
3	2D LC-Chip MS/MS (Plasma)	Xu et al. (2012)	Apolipoprotein D, afamin, apolipoprotein-B-100, glycoprotein, vitamin-D-binding protein; ceruloplasmin, histidine-rich glycoprotein, semaphorin, α-2-macroglobulin	Treatment-naive vs. controls	N = 21 MDD and 21 healthy controls
4	Multiplex (Serum)	Bot et al. (2015)	Prostasin, luteinizing hormone, alpha-1-antitrypsin, urokinase-type plasminogen activator receptor, cathepsin D, hepsin, matrix metalloproteinase-10, interleukin-1 receptor antagonist, von Willebrand factor and fatty acid-binding protein adipocyte	Current MDD and remitted MDD vs. controls	N = 482 MDD and N = 480 controls

#	Method/platform	Protein markers detected	Comparison	N
5	Multiplex (Plasma)	Apolipoprotein A, macrophage colony-stimulating factor, neutrophil gelatinase-associated lipocalin, vitronectin, glutathione S-transferase alpha, myeloperoxidase, N-terminal prohormone of brain natriuretic peptide, receptor tyrosine protein kinase erbB, FASLG receptor, luteinizing hormone, neuropilin 1	Late-life depression vs. controls	N = 80 MDD with MCI
6	Multiplex (Plasma)	Eotaxin, interferon-γ	Remitters vs. non-remitters	n = 274 baseline and exit
7	Multiplex (Plasma)	Platelet-derived growth factor, basic fibroblast growth factor, and granulocyte colony-stimulating factor	Baseline depression severity	n = 274 baseline and exit
8	Multiplex (Plasma)	IL-17	Baseline depression severity	n = 274 baseline and exit
9	Multiplex (Plasma)	C-reactive protein	Baseline depression severity	n = 274 baseline and exit

Diniz et al. (2015) — row 5
Gadad et al. (2017) — row 6
Jha et al. (2017) — rows 7, 8, 9

Listed are the protein markers detected based on the treatment and the methods/platform used from the previous studies.

IL-10 and observed that all three antidepressants significantly increased the IFN- γ/ IL-10 ratio [121]. Several studies have evaluated peripheral blood levels of neuro-trophic factors to predict treatment response and found no evidence for their utility as a biomarker of differential antidepressant response [122–127]. Lee et al., for the first time, showed in five MDD patients that quantitative proteomic studies identified 10 proteins that were consistently upregulated or downregulated [128]. ELISA yielded results consistent with the proteomic analysis for ceruloplasmin, inter-alpha-trypsin inhibitor heavy chain H4, and complement component 1qC [128]. In addition, Stelzhammaer et al. performed molecular profiling using multiplex immunoassay and LC-MS on serum samples from cohorts of first-onset and antidepressant-naive patients ($n = 23$ and 15) and matched controls ($n = 42$ and 21) independently. The results were biomarkers related to inflammatory-like cytokines and interleukins, BDNF, cortisol, angiotensin-converting enzyme, and enzymes related to oxidative stress response [129]. The latest two papers published recently based on the RBM multiplex discovery platform [130, 131] on the plasma biomarkers were truly based on immune markers like cytokines, interleukins, growth factors, and lipids ($n = 78$ MDD and 156 controls and $n = 36$ mild cognitive impairment (MCI) with depression and $n = 44$ controls) [130, 131].

Recently, using CO-MED clinical trial samples, we have found some leading observations related to proteomic biomarkers that can predict antidepressant treat-ment response. Jha et al. observed that higher baseline platelet-derived growth factor level was associated with greater reduction in depression severity in the bupropion/ SSRI arm but not the other two treatment arms [132]. Jha et al., in the same CO-MED subjects, found that higher baseline IL-17 level was associated with a greater reduction in depression severity in the bupropion/SSRI subjects [133]. Jha et al. also found that higher baseline CRP levels were associated with lower depression severity with a bupropion/SSRI combination but not with SSRI monotherapy [134]. Finally, Gadad et al. observed that increased levels of eotaxin-1/CCL11 correlated with re-mission at week 12, whereas decreased levels of IFN-γ correlated with nonremission at week 12 [135].

5.2.7. Metabolomics

Metabolic analytes screened so far in the antidepressant treatment outcome clin-ical trials are summarized in Table 5.3. Metabolomic tools enable identification and quantification of molecules that can report on changes in biochemical pathways. In a small study, Paige et al. found a pattern of reduced levels of metabolites such as glycerate, citrate, glycerol, and octadecadienoate in plasma of currently depressed MDD patients versus healthy controls and remitted MDD patients [136]. Metabolite profiling of tryptophan metabolism in a four-week-long double-blind placebo-controlled study showed that response to either sertraline or placebo was associ-ated with increases in 5-methoxytryptophol and melatonin levels and decreases in kynurenine/melatonin and 3-hydroxykynurenine/ melatonin ratios post-treatment

TABLE 5.3. Metabolomic Markers Associated with Antidepressant Response

	Method/Sample	Author and Year	Biomarkers Discovered	Drug/Context	N
1	^{1}H-NMR (Urine)	Tian et al. (2014)	Creatinine, taurine, 2-oxo-glutarate, xanthurenic acid, glutathione, prostaglandins, malondialdehyde	*Xiaoyaosan*	N = 21 MDD and N = 21 controls
2	LC-MS (Plasma)	Davies et al. (2014)	Tryptophan, serotonin, taurine, 8 acylcarnitines, 13 glycerophospholipids, 3 sphingolipids.	-	N = 21 MDD and N = 21 controls
3	LCEA (Serum)	Zhu et al. (2013)	5-methoxytryptamine, 5-methoxytryptophol, mela-tonin, kyneurinine, 3-hydroxy kyneurenine.	Sertraline	N = 35 MDD and N = 40 controls
4	GC-MS (Serum)	Kaddurah-Daouk et al. (2013)	α-ketoglutarate, glutamine and glutamic acid, homoserine, proline, GABA, glutamic acid, creatinine	Sertraline	N = 46 MDD and N = 46 controls
5	LCEA (Serum)	Kaddurah-Daouk et al. (2011)	Dihydroxyphenylacetic acid, 4-hydroxyphenyllactic acid, serotonin gamma tocopherol, hypoxanthine, xanthine and uric acid, 5-methoxytryptophol, 3-hydroxykynurenine, 5-hydroxyindoleactic acid	Sertraline	N = 46 MDD and N = 46 controls
6	GC-MS and LC-MS (Plasma)	Steffens et al. (2010)	Phenylalanine, aspartate acid, serine, γ-glutamyl amino acids, 3-methyl-2-oxobutyrate, 3-methyl-2-oxovalerate, 4-methyl-2-oxopentanoate.	Sertraline	N = 10 MDD and N = 9 controls
7	LC-MS/MS (Plasma)	Cysyz et al. (2019)	Sphingomyelins, lysophosphatidylcholines, phosphatidylcholines, acylcarnitines	Escitalopram, venlafaxine, mirtazapine, bupropion	N = 159
8	LC-MS/MS (Plasma)	Moaddel et al. (2018)	Circulating sphingomyelins, kynurenine pathway, arginine pathway	Ketamine	Treatment-resisstant MDD (29 subjects) and healthy controls (25 subjects)

Listed are small metabolites associated with the antidepressant treatment.

compared to pretreatment [137]. Using samples from the same study, Kaddurah-Daouk et al. found that pretreatment levels of metabolites of tryptophan, phenylalanine, purine, and tocopherol can be used to predict responders versus nonresponders to sertraline or placebo [138]. In a subsequent study, they found that pretreatment to post-treatment decreases in levels of branched chain amino acids (valine, leucine, and isoleucine) had a moderate to strong correlation with improvement in depression severity in patients taking sertraline [139]. Use of antidepressants alters energy metabolism, as suggested by two- to four-fold higher levels of glucose-6-phosphate and fructose-6-phosphate in mice treated with paroxetine[139]. Kaddurah-Daouk et al. found that pretreatment metabotype predicted response to sertraline or placebo in 46 outpatients with MDD and 46 control subjects. The metabolites were allied to tryptophan metabolism and some organic acids. In a study by Tian et al. (2014) [140] in 21 MDD patients and 21 control subjects, small endogenous metabolites present in urine samples were measured by nuclear magnetic resonance (NMR) and analyzed by multivariate statistical methods. The researchers found that creatinine, taurine, 2-oxoglutarate, and xanthurenic acid increased significantly after the administration of *xiaoyaosan*, a traditional Chinese drug treatment for MDD ($p \leq 0.05$). Zhu et al. (2018) [137] conducted the study on ($n = 35$) or placebo ($n = 40$) in a double-blind four-week trial; response to sertraline treatment was measured using the 17-item Hamilton Rating Scale for Depression (HAMD17). A targeted electrochemistry-based metabolomics platform (LCECA) was used to profile serum samples from MDD patients and showed that metabolites were related to the kyneurinine and tryptophan metabolism pathway. Recently, in our laboratory, Czysz et al. used the AbsoluteIDQ™ p180 kit to investigate plasma metabolites (sphingomyelins, lysophosphatidylcholines, phosphatidylcholines, and acylcarnitines) from a subset of participants in the CO-MED trial [141]. Metabolite concentrations were measured in 159 plasma samples and combined with clinical and sociodemographic variables using the hierarchical lasso. Czysz et al. also found that patients with increased baseline concentrations of phosphatidylcholine C38:1 showed poorer outcome based on a change in the Quick Inventory of Depressive Symptomatology (QIDS) score [141]. However, an increased ratio of hydroxylated sphingomyelins compared to non-hydroxylated sphingomyelins at baseline and a change from baseline to exit were detected. Moaddel et al. found that ketamine treatment in patients with treatment-resistant MDD ($n = 29$) and healthy control subjects ($n = 25$) showed enhancement in metabolites such as circulating sphingomyelins, the kynurenine pathway, and the arginine pathway by LC-MS/MS [142].

5.3. CONCLUSION

Although the field for treating MDD is advancing, there are still ambiguities that need to be addressed if we are to optimize treatment for individual patients (personalized medicine treatment approach). As such, there is not a single clinical assessment that is useful to detect early treatment options (whether a patient responds well to a particular antidepressant medication or not). Nevertheless, there are several factors, such as severity of illness, duration, comorbidity, and older age of onset, can help in predicting treatment response [17]. However, The advancement of research in the area of MDD and antidepressant treatment in recent years has enabled us to identify genetic, proteomic, metabolomics, and any biological predictors that could be used in the near future in a clinical setting [17, 111]. Therefore, identifying an individual factor or set of factors is a pressing need in the treatment of MDD. A biomarker that can predict a priori if an individual patient will respond to a particular treatment of choice, as well as the early distinction between responders and nonresponders, would significantly impact the current situation of treatment. Biomarkers not only allow us to monitor the treatment but also assist in understanding the mechanism of action of drugs in the early stage of clinical trials. Biomarkers could be pathologic, therapeutic, pharmacological, etc., are objectively measured and evaluated to understand the biological phenomenon [135]. Despite decades of research, the neurochemistry, neurobiology, and neuropathology of MDD remain elusive. Therefore, researchers in the recent past have tried to identified the neurobiological process by measuring "endophenotype" using several different advanced methods: pharmacogenomics, genomics, proteomics, metabolomics, hormone, and stress signaling pathways [14]. In a highly heterogeneous disease like MDD, a single biomarker may not be the sole cause for the disease or treatment, and thus a panel of biomarkers/biosignatures is considered to play a promising role for future.

REFERENCES

1. Burton C, Cochran AJ, Cameron IM. Restarting antidepressant treatment following early discontinuation: a primary care database study. Fam Pract 2015;32(5):520–524.
2. Rush AJ, Wisniewski SR, Warden D, et al. Selecting among second-step antidepressant medication monotherapies: predictive value of clinical, demographic, or first-step treatment features. Arch Gen Psychiatry 2008;65(8):870–880.
3. Warden D, Trivedi MH, Wisniewski SR, et al. Predictors of attrition during initial (citalopram) treatment for depression: a STAR*D report. Am J Psychiatry 2007;164(8):1189–1197.
4. Warden D, Rush AJ, Trivedi MH, et al. The STAR*D Project results: a comprehensive review of findings. Curr Psychiatry Rep 2007;9(6):449–459.
5. Trivedi MH, Rush AJ, Wisniewski SR, et al. Evaluation of outcomes with citalopram for depression using measurement-based care in STAR*D: implications for clinical practice. Am J Psychiatry 2006;163(1):28–40.
6. Rush AJ, Trivedi MH, Stewart JW, et al. Combining medications to enhance depression outcomes (CO-MED): acute and long-term outcomes of a single-blind randomized study. Am J Psychiatry 2011;168(7):689–701.
7. Taylor WD, McQuoid DR, Ashley-Koch A, et al. BDNF Val66Met genotype and 6-month remission rates in late-life depression. Pharmacogenomics J 2011;11(2):146–154.
8. Dowsett M, Dunbier AK. Emerging biomarkers and new understanding of traditional markers in personalized therapy for breast cancer. Clin Cancer Res 2008;14(24):8019–8026.
9. Lima JJ, Blake KV, Tantisira KG, Weiss ST. Pharmacogenetics of asthma. Curr Opin Pulm Med 2009;15(1):57–62.

10. Lee AY, Raya AK, Kymes SM, et al. Pharmacogenetics of complement factor H (Y402H) and treatment of exudative age-related macular degeneration with ranibizumab. Br J Ophthalmol 2009;**93**(5):610–613.

11. Vosslamber S, van Baarsen LG, Verweij CL. Pharmacogenomics of IFN-beta in multiple sclerosis: towards a personalized medicine approach. Pharmacogenomics 2009;**10**(1): 97–108.

12. Kessler RC, Berglund P, Demler O, et al. The epidemiology of major depressive disorder. JAMA 2003;**289**(23):3095–3105.

13. Murray CJ, Atkinson C, Bhalla K, et al. The state of US health, 1990–2010: burden of diseases, injuries, and risk factors. JAMA 2013;**310**(6):591–608.

14. Hasler G, Drevets WC, Manji HK, Charney DS. Discovering endophenotypes for major depression. Neuropsychopharmacology 2004;**29**(10):1765–1781.

15. Insel T, Cuthbert B, Garvey M, et al. Research domain criteria (RDoC): toward a new classification framework for research on mental disorders. Am J Psychiatry 2010;**167**(7):748–751.

16. Young EA, Kornstein SG, Marcus SM, et al. Sex differences in response to citalopram: a STAR*D report. J Psychiatr Res 2009;**43**(5):503–511.

17. Friedman ES, Wisniewski SR, Gilmer W, et al. Sociodemographic, clinical, and treatment characteristics associated with worsened depression during treatment with citalopram: results of the NIMH STAR(*)D trial. Depress Anxiety 2009;**26**(7):612–621.

18. Friedman ES, Davis LL, Zisook S, et al. Baseline depression severity as a predictor of single and combination antidepressant treatment outcome: results from the CO-MED trial. Eur Neuropsychopharmacol 2012;**22**(3):183–199.

19. Rush AJ, Wisniewski SR, Zisook S, et al. Is prior course of illness relevant to acute or longer-term outcomes in depressed out-patients? A STAR*D report. Psychol Med 2012;**42**(6):1131–1149.

20. Trivedi MH, Morris DW, Pan JY, et al. What moderator characteristics are associated with better prognosis for depression? Neuropsychiatr Dis Treat 2005;**1**(1):51–57.

21. Zisook S, Lesser I, Stewart JW, et al. Effect of age at onset on the course of major depressive disorder. Am J Psychiatry 2007;**164**(10):1539–1546.

22. Fava M, Rush AJ, Alpert JE, et al. Difference in treatment outcome in outpatients with anxious versus nonanxious depression: a STAR*D report. Am J Psychiatry 2008;**165**(3):342–351.

23. Arnow BA, Blasey C, Williams LM, et al. Depression subtypes in predicting antidepressant response: a report from the iSPOT-D trial. Am J Psychiatry 2015;**172**(8):743–750.

24. Vittengl JR, Clark LA, Jarrett RB. Deterioration in psychosocial functioning predicts relapse/recurrence after cognitive therapy for depression. J Affect Disord 2009;**112**(1):135–143.

25. Lesser I, Rosales A, Zisook S, et al. Depression outcomes of Spanish- and English-speaking Hispanic outpatients in STAR*D. Psychiatr Serv 2008;**59**(11):1273–1284.

26. Bobo WV, Chen H, Trivedi MH, et al. Randomized comparison of selective serotonin reuptake inhibitor (escitalopram) monotherapy and antidepressant combination pharmacotherapy for major depressive disorder with melancholic features: a CO-MED report. J Affect Disord 2011;**133**(3):467–476.

27. Chan HN, Rush AJ, Nierenberg AA, et al. Correlates and outcomes of depressed out-patients with greater and fewer anxious symptoms: a CO-MED report. Int J Neuropsychopharmacol 2012;**15**(10):1387–1399.

28. Sung SC, Haley CL, Wisniewski SR, et al. The impact of chronic depression on acute and long-term outcomes in a randomized trial comparing selective serotonin reuptake inhibitor monotherapy versus each of 2 different antidepressant medication combinations. J Clin Psychiatry 2012;**73**(7):967–976.

29. Sung SC, Wisniewski SR, Balasubramani GK, et al. Does early-onset chronic or recurrent major depression impact outcomes with antidepressant medications? A CO-MED trial report. Psychol Med 2013;**43**(5):945–960.

30. Sung SC, Wisniewski SR, Luther JF, et al. Pre-treatment insomnia as a predictor of single and combination antidepressant outcomes: a CO-MED report. J Affect Disord 2015;**174**: 157–164.

31. Jha MK, Wakhlu S, Dronamraju N, et al. Validating pre-treatment body mass index as moderator of antidepressant treatment outcomes: findings from CO-MED trial. J Affect Disord 2018;**234**:34–37.

32. Biomarkers and surrogate endpoints: preferred definitions and conceptual framework. Clin Pharmacol Ther 2001;**69**(3):89–95.

33. Strimbu K, Tavel JA. What are biomarkers? Curr Opin HIV AIDS 2010;**5**(6):463–466.

34. Garriock HA, Kraft JB, Shyn SI, et al. A genomewide association study of citalopram response in major depressive disorder. Biol Psychiatry 2010;**67**(2):133–138.

35. Ising M, Lucae S, Binder EB, et al. A genomewide association study points to multiple loci that predict antidepressant drug treatment outcome in depression. Arch Gen Psychiatry 2009;**66**(9):966–975.

36. Uher R, Perroud N, Ng MY, et al. Genome-wide pharmacogenetics of antidepressant response in the GENDEP project. Am J Psychiatry 2010;**167**(5):555–564.

37. Ji Y, Biernacka JM, Hebbring S, et al. Pharmacogenomics of selective serotonin reuptake inhibitor treatment for major depressive disorder: genome-wide associations and functional genomics. Pharmacogenom J 2013;**13**(5):456–463.

38. Abo R, Hebbring S, Ji Y, et al. Merging pharmacometabolomics with pharmacogenomics using "1000 Genomes" single-nucleotide polymorphism imputation: selective serotonin reuptake inhibitor response pharmacogenomics. Pharmacogenet Genomics 2012;**22**(4):247–253.

39. Martins-de-Souza D, Harris LW, Guest PC, et al. The role of proteomics in depression research. Eur Arch Psychiatry Clin Neurosci 2010;**260**(6):499–506.

40. Lista S, Faltraco F, Prvulovic D, Hampel H. Blood and plasma-based proteomic biomarker research in Alzheimer's disease. Prog Neurobiol 2013;**101-102**:1–17.

41. Schirle M, Bantscheff M, Kuster B. Mass spectrometry-based proteomics in preclinical drug discovery. Chem Biol 2012;**19**(1):72–84.

42. Xu HB, Zhang RF, Luo D, et al. Comparative proteomic analysis of plasma from major depressive patients: identification of proteins associated with lipid metabolism and immunoregulation. Int J Neuropsychopharmacol 2012;**15**(10):1413–1425.

43. Chen CS, Zhu H. Protein microarrays. Biotechniques 2006;**40**(4):423–427.

44. Uhr M, Tontsch A, Namendorf C, et al. Polymorphisms in the drug transporter gene ABCB1 predict antidepressant treatment response in depression. Neuron 2008;**57**(2):203–209.

45. Kato M, Fukuda T, Serretti A, et al. ABCB1 (MDR1) gene polymorphisms are associated with the clinical response to paroxetine in patients with major depressive disorder. Progr Neuropsychopharmacol Biol Psychiatry 2008;**32**(2):398–404.

46. Gex-Fabry M, Eap CB, Oneda B, et al. CYP2D6 and ABCB1 genetic variability: influence on paroxetine plasma level and therapeutic response. Ther Drug Monit 2008;**30**(4):474–482.

47. Nikisch G, Eap CB, Baumann P. Citalopram enantiomers in plasma and cerebrospinal fluid of ABCB1 genotyped depressive patients and clinical response: a pilot study. Pharmacol Res 2008;**58**(5-6):344–347.

48. Dong C, Wong ML, Licinio J. Sequence variations of ABCB1, SLC6A2, SLC6A3, SLC6A4, CREB1, CRHR1 and NTRK2: association with major depression and antidepressant response in Mexican-Americans. Mol Psychiatry 2009;**14**(12):1105–1118.

49. Peters EJ, Slager SL, Kraft JB, et al. Pharmacokinetic genes do not influence response or tolerance to citalopram in the STAR*D sample. PLoS One 2008;**3**(4):e1872.

50. Laika B, Leucht S, Steimer W. ABCB1 (P-glycoprotein/MDR1) gene G2677T/a sequence variation (polymorphism): lack of association with side effects and therapeutic response in depressed inpatients treated with amitriptyline. Clin Chem 2006;**52**(5):893–895.

51. Mihaljevic Peles A, Bozina N, Sagud M, et al. MDR1 gene polymorphism: therapeutic response to paroxetine among patients with major depression. Prog Neuropsychopharmacol Biol Psychiatry 2008;**32**(6):1439–1444.

52. Kraft JB, Peters EJ, Slager SL, et al. Analysis of association between the serotonin transporter and antidepressant response in a large clinical sample. Biol Psychiatry 2007;**61**(6):734–742.

53. Mrazek DA, Rush AJ, Biernacka JM, et al. SLC6A4 variation and citalopram response. Am J Med Genet B Neuropsychiatr Genet 2009;**150B**(3):341–351.

54. Porcelli S, Fabbri C, Serretti A. Meta-analysis of serotonin transporter gene promoter polymorphism (5-HTTLPR) association with antidepressant efficacy. Eur Neuropsychopharmacol 2012;**22**(4):239–258.

55. Peters EJ, Slager SL, Jenkins GD, et al. Resequencing of serotonin-related genes and association of tagging SNPs to citalopram response. Pharmacogenet Genomics 2009;**19**(1):1–10.

56. McMahon FJ, Buervenich S, Charney D, et al. Variation in the gene encoding the serotonin 2A receptor is associated with outcome of antidepressant treatment. Am J Hum Genet 2006;**78**(5):804–814.

57. Lucae S, Ising M, Horstmann S, et al. HTR2A gene variation is involved in antidepressant treatment response. Eur Neuropsychopharmacol 2010;**20**(1):65–68.

58. Uher R, Huezo-Diaz P, Perroud N, et al. Genetic predictors of response to antidepressants in the GENDEP project. Pharmacogenomics J 2009;**9**(4):225–233.

59. Uher R, Huezo-Diaz P, Perroud N, et al. Genetic predictors of response to antidepressants in the GENDEP project. Pharmacogenomics J 2009;**9**(4):225–233.

60. Horstmann S, Lucae S, Menke A, et al. Polymorphisms in GRIK4, HTR2A, and FKBP5 show interactive effects in predicting remission to antidepressant treatment. Neuropsychopharmacology 2010;**35**(3):727–740.

61. Tiwari AK, Zai CC, Sajeev G, et al. Analysis of 34 candidate genes in bupropion and placebo remission. Int J Neuropsychopharmacol 2013;**16**(4):771–781.

62. Maron E, Tammiste A, Kallassalu K, et al. Serotonin transporter promoter region polymorphisms do not influence treatment response to escitalopram in patients with major depression. Eur Neuropsychopharmacol 2009;**19**(6):451–456.

63. Serretti A, Fabbri C, Pellegrini S, et al. No effect of serotoninergic gene variants on response to interpersonal counseling and antidepressants in major depression. Psychiatry Investig 2013;**10**(2):180–189.

64. Perlis RH, Fijal B, Dharia S, et al. Failure to replicate genetic associations with antidepressant treatment response in duloxetine-treated patients. Biol Psychiatry 2010;**67**(11):1110–1113.

65. Hong CJ, Chen TJ, Yu YW, Tsai SJ. Response to fluoxetine and serotonin 1A receptor (C-1019G) polymorphism in Taiwan Chinese major depressive disorder. Pharmacogenomics J 2006;**6**(1):27–33.

66. Chen J, Lipska BK, Halim N, et al. Functional analysis of genetic variation in catechol-O-methyltransferase (COMT): effects on mRNA, protein, and enzyme activity in postmortem human brain. Am J Hum Genet 2004;**75**(5):807–821.

67. Lachman HM, Papolos DF, Saito T, et al. Human catechol-O-methyltransferase pharmacogenetics: description of a functional polymorphism and its potential application to neuropsychiatric disorders. Pharmacogenetics 1996;**6**(3):243–250.

68. Gogos JA, Morgan M, Luine V, et al. Catechol-O-methyltransferase-deficient mice exhibit sexually dimorphic changes in catecholamine levels and behavior. Proc Natl Acad Sci USA 1998;**95**(17):9991–9996.

69. Kaenmaki M, Tammimaki A, Myohanen T, et al. Quantitative role of COMT in dopamine clearance in the prefrontal cortex of freely moving mice. J Neurochemistry 2010;**114**(6):1745–1755.

70. Sesack SR, Hawrylak VA, Guido MA, Levey AI. Cellular and subcellular localization of the dopamine transporter in rat cortex. Adv Pharmacol 1998;**42**:171–174.

71. Benedetti F, Colombo C, Pirovano A, et al. The catechol-O-methyltransferase Val(108/158) Met polymorphism affects antidepressant response to paroxetine in a naturalistic setting. Psychopharmacology 2009;**203**(1):155–160.

72. Benedetti F, Dallaspezia S, Colombo C, et al. Effect of catechol-O-methyltransferase Val(108/158)Met polymorphism on antidepressant efficacy of fluvoxamine. Eur Psychiatry 2010;**25**(8):476–478.

73. Spronk D, Arns M, Barnett KJ, et al. An investigation of EEG, genetic and cognitive markers of treatment response to antidepressant medication in patients with major depressive disorder: a pilot study. J Affect Disord 2011;**128**(1-2):41–48.

74. Baune BT, Hohoff C, Berger K, et al. Association of the COMT val158met variant with antidepressant treatment response in major depression. Neuropsychopharmacology 2008;**33**(4):924–932.

75. Tsai SJ, Gau YT, Hong CJ, et al. Sexually dimorphic effect of catechol-O-methyltransferase val158met polymorphism on clinical response to fluoxetine in major depressive patients. J Affect Disord 2009;**113**(1-2):183–187.

76. Kocabas NA, Faghel C, Barreto M, et al. The impact of catechol-O-methyltransferase SNPs and haplotypes on treatment response phenotypes in major depressive disorder: a case-control association study. Int Clin Psychopharmacol 2010;**25**(4):218–227.

77. Houston JP, Kohler J, Ostbye KM, et al. Association of catechol-O-methyltransferase variants with duloxetine response in major depressive disorder. Psychiatry Res 2011;**189**(3):475–477.

78. Szegedi A, Rujescu D, Tadic A, et al. The catechol-O-methyltransferase Val108/158Met polymorphism affects short-term treatment response to mirtazapine, but not to paroxetine in major depression. Pharmacogenomics J 2005;**5**(1):49–53.

79. Arias B, Serretti A, Lorenzi C, et al. Analysis of COMT gene (Val 158 Met polymorphism) in the clinical response to SSRIs in depressive patients of European origin. J Affect Disord 2006;**90**(2-3):251–256.

80. Perlis RH, Fijal B, Adams DH, et al. Variation in catechol-O-methyltransferase is associated with duloxetine response in a clinical trial for major depressive disorder. Biol Psychiatry 2009;**65**(9):785–791.

81. Anttila S, Huuhka K, Huuhka M, et al. Catechol-O-methyltransferase (COMT) polymorphisms predict treatment response in electroconvulsive therapy. Pharmacogenomics J 2007;**8**(2):113–116.

82. Domschke K, Zavorotnyy M, Diemer J, et al. COMT val158met influence on electroconvulsive therapy response in major depression. Am J Med Genet B Neuropsychiatr Genet 2010;**153B**(1):286–290.

83. Paddock S, Laje G, Charney D, et al. Association of GRIK4 with outcome of antidepressant treatment in the STAR*D cohort. Am J Psychiatry 2007;**164**(8):1181–1188.

84. Pu M, Zhang Z, Xu Z, et al. Influence of genetic polymorphisms in the glutamatergic and GABAergic systems and their interactions with environmental stressors on antidepressant response. Pharmacogenomics 2013;**14**(3):277–288.

85. Serretti A, Chiesa A, Crisafulli C, et al. Failure to replicate influence of GRIK4 and GNB3 polymorphisms on treatment outcome in major depression. Neuropsychobiology 2012;**65**(2):70–75.

86. Xu G, Lin K, Rao D, et al. Brain-derived neurotrophic factor gene polymorphism (Val66Met) and the early response to antidepressant in Chinese Han population. Psychiatr Genet 2012;**22**(4):214–215.

87. Choi MJ, Kang RH, Lim SW, et al. Brain-derived neurotrophic factor gene polymorphism (Val66Met) and citalopram response in major depressive disorder. Brain Res 2006;**1118**(1):176–182.

88. Katsuki A, Yoshimura R, Kishi T, et al. Serum levels of brain-derived neurotrophic factor (BDNF), BDNF gene Val66Met polymorphism, or plasma catecholamine metabolites, and response to mirtazapine in Japanese patients with major depressive disorder (MDD). CNS Spectr 2012;**17**(3):155–163.

89. Yoshimura R, Kishi T, Suzuki A, et al. The brain-derived neurotrophic factor (BDNF) polymorphism Val66Met is associated with neither serum BDNF level nor response to selective serotonin reuptake inhibitors in depressed Japanese patients. Prog Neuropsychopharmacol Biol Psychiatry 2011;**35**(4):1022–1025.

90. Kang RH, Chang HS, Wong ML, et al. Brain-derived neurotrophic factor gene polymorphisms and mirtazapine responses in Koreans with major depression. J Psychopharmacol 2010;**24**(12):1755–1763.

91. Domschke K, Lawford B, Laje G, et al. Brain-derived neurotrophic factor (BDNF) gene: no major impact on antidepressant treatment response. Int J Neuropsychopharmacol 2010;**13**(1): 93–101.

92. Hennings JM, Kohli MA, Czamara D, et al. Possible associations of NTRK2 polymorphisms with antidepressant treatment outcome: findings from an extended tag SNP approach. PLoS One 2013;**8**(6):e64947.

93. Murphy GM Jr, Sarginson JE, Ryan HS, et al. BDNF and CREB1 genetic variants interact to affect antidepressant treatment outcomes in geriatric depression. Pharmacogenet Genomics 2013;**23**(6):301–313.

94. Kocabas NA, Antonijevic I, Faghel C, et al. Brain-derived neurotrophic factor gene polymorphisms: influence on treatment response phenotypes of major depressive disorder. Int Clin Psychopharmacol 2011;**26**(1):1–10.

95. Gratacos M, Soria V, Urretavizcaya M, et al. A brain-derived neurotrophic factor (BDNF) haplotype is associated with antidepressant treatment outcome in mood disorders. Pharmacogenomics J 2008;**8**(2):101–112.

96. Hall-Flavin DK, Winner JG, Allen JD, et al. Utility of integrated pharmacogenomic testing to support the treatment of major depressive disorder in a psychiatric outpatient setting. Pharmacogenet Genomics 2013;**23**(10):535–548.

97. Porcelli S, Fabbri C, Spina E, et al. Genetic polymorphisms of cytochrome P450 enzymes and antidepressant metabolism. Expert Opin Drug Metab Toxicol 2011;**7**(9):1101–1115.

98. D'Empaire I, Guico-Pabia CJ, Preskorn SH. Antidepressant treatment and altered CYP2D6 activity: are pharmacokinetic variations clinically relevant? J Psychiatr Pract 2011;**17**(5):330–339.

99. Lim S-W, Won H-H, Kim H, et al. Genetic prediction of antidepressant drug response and nonresponse in Korean patients. PLoS One 2014;**9**(9):e107098.

100. Hodgson K, Tansey KE, Uher R, et al. Exploring the role of drug-metabolising enzymes in antidepressant side effects. Psychopharmacology 2015;**232**(14):2609–2617.

101. Hodgson K, Tansey K, Dernovsek MZ, et al. Genetic differences in cytochrome P450 enzymes and antidepressant treatment response. J Psychopharmacol 2014;**28**(2):133–141.

102. Serretti A, Calati R, Massat I, et al. Cytochrome P450 CYP1A2, CYP2C9, CYP2C19 and CYP2D6 genes are not associated with response and remission in a sample of depressive patients. Int Clin Psychopharmacol 2009;**24**(5):250–256.

103. Shams ME, Arneth B, Hiemke C, et al. CYP2D6 polymorphism and clinical effect of the antidepressant venlafaxine. J Clin Pharm Ther 2006;**31**(5):493–502.

104. Grasmader K, Verwohlt PL, Rietschel M, et al. Impact of polymorphisms of cytochrome-P450 isoenzymes 2C9, 2C19 and 2D6 on plasma concentrations and clinical effects of antidepressants in a naturalistic clinical setting. Eur J Clin Pharmacol 2004;**60**(5): 329–336.

105. Lobello KW, Preskorn SH, Guico-Pabia CJ, et al. Cytochrome P450 2D6 phenotype predicts antidepressant efficacy of venlafaxine: a secondary analysis of 4 studies in major depressive disorder. J Clin Psychiatry 2010;**71**(11):1482–1487.

106. Tzvetkov MV, Brockmoller J, Roots I, Kirchheiner J. Common genetic variations in human brain-specific tryptophan hydroxylase-2 and response to antidepressant treatment. Pharmacogenet Genomics 2008;**18**(6):495–506.

107. Peters EJ, Slager SL, McGrath PJ, et al. Investigation of serotonin-related genes in antidepressant response. Mol Psychiatry 2004;**9**(9):879–889.

108. Ellsworth KA, Moon I, Eckloff BW, et al. FKBP5 genetic variation: association with selective serotonin reuptake inhibitor treatment outcomes in major depressive disorder. Pharmacogenet Genomics 2013;**23**(3):156–166.

109. Gadad BS, Raj P, Jha MK, Carmody T, Dozmorov I, Mayes TL, Wakeland EK, Trivedi MH. Association of Novel ALX4 Gene Polymorphisms with Antidepressant Treatment Response: Findings from the CO-MED Trial. Mol Neuropsychiatry 2018 Jun;**4**(1):7–19.

110. Hennings JM, Uhr M, Klengel T, et al. RNA expression profiling in depressed patients suggests retinoid-related orphan receptor alpha as a biomarker for antidepressant response. Transl Psychiatry 2015;**5**:e538.

111. Le-Niculescu H, Kurian SM, Yehyawi N, et al. Identifying blood biomarkers for mood disorders using convergent functional genomics. Mol Psychiatry 2008;**14**(2):156–174.

112. Kéri S, Szabó C, Kelemen O. Blood biomarkers of depression track clinical changes during cognitive-behavioral therapy. J Affect Disord 2014;**164**:118–122.

113. Domschke K, Tidow N, Schwarte K, et al. Serotonin transporter gene hypomethylation predicts impaired antidepressant treatment response. Int J Neuropsychopharmacol 2014;**17**(8):1167–1176.

114. Hannestad J, DellaGioia N, Bloch M. The effect of antidepressant medication treatment on serum levels of inflammatory cytokines: a meta-analysis. Neuropsychopharmacology 2011;**36**(12):2452–2459.

115. Eller T, Vasar V, Shlik J, Maron E. Effects of bupropion augmentation on proinflammatory cytokines in escitalopram-resistant patients with major depressive disorder. J Psychopharmacol 2009;**23**(7):854–858.

116. Yoshimura R, Hori H, Ikenouchi-Sugita A, et al. Higher plasma interleukin-6 (IL-6) level is associated with SSRI- or SNRI-refractory depression. Prog Neuropsychopharmacol Biol Psychiatry 2009;**33**(4):722–726.

117. Uher R, Tansey KE, Dew T, et al. An inflammatory biomarker as a differential predictor of outcome of depression treatment with escitalopram and nortriptyline. Am J Psychiatry 2014;**171**(12):1278–1286.

118. Raison CL, Rutherford RE, Woolwine BJ, et al. A randomized controlled trial of the tumor necrosis factor antagonist infliximab for treatment-resistant depression: the role of baseline inflammatory biomarkers. JAMA Psychiatry 2013;**70**(1):31–41.

119. Svenningsson P, Berg L, Matthews D, et al. Preliminary evidence that early reduction in p11 levels in natural killer cells and monocytes predicts the likelihood of antidepressant response to chronic citalopram. Mol Psychiatry 2014;**19**(9):962–964.

120. Janssen DG, Caniato RN, Verster JC, Baune BT. A psychoneuroimmunological review on cytokines involved in antidepressant treatment response. Hum Psychopharmacol 2010;**25**(3):201–215.

121. Maes M. The immunoregulatory effects of antidepressants. Hum Psychopharmacol 2001;**16**(1):95–103.

122. Buttenschon HN, Foldager L, Elfving B, et al. Neurotrophic factors in depression in response to treatment. J Affect Disord 2015;**183**:287–294.

123. Matrisciano F, Bonaccorso S, Ricciardi A, et al. Changes in BDNF serum levels in patients with major depression disorder (MDD) after 6 months treatment with sertraline, escitalopram, or venlafaxine. J Psychiatr Res 2009;**43**(3):247–254.

124. Gorgulu Y, Caliyurt O. Rapid antidepressant effects of sleep deprivation therapy correlates with serum BDNF changes in major depression. Brain Res Bull 2009;**80**(3):158–162.

125. Ninan PT, Shelton RC, Bao W, Guico-Pabia CJ. BDNF, interleukin-6, and salivary cortisol levels in depressed patients treated with desvenlafaxine. Prog Neuropsychopharmacol Biol Psychiatry 2014;**48**:86–91.

126. Brunoni AR, Machado-Vieira R, Zarate CA Jr, et al. BDNF plasma levels after antidepressant treatment with sertraline and transcranial direct current stimulation: results from a factorial, randomized, sham-controlled trial. Eur Neuropsychopharmacol 2014;**24**(7):1144–1151.

127. Molendijk ML, Spinhoven P, Polak M, et al. Serum BDNF concentrations as peripheral manifestations of depression: evidence from a systematic review and meta-analyses on 179 associations (N=9484). Mol Psychiatry 2014;**19**(7):791–800.

128. Lee J, Joo EJ, Lim HJ, et al. Proteomic analysis of serum from patients with major depressive disorder to compare their depressive and remission statuses. Psychiatry Investig 2015;**12**(2):249–259.

129. Stelzhammer V, Haenisch F, Chan MK, et al. Proteomic changes in serum of first onset, antidepressant drug-naive major depression patients. Int J Neuropsychopharmacol 2014;**17**(10):1599–1608.

130. Bot M, Chan MK, Jansen R, et al. Serum proteomic profiling of major depressive disorder. Transl Psychiatry 2015;**5**:e599.

131. Diniz BS, Sibille E, Ding Y, et al. Plasma biosignature and brain pathology related to persistent cognitive impairment in late-life depression. Mol Psychiatry 2015;**20**(5):594–601.

132. Jha MK, Minhajuddin A, Gadad BS, Trivedi MH. Platelet-derived growth factor as an antidepressant treatment selection biomarker: higher levels selectively predict better outcomes with bupropion-SSRI combination. Int J Neuropsychopharmacol 2017;**20**(11):919–927.

133. Jha MK, Minhajuddin A, Gadad BS, et al. Interleukin 17 selectively predicts better outcomes with bupropion-SSRI combination: novel T cell biomarker for antidepressant medication selection. Brain Behav Immun 2017;**66**:103–110.

134. Jha MK, Minhajuddin A, Gadad BS, et al. Can C-reactive protein inform antidepressant medication selection in depressed outpatients? Findings from the CO-MED trial. Psychoneuroendocrinology 2017;**78**:105–113.

135. Gadad BS, Jha MK, Grannemann BD, et al. Proteomics profiling reveals inflammatory biomarkers of antidepressant treatment response: findings from the CO-MED trial. J Psychiatr Res 2017;**94**:1–6.

136. Paige LA, Mitchell MW, Krishnan KR, et al. A preliminary metabolomic analysis of older adults with and without depression. Int J Geriatr Psychiatry 2007;**22**(5):418–423.

137. Zhu H, Bogdanov MB, Boyle SH, et al. Pharmacometabolomics of response to sertraline and to placebo in major depressive disorder: possible role for methoxyindole pathway. PLoS One 2013;**8**(7):e68283.

138. Kaddurah-Daouk R, Boyle SH, Matson W, et al. Pretreatment metabotype as a predictor of response to sertraline or placebo in depressed outpatients: a proof of concept. Transl Psychiatry 2011;**1**:e26.

139. Kaddurah-Daouk R, Bogdanov MB, Wikoff WR, et al. Pharmacometabolomic mapping of early biochemical changes induced by sertraline and placebo. Transl Psychiatry 2013;**3**:e223.

140. Tian JS, Peng GJ, Gao XX, Zhou YZ, Xing J, Qin XM, Du GH. Dynamic analysis of the endogenous metabolites in depressed patients treated with TCM formula Xiaoyaosan using urinary (1)H NMR-based metabolomics. J Ethnopharmacol 2014;**158**:1–10.

141. Czysz AH, South C, Gadad BS, et al. Can targeted metabolomics predict depression recovery? Results from the CO-MED trial. Transl Psychiatry 2019;**9**(1):11.

142. Moaddel R, Shardell M, Khadeer M, et al. Plasma metabolomic profiling of a ketamine and placebo crossover trial of major depressive disorder and healthy control subjects. Psychopharmacology 2018;**235**(10):3017–3030.

Comorbidities and Differential Diagnoses of Depression

/// 6 /// ANXIETY DISORDERS

CARLY YASINSKI, BONNIE SEIFERT, CALLAN M. COGHLAN, AND BARBARA O. ROTHBAUM

6.1. INTRODUCTION

Anxiety and fear-based disorders are highly comorbid with depression, and rates of co-occurrence are greater than with any other category of psychiatric disorder, including substance use and impulse control disorders.[1,2] Comorbidity with one or more anxiety disorders is strongly associated with greater severity and functional impairment of major depressive disorder (MDD).[2–4] Perhaps related to this greater severity, individuals with anxiety in addition to depression are significantly more likely to seek treatment than those with depression alone but are less likely to respond to treatment.[5] It is therefore vitally important that practitioners, students, and researchers have some understanding of the mechanisms, correlates, and consequences of comorbidity or lack thereof, as a substantial portion of depression patients are likely to have a concurrent anxiety disorder or history of an anxiety disorder. This chapter will review rates of comorbidity of depression with anxiety- and fear-based disorders and the recent major theories of what makes depression and anxiety similar and different from each other. We will also review research on the psychological and neurobiological mechanisms of the overlap between anxiety and depression and the influences of comorbidity on diagnosis, treatment, and prognosis.

6.2. RATES AND PREVALENCE

In the World Health Organization (WHO)'s World Mental Health (WMH) Surveys,[2] 45.7% of those with a lifetime MDD diagnosis (i.e., a diagnosis of MDD at any point currently or in the past) also met criteria for one or more lifetime anxiety disorders as diagnosed by the WHO Composite International Diagnostic Interview (CIDI).[6] These disorders, which align with the fourth edition of the *Diagnostic and Statistical Manual of Mental Disorders* (DSM-IV)[7] anxiety disorders, include generalized anxiety, panic, agoraphobia, specific phobia, social phobia, post-traumatic stress disorder (PTSD), and separation anxiety disorders. An even higher percentage of respondents (51.7%) with 12-month MDD (i.e., a diagnosis of MDD at any time in the past 12 months) reported a lifetime diagnosis of an anxiety disorder, while a slightly lower percentage (41.6%) with 12-month MDD met criteria for an anxiety disorder during the same 12-month period.[a] Together, these percentages suggest that anxiety comorbidity is associated not only with MDD severity, but also with MDD persistence, which is consistent with other large epidemiological studies.[8] The majority of individuals (68%) with a comorbid anxiety disorder and depression tend to report an earlier age of onset of their first anxiety disorder than of their first depressive episode, whereas only 13.5% report an earlier age of onset of depression, and the remaining report simultaneous onset.[9] Social anxiety disorder and separation anxiety disorder are the most likely to precede depression onset, whereas generalized anxiety disorder (GAD) is the most likely to occur simultaneously.[10] Overall, GAD tends to have the greatest rates of comorbidity with MDD out of the anxiety disorders.[11,12]

In the WHO's WMH Surveys, a majority of individuals with MDD and a comorbid anxiety disorder in the past year reported severe role impairment (64.4%), which was defined as interference in their ability to function at home, work, socially, or in their close relationships. This proportion was substantially higher than what was reported by those without a comorbid 12-month anxiety disorder (46.0%). Furthermore, respondents with a 12-month diagnosis of MDD and an anxiety disorder were more likely to report they had "seriously thought about committing suicide" in the past 12 months (19.5%) in comparison to those with MDD without a comorbid anxiety disorder (8.9%).[4] Higher rates of comorbidity between MDD and anxiety were found in women compared to men and previously married (including separated, divorced, and widowed) than currently or never married people. People with MDD and a comorbid anxiety disorder were more likely to report seeking any type of treatment for their condition in the past year (56.2%) than those without an anxiety disorder (37.3%), regardless of country. Despite this higher rate of treatment-seeking, other studies have demonstrated that comorbid anxiety is associated with lower rates of treatment completion and treatment response.[13,14]

---

[a] Obsessive-compulsive disorder (OCD) was not included in reports on prevalence and comorbidity in the WMH Surveys. Reasons for this are not described in articles on the WMH; however, in the National Comorbidity Survey-Replication (NCS-R), the US arm of the WMH, problematic skip logic during assessment of OCD caused the prevalence to be underestimated (see https://www.hcp.med.harvard.edu/ncs/faqncsr.php). A reassessment was completed on a portion of respondents and the resulting publication estimated prevalence and comorbidity of OCD in the NCS-R,[8] which indicated similar rates of comorbidity with MDD as other anxiety disorders (40.7%).

6.3. THEORETICAL MODELS AND CLASSIFICATION

In the major diagnostic systems, including the DSM-IV, the DSM-5,[7,15] and the International Classification of Disorders 9 and 10,[16] anxiety disorders have been classified separately from depressive or mood disorders. Despite these distinctions, recent psychopathological, genetic, and treatment research has emphasized the overlap between these categories of disorders and noted that all anxiety disorders share some commonalities with depression.[17–19] Furthermore, researchers have contended that certain anxiety disorders, such as GAD and PTSD, are better classified with depression as distress or "anxious-misery" disorders than in a category with disorders better characterized by fear, such as panic disorder.[20,21] Below we review the major theories of shared and distinct psychopathology among depression and anxiety disorders, review the neurobiological and genetic underpinnings of these similarities and distinctions, and discuss the implications of overlap and comorbidity for treatment.

6.3.1. Two-Factor Models

The simplest and arguably the most parsimonious models of anxiety and depression are two-factor models, which characterize anxiety and depression as having overlapping but distinct relationships to two domains of general affect: positive affect (PA), which includes positive feelings such as enthusiasm, energy, joy, and alertness, and negative affect (NA), which includes sadness, fear, anger, and guilt. Tellegen and Watson's seminal work during the 1980s and 1990s provided evidence for the replicability and importance of these two overarching factors[22–24] and established that both anxiety and depression are highly correlated with measures of NA, but that only depression is correlated with (low) PA. These two factors have been linked to the behavioral inhibition system (BIS) and behavioral activation system (BAS)[25,26] and to the positive and negative valence systems proposed by the National Institute of Mental Health's research domain criteria (RDoC).[27] Significant empirical support for the distinct nature of PA and NA and related factors has been built over the past three decades.[19,25] Importantly, these factors have been linked to two separate dimensions of early emerging temperament, positive and negative affectivity,[28] and to distinct neurobiological mechanisms.[29,30]

6.3.2. Tripartite Model

Clark and Watson in 1991[29] expanded on two-factor approaches by proposing the tripartite model, in which NA is a common construct shared by anxiety and depression, and the constructs of PA and physiological hyperarousal (PH) are the distinguishing features of depression and anxiety, respectively.[31] In this model, low levels of PA differentiate depressive disorders and physiological hyperarousal differentiates anxiety disorders. Studies suggest that focusing on symptoms unique to each construct, versus those that are shared, aids in differential diagnosis; however, discriminant validity among measures has been problematic at times and results seem to vary significantly across studies.[29]

Chorpita and colleagues'[32] alternate conceptualization of the tripartite model asserts that anxiety manifests solely from NA, that low PA is associated with depression, and that the addition of fear to the third construct of PH is more accurate than physiological hyperarousal alone. Their model asserts that tension, apprehension, worry, and general distress correspond with anxiety; anhedonia and hopelessness correspond with depression. Results using this modified model indicate that, even though the constructs of fear, anxiety, and depression are correlated, they are also distinct.[29]

This revised tripartite model improves differential diagnosis, but limitations of this approach remain, including a lack of ability to account for the broad diversity found among anxiety disorders, the differential correlations shown with depressive symptoms and diagnoses, and observed contradictions regarding the constructs of NA, PA, and PH. For instance, the construct of NA is not necessarily a shared component between all anxiety and depressive disorders, and there is some evidence that indicates NA is more weakly correlated to disorders characterized by avoidance behaviors; furthermore, some research suggests that low PA is characteristic not only of depression but of social phobia as well. In regard to physiological hyperarousal, research has raised questions about how adequately PH discriminates between anxiety and mood disorders, considering that it often presents as a distinguishing feature of panic disorder and does not generalize across the broad spectrum of anxiety.[31–33]

6.3.3. Hierarchical Models

Various hierarchical models of anxiety and depression have attempted to address the diversity of anxiety disorders[34–37] by positing that each individual syndrome or disorder is characterized by a common shared component (general distress or NA), similarly to the tripartite model, but that each disorder also has a unique component that makes it distinct from depression and all the other anxiety disorders. While these models have many similarities to the tripartite model, they diverge in their view of anxious or physiological hyperarousal as a specific component of panic disorder (or in some cases a few but not all anxiety disorders) rather than a factor shared across anxiety disorders. Minkea and colleagues' integrative hierarchical model[35] emphasizes that the anxiety and depressive disorders all differ regarding the size of both the general and specific components; for example, depression and GAD are both characterized by high levels of general distress or NA, whereas OCD and specific phobia involve high levels of specific distress (e.g., contamination concerns or animal fears) and lower levels of general distress. Prenoveau and colleagues' trilevel model[36] further differentiates anxiety and depression symptoms by proposing three hierarchical levels at which each syndrome or diagnosis can be characterized according to a broad general distress factor, two factors of intermediate breadth (anxious-misery and fears), and five narrow group factors (depression, fears of specific stimuli, anxious arousal/somatic tension, social fears, and interoceptive/agoraphobic fears). Each of these models has at least some empirical support, but the quadripartite model we discuss next may represent the most comprehensive and best-fitting model given recent research.

6.3.4. Quadripartite Model

By combining the explicit symptom focus of the tripartite model, the modeling of specific symptom dimensions and explicit quantitative focus of the integrative hierarchical model, and the DSM-IV as the basis for its organizational framework, the quadripartite model focuses on the interconnectivity among specific symptom dimensions within each diagnosis.[33] The quadripartite model is based on the principle that symptoms can be classified and grouped across two distinct quantitative dimensions: their magnitude of general distress and their level of specificity (i.e., whether they are more associated with anxiety or depression). These two dimensions result in four basic symptom classification types: (1) high distress (i.e., NA) symptoms with limited specificity; (2) high distress symptoms with greater specificity; (3) low distress symptoms with greater specificity; and (4) low distress symptoms with limited specificity. Unlike the tripartite model in which only symptoms associated with high NA or distress are categorized as "nonspecific," the quadripartite model contends that there are symptoms of low specificity to anxiety or depression that are *not* associated with high distress, such as insomnia. This organization of symptoms into four categories can aid clinicians and researchers in focusing more on those symptom dimensions that have greater specificity, regardless of their level of NA, for the purposes of differential diagnosis. However, the quadripartite model still emphasizes the importance of evaluating and treating symptoms that are common across depression and anxiety. Figure 6.1 provides a visual organizational framework for conceptualizing the quadripartite model.

6.4. NEUROPHYSIOLOGICAL PATTERNS IN ANXIETY AND DEPRESSION

Underscoring the overlap in mechanisms of anxiety and depression, translational and neurobiological research has identified a few common neural pathways disrupted in these disorders, although the exact nature of this disruption differs somewhat between them. Both anxiety and depression have been associated with hyperactivation of the amygdala, part of the brain's limbic system involved in detecting and interpreting emotional stimuli[38,39] in response to both masked threat stimuli[40] and disorder-specific stimuli, for example phobic stimuli (in specific phobia), negative social cues (social anxiety disorder), and sad faces (in depression).[39,40] These neurological findings have been bolstered by psychophysiological findings suggesting exaggerated responses to threat and more biased attention toward and faster processing of negative stimuli.[38,39] For example, individuals with depression and anxiety

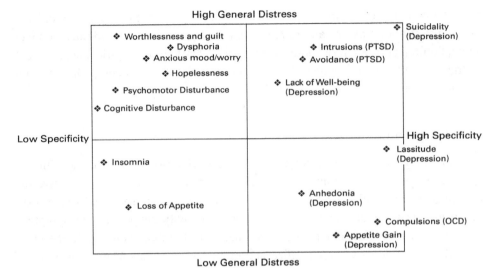

FIGURE 6.1. Distribution of major anxiety and depression symptoms according to the quadripartite model. Based approximately on data reported in reference 19. High-specificity symptoms have the disorder they are associated with in parentheses to their right.

disorders have differed from healthy controls in startle reactivity, both at "baseline" (i.e., overall) and specifically in response to feared stimuli, a reaction linked to the amygdala.[41] However, the exact nature of these differences in startle reactivity differ somewhat across disorders. In line with many of the theoretical models, including the quadripartite and tripartite models, neurophysiological research has generally found distinct patterns of response depending on whether disorders are characterized more by fear (i.e., responses to imminent or immediate threat) or anxious distress (i.e., responses to distal or uncertain threats).[38,42] Exaggerated responses to disorder-specific stimuli as evidenced by increased amygdala responses have been found across anxiety disorders and depression,[38] but fear-potentiated startle (i.e., exaggerated startle response to disorder-specific stimuli) has been found primarily in fear disorders (e.g., specific phobia, panic disorder, and PTSD in some studies).[41] Increased general or baseline startle response, as well as increased responding to *safe* or *nonthreatening* cues when presented in the context of threat, have been linked to disorders of anxious distress such as GAD, but not with depression.[41] In contrast, depression has been associated with *decreased* fear-potentiated startle[37] and slower attention bias to threat.[41] These discrepant patterns of startle responses may represent differential hyper- or hypoactivation of various parts of the amygdala depending on the disorder.[38,41]

Anxiety and depression have been linked not only to hyperactivity of brain areas associated with initial emotional response, but with hypoactivity of brain areas associated with cognitive control and flexibility in response to emotional reactivity, including the dorsolateral prefrontal cortex (DLPFC), the ventromedial prefrontal cortex (VMPFC), and the anterior cingulate cortex (ACC).[38,40] Hypoactivation of the DLPFC and the dorsal ACC has been observed across anxiety disorders and depression and has been associated with difficulty inhibiting irrelevant stimuli.[40] This difficulty with inhibition has been linked with prolonged processing of emotional experiences and with repetitive negative thought patterns that have been identified as transdiagnostic, such as rumination and worry.[39,40] Such irregularities may be associated with the general distress and NA that cuts across many emotional disorders. Psychophysiological research has linked depression and some anxiety disorders to greater error-related negativity (ERN), an event-related potential (ERP) response thought to reflect the brain's detection of errors, which originates in the ACC. Enhanced ERN amplitude, signifying higher levels of error detection, has been consistently found in people with disorders characterized by high levels of NA and anxious distress/misery, such as depression, GAD, and OCD, but not in disorders more associated with fear, such as specific phobia.[41]

Consistent with the tripartite and quadripartite models, some neurobiological findings have been linked only to those disorders characterized by low PA. Reduced amygdala activation in response to positive stimuli has been consistently reported among people with major depression,[40] as has reduced activation in neural circuits associated with reward during reward learning paradigms.[38] Similarly, reduced electroencephalographic (EEG) activity in the left frontal lobe has been associated with both reduced approach motivation and depression, and hypothesized to be one mechanism of anhedonia.[43] Decreased nucleus accumbens and prefrontal cortex (PFC) activity in depressed individuals compared to controls has been associated with reduced ability to upregulate or sustain positive mood, suggesting difficulties in cognitive control and maintenance of positive affect.[39] Similar results have not been found in individuals with anxiety disorders without comorbid depression, underscoring this diagnostic distinction.

6.5. GENETIC AND ENVIRONMENTAL CONTRIBUTIONS TO COMORBIDITY

Large studies investigating the genetics of anxiety and depression have suggested that 30% to 40% of the variability in these disorders is attributable to cumulative genetic influences, with most of the remaining influence attributable to the non-shared environment, rather than the shared or familial environment.[44–46] GAD is the anxiety disorder shown to share the most genetic risk with depression.[47] Genetic variation appears to play a particularly strong role in explaining the comorbidity between MDD, and GAD or PTSD, although genetics also accounts for some of the comorbidity between depression and anxiety more broadly.[47] Childhood adversity, including abuse, neglect, poverty, family chaos, and maladaptive parenting, is a consistent environmental predictor of depression, PTSD, and some anxiety disorders.[48,49] Twin studies and other studies that parse heritability, environmental risk factors, and their interaction have provided relatively consistent estimates of the magnitude of these influences, but attempts to identify specific genetic variants associated with these disorders have not revealed many consistent results. Candidate genes related to serotonergic and dopaminergic functioning in the central nervous system have been linked to a number of anxiety disorders and depression, but replicable patterns have been difficult to identify. Perhaps the most consistent convergent biological and genetic evidence has arisen for the effect of variations in the *FKBP5* gene, which have been shown to interact with early life adversity to predict PTSD and depression, most likely via alterations in the stress responses of the hypothalamic–pituitary–adrenal (HPA) axis.[50] Overall, though, anxious and depressive disorders are highly heterogeneous and phenotypically complex, so large sample sizes and more sophisticated studies (including gene-environment interaction studies and genome-wide association studies [GWAS]) are needed to identify reliably additional genetic patterns or markers.[50]

6.6. TREATMENT

The significant overlap in anxiety disorders and depression suggests that treatment should target at least some of the same pathological mechanisms. Selective serotonin reuptake inhibitors (SSRIs) and related medications are the most common pharmacological treatment for both anxious and depressive disorders and have demonstrated significant therapeutic effects across these disorders.[51] In contrast, other medications, such as benzodiazepines, have been shown to have positive effects on anxiety, including GAD and anxious depression, but not on depression without anxious features[52] or PTSD.[53] Studies examining moderators of antidepressant medication treatment have found that depressed patients with significant comorbid anxiety (a comorbid anxiety disorder and/or a high score on an established anxiety measure) demonstrate lower response and remission rates than those without significant anxiety.[13,54,55] Studies examining cognitive behavioral therapy (CBT) for depression have not as consistently found a moderating effect of anxiety on outcomes,[56,57] although some studies have.[55] Research examining the effects of anxiety-focused psychotherapeutic treatments on depression have generally demonstrated concomitant reductions in both anxiety and depressive symptoms, and meta-analyses of depression therapy have shown that anxious and depressive symptoms both reduce over treatment.[57,58] The state of current research on moderators of treatment outcome does not provide a basis for recommending specific treatments for depression with versus without anxious features. However, recent studies examining patients with treatment-resistant (or not fully responsive) depression, many of whom experience significant anxiety, suggest that adding either an SSRI or CBT for those who are not responding to monotherapy with the other treatment leads to significantly improved rates of response and remission of depression.[55,59] Together, these results suggest that patients with anxious depression or depression comorbid with an anxiety disorder are likely to benefit from combined medication and psychotherapy treatment if they do not fully respond to one or the other. Another large randomized controlled trial on the treatment of chronic depression found that combining the antidepressant nefazadone with cognitive behavioral analysis system of psychotherapy (CBASP) led to larger reductions in anxiety than either treatment alone, also suggesting the benefit of combined treatment for comorbid anxiety.[60]

Recent research into transdiagnostic cognitive-behavioral treatments has demonstrated that comorbid depression and anxiety both respond to transdiagnostic CBTs, such as the Unified Protocol for the Transdiagnostic Treatment of Emotional Disorders (i.e., the Unified Protocol),[17] and that such treatment may lead to equivalent outcomes, and possibly better retention, than disorder-specific protocols.[61] Both SSRIs and CBT target increased NA and difficulties with cognitive control of negative material (e.g., rumination and perseveration).[62] However, neither type of treatment directly targets difficulties with PA and anhedonia, which may explain why these treatments have generally shown larger effects sizes on anxiety than on depression. Studies have demonstrated that difficulties with PA are associated with a poorer outcome of both types of treatment and worse long-term prognosis.[63] Therefore, recent treatment research has begun to explore ways to enhance PA and reward sensitivity directly across both depression and anxiety disorders through cognitive-behavioral treatments such as positive affect treatment (PAT)[63] and medication treatments such as ketamine for treatment-resistant depression.[64]

Examination of the prescribing practices of real-world psychiatrists has revealed that most based their prescribing on symptom profiles rather than diagnostic category or specific disorder.[65,66] Likewise, some leaders in the field of CBT have recently advocated for a focus on treating psychopathological processes, such as rumination, negative attention bias, or anhedonia, through "process-focused CBT" rather than relying on protocols for specific disorders, which often do not fully capture what is needed to target the heterogeneous nature of anxiety and depression.[67] In line with this focus, past treatment research has demonstrated that disorders such as GAD and depression both benefit from therapeutic techniques focused on reducing perseveration and repetitive negative thought, whereas depression and social anxiety disorder both benefit from enhancing approach motivation and PA. In contrast, panic disorder, OCD, specific phobias, and PTSD all respond well to exposure-based approaches as they all have significant fear components.

6.7. CONCLUSION

Depressive and anxiety disorders are significantly comorbid, particularly in clinical populations. When depression co-occurs with anxiety, it often results in higher severity, functional impairment, and suicide risk, as well as lower response to treatment. Both anxiety and depression are characterized by high levels of NA, although the nature and specificity of this distress vary across disorders, with depression, GAD, and PTSD associated with higher levels of general NA and distress, and panic disorder and specific phobias associated with more specific NA responses and physiological hyperarousal. Anhedonia and low levels of positive affect are most prominent in depression, although they also are found in social anxiety disorder to a lesser degree. The similarities and differences across anxiety and depression have been reflected in neurobiological and psychophysiological research, with an overactive amygdala response to negative stimuli and underactive cognitive control through areas of the PFC being common across all. Both types of disorders have been shown to be influenced by genetics, environment, and their interaction, but reliable genetic patterns that explain their overlap and distinctions still need to be established. Anxiety and depression respond to many of the same treatments, and recent treatment research has emphasized the importance of treating specific symptoms and pathological processes rather than taking a disorder-specific or syndromal approach. Future research should aim toward better establishing genetic, biological, and psychological underpinnings of these two pathologies, which will ideally lead to more effective treatment approaches.

AUTHOR NOTE

Dr. Rothbaum has funding from Wounded Warrior Project, Department of Defense Clinical Trial Grant No. W81XWH-10-1-1045, National Institute of Mental Health Grant No. 1R01MH094757-01, and McCormick Foundation. Dr. Rothbaum receives royalties from Oxford University Press, Guilford, APPI, and Emory University and received one advisory board payment from Genentech, Jazz Pharmaceuticals, and Aptinyx.

REFERENCES

1. Kessler RC, Berglund P, Demler O, et al. The epidemiology of major depressive disorder: Results from the National Comorbidity Survey Replication (NCS-R). JAMA. 2003; 289(23):3095–3105.
2. Kessler RC, Sampson NA, Berglund P, et al. Anxious and non-anxious major depressive disorder in the World Health Organization World Mental Health Surveys. Epidemiol Psychiatr Sci. 2015; 24(3):210–226.
3. McLaughlin TP, Khandker RK, Kruzikas DT, Tummala R. Overlap of anxiety and depression in a managed care population: Prevalence and association with resource utilization. J Clin Psychiatry. 2000; 67(8):1187–1193.
4. Roy-Byrne PP, Stang P, Wittchen HU, et al. Lifetime panic–depression comorbidity in the National Comorbidity Survey: Association with symptoms, impairment, course and help-seeking. Br J Psychiatry. 2000; 176(3):229–235.
5. Jakubovski E, Bloch MH. Prognostic subgroups for citalopram response in the STAR* D trial. J Clin Psychiatry. 2014; 75(7):738.
6. Kessler RC, Üstün TB. The World Mental Health (WMH) survey initiative version of the World Health Organization (WHO) Composite International Diagnostic Interview (CIDI). Int J Methods Psychiatr Res. 2004; 13(2):93–121.
7. American Psychiatric Association. *Diagnostic and Statistical Manual of Mental Disorders.* 4th ed. Washington, DC: American Psychiatric Association; 2000.
8. Ruscio AM, Stein DJ, Chiu WT, Kessler RC. The epidemiology of obsessive-compulsive disorder in the National Comorbidity Survey Replication. Mol Psychiatry. 2010; 15(1):53–63.
9. Spinhoven P, van Balkom AJ, Nolen WA. Comorbidity patterns of anxiety and depressive disorders in a large cohort study: The Netherlands Study of Depression and Anxiety (NESDA). J Clin Psychiatry. 2011; 72:341–348.

10. Cummings CM, Caporino NE, Kendall PC. Comorbidity of anxiety and depression in children and adolescents: 20 years after. Psychol Bull. 2014; 140(3):816–845.
11. King-Kallimanis B, Gum AM, Kohn R. Comorbidity of depressive and anxiety disorders for older Americans in the National Comorbidity Survey-Replication. Am J Geriatr Psychiatry. 2009; 17(9):782–792.
12. Hofmeijer-Sevink MK, Batelaan NM, van Megen HJ, et al. Clinical relevance of comorbidity in anxiety disorders: A report from the Netherlands Study of Depression and Anxiety (NESDA). J Affect Disord. 2012; 137(1):106–112.
13. Saveanu R, Etkin A, Duchemin AM, et al. The International Study to Predict Optimized Treatment in Depression (iSPOT-D): Outcomes from the acute phase of antidepressant treatment. J Psychiatr Res. 2015; 61:1–2.
14. Shippee ND, Rosen BH, Angstman KB, et al. Baseline screening tools as indicators for symptom outcomes and health services utilization in a collaborative care model for depression in primary care: A practice-based observational study. Gen Hosp Psychiatry. 2014; 36(6):563–569.
15. American Psychiatric Association. *Diagnostic and Statistical Manual of Mental Disorders: DSM-5*. Arlington, VA: American Psychiatric Association; 2013.
16. World Health Organization. The ICD-10 classification of mental and behavioural disorders: Clinical descriptions and diagnostic guidelines.1992. https://www.who.int/classifications/icd/en/bluebook.pdf.
17. Barlow DH, Farchione TJ, Sauer-Zavala S, et al. *Unified Protocol for Transdiagnostic Treatment of Emotional Disorders: Therapist Guide*. New York: Oxford University Press; 2017.
18. Mineka S, Watson D, Clark LA. Comorbidity of anxiety and unipolar mood disorders. Annu Rev Psychol. 1998; 49(1):377–412.
19. Watson D. Differentiating the mood and anxiety disorders: A quadripartite model. Annu Rev Clin Psychol. 2009; 5:221–247.
20. Watson D. Rethinking the mood and anxiety disorders: A quantitative hierarchical model for DSM-V. J Abnorm Psychol. 2005; 114(4):522.
21. Kotov R, Krueger RF, Watson D, et al. The Hierarchical Taxonomy of Psychopathology (HiTOP): A dimensional alternative to traditional nosologies. J Abnorm Psychol. 2017; 126(4):454.
22. Tellegen A. Structures of mood and personality and their relevance to assessing anxiety, with an emphasis on self-report. In Tuma AH, Maser JD, eds. *Anxiety and the Anxiety Disorders*. Hillsdale, NJ: Lawrence Erlbaum; 1985:681–706.
23. Watson D, Clark LA. Measurement and mismeasurement of mood: Recurrent and emergent issues. J Pers Assess. 1997; 68(2):267–296.
24. Watson D, Tellegen A. Toward a consensual structure of mood. Psychol Bull. 1985;98(2): 219–235.
25. Busseri MA. Examining the structure of subjective well-being through meta-analysis of the associations among positive affect, negative affect, and life satisfaction. Pers Individ Dif. 2018; 122:68–71.
26. Carver CS, White TL. Behavioral inhibition, behavioral activation, and affective responses to impending reward and punishment: The BIS/BAS scales. J Pers Soc Psychol. 1994; 67(2):319.
27. Jorm AF, Christensen H, Henderson AS, et al. Using the BIS/BAS scales to measure behavioural inhibition and behavioural activation: Factor structure, validity and norms in a large community sample. Pers Individ Dif. 1998; 26(1):49–58.
28. Sanislow CA, Pine DS, Quinn KJ, et al. Developing constructs for psychopathology research: Research domain criteria. J Abnorm Psychol. 2010; 119(4):631.
29. Clark LA, Watson D. Tripartite model of anxiety and depression: Psychometric evidence and taxonomic implications. J Abnorm Psychol. 1991; 100(3):316.

30. Watson D, Stasik SM. Examining the comorbidity between depression and the anxiety disorders from the perspective of the quadripartite model. In Richards CS, O'Hara MW, eds. *The Oxford Handbook of Depression and Comorbidity.* New York: Oxford University Press; 2014:46–65.

31. Anderson ER, Hope DA. A review of the tripartite model for understanding the link between anxiety and depression in youth. Clin Psychol Rev. 2008; 28(2):275–287.

32. Chorpita BF, Plummer CM, Moffitt CE. Relations of tripartite dimensions of emotion to childhood anxiety and mood disorders. J Abnorm Child Psychol. 2000; 28(3):299–310.

33. Watson D. Differentiating the mood and anxiety disorders: A quadripartite model. Annu Rev Clin Psychol. 2009; 5:221–247.

34. Barlow DH. The nature of anxiety: Anxiety, depression, and emotional disorders. In Rapee RM, Barlow DH, eds. *Chronic Anxiety: Generalized Anxiety Disorder and Mixed Anxiety-Depression.* New York: Guilford Press; 1991:1–28.

35. Mineka S, Watson D, Clark LA. Comorbidity of anxiety and unipolar mood disorders. Annu Rev Psychol. 1998; 49(1):377–412.

36. Prenoveau JM, Zinbarg RE, Craske MG, et al. Testing a hierarchical model of anxiety and depression in adolescents: A tri-level model. J Anxiety Disord. 2010; 24(3):334–344.

37. Zinbarg RE, Barlow DH. Structure of anxiety and the anxiety disorders: A hierarchical model. J Abnorm Psychol. 1996; 105(2):181.

38. Craske MG, Rauch SL, Ursano R, et al. What is an anxiety disorder? Depress Anxiety. 2009; 26(12):1066–1085.

39. Disner SG, Beevers CG, Haigh EA, Beck AT. Neural mechanisms of the cognitive model of depression. Nat Rev Neurosci. 2011; 12(8):467–477.

40. Williams LM, Goldstein-Piekarski AN, Chowdhry N, et al. Developing a clinical translational neuroscience taxonomy for anxiety and mood disorder: Protocol for the baseline–follow-up Research Domain Criteria Anxiety and Depression ("RAD") project. BMC Psychiatry. 2016; 16:68.

41. Vaidyanathan U, Nelson LD, Patrick CJ. Clarifying domains of internalizing psychopathology using neurophysiology. Psychol Med. 2012; 42(3):447–459.

42. LeDoux JE, Pine DS. Using neuroscience to help understand fear and anxiety: A two-system framework. Am J Psychiatry. 2016; 173(11):1083–1093.

43. Nusslock R, Walden K, Harmon-Jones E. Asymmetrical frontal cortical activity associated with differential risk for mood and anxiety disorder symptoms: An RDoC perspective. Int J Psychophysiol. 2015; 98(2):249–261.

44. Mosing MA, Gordon SD, Medland SE, et al. Genetic and environmental influences on the comorbidity between depression, panic disorder, agoraphobia, and social phobia: A twin study. Depress Anxiety. 2009; 26(11):1004–1011.

45. Hettema JM, Neale MC, Kendler KS. A review and meta-analysis of the genetic epidemiology of anxiety disorders. Am J Psychiatry. 2001; 158(10):1568–1578.

46. Sullivan PF, Neale MC, Kendler KS. Genetic epidemiology of major depression: Review and meta-analysis. Am J Psychiatry. 2000; 157(10):1552–1562.

47. Cummings CM, Caporino NE, Kendall PC. Comorbidity of anxiety and depression in children and adolescents: 20 years after. Psychol Bull. 2014; 140(3):816–845.

48. Cerdá M, Sagdeo A, Johnson J, Galea S. Genetic and environmental influences on psychiatric comorbidity: A systematic review. J Affect Disord. 2010; 126(1):14–38.

49. Melton TH, Croarkin PE, Strawn JR, Mcclintock SM. Comorbid anxiety and depressive symptoms in children and adolescents: A systematic review and analysis. J Psychiatr Pract. 2016; 22(2):84–98.

50. Smoller JW. The genetics of stress-related disorders: PTSD, depression, and anxiety disorders. Neuropsychopharmacology. 2016; 41(1):297–319.

51. Cuijpers P, Sijbrandij M, Koole SL, et al. Adding psychotherapy to antidepressant medication in depression and anxiety disorders: A meta-analysis. World Psychiatry. 2014; 13(1):56–67.

52. Dunlop BW, Davis PG. Combination treatment with benzodiazepines and SSRIs for co-morbid anxiety and depression: A review. Prim Care Companion J Clin Psychiatry. 2008; 10(3):222–228.

53. Rothbaum BO, Price M, Jovanovic T, et al. A randomized, double-blind evaluation of D-cycloserine or alprazolam combined with virtual reality exposure therapy for posttraumatic stress disorder in Iraq and Afghanistan War veterans. Am J Psychiatry. 2014; 171(6):640–648.

54. Fava M, Rush AJ, Alpert JE, et al. Difference in treatment outcome in outpatients with anx-ious versus nonanxious depression: A STAR*D report. Am J Psychiatry. 2008; 165:342–351.

55. Dunlop BW, LoParo D, Kinkead B, et al. Benefits of sequentially adding cognitive-behavioral therapy or antidepressant medication for adults with nonremitting depression. Am J Psychiatry. 2019; 176(4):275–286.

56. Fournier JC, DeRubeis RJ, Shelton RC, et al. Prediction of response to medication and cogni-tive therapy in the treatment of moderate to severe depression. J Consult Clin Psychol. 2009; 77:775–787.

57. McEvoy PM, Nathan P. Effectiveness of cognitive behavior therapy for diagnostically heter-ogeneous groups: A benchmarking study. J Consult Clin Psychol. 2007; 75:344–350

58. Weisz JR, McCarty CA, Valeri SM. Effects of psychotherapy for depression in children and adolescents: A meta-analysis. Psychol Bull. 2006; 132(1):132–149.

59. Wiles N, Thomas L, Abel A, et al. Cognitive behavioural therapy as an adjunct to pharma-cotherapy for primary care based patients with treatment-resistant depression: Results of the CoBalT randomised controlled trial. Lancet. 2013; 381(9864):375–384.

60. Ninan PT, Rush AJ, Kornstein SG, et al. Symptomatic and syndromal anxiety in outpatients with chronic forms of major depression: Effect of nefazodone, cognitive behavioral analysis system of psychotherapy, and their combination. J Clin Psychiatry. 2002; 63:434–441.

61. Steele SJ, Farchione TJ, Cassiello-Robbins C, et al. Efficacy of the Unified Protocol for transdiagnostic treatment of comorbid psychopathology accompanying emotional disorders compared to treatments targeting single disorders. J Psychiatr Res. 2018; 104:211–216.

62. Craighead WE, Dunlop BW. Combination psychotherapy and antidepressant medication treatment for depression: For whom, when, and how. Annu Rev Psychol. 2014; 65:267–300.

63. Craske MG, Meuret AE, Ritz T, et al. Treatment for anhedonia: A neuroscience-driven ap-proach. Depress Anxiety. 2016; 33(10):927–38.

64. Newport DJ, Carpenter LL, McDonald WM, et al. Ketamine and other NMDA antagonists: Early clinical trials and possible mechanisms in depression. Am J Psychiatry. 2015; 172(10):950–966.

65. Bostic JQ, Rho Y. Target-symptom psychopharmacology: Between the forest and the trees. Child Adolesc Psychiatr Clin North Am. 2006; 15(1):289–302.

66. Mohamed S, Rosenheck RA. Pharmacotherapy of PTSD in the US Department of Veterans Affairs: Diagnostic- and symptom-guided drug selection. J Clin Psychiatry. 2008; 69(6):959–965.

67. Hayes SC, Hofmann SG. *Process-Based CBT: The Science and Core Clinical Competencies of Cognitive Behavioral Therapy.* Oakland, CA: Context Press; 2018.

/// 7 /// BIPOLAR DISORDER

SABRINA C. DA COSTA, MARSAL SANCHES, AND JAIR C. SOARES

7.1. INTRODUCTION

Bipolar disorder (BD) is a chronic and severe mental illness with a lifetime prevalence of 2.1% and subthreshold forms affecting another 2.4% of the US population.[1] It is among the 10 leading causes of disability in young adults worldwide,[2,3] with significant morbidity arising from acute affective episodes and subacute states. Subjects with BD tend to remain symptomatic for a significant amount of their lifetime, with estimates of more than one-third of patients relapsing into an acute episode within one year, even with proper treatment.[4-7] Depressive symptoms prevail in the course of illness,[8,9] and treatment resistance in bipolar depression seems to be the rule rather than the exception.

Phenotypically, unipolar and bipolar depression seem to share several clinical features, making the differential diagnosis often challenging. Evidence suggests that there is an average delay of 10 years between initial symptoms and diagnosis.[10,11] Moreover, a significantly higher prevalence of major depressive disorder (MDD; 16.2%)[12] compared to bipolar spectrum disorders (4.5%)[1], similarities in the clinical presentation, and an often unclear history of manic or hypomanic episodes seem to contribute to the misdiagnosis of BD as unipolar depression.

Multidimensional approaches have been proposed to better predict BD in high-risk populations, based on comprehensive clinical assessments along with a combination of neuroimaging studies and biological markers. Screening instruments, such as the Mood Disorders Questionnaire (MDQ)[13] and the Hypomania/Mania Symptom Checklist (HCL-32),[14] are available for the clinician; however, recent evidence suggests that most individuals who screened positive for BD had never received further investigation.[15] Since early diagnosis and prompt interventions have the potential to decelerate illness progression and reduce the burden associated with BD,[16,17] there is certainly a need for interventions aiming at increasing the awareness on the part of healthcare professionals of the proper detection of BD among depressed individuals.

Therefore, this chapter aims to provide a critical overview of different aspects involving the differential diagnosis of MDD and BD, emphasizing major dissimilarities between bipolar and unipolar depression. The goal is to highlight psychopathological, sociodemographic, and neurobiological features to further assist the clinician in distinguishing these disorders. Pathological and therapeutic implications of misdiagnosing BD are also briefly discussed.

7.2. PSYCHOPATHOLOGICAL AND SOCIODEMOGRAPHIC ASPECTS IN THE DIFFERENTIAL DIAGNOSIS

BD and related disorders are separated from depressive disorders in the fifth edition of the *Diagnostic and Statistical Manual of Mental Disorders* (DSM-5; Table 7.1).[18] While BD I represents the classic manic-depressive illness, usually characterized by dramatic clinical presentations, particularly during manic episodes, bipolar II disorder is usually more challenging to differentiate from MDD.[19] According to the DSM-5 classification, episodes of major depression are characterized by discrete periods of at least two weeks' duration involving changes in affect, cognition, and neurovegetative functions, with interepisode remission of symptoms.[18] BD criteria include (a) at least one manic episode, regardless of prior depressive, manic, or hypomanic episodes for BD I; (b) lifetime experience of at least one major depressive episode and at least one hypomanic episode for BD II; (c) and the presence of at least two years (one year for children and adolescents) of both depressive and hypomanic symptoms without satisfying full criteria for manic, hypomanic, or depressive episodes for cyclothymic disorder (see Table 7.1).[18] It is noteworthy

TABLE 7.1. New Classification of Mood Disorders According to DSM-5

Bipolar and Related Disorders	Depressive Disorders
Bipolar I disorder	Disruptive mood dysregulation disorder
Bipolar II disorder	Major depressive disorder
Cyclothymic disorder	Persistent depressive disorder (dysthymia)
Substance/medication-induced bipolar and related disorder	Premenstrual dysphoric disorder
	Substance/medication-induced depressive disorder
Bipolar and related disorder due to another medical condition	Depressive disorder due to another medical condition
Other specified bipolar and related disorder	Other specified depressive disorder
Unspecified bipolar and related disorder	Unspecified depressive disorder

that, according to DSM-5 criteria, a manic episode is characterized by a distinct period of abnormally or persistently elevated, expansive or irritable mood, increased goal-directed activity or energy, lasting at least one week and present most of the day, nearly every day (or any duration if hospitalization is required). During this period, three or more of the following symptoms are also present: grandiosity or inflated self-esteem, decreased need for sleep, pressured speech, flight of ideas, distractibility, and high risk-taking behaviors. Hypomanic episodes share clinical features and diagnostic criteria, except for shorter duration (at least four consecutive days) and lesser severity of impairment. Compared to manic episodes, hypomanic episodes are usually not severe enough to require hospitalization or cause marked functional impairment. Lastly, if psychotic symptoms are present, the episode is considered manic by definition.[18]

Delays of about 10 years between initial symptoms and formal diagnosis of BD have been described in the literature, usually as a consequence of depressive polarity at the onset of illness, the predominance of depressive symptoms during early stages and throughout the course of BD, and phenotypical similarities between unipolar and bipolar depression.[10,11] Evidence suggest that medical attention is frequently sought during depressive episodes, and a significant number of individuals suffering from BD seem to be unaware of and/or unable to retrospectively recall or recognize manic or hypomanic symptoms as problematic. Since major depressive episodes may be accompanied by increased irritability, psychotic symptoms, and even subthreshold hypomanic features, predicting BD on the basis of clinical phenomenology may be challenging. There is still debate over whether treatment-resistant unipolar depression (TR-UD) should be considered within the bipolar spectrum disorders;[20–22] thus, psychopathological and sociodemographic features may help in the differential diagnosis of bipolar versus unipolar depression (Table 7.2).

A recent comparative study of 194 patients (n =100 with TR-UD and 94 with BD) suggested that TR-UD may constitute a distinct psychopathological entity and not necessarily a prodromal state for bipolar depression.[21,22] In this study, subjects with TR-UD exhibited greater severity of depression, higher prevalence of anxiety and panic disorders, melancholic features, cluster C personality disorders, later age of onset of depression, and fewer hospitalizations compared to the BD group.[21,22] Another study assessing predictors of conversion to BD in 287 high-risk young participants (aged 12–30) found that specific depressive features, such as psychomotor retardation and at least five major depressive episodes, were associated with higher risks of further development of BD.[23] Multiple major depressive episodes and disruptive behaviors in high-risk youngsters also warrant close monitoring about possible evolving bipolarity, since these individuals tend to display higher rates of subthreshold mania or hypomania; manic, mixed, or hypomanic episodes; and major depressive episodes compared with non-high risk offspring.[24] Higher rates of attention-deficit/hyperactivity disorder, disruptive behavior disorders, anxiety disorders, and substance use disorders were also seen in at-risk individuals (offspring of parents with BD).[24] Additionally, symptoms of anxiety, irritability, and

TABLE 7.2. Psychopathological and Sociodemographic Features in Bipolar Versus Unipolar Depression

Bipolar Spectrum Disorders	Depressive Disorders
Early age at onset (<25 years)	Late age at onset (> 25 years)
Multiple/recurrent depressive episodes (≥5)	Fewer depressive episodes/ hospitalizations
Disruptive behaviors and history of aggression	Longer duration of episodes and greater severity
Subthreshold mania, hypomania, manic, mixed, or hypomanic episodes	Initial insomnia, appetite/weight loss, somatic complaints
Anxiety, irritability, and agitation	Worthlessness, low self-esteem
Non-suicidal self-injurious behaviors	Less suicidality
Suicidal behaviors and multiple suicide attempts	No family history of BD
Family history of BD	Less likely to have atypical symptoms
Atypical depressive symptoms	Social withdrawal
Antidepressant-induced expansive/ irritable affect	Melancholic features
Mood reactivity	Higher prevalence of cluster C personality disorders
History of treatment-resistant depression	

agitation are usually more prevalent among patients with BD I experiencing depressive symptoms and could be used to aid the clinician in recognizing more severe forms of BD I.[25] Similarly, symptoms of overt irritability and/or psychomotor agitation should also be closely monitored, since they might represent subthreshold manic symptoms.[26]

Aggressiveness in depression is significantly associated with bipolar spectrum disorders. That association seems to be independent from other factors, such as substance use disorders and comorbid borderline personality disorder.[27] Rates of nonsuicidal self-injurious behaviors, emotional dysregulation, motor hyperactivity, distractibility, and pressured speech were also significantly higher among youngsters with bipolar depression compared with unipolar depression.[28] Moreover, subthreshold mania, cyclothymia, family history of BD, atypical depressive symptoms, and antidepressant-induced elated, expansive, or irritable mood seem to be significantly more frequent among youngsters with bipolar depression compared with unipolar depression.[29] Additional demographic risk factors for the transition from MDD to BD include younger age at onset, black race/ethnicity, and low socioeconomic status (less than high school education), according to the National Epidemiologic Survey on Alcohol and Related Conditions).[30]

A study comprising 1,228 subjects (n = 386 BD I, 158 BD II, and 684 MDD) found that seven clinical features showed significant association with BD I compared with MDD: psychotic symptoms (particularly delusions), psychomotor retardation, incapacitation (higher severity of functional impairment), higher number of mixed symptoms, higher number of episodes, shorter episode length, and a history of antidepressant-induced expansive or elated affect. Moreover, in the same study, greater number of mixed symptoms and a history of elation after receiving antidepressant treatment also showed an association with BD II compared with MDD.[31] Onset characteristics in BD have been associated with subsequent predominant polarity, suicidal behaviors, and substance use in BD I.[32,33] Depressive onset seems to be particularly relevant as a predictor of suicidal behaviors and higher risk of suicide attempts,[32] multiple depressive episodes, and alcohol misuse in the course of BD.[33] Additionally, a study comparing mixed, melancholic, and anxious features in depression as a predictor of bipolar versus unipolar depression found that mixed depressive symptoms were significantly associated with hallmarks of bipolarity, while melancholic features were more frequently diagnosed in patients with unipolar depression.[34]

Self-administered and clinician-rated clinical instruments are widely available for screening of BD in individuals with depression (Table 7.3), with a goal of improving early detection of bipolar spectrum disorders; however, only about 20% of bipolar patients experiencing depressive symptoms will be properly diagnosed with BD.[35] The most commonly used rating scales in clinical practice include the Mood Disorder Questionnaire (MDQ),[13] the Hypomania/Mania Symptom Checklist (HCL-32),[14] the Screening Assessment of Depression-Polarity (SAD-P),[36] the Bipolar Inventory Symptom Scale (BISS),[37] the Bipolar Spectrum Diagnostic Scale (BSDS),[38] the Bipolar Prodrome Symptom Interview and Scale-Prospective (BPSS-P),[39] and the Probabilistic Approach for Bipolar Depression.[40] Although these rating scales have utility in clinical practice, comprehensive clinical evaluation and collateral information are indispensable for diagnostic accuracy in BD.

7.3. NEUROBIOLOGICAL, STRUCTURAL, AND FUNCTIONAL DIFFERENCES BETWEEN BD AND MDD

Despite phenotypical resemblance, unipolar and bipolar depression seem to have distinct underlying pathophysiological mechanisms. Over the past decades, theories about and evidence on neurobiological aspects have evolved into more complex models of disease where signal transduction pathways from monoamine neurotransmitters, second messengers, enzymatic systems, transcription factors and epigenetic modifications, immune-inflammatory and oxidative stress pathways, and neurotrophin-regulation systems seem to play a role in illness development and progression.[41,42] Recent imaging studies have shown distinct structural and functional brain abnormalities in BD and MDD, particularly involving neural systems that control emotion, reward processing, and emotion regulation.[43–49] These neural circuitries involve cortico-limbic systems and subcortical areas (amygdala and ventral striatum for emotion and reward processing), ventromedial and dorsomedial prefrontal areas and anterior cingulate cortical regions (emotion regulation), and lateral prefrontal cortex (cognitive and impulse control and top-down regulation of emotion).[43–49]

TABLE 7.3. Rating Scales for BD Screening

Rating Scale	Type of Scale	Description	Comments
Mood Disorder Questionnaire (MDQ)[13]	Self-report	15 questions; first 13 questions are designed to identify lifetime manic or hypomanic symptoms; 2 last questions will measure severity and level of functional impairment	Sensitivity 0.73 Specificity 0.90
Hypomania/mania Checklist (HCL-32)[14]	Self-report	2 introductory questions on current emotional state; 32 questions designed to identify manic and hypomanic symptoms	Sensitivity 0.8 Specificity 0.51
Bipolar Spectrum Diagnostic Scale (BSDS)[38]	Self-report	Designed to identify bipolar II and other forms of bipolar spectrum disorders; composed of two parts: the first part is a paragraph containing 19 sentences describing symptoms of bipolar disorder; the second part is one simple multiple-choice question, asking subjects to rate how well the story describes them overall.	Sensitivity 0.76 Specificity 0.85–0.93
Screening Assessment of Depression-Polarity (SAD-P)[36]	Clinician-rated	3-item scale: (1) presence of delusions, (2) number of prior episodes of major depression, and (3) family history of major depression or mania.	Sensitivity of 0.82 (bipolar I index sample), 0.72 (bipolar I cross-validation sample), and 0.58 (bipolar II cross-validation sample)
Bipolar Inventory Symptom Scale (BISS)[37]	Clinician-rated	44-item scale designed to assess behavioral disturbances in BDs; divided into clusters of symptoms/behaviors (depressed, manic/hypomanic, mixed manic or recovered status)	Interrater reliability >0.61; internal consistency 0.63–0.93

(continued)

TABLE 7.3. Continued

Rating Scale	Type of Scale	Description	Comments
Bipolar Prodrome Symptom Interview and Scale-Prospective (BPSS-P)[39]	Clinician-rated	Semi-structured interview developed based on the DSM-IV criteria for BD and MDD, clusters of symptoms (mania, depression and general symptom index)	Internal consistency: BPSS-P Mania (Cronbach's α = 0.87), Depression (Cronbach's α = 0.89), and General Symptom Index (Cronbach's α = 0.74).
Probabilistic Approach for Bipolar Depression[40]	Clinician-rated	1. **Symptomatology and Mental State Signs:** hypersomnia/ increased daytime napping; hyperphagia/ increased weight; other atypical depressive symptoms; psychomotor retardation; psychotic features; mood lability/manic symptoms. 2. **Course of Illness:** early onset of depression (<25 years); multiple prior episodes. 3. **Family History:** positive for BD	Higher odds of BD-I depression if positive for $\geq$5 items

In a recent functional magnetic resonance imaging (fMRI) study assessing neural correlates and functional interactions underlying reward processing in BD patients (n = 16) compared to healthy controls (HC; n = 16), individuals with BD showed reduced neural responses of the ventral striatum to reward stimuli (possibly related to anhedonia) and decreased suppression of the reward-related activation of the mesolimbic reward system while having to reject immediate reward in favor of the long-term goal (which seems to be consistent with impulsivity, one of the clinical hallmarks in BD).[50] Interestingly, another fMRI study assessing brain activation in unipolar (n = 25) and bipolar (n = 25) depressed subjects compared with HC (n = 25) found no differences in cortico-limbic regions between subjects (BD vs. MDD).[51] In this study, major differences occurred in primary and secondary visual processing regions, where subjects with BD I showed decreased in activation of the middle occipital gyrus, lingual gyrus, and middle temporal gyrus during emotional processing compared to both MDD and HC, whereas MDD subjects showed increased activation in the parahippocampus, parietal lobe, and postcentral gyrus during attentional processing, with significance only in the postcentral gyrus between MDD and HC.[51]

An MRI study comparing neurobiological commonalities and distinctions among individuals with schizophrenia (n = 185), BD (n = 86), MDD (n = 108), and HC (n = 156) found significant differences in gray matter (GM) volumes primarily in paralimbic and heteromodal cortices in addition to differences in white matter integrity in five clusters: callosal, limbic-paralimbic-heteromodal, cortico-cortical, thalamocortical, and cerebellar white matter.[52] Here, significant GM decreases in right orbital frontal cortex and left inferior parietal cortex were found in the schizophrenia and BD groups compared to the HC group, but not MDD. The schizophrenia and MDD groups, but not the BD group, showed decreases in the right inferior occipital cortex compared to HC. Also, the BD and MDD groups had decreases in left dorsolateral prefrontal cortex and right supplementary motor area compared to HC.[52] There were significant GM decreases in the right precentral gyrus in the BD group only when compared to the HC. Lastly, in this study, post hoc analyses revealed significantly decreased fractional anisotropy (FA) values in all five clusters (callosal, limbic-paralimbic-heteromodal, cortico-cortical, thalamocortical, and cerebellar white matter) in the schizophrenia and BD groups, with no significant differences between the MDD and HC groups.[52]

A voxel-based diffusion tensor imaging (DTI) study on unmedicated unipolar (n = 36) and bipolar (n = 36) depressed individuals and HC (n = 45) found abnormal segments of the right uncinated fasciculus (insular and prefrontal cortex) in BD and left anterior thalamic radiation in MDD.[53] Another voxel-based DTI study (n = 39 BD, n = 43 MDD, n = 42 HC) revealed decreased FA in BD versus MDD in the corpus callosum and the cingulum. GM exploratory analysis revealed decreased FA in the left middle frontal gyrus and in the right inferior frontal gyrus in MDD compared to HC, and in the left superior medial gyrus in BD versus HC.[54] Lower resting-state functional connectivity between the left insula and left mid-dorsolateral prefrontal cortex and between bilateral insula and right frontopolar prefrontal cortex were also observed in BD (n = 36) compared to MDD (n = 40) and HC (n = 40), while lower resting-state functional connectivity between the right amygdala and the left anterior hippocampus was observed in MDD compared to BD and HC.[55]

In addition to neuroimaging studies, abnormalities in the immune-inflammatory pathways have been more extensively studied in psychiatric disorders over the past decade. A recent meta-analysis on cytokine alterations on schizophrenia, BD, and MDD found that there were similarities in the patterns of cytokine abnormalities during acute and chronic phases of these three illnesses, suggesting possible common underlying pathways for immune dysfunction during acute episodes of schizophrenia, MDD, and BD. Effects of treatment on cytokines were more significant for schizophrenia and MDD, although less frequently studied in acute mania. In this study, levels of interleukin-6 (IL-6), tumor necrosis factor-α, one soluble cytokine receptor (sIL-2R), and one cytokine receptor antagonist (IL-1RA) were significantly increased in subjects with schizophrenia, bipolar mania, and MDD compared to HC. Following treatment, IL-6 levels significantly decreased in both schizophrenia and MDD, sIL-2R levels increased in schizophrenia, and IL-1RA levels decreased in bipolar mania.[56]

Similarly, a recent study comparing the ratio of mature brain-derived neurotrophic factor (mBDNF), a marker of neuronal growth and resilience, to pro-BDNF in MDD and BD patients and HC found that both plasma mBDNF levels and the mBDNF-to-proBDNF (M/P) ratio at baseline were significantly decreased in BD individuals compared to the MDD group and HC.[57] interestingly, the M/P ratio was restored to normal levels after antidepressant treatment in the MDD group, but not in the BD group.[57] Moreover, in a different study, serum levels of neuron-specific enolase, a marker of neuronal damage, were significantly decreased in MDD and BD subjects compared to the HC group, although its pathophysiological significance and response to treatment warrant further investigation.[58] Lastly, growing body of evidence has also proposed genetic biomarkers for differential diagnosis of MDD and BD. A recent systematic review of 27 studies comprising 3,086 subjects ($n = 486$ BD, $n = 1,212$ MDD, $n = 1,388$ HC) assessing abnormalities in genes that play a role in immune-inflammatory processes and oxidative stress, neurogenesis, and synaptic plasticity found that BDNF gene expression was one of the genetic biomarkers of relevance in differentiating BD and MDD.[59] Additionally, a recent study assessing the role of microRNAs (miRNAs) abnormalities in the pathogenesis of neuropsychiatric disorders (MDD, $n = 20$; BD, $n = 20$; HC, $n = 20$) found that five miRNAs were specifically altered in MDD (hsa-let-7a-5p, hsa-let-7d-5p, hsa-let-7f-5p, hsa-miR-24-3p. and hsa-miR-425-3p) and five miRNAs (hsa-miR-140-3p, hsa-miR-30d-5p, hsa-miR-330-5p, hsa-miR-378a-5p. and hsa-miR-21-3p) were altered in BD patients, whereas two miRNAs (hsa-miR-330-3p and hsa-miR-345-5p) were dysregulated in both disorders.[60]

7.4. COMMON PITFALLS: PATHOLOGICAL AND THERAPEUTIC IMPLICATIONS OF MISDIAGNOSING BIPOLAR DEPRESSION

Evidence-based treatments for BD include psychotropic medications, somatic and neuromodulatory approaches (e.g., electroconvulsive therapy, repetitive transcranial magnetic stimulation, deep brain stimulation), and psychosocial interventions (cognitive–behavioral therapy, enhanced relapse prevention and individual psychoeducation, interpersonal and social rhythm therapy, group therapy, functional remediation, systematic care management, and family-focused therapy).[61–64]

Whereas options for the treatment of acute mania, such as lithium, valproate, and atypical antipsychotics, are usually effective, the treatment of bipolar depression remains a clinical challenge. Treatment resistance seems to be the general rule in bipolar depression. Lithium, lamotrigine, and quetiapine monotherapy remain the first-line drugs of choice, as well as olanzapine-fluoxetine, or lithium or divalproex in combination with a selective serotonin reuptake inhibitor (SSRI) or bupropion. Manic or hypomanic switch, mood lability, mixed states, and frequent cycling are of particular concern with antidepressant treatment in BD, especially in monotherapy. Although the risks of manic switch and other mood and behavioral disturbances seem to be lower with SSRIs, the use of antidepressants in BD remains highly controversial; therefore, close clinical monitoring is necessary while prescribing antidepressants to individuals with BD, and concomitant use of traditional mood stabilizers, anticonvulsants, or second-generation antipsychotic medications is generally warranted.[61–64] Moreover, emerging evidence from experimental and clinical use of drugs targeting glutamatergic and nonglutamatergic systems holds promise in unipolar and bipolar depression.[65–70]

Earlier age of onset of BD seems to be associated with longer delays to adequate treatment, greater severity of depressive symptoms, and higher levels of comorbid anxiety and substance use.[71] Moreover, high latencies between the first affective episode and the eventual diagnosis of BD have been associated with overall adverse clinical outcomes and poor long-term prognosis. Misdiagnosing BD leads to delays in proper treatment, protracted mood symptoms and prolonged affective episodes, increased suicidality, higher rates of disability, functional impairment, comorbid psychiatric and nonpsychiatric disorders, cognitive decline, and increased morbidity and mortality, the later as a result of high rates of suicide and other causes of premature death.[26,72,73] For instance, evidence suggests that residual depressive symptoms, sleep disturbance, and perceived cognitive impairment may represent determinants of psychosocial functioning in BD.[74]

Significant burden seems to result from misdiagnosis, delayed diagnosis, and/ or poorly controlled BD. Similarly to other chronic conditions, such as autoimmune disorders or diabetes mellitus, for example, where a chronic low degree of inflammation, microvascular and macrovascular complications, etc., lead to illness progression and end-stage disease, it has recently been proposed that BD is also a progressive disorder, including asymptomatic states in at-risk individuals, prodromal symptoms, episodicity, and finally end-stage disease, characterized by treatment refractoriness and low remission rates.[75] Multiple affective episodes seem to result in neurobiological and anatomical brain abnormalities that accelerate illness progression, with subsequent reduction in interepisode interval and treatment resistance.[76,77] Extensive data suggest that the majority of patients with bipolar depression will fail to respond or respond only insufficiently to traditional therapies. Existing psychotropic medications, primarily antidepressants, mood stabilizers, and atypical antipsychotics, have been associated with only limited efficacy in bipolar depression, along with delayed onset of action and a significant burden of side effects.[78–82] Therefore, strategies to improve diagnosis accuracy, ideally during early stages of illness, are pivotal, since early diagnosis of this condition may enable prompt interventions aiming at modifying the illness progression, with consequent more favorable clinical outcomes and better long-term prognosis.

7.5. FINAL REMARKS

Since, phenotypically, unipolar and bipolar depression seem to share clinical characteristics that make the differential diagnosis often challenging, strategies to improve diagnostic accuracy are critical. In view of the limitations of existing diagnostic models, integrative approaches have been proposed to improve early detection of BD in at-risk populations. In 2010, the National Institute of Mental Health proposed the Research Domain Criteria (RDoC), a framework to address the need for new approaches on the classification of mental disorders. Although the RDoC is a framework fundamentally designed for research purposes, the goal is to attain precision medicine for psychiatry through a diagnostic system based on a deeper understanding of the pathophysiological and psychosocial underpinnings of psychiatric conditions.[83]

Although recent evidence on neurobiological markers holds promise, there is certainly a need for larger prospective studies to replicate the existing findings and elucidate their clinical and therapeutic implications. As of now, the differential diagnosis of unipolar and bipolar disorders still relies mostly on clinical findings, so a comprehensive clinical evaluation is indispensable to improve the diagnostic accuracy of BD. The awareness of healthcare professionals of the possible differential diagnosis with BD among patients with depression needs to be increased. Given the extensive clinical, pathophysiological, and therapeutic implications of misdiagnosing BD, close monitoring of at-risk individuals should also be warranted. Unraveling the biological mechanisms underlying neuropsychiatric conditions will possibly enable a paradigm shift in the diagnosis of affective disorders, transitioning from phenotypical criteria, where diagnoses are based on clusters of behavioral signs and symptoms, to integrative approaches, where neurobiological markers will also play an important role as specific biosignatures in psychiatric conditions to more precisely establish psychiatric diagnoses.

REFERENCES

1. Merikangas KR, Akiskal HS, Angst J, et al. Lifetime and 12-month prevalence of bipolar spectrum disorder in the National Comorbidity Survey replication. *Arch Gen Psychiatry*. 2007;64(5):543–552. doi:10.1001/archpsyc.64.5.543

2. Mathers CD, Iburg KM, Begg S. Adjusting for dependent comorbidity in the calculation of healthy life expectancy. *Popul Health Metr.* 2006;4:4. doi:10.1186/1478-7954-4-4

3. Whiteford H, Degenhardt L, Rehm J, et al. Global burden of disease attributable to mental and substance use disorders: findings from the Global Burden of Disease Study 2010. *Lancet.* 2013;382(9904):1575–1586. doi:10.1016/S0140-6736(13)61611-6

4. Gitlin MJ, Swendsen J, Heller TL, Hammen C. Relapse and impairment in bipolar disorder. *Am J Psychiatry.* 1995;152(11):1635–1640.

5. Frye MA, Yatham L, Ketter TA, et al. Depressive relapse during lithium treatment associated with increased serum thyroid-stimulating hormone: Results from two placebo-controlled bipolar I maintenance studies. *Acta Psychiatr Scand.* 2009;120(1):10–13. doi:10.1111/j.1600-0447.2008.01343.x

6. McAllister-Williams RH. Relapse prevention in bipolar disorder: a critical review of current guidelines. *J Psychopharmacol.* 2006;20(2 suppl):12–16. doi:10.1177/1359786806063071

7. Perlis RH, Ostacher MJ, Marangell LB, et al. Predictors of recurrence in bipolar disorder: primary program for bipolar disorder (STEP-BD). *Am J Psychiatry.* 2006;163(4):217–224.

8. Judd LL, Akiskal HS, Schettler PJ, et al. The long-term natural history of the weekly symptomatic status of bipolar I disorder. *Arch Gen Psychiatry.* 2002;59(6):530–537. doi:10.1001/archpsyc.59.6.530

9. Judd LL, Akiskal HS, Schettler PJ, et al. A prospective investigation of the natural history of the long-term weekly symptomatic status of bipolar II disorder. *Arch Gen Psychiatry.* 2003;60(3):261–269.

10. Lish JD, Dime-Meenan S, Whybrow PC, et al. The National Depressive and Manic-Depressive Association (DMDA) survey of bipolar members. *J Affect Disord.* 1994;31(4):281–294.

11. Baldessarini RJ, Tondo L, Baethge CJ, et al. Effects of treatment latency on response to maintenance treatment in manic-depressive disorders. *Bipolar Disord.* 2007;9(4):386–393. doi:10.1111/j.1399-5618.2007.00385.x

12. Kessler RC, Berglund P, Demler O, et al. The epidemiology of major depressive disorder: results from the National Comorbidity Survey Replication (NCS-R). *JAMA.* 2003;289(23):3095–3105. doi:10.1097/00132578-200310000-00002

13. Hirschfeld RM, Williams JB, Spitzer RL, et al. Development and validation of a screening instrument for bipolar spectrum disorder: the Mood Disorder Questionnaire. *Am J Psychiatry.* 2000;157(11):1873–1875. doi:10.1176/appi.ajp.157.11.1873

14. Angst J, Adolfsson R, Benazzi F, et al. The HCL-32: towards a self-assessment tool for hypomanic symptoms in outpatients. *J Affect Disord.* 2005;88(2):217–233. doi:10.1016/j.jad.2005.05.011

15. Hirschfeld RM, Calabrese JR, Weissman MM, et al. Screening for bipolar disorder in the community. *J Clin Psychiatry.* 2003;64(1):53–59.

16. Fernandes BS, Dean OM, Dodd S, et al. N-acetylcysteine in depressive symptoms and functionality: A systematic review and meta-analysis. *J Clin Psychiatry.* 2016;77(4):e457–e466. doi:10.4088/JCP.15r09984

17. Post RM, Leverich GS, Kupka RW, et al. Early-onset bipolar disorder and treatment delay are risk factors for poor outcome in adulthood. *J Clin Psychiatry.* 2010;71(7):864–872. doi:10.4088/JCP.08m04994yel

18. American Psychiatric Association. *Diagnostic and Statistical Manual of Mental Disorders,* fifth ed. Washington, DC: APA; 2013.

19. Benazzi F. Bipolar disorder-focus on bipolar II disorder and mixed depression. *Lancet.* 2007;369(9565):935–945. doi:10.1016/S0140-6736(07)60453-X

20. Correa R, Akiskal H, Gilmer W, et al. Is unrecognized bipolar disorder a frequent contributor to apparent treatment resistant depression? *J Affect Disord.* 2010;127(1-3):10–18. doi:10.1016/j.jad.2010.06.036

21. Nuñez NA, Comai S, Dumitrescu E, et al. Psychopathological and sociodemographic features in treatment-resistant unipolar depression versus bipolar depression: a comparative study. *BMC Psychiatry*. 2018;18(1). doi:10.1186/s12888-018-1641-y

22. Nuñez NA, Comai S, Dumitrescu E, et al. Psychopathological and sociodemographic features in treatment resistant unipolar, bipolar I and II depression: a comparative study. *Neuropsychopharmacology*. 2017;43(Supp 1):S343. doi:http://dx.doi.org/10.1038/npp.2017.265

23. Frankland A, Roberts G, Holmes-Preston E, et al. Clinical predictors of conversion to bipolar disorder in a prospective longitudinal familial high-risk sample: focus on depressive features. *Psychol Med*. 2017:1–9.

24. Axelson D, Goldstein B, Goldstein T, et al. Diagnostic precursors to bipolar disorder in offspring of parents with bipolar disorder: a longitudinal study. *Am J Psychiatry*. 2015;172(7):638–646. doi:10.1176/appi.ajp.2014.14010035

25. Suppes T, Eberhard J, Lemming O, et al. Anxiety, irritability, and agitation as indicators of bipolar mania with depressive symptoms: a post hoc analysis of two clinical trials. *Int J Bipolar Disord*. 2017;5(1):36. doi:10.1186/s40345-017-0103-7

26. Judd LL, Schettler PJ, Akiskal H, et al. Prevalence and clinical significance of subsyndromal manic symptoms, including irritability and psychomotor agitation, during bipolar major depressive episodes. *J Affect Disord*. 2012;138(3):440–448. doi:10.1016/j.jad.2011.12.046

27. Verdolini N, Perugi G, Samalin L, et al. Aggressiveness in depression: a neglected symptom possibly associated with bipolarity and mixed features. *Acta Psychiatr Scand*. 2017;136(4):362–372. doi:10.1111/acps.12777

28. Diler RS, Goldstein TR, Hafeman D, et al. Distinguishing bipolar depression from unipolar depression in youth: preliminary findings. *J Child Adolesc Psychopharmacol*. 2017;27(4):310–319. doi:10.1089/cap.2016.0154

29. Scott J, Marwaha S, Ratheesh A, et al. Bipolar at-risk criteria: an examination of which clinical features have optimal utility for identifying youth at risk of early transition from depression to bipolar disorders. *Schizophr Bull*. 2017;43(4):737–744. doi:10.1093/schbul/sbw154

30. Gilman SE, Dupuy JM, Perlis RH. Risks for the transition from major depressive disorder to bipolar disorder in the National Epidemiologic Survey on Alcohol and Related Conditions. *J Clin Psychiatry*. 2012;73(6):829–836. doi:10.4088/JCP.11m06912

31. Leonpacher AK, Liebers D, Pirooznia M, et al. Distinguishing bipolar from unipolar depression: the importance of clinical symptoms and illness features. *Psychol Med*. 2015;45(11):2437–2446. doi:10.1017/S0033291715000446

32. Cremaschi L, Dell'Osso B, Vismara M, et al. Onset polarity in bipolar disorder: a strong association between first depressive episode and suicide attempts. *J Affect Disord*. 2017;209:182–187. doi:10.1016/j.jad.2016.11.043

33. Etain B, Lajnef M, Bellivier F, et al. Clinical expression of bipolar disorder type I as a function of age and polarity at onset: convergent findings in samples from France and the United States. *J Clin Psychiatry*. 2012;73(4). doi:10.4088/JCP.10m06504

34. Zaninotto L, Souery D, Calati R, et al. Mixed, melancholic, and anxious features in depression: a cross-sectional study of sociodemographic and clinical correlates. *Ann Clin Psychiatry*. 2014;26(4):243–253.

35. Goldberg JF, Harrow M, Whiteside JE. Risk for bipolar illness in patients initially hospitalized for unipolar depression. *Am J Psychiatry*. 2001;158(8):1265–1270.

36. Solomon DA, Leon AC, Maser JD, et al. Distinguishing bipolar major depression from unipolar major depression with the Screening Assessment of Depression-Polarity (SAD-P). *J Clin Psychiatry*. 2006;67(3):434–442. doi:10.4088/JCP.v67n0315

37. Bowden CL, Singh V, Thompson P, et al. Development of the Bipolar Inventory of Symptoms Scale. *Acta Psychiatr Scand*. 2007;116(3):189–194. doi:10.1111/j.1600-0447.2006.00955.x

38. Ghaemi SN, Miller CJ, Berv DA, et al. Sensitivity and specificity of a new bipolar spectrum diagnostic scale. *J Affect Disord*. 2005;84(2-3):273–277. doi:10.1016/S0165-0327(03)00196-4

39. Correll CU, Olvet DM, Auther AM, et al. The Bipolar Prodrome Symptom Interview and Scale-Prospective (BPSS-P): description and validation in a psychiatric sample and healthy controls. *Bipolar Disord*. 2014;16(5):505–522. doi:10.1111/bdi.12209

40. Mitchell PB, Goodwin GM, Johnson GF, Hirschfeld RMA. Diagnostic guidelines for bipolar depression: a probabilistic approach. *Bipolar Disord*. 2008;10(1 pt 2):144–152. doi:10.1111/j.1399-5618.2007.00559.x

41. Post RM. Mechanisms of illness progression in the recurrent affective disorders. *Neurotox Res*. 2010;18(3-4):256–271. doi:10.1007/s12640-010-9182-2

42. Post RM, Fleming J, Kapczinski F. Neurobiological correlates of illness progression in the recurrent affective disorders. *J Psychiatr Res*. 2012;46(5):561–573. doi:10.1016/j.jpsychires.2012.02.004

43. Benedetti F, Yeh PH, Bellani M, et al. Disruption of white matter integrity in bipolar depression as a possible structural marker of illness. *Biol Psychiatry*. 2011;69(4):309–317. doi:10.1016/j.biopsych.2010.07.028

44. Bora E, Fornito A, Yücel M, Pantelis C. Voxelwise meta-analysis of gray matter abnormalities in bipolar disorder. *Biol Psychiatry*. 2010;67(11):1097–1105. doi:10.1016/j.biopsych.2010.01.020

45. Strakowski SM, DelBello MP, Sax KW, et al. Brain magnetic resonance imaging of structural abnormalities in bipolar disorder. *Arch Gen Psychiatry*. 1999;56(3):254–260.

46. Adler CM, DelBello MP, Jarvis K, et al. Voxel-based study of structural changes in first-episode patients with bipolar disorder. *Biol Psychiatry*. 2007;61(6):776–781. doi:10.1016/j.biopsych.2006.05.042

47. Kupfer DJ, Frank E, Phillips ML. Major depressive disorder: new clinical, neurobiological, and treatment perspectives. *Lancet*. 2012;379(9820):1045–1055. doi:10.1016/S0140-6736(11)60602-8

48. De Almeida JRC, Phillips ML. Distinguishing between unipolar depression and bipolar depression: current and future clinical and neuroimaging perspectives. *Biol Psychiatry*. 2013;73(2):111–118. doi:10.1016/j.biopsych.2012.06.010

49. Strakowski SSM, Adler CMC, Almeida J, et al. The functional neuroanatomy of bipolar disorder: a consensus model. *Bipolar Disord*. 2012;14(4):313–325. doi:10.1111/j.1399-5618.2012.01022.x

50. Trost S, Diekhof EK, Zvonik K, et al. Disturbed anterior prefrontal control of the mesolimbic reward system and increased impulsivity in bipolar disorder. *Neuropsychopharmacology*. 2014;39(8):1914–1923. doi:10.1038/npp.2014.39

51. Cerullo MA, Eliassen JC, Smith CT, et al. Bipolar I disorder and major depressive disorder show similar brain activation during depression. *Bipolar Disord*. 2014;16(7):703–712. doi:10.1111/bdi.12225

52. Chang M, Womer FY, Edmiston EK, et al. Neurobiological commonalities and distinctions among three major psychiatric diagnostic categories: a structural MRI study. *Schizophr Bull*. 2018;44(1):65–74. doi:10.1093/schbul/sbx028

53. Deng F, Wang Y, Huang H, et al. Abnormal segments of right uncinate fasciculus and left anterior thalamic radiation in major and bipolar depression. *Prog Neuropsychopharmacology Biol Psychiatry*. 2018;81:340–349. doi:10.1016/j.pnpbp.2017.09.006

54. Repple J, Meinert S, Grotegerd D, et al. A voxel-based diffusion tensor imaging study in unipolar and bipolar depression. *Bipolar Disord*. 2017;19(1):23–31. doi:10.1111/bdi.12465

55. Ambrosi E, Arciniegas DB, Madan A, et al. Insula and amygdala resting-state functional connectivity differentiate bipolar from unipolar depression. *Acta Psychiatr Scand*. 2017;136(1):129–139. doi:10.1111/acps.12724

56. Goldsmith DR, Rapaport MH, Miller BJ. A meta-analysis of blood cytokine network alterations in psychiatric patients: comparisons between schizophrenia, bipolar disorder and depression. *Mol Psychiatry*. 2016;21:1696–1709. doi:10.1038/mp.2016.3

57. Zhao G, Zhang C, Chen J, et al. Ratio of mBDNF to proBDNF for differential diagnosis of major depressive disorder and bipolar depression. *Mol Neurobiol.* 2016;54(7):1–10. doi:10.1007/s12035-016-0098-6

58. Wiener CD, Jansen K, Ghisleni G, et al. Reduced serum levels of neuron specific enolase (NSE) in drug-naïve subjects with major depression and bipolar disorder. *Neurochem Res.* 2013;38(7):1394–1398. doi:10.1007/s11064-013-1036-x

59. Menezes IC, von Werne Baes C, Lacchini R, Juruena MF. Genetic biomarkers for differential diagnosis of major depressive disorder and bipolar disorder: a systematic and critical review. *Behav Brain Res.* 2018. doi:10.1016/j.bbr.2018.01.008

60. Maffioletti E, Cattaneo A, Rosso G, et al. Peripheral whole blood microRNA alterations in major depression and bipolar disorder. *J Affect Disord.* 2016;200:250–258. doi:10.1016/j.jad.2016.04.021

61. Geddes JR, Miklowitz DJ. Treatment of bipolar disorder. *Lancet.* 2013;381(9878):1672–1682. doi:10.1016/S0140-6736(13)60857-0

62. Yatham LN, Kennedy SH, Parikh SV, et al. Canadian Network for Mood and Anxiety Treatments (CANMAT) and International Society for Bipolar Disorders (ISBD) 2018 guidelines for the management of patients with bipolar disorder. *Bipolar Disord.* 2018;20(2):97–170. doi:10.1111/bdi.12609

63. Pacchiarotti I, Bond DJ, Baldessarini RJ, et al. The International Society for Bipolar Disorders (ISBD) task force report on antidepressant use in bipolar disorders. *Am J Psychiatry.* 2013;170(11):1249–1262. wos:000326724300008.

64. Goodwin GM, Anderson I, Arango C, et al. ECNP consensus meeting, bipolar depression, Nice, March 2007. *Eur Neuropsychopharmacol.* 2008;18(7):535–549. doi:10.1016/j.euroneuro.2008.03.003

65. Machado-Vieira R, Henter ID, Manji HK, Zarate CA. Potential novel treatments in bipolar depression. In Zarate CA Jr, Manji HK, eds. *Bipolar Depression: Molecular Neurobiology, Clinical Diagnosis, and Pharmacotherapy.* Basel: Birkhäuser Verlag, 2009:259–285. doi:10.1007/978-3-319-31689-5_12

66. Iadarola ND, Niciu MJ, Richards EM, et al. Ketamine and other N-methyl-D-aspartate receptor antagonists in the treatment of depression: a perspective review. *Ther Adv Chronic Dis.* 2015;6(3):97–114. doi:10.1177/2040622315579059

67. Niciu MJ, Luckenbaugh DA, Ionescu DF, et al. Clinical predictors of ketamine response in treatment-resistant major depression. *J Clin Psychiatry.* 2014;75(5). doi:10.4088/JCP.13m08698

68. Sanacora G, Zarate CA, Krystal JH, Manji HK. Targeting the glutamatergic system to develop novel, improved therapeutics for mood disorders. *Nat Rev Drug Discov.* 2008;7(5):426–437. doi:10.1038/nrd2462

69. Henter ID, de Sousa RT, Gold PW, et al. Mood therapeutics: novel pharmacological approaches for treating depression. *Expert Rev Clin Pharmacol.* 2017;10(2):153–166. doi:10.1080/17512433.2017.1253472

70. da Costa SC, Machado-Vieira R, Soares JC. Novel therapeutics in bipolar disorder. *Curr Treat Options Psychiatry.* 2018;5(1):162–181. doi:10.1007/s40501-018-0140-6

71. Joslyn C, Hawes DJ, Hunt C, Mitchell PB. Is age of onset associated with severity, prognosis, and clinical features in bipolar disorder? A meta-analytic review. *Bipolar Disord.* 2016;18(5):389–403. doi:10.1111/bdi.12419

72. Nordentoft M, Mortensen PB, Pedersen CB. Absolute risk of suicide after first hospital contact in mental disorder. *Arch Gen Psychiatry.* 2011;68(10):1058–1064. doi:10.1001/archgenpsychiatry.2011.113

73. Crump C, Sundquist K, Winkleby MA, Sundquist J. Comorbidities and mortality in bipolar disorder: a Swedish national cohort study. *JAMA Psychiatry.* 2013;70(9):931–939. doi:10.1001/jamapsychiatry.2013.1394

74. Samalin L, Boyer L, Murru A, et al. Residual depressive symptoms, sleep disturbance and perceived cognitive impairment as determinants of functioning in patients with bipolar disorder. *J Affect Disord.* 2017;210:280–286. doi:10.1016/j.jad.2016.12.054

75. Berk M, Kapczinski F, Andreazza AC, et al. Pathways underlying neuroprogression in bipolar disorder: focus on inflammation, oxidative stress and neurotrophic factors. *Neurosci Biobehav Rev.* 2011;35(3):804–817. doi:10.1016/j.neubiorev.2010.10.001

76. Post RM. Transduction of psychosocial stress into the neurobiology of recurrent affective disorder. *Am J Psychiatry.* 1992;149(8):999–1010.

77. da Costa SC, Passos IC, Lowri C, et al. Refractory bipolar disorder and neuroprogression. *Prog Neuropsychopharmacol Biol Psychiatry.* 2016;70:103–110. doi:10.1016/j.pnpbp.2015.09.005

78. Poon SH, Sim K, Sum MY, et al. Evidence-based options for treatment-resistant adult bipolar disorder patients. *Bipolar Disord.* 2012;14(6):573–584. doi:10.1111/j.1399-5618.2012.01042.x

79. Marc M, Chantal H. Treatment-resistant bipolar depression (TRBD): Definition and therapeutic strategies. *Bipolar Disord.* 2012;14:101–102.

80. Sienaert P, Lambrichts L, Dols A, De Fruyt J. Evidence-based treatment strategies for treatment-resistant bipolar depression: a systematic review. *Bipolar Disord.* 2013;15(1):61–69. doi:10.1111/bdi.12026

81. Tondo L, Vázquez GH, Baldessarini RJ. Options for pharmacological treatment of refractory bipolar depression. *Curr Psychiatry Rep.* 2014;16(2):431. doi:10.1007/s11920-013-0431-y

82. Goodwin GM. Bipolar depression and treatment with antidepressants. *Br J Psychiatry.* 2012;200(1):5–6. doi:10.1192/bjp.bp.111.095349

83. Insel T, Cuthbert B, Garvey M, et al. Research domain criteria (RDoC): toward a new classification framework for research on mental disorders. *Am J Psychiatry.* 2010;167(7):748–751. doi:10.1176/appi.ajp.2010.09091379

/// 8 /// PRIMER ON DEPRESSION

Suicide, Suicidal Behavior, and Suicidal Ideation

JENNIFER L. HUGHES

8.1. INTRODUCTION

Suicide is a serious, and growing, public health problem worldwide, with approximately 800,000 people dying by suicide per year.[1] Suicide is one of the leading causes of death in the United States, and rates increased in almost every state from 1999 through 2016.[2] In addition to completed suicides, suicidal behavior is problematic. More than 1 million people per year attempt suicide in the United States.[3] Beyond the impact on the suicidal individual and others affected, suicide contributes to early death, morbidity, lost productivity, and healthcare costs.[1,4]

The National Strategy for Suicide Prevention highlights the national importance of addressing this mental health issue.[4] There are a number of detailed resources for additional information about suicide, suicidal behavior, and suicidal ideation (Table 8.1). This chapter outlines the risk and protective factors related to suicide, research findings about the mechanisms and functions of suicidal behavior, principles of crisis intervention, and treatments to address suicidal behavior and offers an overview of suicide risk and treatment in special populations, and an overview of postvention efforts.

8.2. HISTORY AND PHILOSOPHY OF SUICIDE

Scientific theory and research on suicide began at the end of the 19th century, but the earliest reference of suicidal thinking appeared in writing in approximately 2000 BC, called "Dialogue of a Man with His Soul." Philosophies of suicide include several perspectives.[5] In the moralistic perspective, espoused by Plato, Aristotle, Plutarch, and Kant, suicide is unacceptable; the overriding moral obligation is to

TABLE 8.1. Additional Resources Specific to Suicide, Suicidal Behavior, and Suicidal Ideation

Organization	Website
American Association of Suicidology	http://www.suicidology.org/
American Foundation for Suicide Prevention	www.afsp.org
CDC	https://www.cdc.gov/violenceprevention/suicide/index.html
National Institute of Mental Health	https://www.nimh.nih.gov/health/topics/suicide-prevention/index.shtml
National Suicide Prevention Lifeline	https://suicidepreventionlifeline.org/
Safety Planning Intervention	http://www.suicidesafetyplan.com
SAVE (Suicide Awareness Voices of Education)	https://save.org/
Substance Abuse and Mental Health Services Administration	https://www.samhsa.gov/suicide-prevention
Suicide Prevention Resource Center	www.sprc.org
Zero Suicide	https://zerosuicide.sprc.org/

Report Name and Agency	Website
Preventing Suicide: A Technical Package of Policy, Programs, and Practices (CDC)	https://www.cdc.gov/violenceprevention/pdf/suicideTechnicalPackage.pdf
National Strategy for Suicide Prevention: Goals and Objectives for Action (US Surgeon General and National Action Alliance for Suicide Prevention)	https://www.surgeongeneral.gov/library/reports/national-strategy-suicide-prevention/index.html
Preventing Suicide: A Global Imperative (WHO)	https://www.who.int/mental_health/suicide-prevention/world_report_2014/en/

protect life and prevent suicide. Aquinas had a more religious philosophy (it was a "sin" to take one's life). In the libertarian perspective, espoused by Zeno, Sir Thomas More, and John Donne, suicide is an individual's "self-indulgent right"; it is a reasonable and calculated act to avoid pain. Hume concludes that the act receives its meaning from the circumstances, characters, and purpose of those committing it and also from the consequences of their act. In the relativist perspective, the "rightness" or "wrongness" of suicide is to be considered given the situation, and thus the corresponding obligation to intervene (or not); in other words, there is a "cost/benefit analysis of utility." Only in recent history have some countries, such as India, decriminalized suicide; it remains illegal in several countries throughout Africa and Asia.[6]

TABLE 8.2. Suicide Nomenclature

Suicide	"Death caused by self-directed injurious behavior with any intent to die as a result of the behavior"[9]
Suicide attempt	"A non-fatal self-directed potentially injurious behavior with any intent to die as a result of the behavior. A suicide attempt may or may not result in injury"[9]
Suicidal ideation	"Thought of engaging in behavior intended to end one's life"[10]
Suicide plan	"The formulation of a specific method through which one intends to die"[10]

8.3. SUICIDE NOMENCLATURE

Over time there has been debate regarding the inconsistent nomenclature of suicidology.[7,8] For example, some studies refer to suicidal ideation, suicidal gestures, suicidal behavior, or suicidal threats. Table 8.2 lists the recommended standard terms across the field of suicidology.[9,10] It is important to distinguish multiple attempters from single attempters, given the high risk of death by suicide in those individuals with a history of self-harm and/or suicidal behavior.[11–14] Recent data suggest utility in assessing individuals for interrupted attempts and aborted attempts.[9] Marzuk and colleagues introduced the category "aborted suicide attempts" to describe an event in which an individual has an intent to injure the self with intent to die but stops prior to enacting any self-harm.[15] Interrupted attempts are those instances in which an individual takes steps to injure the self with intent to die but is stopped by another person prior to the fatal injury.[9] Both aborted and interrupted attempts have been associated with future suicide attempts.[15,16] The term "suicidality" has been used to describe all types of suicide-related events, ranging from death by suicide to suicidal ideation. This term, however, has been deemed less useful given its nonspecificity, and the use of more specific terminology is recommended.[9,17]

8.4. EPIDEMIOLOGY OF SUICIDAL BEHAVIOR

The true rates of death by suicide and suicide attempts are difficult to ascertain. Deaths by suicide may be recorded as accidental deaths due to legal issues and/or complicated procedures related to classifying a death as a suicide.[1] In addition, individuals may not disclose suicide attempts to others, and low-lethality attempts may not always require medical attention. The distribution of suicide deaths by gender differs globally; in low- and middle-income countries, the male/female ratio is 1.5, whereas in richer countries the ratio is 3.0.[1] A review placed the lifetime prevalence in 17 countries as follows: suicidal ideation, 9.2%; suicide plans, 3.1%; and nonlethal attempts, 2.7%.[18] Cross-nationally, about one-third of those who think about suicide will go on to make an attempt.[18] Intentional ingestion of pesticides, hanging, and death by firearm are the most common suicide attempt methods across the world.[1]

Suicide is the tenth leading cause of death in the United States.[2] Suicide affects individuals of all ages; it is the second leading cause of death in those aged 10 to 34, the fourth leading cause of death in those aged 35 to 54, and the eighth leading cause of death in those aged 55 to 64.[2] In 2017, men died by suicide 3.54 times more often than women. The highest suicide rates in the United States are among non-Hispanic American Indian/Alaska Native and non-Hispanic white populations.[19] In 2017, firearms accounted for 50.57% of all suicide deaths, making it the most common mean of suicide in the United States, followed by suffocation and poisoning.[2]

8.5. RISK AND PROTECTIVE FACTORS

There is no single cause of suicide. The reasons for and predictors of suicide and suicidal behavior vary across individuals. Most risk factors account for a small proportion of the variance in predicting suicide deaths. A previous history of suicidal behavior or self-harm is the most consistently replicated risk factor for death by suicide. This history is also a strong predictor of premature death by unnatural causes (e.g., drug overdose, car accidents, homicide) and of nonfatal suicidal behavior. In a meta-review that included 20 systematic reviews and meta-analyses to report mortality risks in 20 different mental disorders, patients with borderline personality disorder (mostly inpatient samples), anorexia nervosa (mostly inpatient samples), depression, and bipolar disorder had the highest suicide risks.[20] Substance abuse; emerging psychosis; schizophrenia; sexual and gender minority status; veteran status; bullying; exposure to suicide; and other forms of psychosocial stress, such as relationship problems, physical health issues, or a crisis in the near past or future are associated with increased risk for fatal and nonfatal suicide attempts. Some medical treatments may also be associated with increased suicide risk (e.g., changes in medication dosing, discontinuation of medications, steroids and steroid withdrawal). Sleep disturbance may be an indicator of imminent suicide risk. See reviews for more information on risk and protective factors in the United States.[4]

Across the world, consistent cross-national risk factors include female, younger, less educated, unmarried, and having a mental disorder. The strongest diagnostic risk factors include having a mood disorder in richer countries and having an impulse control disorder in low- to middle-income countries. There is no group difference until mid-adolescence, when rates among males increase relative to females, and the rise for males is greatest among Native American/Alaskan Natives.[10]

The World Health Organization recommends an approach to understanding suicide risk that includes (1) health system and societal risk factors, such as barriers to accessing healthcare, access to means, suicide contagion related to inappropriate media reporting and social media use, stigma of help-seeking behavior; (2) community and relationship factors, such as disaster, war and conflict, stress related to acculturation or dislocation, discrimination, trauma, and abuse, sense of isolation, lack of support, and relationship conflict or discord; and (3) individual risk factors such as previous suicide attempt, current or lifetime psychopathology (mood disorders most common), substance use/abuse, recent loss (job or financial), hopelessness, chronic pain, chronic illness, family history of suicide, parental psychiatric conditions (in youth), and other biological/genetic risk.[1] Protective factors include strong personal relationships, religious or spiritual beliefs, positive coping strategies, fair number of reasons for living, future goals, and treatment adherence. The report by the Centers for Disease Control and Prevention (CDC), "Preventing Suicide: A Technical Package of Policy, Programs, and Practices," includes a detailed discussion of a core set of strategies to help communities and states develop prevention activities to address these risk and protective factors.[19]

But does knowing about risk and protective factors make a difference? In a meta-analysis of 365 studies from past 50 years, across odds ratios, hazard ratios, and diagnostic accuracy analyses, prediction was only slightly better than chance for all outcomes.[21] No broad category or subcategory accurately predicted far-above-chance levels, suggesting that predictive validity has not improved across 50 years of research. Franklin and colleagues noted that studies rarely examined the combined effect of multiple risk factors and risk factors have been homogenous over time, with five broad categories accounting for nearly 80% of all risk-factor tests.[21]

The variation in risk and protective factors across individuals has led to interest in machine learning and related approaches to identify individuals with a heightened imminent risk for suicide.[22] By analyzing the full spectrum of the electronic health record, computerized risk screening approaches can identify risk and protective factors beyond what individual clinicians can see.[23] In a recent examination of an electronic health record, the strongest predictors remained (e.g., substance abuse, psychiatric disorder), but also less conventional predictors were identified (e.g., certain injuries, chronic conditions).[23] However, this does not mean existing risk guidelines are invalid or useless; these have been widely used in clinical settings and often have been rationally derived by expert consensus.

8.6. MODELS OF SUICIDE

Many theories and models of suicide have been proposed. Shneidman explained suicide as a response to overwhelming pain (i.e., psychache).[24,25] An early model of understanding suicide, based on a frequently used model of mental illness, was the stress-diathesis model.[26–28] In an examination of risk factors in 347 consecutive patients admitted to a university psychiatric hospital, Mann and colleagues (1999) tested a stress-diathesis model of suicidal behavior.[26] They found that higher levels of subjective depression, higher levels of suicidal ideation, fewer reasons for living, lifetime history of impulsivity, and lifetime history of aggression separated suicide attempters from non-attempters.[26] In conclusion, it appears that a psychiatric diagnosis acts as the stress in the model, while other preexisting factors such as a tendency to experience suicidal thoughts or to be more impulsive make up the diathesis.[26]

The cognitive model of suicide points to maladaptive cognitions, including suicidal thoughts, as the fundamental pathway to suicidal behavior.[29–31] To conceptualize the suicide attempt, one must examine the automatic thoughts and core beliefs that were activated just prior to the suicidal behavior.[32] These cognitions often include hopelessness, helplessness, unlovability, and perceived inability to tolerate distress. Rudd and colleagues referred to the "suicidal mode," which includes suicide-related thoughts, negative affect, physical or physiological symptoms, and intent (behavior and motivation).[30] It has been hypothesized that once an individual has engaged in suicidal behavior, the "suicidal mode" becomes more available and thus is more easily activated. Rudd elaborated that the "suicidal mode" contains the "suicidal belief system" or the maladaptive meaning that is constructed (including compensatory strategies and the conditional rules or assumptions) and assigned to the self, the environment, and the future.[29] Other skills deficits in individuals struggling with suicide often include rigid, dichotomous thinking about the self and others, poor problem solving, and a view of suicide as a coping strategy.[31]

A highly studied intervention to address suicide, dialectical behavioral therapy (DBT), is founded on the biosocial theory of borderline personality disorder.[33] This theory posits that borderline personality disorder develops as a result of biological vulnerabilities to emotional dysregulation and repeated exposure to an invalidating environment. Within this model, suicide attempts are conceptualized as a maladaptive problem-solving behavior with the intent to escape unbearable emotional pain.[33]

A newer model of understanding suicide is that of the interpersonal-psychological theory of suicide;[34,35] this model has also been conceptualized as applying to youth.[36] This theory is based on three major tenets.[37] First, they propose that people who die by suicide have developed a pain tolerance through life experiences, thereby habituating toward violence and pain. This desensitization, coupled with a sense of burdensomeness and a decreased sense of belongingness, contribute to one's suicide risk.[34,37,38] Early tests of this model have shown promise in predicting suicide, above and beyond previously identified risk factors.[39] Joiner's work was pivotal in pointing theorists to consider suicide across the continuum; that is, how suicidal ideation might progress to suicidal behavior. This has become known as the ideation-to-action framework.[40] Examples of newer theories under this framework, which need to be tested, include the three-step theory[41] and the integrated motivational-volitional model.[42]

8.7. DETECTION AND ASSESSMENT

There is increasing recognition that both suicide risk detection and suicide risk assessment are needed in suicide prevention efforts. Assessment of risk is very different from detection of risk; detection often involves screening. One must consider the role of community, school, and healthcare organizations in detection, while healthcare professionals and mental health professionals are vital in risk assessment.

Detection through screening for suicide risk is the first step in any suicide prevention program, as it helps to raise awareness and provides for a common language about suicide within a specific setting, agency, health system, or institution. Screening helps to ensure that staff are following a standardized, evidence-based protocol to identify individuals at risk and offers guidance for developing an action plan to manage risk (Zero Suicide, https://zerosuicide.sprc.org/toolkit/identify/screening-and-assessing-suicide-risk).

Detection may occur through screening with a brief measure. In youth populations, the most studied screening detection tool is the Ask Suicide-Screening Questions (ASQ).[43,44] The ASQ comprises four questions of escalating severity about suicidal thoughts and behavior, which includes a fifth question to assess imminent risk if any of the first four are endorsed. A commonly used tool that has been used by the US Food and Drug Administration (FDA), as well as in medical, inpatient, and outpatient settings, is the Columbia Suicide Severity Rating Scale (C-SSRS; http://cssrs.columbia.edu/), a semi-structured clinician-rated interview.[8,45] Both suicidal behavior and suicidal ideation are rated on a 0-to-5 scale, with suicidal ideation ratings ranging from 0 ("no ideation") to 5 ("suicidal ideation with intent and a clear plan") and suicidal behavior ratings ranging from 0 ("no behavior") to 5 ("multiple attempts during the assessment period"). In addition, because suicidal ideation fluctuates over time, the modal and most severe since the past assessment are rated. A recent quality improvement program for universal suicide screening used this measure successfully in a large healthcare system.[46]

An additional strategy for detection is to train key "gatekeepers" (e.g., schoolteachers, nursing home staff, religious leaders) in the signs of depression and suicide risk so that they might know how to ask those individuals with whom they interact about suicide. Most programs show evidence of helping the gatekeepers feel more confident in asking about suicide and/or in increasing their knowledge about mental health. Examples of detection programs include Mental Health First Aid[47–49] and Question, Persuade, Refer (QPR).[50–51]

Suicide risk assessment involves the detailed assessment of suicide risk by a healthcare or mental health professional. Pisani, Murrie, and Silverman propose risk formulations that synthesize data into four distinct judgments to directly inform intervention plans: risk status (the patient's risk relative to a specified subpopulation), risk state (the patient's risk compared to baseline or other specified time points), available resources from which the patient can draw in crisis, and foreseeable changes that may exacerbate risk.[52]

The use of systematic assessment approaches is critical. The Suicide Assessment Five-Step Evaluation and Triage (SAFE-T; https://www.integration.samhsa.gov/images/res/SAFE_T.pdf) was first developed to address the Joint Commission's 2007 Patient Safety Goals on Suicide. It was intended for use by mental health professionals, though it has also been used by other healthcare professionals, and includes five steps:

1. Identify risk factors.
2. Identify protective factors.
3. Conduct suicide inquiry.
4. Determine risk level/intervention.
5. Document.

The C-SSRS has also been used as a risk assessment tool. [8,45] Just as important as its ability to identify who might attempt suicide, it was the first scale to assess the full range of a person's suicidal ideation and behavior, including intensity, frequency, and changes over time. In 2011, the CDC adopted the scale's definitions for suicidal behavior and recommended the use of the C-SSRS for data collection. In 2012, the FDA declared the C-SSRS the standard for measuring suicidal ideation and behavior in clinical trials. A new measure, the Concise Health Risk Tracking (CHRT) scale, has shown promise in monitoring suicidal ideation and behavior in patients.[53] This measure includes both a clinician rating and self-report. It is unique as it includes not only questions about suicidal ideation and behavior, but also questions about common risk factors associated with suicide, such as perceived lack of social support and hopelessness. Other frequently used clinician-rated measures include the Scale for Suicidal Ideation,[54] the Beck Scale for Suicidal Ideation,[55] and the Parasuicide History Interview.[56] (For a review of self-report measures of suicidal ideation and behavior, see reference 57.)

8.8. SUICIDE CRISIS INTERVENTION

One important crisis intervention is creating an environment that protects against suicide; this is often referred to as lethal means restriction. Studies have shown that the average interval between deciding to make a suicide attempt and making an attempt is 5 to 10 minutes,[58,59] so every effort that can delay the person's ability to act on this decision can potentially make the difference in thought versus action. Public health efforts to address this have included erecting barriers or putting up nets to prevent individuals from jumping; putting up signs about how to seek help in places that are known to be environments where suicide attempts occur; and organizing campaigns to support safe medication, household product, and firearm storage.[19] There is evidence that these efforts do reduce suicide attempts.[60,61] Another approach to lethal means restriction involves training healthcare and mental healthcare providers to engage the suicidal individual and/or family to create a safe living environment, free from easy access to lethal means. The Emergency Department Counseling on Access to Lethal Means (ED-CALM) quality improvement project demonstrated effectiveness in improving parents' follow-through on locking up medications and firearms after receiving counseling from trained psychiatric emergency clinicians on presenting to the hospital with a suicidal youth.[62] The Suicide Prevention Resource Center offers training in the CALM approach (https://www.sprc.org/resources-programs/calm-counseling-access-lethal-means-0).

Additional strategies for crisis intervention include crisis support services, such as the National Suicide Prevention Lifeline. More recently, these efforts have expanded to include online chat services and text messaging, with the goal of delaying the individual from acting on the suicidal urges and encouraging the individual to seek additional support or intervention.[19]

Often the first point of contact for a suicidal person is the emergency department. Fleischmann and colleagues developed a brief intervention and contact for suicide attempters, which was delivered in the emergency department as part of discharge.[63] This one-hour information session (plus nine follow-up phone calls or visits) included understanding suicidal behavior as a sign of psychological or social distress, risk and protective factors, basic epidemiology, repetition, alternatives to suicidal behavior, and referral options. It was delivered by a person who was part of the clinical experience (e.g., doctor, nurse, and psychologist). In a randomized controlled trial in five countries, there were fewer deaths in the intervention group (0.2% vs. 2.2% in the treatment-as-usual group) at the 18-month follow-up.[63]

More recently, Stanley and Brown tested a model of safety planning. This intervention, called the Safety Plan Intervention, was delivered in emergency departments and included a brief clinical intervention with safety plan approach plus two follow-up calls to monitor suicide risk, review and revise the safety plan, and support treatment engagement.[64] In a study of 1,640 total patients, with 1,186 in the intervention group and 454 in the control group, patients who received the intervention were less likely to engage in suicidal behavior (3.03%) versus usual care (5.29%) during 6 months of follow-up.[64]

A "no harm contract" or "no suicide contract" is not advised, as there is evidence these are not effective.[65–67] In contrast, a safety plan is an agreement and commitment to use skills or the safety plan or seek support before trying to hurt oneself.

8.9. PSYCHOSOCIAL TREATMENT OF SUICIDAL BEHAVIOR

The original treatments for suicide were designed to address depression. This was limiting, as (1) not all suicidal patients are depressed and (2) treatments might not address psychological mechanisms related to suicide, may not address other modifiable risk factors for future suicidal behavior, and may not allow patients to develop strategies to help in future suicidal crisis, and (3) there was no evidence this was efficacious, as suicidal patients were often excluded from depression trials.[68] More recently, treatment efforts have included suicide-specific interventions.

Several approaches to the treatment of suicide have been empirically examined, including cognitive–behavioral therapy (CBT), interpersonal psychotherapy (IPT), DBT, and family treatment.[32,69–74] DBT was the first intervention to show efficacy in the treatment of suicidal behavior; however, this intensive treatment often involves

100 sessions per year and requires extensive training and certification of therapists. This treatment may be most appropriate for individuals with borderline personality disorder. IPT has also exhibited efficacy in the treatment of suicide attempters and may prove to be a promising intervention as well.[69] A randomized, controlled trial of a CBT approach for the prevention of suicide attempts established efficacy for this intervention.[75] CBT may be an especially useful treatment as it is brief, focused, and problem-oriented and able to address the maladaptive cognitions, including hopelessness, that are often related to suicidal behavior.[32] In addition, a major treatment goal in CBT is building the patient's support system, including mental health systems, family, and friends.[32]

8.10. BIOLOGICAL UNDERSTANDING AND TREATMENT OF SUICIDAL BEHAVIOR

Statistically, it was estimated that the heritability for suicide reached 30% to 55% for suicidal behavior and ideation.[76,77] Genetic factors and early life adversity appear to shape suicide risk through affecting brain circuitry and chemistry involved in reactivity to stressors. Genome-wide association studies (GWAS) have been nonspecific. In a study using polygenic risk score (PRS) association tests to examine family-based sample of 660 trios with suicide attempt outcome in the offspring, polygenic association of single nucleotide polymorphisms (SNPs) in 750 neurodevelopmental genes was driven by suicide attempt phenotype (*not* psychiatric diagnosis), thus suggesting a "polygenic and neurodevelopmental 'trait' ".[78]

Among the first to be described was the altered levels of serotonin and serotonin signaling in individuals exhibiting suicidal behaviors.[79] There are fewer presynaptic serotonin transmitter sites in the prefrontal cortex, hypothalamus, occipital cortex, and brainstem of suicide victims. Thus, less serotonin (which is related to inhibition) reaches the areas of the brain involved in personality, decision making, appropriate social behavior, and hormone control. Low levels of 5-HIAA in the cerebrospinal fluid (CSF) predict suicide attempts and completions, with lower CSF 5-HIAA levels related to more lethal attempts. There is evidence that individuals exhibiting suicidal behaviors have unique serotonin genotype and expression patterns, and low serotonin levels are associated with personality traits linked to suicide, such as impulsive aggression.[79,80]

Inflammatory responses have been linked to suicidal behavior. Some evidence suggests that inflammation linked to suicide might occur both in the central nervous system and in peripheral tissues, as detected in blood samples. Consistent with the data from studies of early life adversity, stress response systems might be altered during suicidal states. Substantial alterations of the polyamine system and the hypothalamic–pituitary–adrenal (HPA) axis have been described in the brains of people who attempt suicide and who die by suicide. Altered responses to stressful social situations might lead to psychopathological disorders and suicidal behavior, for example, a noted deficiency of noradrenergic neurons in the locus coeruleus could be in response to too much noradrenaline release in response to pre-suicide stress. Multilevel HPA axis dysfunction appears to be strongest biomarker.[80] The serotonergic system has a bidirectional relationship to the HPA axis and is linked to inflammatory processes.

There are no direct studies of the antisuicide effect of selective serotonin reuptake inhibitors (SSRIs). Some postmortem studies show differences in treated depression and untreated depression in those who die by suicide: Those who had untreated depression had fewer mature granule neurons in the hippocampus and a smaller volume of the dentate gyrus.[79] One pilot study demonstrated a "modest" advantage of the SSRI paroxetine compared to bupropion (a noradrenergic-dopaminergic medication) when used in depressed patients with greater baseline suicidal ideation.[81] Lithium reduces the risk of suicide and suicidal behavior.[82] Treatments targeting the glutamate pathway, such as ketamine, have yielded some promising initial results in the treatment of severe depression and suicidal ideation. Ketamine led to a greater reduction in suicidal ideation following a single intravenous infusion compared with placebo controls in individuals with suicidal ideation and treatment-refractory major depressive disorder, bipolar disorder, or post-traumatic stress disorder; this reduction was immediate (by day 1), and it persisted up to seven days after a single infusion.[83]

8.11. SPECIAL POPULATIONS

8.11.1. Youth

Unfortunately, adolescent suicidal behavior is common; it is the second leading cause of death for 15- to 24-year-olds and the fourth for 5- to 14-year-olds.[2] Additionally, for every one adolescent death by suicide in the United States, there are an estimated 100 to 200 nonlethal suicide attempts made by adolescents. Adolescent suicidal ideation and behavior is somewhat common: 17.2% of high school students reported that they had seriously considered attempting suicide over the course of the year, 7.4% reported attempting suicide one or more times, and 2.4% reported making a suicide attempt that required medical attention.[84]

Psychological treatments with the strongest support of efficacy for reducing suicidal behavior among youth include behavior change, skill enhancement, family engagement, and strengthening of interpersonal bonds.[85] Integrated cognitive–behavioral therapy has demonstrated efficacy in youth with co-occurring substance dependence and suicidal behavior.[86] Attachment-based family therapy, an approach that focuses on strengthening the quality of attachment between the suicidal youth and family, has also shown promise.[87] DBT for adolescents, an intervention that includes the youth, parents, and a skills group component as well as phone coaching, has recently been validated in two randomized controlled trials.[88,89] Lastly, the SAFETY program, a cognitive–behavioral family intervention designed to increase safety and reduce suicide attempt, has shown promise in reducing repeat suicidal behavior.[90,91] No medication studies have focused explicitly on suicidal youth.

8.11.2. Geriatric

In 2016, the second highest rate of death by suicide occurred in those 85 and older (18.98 per 100,000), with 18.2 in those age 75 to 84 and 15.38 in those aged 65 to 74.[2] In geriatric populations, the risk of death on the first attempt is greater, with the ratio of attempts to deaths being 4:1. Specific risk factors related to this population include becoming a widow/widower, the presence of other mental disorders, physical illness, bereavement, and social isolation.[92–94] Seventy percent of all suicide deaths by older adults are by firearm.

Primary care screening for suicidal ideation and behavior is vital in this population, as most older patients visit their physician due to other health problems. Depression screeners, such as the Geriatric Depression Scale, may be useful. There is a lack of research in treatments specifically for older suicidal patients, but some promising approaches include DBT skills training and phone coaching,[95] a primary care version of problem-solving therapy and medication,[96] and IPT.[97]

8.11.3. Sexual and Gender Minorities

Sexual minority youth seriously contemplate suicide at almost three times the rate of non-sexual minority youth.[98] Sexual minority youth are almost five times as likely to have attempted suicide compared to non-sexual minority youth.[98] In a national study, 40% of transgender adults reported having made a suicide attempt, and 92% of these individuals reported having attempted suicide before the age of 25.[99] Sexual and gender minority youth who come from highly rejecting families are 8.4 times as likely to have attempted suicide as LGB peers who reported no or low levels of family rejection.[100] Individual and institutional discrimination related to social isolation, low self-esteem, negative sexual and gender identity, depression, anxiety, other mental disorders may be related to the increased risk in this population.[101] No studies to date have examined interventions specifically targeting suicidal behavior in sexual and gender minority youth populations.

8.12. AFTER A SUICIDE: POSTVENTION, POSTTRAUMATIC GROWTH, LIVED EXPERIENCE, SURVIVORS OF SUICIDE

The definition of postvention is from the US National Guidelines developed by the Survivors of Suicide Loss Task Force: "An organized response in the aftermath of a suicide to accomplish any one or more of the following: to facilitate the healing of individuals from the grief and distress of suicide loss, to mitigate other negative effects of exposure to suicide, and/or to prevent suicide among people who are at high risk after exposure to suicide."[102] Per the Suicide Prevention Resource Center (SPRC), the key principles for creating a comprehensive postvention effort include (1) planning ahead to address individual and community needs, (2) providing immediate and long-term support, (3) tailoring responses and services to the unique needs of suicide loss survivors, and (4) involving survivors of suicide loss in planning and implementing postvention efforts. An additional important aspect of postvention is safe reporting and messaging about suicide; news media are encouraged to follow the Recommendations on Reporting on Suicide (http://www.reportingonsuicide. org), as studies have shown that changes in reporting after a death by suicide can result in reductions in future suicides.[19]

Suicide "survivors," a self-defined condition of a person who has been exposed to suicide and feels affected by the death, are at risk for grief, mental illness, impaired social functioning, and fatal and nonfatal suicidal behavior.[103] In a meta-analysis of population-based studies ($n = 18$) to examine exposure to suicide, the pooled past-year prevalence of exposure to suicide was 4.31% and the pooled lifetime prevalence of exposure to suicide was 21.83%.[104]

8.13. CONCLUSION

Suicide is a multiply determined phenomenon, occurring because of a convergence of genetic, environmental, psychological, social, cultural, and systemic risk and protective factors. Suicide prevention efforts must include interventions across the spectrum, including public health, primary care, psychiatry and mental health subspecialties, hospital systems, school, and community prevention efforts. To date, no single strategy has addressed this public health problem, but combinations of strategies at the individual level and the population level are needed.[105]

REFERENCES

1. World Health Organization. *Suicide Prevention: A Global Imperative*. Geneva, Switzerland: WHO Press; 2014.
2. CDC. Web-based Injury Statistics Query and Reporting System (WISQARS): 2018. Atlanta, GA: National Center for Injury Prevention and Control. https://www.cdc.gov/injury/wisqars/index.html
3. Drapeau CW, McIntosh JL; American Association of Suicidology. USA suicide: 2017 official final data. https://dmh.mo.gov/mentalillness/suicide/docs/2017Nationaldatapgsv1-FINAL.pdf. Accessed March 1, 2019.
4. U.S. Department of Health and Human Services (HHS) Office of the Surgeon General and National Action Alliance for Suicide Prevention. *2012 National Strategy for Suicide Prevention: Goals and Objectives for Action*. Washington, DC: HHS, 3012.
5. Khan, M.M., & Mian, A.I. The one truly serious philosophical problem: ethical aspects of suicide. *Int Rev Psychiatry*. 2010; 22:288–293.
6. Behere, P.B., Sathyanarayana Rao, T.S., & Mulmule, A.N. Decriminalization of attempted suicide law: journey of fifteen decades. *Indian J Psychiatry*. 2015; 57(2):122–124.

7. O'Carroll, P., Berman, A., Maris, R., et al. Beyond the Tower of Babel: a nomenclature for suicidology. *Suicide Life Threat Behav.* 1996; 26:237–252.

8. Posner, K., Oquendo, M.A., Gould, M., et al. Columbia Classification Algorithm of Suicide Assessment (C-CASA): classification of suicidal events in the FDA's pediatric suicidal risk analysis of antidepressants. *Am J Psychiatry.* 2007; 164:1035–1043.

9. Crosby, A.E., Ortega, L., & Melanson, C. *Self-Directed Violence Surveillance: Uniform Definitions and Recommended Data Elements, version 1.0.* Atlanta, GA: Centers for Disease Control and Prevention, National Center for Injury Prevention and Control; 2011.

10. Nock, M.K., Borges, G., Bromet, E.J., et al. Suicide and suicidal behavior. *Epidemiol Rev.* 2008; 30:133–154.

11. Miranda, R., Scott, M., Hicks, R., et al. Suicide attempt characteristics, diagnoses, and future attempts: comparing multiple attempters to single attempters and ideators. *J Am Acad Child Adolesc Psychiatry.* 2008; 47:32–40.

12. Neeleman, J. A continuum of premature death: meta-analysis of competing mortality in the psychosocially vulnerable. *Int J Epidemiol.* 2001; 30(1):154–162.

13. Owens, D., Horrocks, J., & House, A. Fatal and non-fatal repetition of self-harm: systematic review. *Br J Psychiatry.* 2002; 181:193–199.

14. Christiansen, E., & Jensen, B.F. Risk of repetition of suicide attempt, suicide or all deaths after an episode of attempted suicide: a register-based survival analysis. *Aust N Z J Psychiatry.* 2007; 41(3):257–265.

15. Marzuk, P. M., Tardiff, K., Leon, A. C., et al. The prevalence of aborted suicide attempts among psychiatric inpatients. *Acta Psychiatr Scand.* 1997; 96:492–496.

16. Barber, M. E., Marzuk, P. M., Leon, A. C., & Portera, L. Aborted suicide attempts: a new classification of suicidal behavior. *Am J Psychiatry.* 1998; 155: 385–389.

17. Meyer, R.E., Salzman, C., Youngstrom, E.A., et al. Suicidality and risk of suicide—definition, drug safety concerns, and a necessary target for drug development: a consensus statement. *J Clin Psychiatry.* 2010; 71(8): e1–e21.

18. Nock, M.K., Borget, G., Bromet, E.J., et al. Cross-national prevalence and risk factors for suicidal ideation, plans and attempts. *Br J Psychiatry.* 2008; 192:98–105.

19. Stone, D.M., Holland, K.M., Bartholow, B., et al. *Preventing Suicide: A Technical Package of Policies, Programs, and Practices.* Atlanta, GA: National Center for Injury Prevention and Control, Centers for Disease Control and Prevention; 2017.

20. Chesney, E., Goodwin, G.M., & Fazel, S. Risks of all-cause and suicide mortality in mental disorders: a meta-review. *World Psychiatry.* 2014; 13(2):153–160.

21. Franklin, J.C., Ribeiro, J.D., Fox, K.R., et al. Risk factors for suicidal thoughts and behaviors: a meta-analysis of 50 years of research. *Psychol Bull.* 2017; 142(2):187–232.

22. Walsh, C.G., Ribeiro, J.D., & Franklin, J.C. Predicting suicide attempts in adolescents with longitudinal clinical data and machine learning. *J Child Psychol Psychiatry Allied Discip.* 2018; 59(12):1261–1270.

23. Barak-Corren, Y., Castro, V.M., Javitt, S., et al. Predicting suicidal behavior from longitudinal electronic health records. *Am J Psychiatry.* 2017; 174(2):154–162.

24. Shneidman, E.S. *Definition of Suicide.* New York: Wiley; 1985.

25. Shneidman, E.S. *Suicide as Psychache: A Clinical Approach to Self-Destructive Behavior.* Northfield, NJ: Jason Aronson; 1993.

26. Mann, J.J., Waternaux, C., Haas, G.L., & Malone, K.M. Toward a clinical model of suicidal behavior in psychiatric patients. *Am J Psychiatry.* 1999; 156:181–189.

27. Rubinstein, D.H. A stress-diathesis theory of suicide. *Suicide Life Threat Behav.* 1986; 16:182–197.

28. Shaffer, D., & Pfeffer, C. Practice parameter for the assessment and treatment of children and adolescents with suicidal behavior. *J Am Acad Child Adolesc Psychiatry.* 2001; 40(Suppl. 7):24S–51S.

29. Rudd, M.D. Cognitive therapy for suicidality: an integrative, comprehensive, and practical approach to conceptualization. *J Contemp Psychother.* 2004; 34:59–72.

30. Rudd, M. D., Joiner, T. F., & Rajab, M. R. *Treating Suicidal Behavior.* New York: Guilford Press; 2001.

31. Weishaar, M., & Beck, A.T. Cognitive approaches to understanding and treating suicidal behavior. In S. Blumenthal & D. Kupfer (Eds.). *Suicide over the Life Cycle.* Washington, DC: American Psychiatric Press; 1990.

32. Berk, M S., Henriques, G. R., Warman, D. M., et al. A cognitive therapy intervention for suicide attempters: an overview of the treatment and case examples. *Cogn Behav Pract.* 2004; 11:265–277.

33. Linehan, M.M. *Cognitive-Behavioral Treatment of Borderline Personality Disorder.* New York: Guilford Press; 1993.

34. Joiner, T.E., Jr. *Why People Die by Suicide.* Cambridge, MA: Harvard University Press; 2005.

35. Van Orden, K.A., Witte, T.K., Cukrowicz, K.C., et al. The interpersonal theory of suicide. *Psychol Rev.* 2010; 117(2):575–600.

36. Stewart, S.M., Eaddy, M., Horton, S.E., et al. The validity of the interpersonal theory of suicide in adolescence: a review. *J Clin Child Adolesc Psychol.* 2017; 46(3):437–449.

37. Joiner, T.E., Jr., Van Orden, K.A., Witte, T.K., & Rudd, M.D. Main predictions of the interpersonal-psychological theory of suicidal behavior: empirical tests in two samples of young adults. *J Abnorm Psychol.* 2009; 118:634–646.

38. Joiner, T.E., Jr., Pettit, J.W., Walker, R.L., et al. Perceived burdensomeness and suicidality: two studies on the suicide notes of those attempting and completing suicide. *J Soc Clin Psychol.* 2002; 21:531–545.

39. Chu, C., Buchman-Schmitt, J.M., Stanley, I.H., et al. The interpersonal theory of suicide: A systematic review and meta-analysis of a decade of cross-national research. *Psychol Bull.* 2017; 143(12):1313–1345.

40. Klonsky, E.D., & May, A.M. Differentiating suicide attempters from suicide ideators: a critical frontier for suicidology research. *Suicide Life Threat Behav.* 2014; 1:1–5.

41. Klonsky, E.D., & May, A.M. The three-step theory (3ST): a new theory of suicide rooted I the "ideation-to-action" framework. *Int J Cogn Ther.* 2015; 8(2):114–129.

42. O'Connor, R.C. The integrated motivational-volitional model of suicidal behavior. *Crisis.* 2011; 32(6):295–298.

43. Horowitz, L., Ballard, E., Teach, S.J., et al. Feasibility of screening patients with nonpsychiatric complaints for suicide risk in a pediatric emergency department: a good time to talk? *Pediatr Emerg Care.* 2010; 26(11):787.

44. Horowitz, L.M., Bridge, J.A., Pao, M., & Boudreaux, E.D. Screening youth for suicide risk in medical settings: time to ask questions. *Am J Prev Med.* 2014; 47(3):S170–S175.

45. Posner, K., Brent, D., Lucas, C., et al. *Columbia-Suicide Severity Rating Scale (C-SSRS).* Unpublished measure. New York: New York State Psychiatric Institute; 2004.

46. Roaten, K., Johnson, C., Genzel, R., et al. Development and implementation of a universal suicide risk screening program in a safety-net hospital system. *Jt Comm J Qual Patient Saf.* 2018; 44:4–11.

47. Kitchener, B.A., & Jorm, A.F. Mental health first aid training in a workplace setting: a randomized controlled trial. *BMC Psychiatry.* 2004; 4(23):1–8.

48. Jorm, A. F., Kitchener, B. A., O'Kearney, R., & Dear, K. Mental health first aid training of the public in a rural area: a cluster randomized trial. *BMC Psychiatry.* 2004; 4(33):1–9.

49. Svensson, B., & Hansson, L. Effectiveness of mental health first aid training in Sweden: a randomized controlled trial with a six-month and two-year follow-up. PLoS ONE. 2014; 9(6): e100911.

50. Quinnett P. *QPR: Ask a Question, Save a Life.* The QPR Institute and Suicide Awareness/ Voices of Education; 1995.

51. Quinnett P. QPR Institute. 1999. http://www.qprinstitute.com/.

52. Pisani, A.R., Murrie, D.C., & Silverman, M.M. Reformulating suicide risk formulation: from prediction to prevention. *Acad Psychiatry.* 2016; 40(4):623–629.

53. Trivedi, M.H., Wisniewski, S.R., Morris, D.W., et al. Concise Health Risk Tracking scale: a brief self-report and clinician rating of suicidal risk. *J Clin Psychiatry.* 2011; 72(6):757–764.

54. Beck, A.T., Kovacs, M., & Weissman, A. Assessment of suicidal intention: the Scale for Suicide Ideation. *J Consult Clin Psychol.* 1979; 47:343–352.

55. Beck, A.T., & Steer, R.A. *Manual for the Beck Scale for Suicide Ideation.* San Antonio, TX: Psychological Corporation; 1991.

56. Linehan, M.M., Wagner, A.W., & Cox, G. *Parasuicide History Interview: Comprehensive Assessment of Parasuicidal Behavior.* Unpublished manuscript. Seattle: University of Washington; 1983.

57. Batterham, P.J., Ftanou, M., Pirkis, J., et al. A systematic review and evaluation of measures for suicidal ideation and behaviors in population-based research. *Psychol Assessment.* 2015; 27(2):501–512.

58. Simon, O.R., Swann, A.C., Powell, K.E., et al. Characteristics of impulsive suicide attempts and attempters. *Suicide Life Threat Behav.* 2001; 32(1 Suppl):49–59.

59. Deisenhammer, E.A., Ing, C.M., Strauss, R., et al. The duration of the suicidal process: how much time is left for intervention between consideration and accomplishment of a suicide attempt? *J Clin Psychiatry.* 2009; 70(1):19–24.

60. Cox, G.R., Owens, C., Robinson, J., et al. Interventions to reduce suicides at suicide hotspots: a systematic review. *BMC Public Health.* 2013; 13(1):1–12.

61. Rowhani-Rahbar, A., Simonetti, J.A., & Rivara, F.P. Effectiveness of interventions to promote safe firearm storage. *Epidemiol Rev.* 2016; 38(1):111–124.

62. Runyan, C.W., Becker, A., Brandspigel, S., et al. Lethal means counseling for parents of youth seeking emergency care for suicidality. *West J Emerg Med.* 2016; 17(1):8–14.

63. Fleishmann, A., Bertolote, J.M., Wasserman, D., et al. Effectiveness of brief intervention and contact for suicide attempters: a randomized controlled trial in five countries. *Bull World Health Organ.* 2008; 86:703–709.

64. Stanley, B., Brown, G.K., Brenner, L.A., et al. Comparison of the Safety Planning Intervention with follow-up vs. usual care of suicidal patients treated in the emergency department. *JAMA Psychiatry.* 2018; 75(9):894–900.

65. Range, L.M., Campbell, C., Kovac, S.H., et al. No-suicide contracts: an overview and recommendations. *Death Stud.* 2002; 26(1):51–74.

66. Stanford, E. J., Goetz, R. R., & Bloom, J. The no harm contract in the emergency assessment of suicidal risk. *J Clin Psychiatry.*1994; 55(8):344–348.

67. Simon, R.I. The suicide prevention contract: clinical, legal, and risk management issues. *J Am Acad Psychiatry Law.* 1999; 27(3):445–450.

68. Wenzel, A., & Jager-Hyman, S. Cognitive therapy for suicidal patients: current status. *Behav Ther.* 2012; 35(7):121–130.

69. Elspeth, G., Kapur, N., Mackway-Jones, K., et al. Predictors of outcome following brief psychodynamic-interpersonal therapy for deliberate self-poisoning. *Aust N Z J Psychiatry.* 2003; 37:532–536.

70. Harrington, R., Kerfoot, M., Dyer, E., et al. Randomized trial of a home-based family intervention for children who have deliberately poisoned themselves. *J Am Acad Child Adolesc Psychiatry.* 1998; 37:512–518.

71. Linehan, M. M., Armstrong, H. E., Suarez, A., et al. Cognitive-behavioral treatment of chronically parasuicidal borderline patients. *Arch Gen Psychiatry.* 1991; 48:1060–1064.

72. Linehan, M. M., Comtois, K. A., Murray, A. M., et al. Two-year randomized controlled trial and follow-up of dialectical behavior therapy vs. therapy by experts for suicidal behaviors and borderline personality disorder. *Arch Gen Psychiatry.* 2006; 63:757–766.

73. Rotheram-Borus, M. J., Piacentini, J., Cantwell, C., et al. The 18-month impact of an emergency room intervention for adolescent female suicide attempters. *J Consult Clin Psychol,* 2000; 68:1081–1093.

74. Salkovskis, P. M., Atha, C., & Storer, D. Cognitive-behavioural problem solving in the treatment of patients who repeatedly attempt suicide: a controlled trial. *Br J Psychiatry.* 1990; 157:871–876.

75. Brown, G. K., Have, T. T., Henriques, G. R., et al. Cognitive therapy for the prevention of suicide attempts: a randomized controlled trial. *JAMA.* 2005; 294:563–570.

76. Brent, D.A., & Mehlem, N. Familial transmission of suicidal behavior. *Psychiatr Clin North Am.* 2008; 31:157.

77. Voracek, M., & Loibl, L.M. Genetics of suicide: a systematic review of twin studies. *Wien Klin Wochenschr.* 2007; 119:463–475.

78. Sokolowski, M., Wasserman, J., & Wasserman, D. Polygenic associations of neurodevelopmental genes in suicide attempt. *Mol Psychiatry.* 2016; 21:1381–1390.

79. Van Heeringen, K., & Mann, J.J. The neurobiology of suicide. *Lancet Psychiatry.* 2014; 1:63–72.

80. Oquendo, M.A., Sullivan, G.M., Sudol, K., et al. Toward a biosignature for suicide. *Am J Psychiatry.* 2014; 171(12):1259–1277.

81. Grunebaum, M.F., Ellis, S.P., Duan, N., et al. Pilot randomized clinical trial of an SSRI vs bupropion: effects on suicidal behavior, ideation, and mood in major depression. *Neuropsychopharmacology.* 2012; 37(3):697–706.

82. Cipriani, A., Pretty, H., Hawton, K., & Geddes, J.R. Lithium in the prevention of suicidal behavior and all-cause mortality in patient with mood disorders: a systematic review of randomized trials. *Am J Psychiatry.* 2005; 162(10):1805–1819.

83. Wilkinson, S.T., Ballard, E.D., Bloch, M.H., et al. The effect of a single dose of intravenous ketamine on suicidal ideation: a systematic review and individual participant data meta-analysis. *Am J Psychiatry.* 2018; 175:150–158

84. Kann, L., McManus, T., Harris, W.A., et al. Youth risk behavior surveillance—United States, 2017. *MMWR Surveill Summ.* 2018; 67(No. SS-8).

85. Cha, C.B., Franz, P.J., Guzman, E.M., et al. Annual research review: suicide among youth – epidemiology, (potential) etiology, and treatment. *J Child Psychol Psychiatry.* 2018; 59(4):460–482.

86. Esposito-Smythers, C., Spirito, A., Kahler, C.W., et al. Treatment of co-occurring substance abuse and suicidality among adolescents: a randomized trial. *J Consult Clin Psychol.* 2011; 79(6):728–739.

87. Diamond, G.S., Wintersteen, M.B., Brown, G.K., et al. Attachment-based family therapy for adolescents with suicidal ideation: a randomized controlled trial. *J Am Acad Child Adolesc Psychiatry.* 2010; 49(2):122–131.

88. Mehlum, L., Tørmoen, A.J., Ramberg, M., et al. Dialectical behavior therapy for adolescents with repeated suicidal and self-harming behavior: a randomized trial. *J Am Acad Child Adolesc Psychiatry.* 2014; 53(10):1082–1091.

89. McCauley, E., Berk, M.S., Asarnow, J.R., et al. Efficacy of dialectical behavior therapy for adolescents at high risk for suicide: a randomized clinical trial. *JAMA Psychiatry.* 2018; 75(8):777–785.

90. Asarnow, J.R., Berk, M., Hughes, J.L., & Anderson, N.L. The SAFETY Program: a treatment-development trial of a cognitive-behavioral family treatment for adolescent suicide attempters. *J Clin Child Adolesc Psychol.* 2015; 44(1):194–203.

91. Asarnow, J.R., Hughes, J.L., Babeva, K.N., & Sugar, C.A. Cognitive-behavioral family treatment for suicide attempt prevention: a randomized controlled trial. *J Am Acad Child Adolesc Psychiatry.* 2017; 56(6):506–514.

92. Sinyor, M., Tan, L.P., Schaffer, A., et al. Suicide in the oldest old: an observational study and cluster analysis. *Int J Geriatr Psychiatry.* 2016; 31(1):33–40.

93. Bonnewyn, A., Shah, A., & Demyttenaere, K. Suicidality and suicide in older people. *Rev Clin Gerontol.* 2009; 19(4):271–294.

94. Conwell, Y., Van Orden, K., & Caine, E.D. Suicide in older adults. *Psychiatr Clin North Am.* 2011; 34(2):451–468.

95. Lynch, T.R., Morse, J.Q., Mendelson, T., & Robins, C.J. Dialectical behavior therapy for depressed older adults: a randomized pilot study. *Am J Geriatr Psychiatry.* 2003; 11(1):33–45.

96. Unutzer, J., Tang, L., Oishi, S., et al. Reducing suicidal ideation in depressed older primary care patients. *J Am Geriatr Soc.* 2006; 54(10):1550–1556.

97. Heisel, M.J., Duberstein, P.R., Talbot, N.L., et al. Adapting interpersonal psychotherapy for older adults at risk for suicide: Preliminary findings. *Prof Psychol Res Pr.* 2009; 40(2):156–164.

98. Kann, L. Olsen, E.O., McManus, T., et al. Sexual identity, sex of sexual contacts, and health-related behaviors among students in grades 9–12—United States and selected sites, 2015. *MMWR Surveill Summ.* 2016; 65(SS-9):1–202.

99. James, S.E., Herman, J.L., Rankin, S., et al. *The Report of the 2015 U.S. Transgender Survey.* Washington, DC: National Center for Transgender Equality; 2016.

100. Family Acceptance Project. Family rejection as a predictor of negative health outcomes in white and Latino lesbian, gay, and bisexual young adults. *Pediatrics.* 2009; 123(1):346–352.

101. Hatzenbuehler, M.L. The social environment and suicide attempts in lesbian, gay, and bisexual youth. *Pediatrics.* 2011; 127(5):896–903.

102. Survivors of Suicide Loss Task Force. *Responding to Grief, Trauma, and Distress After a Suicide: U.S. National Guidelines.* Washington, DC: National Action Alliance for Suicide Prevention. 2015. http://www.sprc.org/resources-programs/responding-grief-trauma-and-distress-after-suicide-us-national-guidelines.

103. Pitman, A., Osborn, D., King, M., & Erlangsen, A. Effects of suicide bereavement on mental health and suicide risk. *Lancet Psychiatry.* 2014; 1:86–94.

104. Andriessen, K., Rahman, B., Draper, B., et al. Prevalence of exposure to suicide: a meta-analysis of population-based studies. *J Psychiatr Res.* 2017; 88: 113–120.

105. Zalsman, G., Hawton, K., Wasserman, D., et al. Suicide prevention strategies revisited: 10-year systematic review. *Lancet Psychiatry.* 2016; 3:646–659.

/// 9 /// # GENERAL MEDICAL CONDITIONS

Comorbidities and Differential Diagnosis

PATRICIA PILKINTON AND LORI L. DAVIS

9.1. INTRODUCTION

Major depression is a systemic illness that is associated with a multitude of comorbid medical conditions.[1] While the point prevalence of depression in the community is about 2% to 4%, the prevalence jumps to 5% to 10% in primary care outpatients. The Sequenced Treatment Alternatives to Relieve Depression (STAR*D) study found that 53% of the enrolled patients with major depression had significant comorbid medical condition and the presence of these general medical conditions influenced the severity and symptom patterns of the depressive episode.[2] Individuals with depression are at elevated risk of developing cardiometabolic disorders, sudden death, and premature death.[3,4] Conversely, many medical illnesses are known to increase the likelihood of developing major depression. Compared to those with chronic medical illness alone, patients with chronic medical illness and concurrent depression or anxiety report significantly more somatic complaints and symptoms. Their somatic symptoms are at least as strongly associated with depression and anxiety as they are with objective physiologic measures for diabetes, pulmonary disease, heart disease, and arthritis. In addition, improvement in their depression is associated with decreased somatic symptoms even without improvement in the physiologic measures.[5] Recent studies examining the overlap of depressive and medical illness have helped to increase our understanding of the complex bidirectional relationship that exists between them.[6] Shared genetic, environmental, psychosocial, physiologic, and immunologic origins of disease explain much of the connection between depression and medical illness. Patients with concurrent major depression and medical illnesses have lower quality of life and higher morbidity and mortality and consume more health care resources that those with depression or medical illness alone. Recognition of comorbid depression and medical illness is essential in that it may affect the workup, treatment options, and expected outcome.[7]

9.2. EVALUATION OF DEPRESSION AT THE INITIAL CLINICAL ENCOUNTER

When evaluating a patient with a chief complaint of depression, the clinician is typically faced with two questions in constructing a differential diagnosis: "Is there an underlying medical reason for this patient's depression?" and "Is this medically ill patient also depressed?" A provider should never assume that the complains of depression and neurovegetative symptoms are a natural part of the medical disease, since a missed opportunity to treat depression can prolong unnecessary suffering. There is also the concern that treatment for major medical conditions may be contributing to the clinical picture in the form of side effects and/or adverse drug–drug interactions, especially in the presence of polypharmacy.[8,9]

Untangling these issues requires a thoughtful and structured approach that includes obtaining a history of both medical and mental health symptoms, with careful attention to the onset and clustering of symptoms as well as the use of medications. This is accomplished by using a review-of-systems checklist for physical and mental health symptoms completed before the interview and supplemented by additional questions during the appointment. For example, the onset of first depressive symptoms later in life concurrent with tremor, "slowness," declining handwriting, decreasing mobility, and falls may prompt a neurologic evaluation for Parkinson's disease. However, if these symptoms were emerging after the start of an antipsychotic medication, the differential diagnosis would include drug-induced parkinsonism. Table 9.1 provides guidance on the laboratory tests that may be warranted in evaluating a major depressive episode, especially for first-onset depression. Table 9.2 lists medications that might have depression as a side effect.

An atypical clinical presentation should prompt the clinician to consider comorbid medical illness as a potential contributor to the clinical picture, such as depression presenting for the first time later in life, somatic or vegetative symptoms without cognitive symptoms (e.g., profound fatigue without hopelessness, guilt, negative ruminations), depression coinciding with a major change in medical status or medications (e.g., after starting interferon), accompanying unusual neurologic symptoms (e.g., olfactory or tactile hallucinations, gait imbalance), or significant impairment in activities of daily living. These scenarios represent an atypical presentation that warrants a careful evaluation of potential comorbid medical problems that are either a cause or contributor to the clinical presentation of depression.

Patients who fail to respond to an adequate dose and duration of antidepressant treatment or those who have improvement in one aspect of depression but complain of ongoing physical or cognitive symptoms may also warrant further investigation. In addition, remission of some depressive symptoms but not others (e.g., mood and

TABLE 9.1. Laboratory Tests in the Evaluation of Depression and Comorbid Medical Conditions

Laboratory Study	Possible Relationship
Complete blood count and differential	Low hemoglobin: GI bleeding, bone marrow suppression
	High hemoglobin: elevated testosterone, smoking, lung disease
	Low mean corpuscular volume: anemia, iron deficiency
	High mean corpuscular volume: B12, folate deficiency, use of anticonvulsants
	Low white blood cell count: often normal but may be HIV, bone marrow suppression
	High white blood cell count: infection, lithium therapy, myeloproliferative disease
Thyroid stimulating hormone	Hypothyroidism
Renal function	Uremia, increasing potential for drug toxicity
Liver function	Alcohol abuse, fatty liver, hepatitis, liver failure, pancreatic disorders
Lipid panel	Elevated risk for vascular disorders and stroke
Blood glucose/HbA1c	Diabetes
Electrolytes	Sodium: polydipsia, syndrome of inappropriate antidiuretic hormone secretion (SIADH), malignancy, SSRIs and antipsychotics, diabetes insipidus, cortisol abnormalities
	Calcium: malignancy, parathyroid disorders, sarcoid, TB
	Magnesium: malnutrition, alcoholism, malabsorption
	Potassium: aldosterone abnormalities, chronic kidney disease
Nutritional status	B12, folate, vitamin D
Sedimentation rate	Nonspecific indicator of inflammation
C-reactive protein	
Antinuclear antibody	Rheumatic diseases, lupus
Rheumatoid factor	
HIV, hepatitis	Important in treatment selection
Pregnancy test	Important in treatment selection
Urinalysis	Urine infection (important in elderly, delirium)
Urine drug screen	Assess illicit and prescription drug use

appetite improve but complaints of memory persist) would also require additional considerations in comorbid or differential diagnosis of the depressive episode.

A positive family history of neurologic conditions (e.g., Huntington's disease, Wilson's disease), family members with death at a young age, and an absence of

TABLE 9.2. Medications That May Contribute to Depression

Medication Class	Examples
Analgesics/muscle relaxants	Opiates, tramadol, pregabalin, ibuprofen, cyclobenzaprine
Antihypertensives	Reserpine, beta blockers, alpha agonists, methyldopa, nifedipine, enalapril
Sedative–hypnotics	Alcohol, benzodiazepines, barbiturates, carisoprodol, z-drugs
Anticonvulsants	Phenytoin, barbiturates, carbamazepine, gabapentin, topiramate
GI agents	Metoclopramide, H2 blockers, proton-pump inhibitors
Hormonal agents	Finasteride, oral contraceptives, leuprolide, anabolic steroids, corticosteroids
Antineoplastic/immune-modifying agents	Cyclosporine, vincristine, methotrexate, mycin drugs (e.g., bleomycin)
Antibiotics/antivirals	Metronidazole, ciprofloxacin, antiretrovirals
Cardiac	Digitalis, quinidine, procainamide
Other	Retinoids, amphotericin, stimulants

family history of depression or mood disorder are also red flags for possible underlying medical causes or confounders of depression. More obvious flags are presentation of a patient with a known medical illness, particularly one with immunologic or neurologic disorders that preceded the development of depression, or with abnormal vital signs, e.g., fever suggests possible infection; low temperature is associated with sepsis, antipsychotic side effect, or hypothalamic injury; tachycardia above 100 is a red flag for hyperthyroidism, cardiac arrhythmia, or a sign of withdrawal from or intoxication with a substance of abuse. Blood pressure elevation is nonspecific but may indicate substance withdrawal, cardiac issues, or endocrine disturbance.

9.3. COMMONLY ENCOUNTERED MEDICAL COMORBIDITIES

9.3.1. Cardiovascular

Depression is a risk factor for the development and progression of cardiovascular disease, coronary heart disease, and myocardial infarction.[10–12] The prevalence of depression in patients with coronary artery disease, heart failure, myocardial infarction, or cerebral vascular accident is substantially greater than in the general population.[13,14] The high rates of depression after cardiac surgery highlight the need for appropriate identification, support, and intervention efforts.[15] The American Heart Association emphasizes depression as a poor prognostic risk factor in patients with acute coronary syndromes.[16] Depressive symptoms are important predictors of cardiovascular morbidity and mortality, so it is critically important to assess for the presence of depression in patients with comorbid cardiovascular disease.[17] Shared biologic mechanisms and genetic variants involving pathways for corticotrophin-releasing hormone signaling, AMPK signaling, cAMP-mediated or G-protein coupled receptor signaling, axonal guidance signaling, serotonin or dopamine receptor signaling, dopamine-DARPP32 feedback in cAMP signaling, circadian rhythm signaling, and leptin signaling may explain the strong association among cardiovascular disease, metabolic diseases, and mood disorders.[18] Individuals with cardiovascular disease can be highly heterogeneous in their presentation of depressive symptoms, including a mix of somatic depressive symptoms such as loss of energy, sleep disturbances, changes in appetite and irritability, and cognitive symptoms such as pessimism, guilt, indecisiveness, worthlessness, and difficulty concentrating.

Following acute myocardial infarction, treatment with cognitive–behavioral therapy (CBT)[19] and antidepressants such as sertraline[20] and mirtazapine[21] can lead to improvement in depression and overall clinical impression. The combination of CBT and supportive stress management has also been shown to be beneficial for patients with depression following coronary bypass surgery.[22] In depressed patients with congestive heart failure, treatment studies with antidepressants such as citalopram[23] or sertraline[24] have had mixed results, perhaps reflecting that chronic disease limits the efficacy of antidepressant medication.

9.3.2. Pulmonary

Chronic obstructive pulmonary disease (COPD) typifies the bidirectional relationship between depression and medical illness.[25] Smoking, depression, and COPD are interrelated risk factors, as individuals with depression are more likely to smoke, and those with COPD are at high risk of depression. Patients with recent COPD exacerbations and those on long-term oxygen therapy are at particularly higher risk for depression. Depressed patients with COPD are more likely to experience mortality and require rehospitalization while having lower quality of life and reduced physical functioning.[26]

Optimal management of COPD includes treatment with medication and pulmonary rehabilitation. Engaging in physical exercise has been shown to improve pulmonary function and depression,[27] although it is often difficult to engage this population in exercise-based treatments as they may provoke anxiety, panic, and dyspnea. Despite vigorous data supporting the interplay of depression and COPD, studies of antidepressant treatment are very limited. Psychotherapies aimed at reducing anxiety and dyspnea and improving quality of life in COPD are promising.

9.3.3. Renal

Depression is the most common mental disorder among individuals with chronic kidney disease, although its exact prevalence varies widely from study to study depending on population and methodology.[28] Overall, approximately 34% of patients with chronic renal disease are positive for depression, with dialysis patients at the greatest risk (39%).[29] Interestingly, these rates were lower (20.3%) using clinical interviews and specified diagnostic criteria, suggesting that screening tools are biased by physical symptoms such as uremia and fatigue.[30] Among patients undergoing dialysis, depression is a significant predictor of mortality.[31] This subpopulation of depressed dialysis patients has been shown to have elevated levels of inflammatory cytokines such as interleukin-6.[32] Increasing the frequency of dialysis to six times per week from three appears to improve measures of well-being, overall mental health, and quality of life but not specific measures of depression.[33] In patients who receive a kidney transplant, the prevalence of depression declines, but it remains higher than the general population at approximately 25%.[34]

Despite the frequency of depression in the chronic renal disease population, there are limited studies of the use of antidepressants and other psychotropics. Small and open-label studies support the use of selective serotonin reuptake inhibitors (SSRIs),[35] particularly sertraline, but larger trials have had inconclusive or equivocal results.[36,37] Most antidepressants require dose adjustment for renal impairment and are highly protein-bound, making them poorly dialyzable. Clinically, SSRIs and mirtazapine are typically prescribed at lower doses to compensate for renal decline and to minimize the side effect burden.[38] The serotonin and norepinephrine reuptake inhibitors (SNRIs) venlafaxine and duloxetine are predominately eliminated by the kidneys, making them unsuitable in patients with moderate to severe renal compromise,[38] although they are often used in patients with mild renal disease who have diabetic neuropathy. The cardiotoxic properties of tricyclic antidepressants make them less suitable for patients on dialysis, particularly since electrolyte disturbances may also predispose to cardiac problems and prolonged QT syndrome. Tricyclics are commonly used in mild renal disease, however, as adjunctive agents for treating neuropathic pain. Fortunately, blood levels are easily obtained and can help to guide dosing, although toxicity can occur even with therapeutic serum levels. Less traditional options, such as monoamine oxidase inhibitors and stimulants, are infrequently used due to potential drug interactions. Lithium, while relatively contraindicated in patients with renal impairment, can be used successfully in patients on hemodialysis by giving a single dose after dialysis and monitoring the dose needed to maintain a therapeutic level until the next dialysis.

Psychiatric consultation services are often integrated into dialysis units and renal transplant programs due to the complex nature of renal care. In concert with concerns about depression, the patient may also have delirium, emerging cognitive impairment, dialysis anxiety, or limited supports, which may ultimately lead to suboptimal adherence and worsening outcome. Clinicians in these settings may also be asked to evaluate the role of depression in patients who decide to decline or terminate dialysis.

9.3.4. Diabetes

Although the relationship between depression and diabetes seems to be bidirectional, diabetes is an independent risk factor for the development of major depression.[39] The prevalence of depression among adults with type 2 diabetes is 12% to 18%[40] and only about a third of diabetic patients ever receive mental health treatment in the United States,[39] with much fewer to nonexistent treatment in many countries. In patients with type 2 diabetes, concurrent major depression is significantly associated with a previous diagnosis of major depressive disorder, female gender, lower level of education, less exercise, and higher diabetes distress levels.[41] Depression contributes to diabetic complications and poor glycemic control through metabolic and behavioral processes, possibly explaining significant correlations in health care use among diabetic patients with depression compared to those without.[42] Shared psychophysiologic mechanisms for stress and inflammation are present in this comorbid population. Major depression is associated with higher cortisol and sympathetic nervous system tone, contributing to an increase in blood glucose levels and downstream insulin resistance, visceral obesity, and metabolic syndrome.[43] However, in somewhat of a mirror image pathology, defective brain insulin signaling and elevated pro-inflammatory markers in diabetic states are associated with depressive behaviors and impairment of stress adaptation in animal models. In addition to low socioeconomic status as a known risk factor, other contributing factors for diabetes and depression are poor sleep, reduced physical exercise, and poor diet.[44] Depression also reduces a patient's motivation to adhere to diet, exercise, and self-care activities that promote better outcomes for the diabetic disease. With the incidence of diabetes on the rise worldwide, it is very important for the clinician to be aware of the concurrent elevated risk of depression in this patient population and need for disease management of both conditions to get the best long-term outcomes.

Medications used to treat diabetes, such as metformin[45] and thiazolidinediones,[46] may have direct antidepressant-like effects. Probiotics may modulate inflammatory markers and insulin signaling and are emerging as a treatment for depression.[47] Antidepressants, such as SSRIs or bupropion, are moderately effective for depression in patients with diabetes, and sertraline has a favorable effect on glycemic control.[48,49] CBT has beneficial effects on glycemic control[50] in addition to a positive impact on depressive symptoms.[51] Collaborative care is a coordinated care management in primary care settings that provides guideline-based management to patients with depression and chronic medical illnesses. Collaborative care for patients with comorbid depression and diabetes yields significant improvement in depression response and remission and higher rates of adherence to antidepressant and oral hypoglycemic agents, but not a substantial reduction in HbA1c values.[52]

9.3.5. Hypothyroidism

One of the great mimics of depression is hypothyroidism. Although hypothyroidism is not the cause of most depression, there is a 2.5-fold risk of depression in adults with hypothyroidism. Patients being evaluated for depression should undergo a thyroid stimulating hormone (TSH) laboratory test to rule out hypothyroidism, as even subclinical hypothyroidism can have a negative impact on depression. A high TSH level indicates a possible low thyroid level and a thyroid profile laboratory test can be ordered to confirm the diagnosis of hypothyroidism. Conversely, a low TSH may indicate hyperthyroidism.

Although research outcomes are mixed, levothyroxine can sometimes ameliorate the symptoms of low energy, depression, and sleep and appetite disturbances in people with subclinical hypothyroidism.[53] However, studies are more consistent in showing that depressive symptoms resolve with a thyroid supplement in patients with overt hypothyroidism. In monitoring treatment, TSH levels need to reach 2.5 µIU/mL or less in order to achieve optimal outcomes.[54] Fortunately, thyroid supplementation is well tolerated and has a low risk of side effects.

9.3.6. Gastrointestinal and Hepatic

Symptoms attributed to the gastrointestinal (GI) tract are often reported by patients with anxious and depressive symptoms. These range from mild "butterflies" or nausea typical of anxiety to anorexia and weight loss that may accompany severe depression. Many of our psychotropic medications are aimed at key neurotransmitters like serotonin, norepinephrine, and dopamine in the brain. Those same receptors are present throughout the human gut, the "gut–brain axis,"[55] which helps explain the impacts that our psychotropic medications may have on gut function. Conversely, proton-pump inhibitors used to treat common GI disorders, such as gastric reflux disease, are known to be associated with depression.[56]

Historically, the most common GI disorders associated with depression were digestive system tumors.[57] About half of patients with pancreatic cancer will experience depressive symptoms prior to receiving their cancer diagnosis; this is a much higher incidence than other GI or abdominal cancers.[58] This has been attributed to the unique role of the pancreas as both an endocrine and exocrine gland with impacts on immunologic and neuroendocrine function.[59]

Irritable bowel, characterized by complaints of diarrhea and/or constipation along with cramping and discomfort, are frequent in this population.[60] The presence of bowel symptoms that awaken one from sleep, fever, weight loss that is disproportionate to the severity of depression, and bloody or tarry stool suggests more serious illness and a GI workup for other causes is needed. Less commonly, weight gain is described by the depressed patient. Typically, this is associated with atypical depression, but it could also signal underlying endocrine dysregulation, decreased exercise due to low energy, food cravings (e.g., carbohydrates and high-fat foods aimed at "improving energy"), or medication side effects.

A meta-analysis of studies looking at the prevalence of depression in patients with inflammatory bowel disease shows that over 15% will meet criteria for a depressive disorder, with higher rates in Crohn's disease compared to ulcerative colitis.[61] Depression is highly associated with clinical recurrence of bowel disease, increased hospitalization, and lower compliance with treatment.[62,63] Among patients with active disease, the prevalence of depressive symptoms exceeds 40%. Chronic inflammatory bowel conditions carry a high burden of disease as they start in early adulthood and have persistent symptoms that contribute to lower quality of life and work disability during prime working years.[29] Many patients require ongoing treatment with anti-inflammatories, pain medications, steroids, and immune modulators that may further impact mood.[64] SSRIs[65] and psychotherapy[66] have both been shown to improve mood and outcome in this population.

Chronic disorders of the liver, including hepatitis B and C, alcoholic liver disease, and non-alcoholic fatty liver disease (NAFLD) have a well-established relationship to depression, with rates of over 40% in those with cirrhosis.[57] While the mechanisms are unclear, studies suggest that there are shared risk factors (alcohol, substance use) and inflammatory and neuroendocrine mediators (obesity, diabetes, cytokines, stress hormones) in addition to direct cognitive effects.[67] The presence of depression in chronic liver disease has been linked with lower quality of life, increased mortality, poorer response to treatment, premature discontinuation, and lower adherence to anti-viral medications.[68-70] In NAFLD, depression has been associated with more severe histologic findings on biopsy.[71] One retrospective study showed that depression increased the likelihood of liver transplant rejection,[72] though prospective studies are lacking.

The high rates of chronic liver disease worldwide mean that most clinicians will treat with patients in varying degrees of hepatic compromise, including those facing liver transplant and undergoing antiviral therapy. Traditional pegylated interferon alpha treatment has a propensity to exacerbate depression, with the greatest risk in individuals with prior depressive history who are undergoing high-dose, long-duration treatment.[73] Prospective studies show that depression scores may escalate during the period of interferon treatment and return to pretreatment baseline after treatment completion.[74] Pretreatment of patients at high risk for depression has been shown to improve treatment response and adherence to interferon therapy.[75] Fortunately, newer direct-acting antivirals appear less likely to provoke depressive symptoms during treatment, in addition to having shorter treatment length and improved tolerability compared to interferon therapy.[76,77] Viral suppression, without regard to the treatment used, results in improved quality of life, better cognition, and less depression.[78]

9.3.7. Immunologic and Dermatologic Disorders

The intricate crosstalk of neuroendocrine and immune systems through chemical mediators is thought to contribute to the high prevalence of depressive disorders in patients with immunologic disorders such as lupus,[79] rheumatoid arthritis, psoriasis,[80] ankylosing spondylitis,[81] and sarcoid. This elevated risk, up to 50% in some studies, has been attributed to the physically disabling, stigmatizing, and often painful symptoms that begin in early adulthood and impact circadian rhythm, social relationships, work performance, and long-term survival. Greater depression is associated with illness that is poorly controlled or nonresponsive to treatment. Suicidal ideation and suicide behaviors are seen with higher frequency in patients with immunologic illness, particularly neuropsychiatric systemic lupus. Patients with psoriasis have increased suicidal ideation compared to patients presenting with allergy or melanoma.[82]

Tumor necrosis factor inhibitors and interleukin inhibitors appear to prompt improvement in the physical disorders, inflammatory markers, and depressive symptoms of many of these disorders.

9.3.8. Neurologic Illness

The prevalence of major depression is high among patients with neurologic disorders, given the persistent and disabling effects of many neurologic illnesses. Furthermore, the recognition of depression is challenging as there can be considerable overlap in symptoms. Depression screening tools need to be carefully reviewed by the clinician to discern whether the score is being influenced by the physical manifestations of the patient's neurologic disease. Questions that elicit the negative cognitive state (i.e., guilt, low self-esteem, feelings of failure, suicidal ideation) may be more reliable indicators of depression than somatically focused items (i.e., moving slowly, fidgeting, appetite or sleep changes, physical fatigue).

In some instances, depression may be the presenting symptom of a developing neurologic disorder, especially those affecting the basal ganglia.[83] Movement disorders, such as Parkinson's,[84] Huntington's, and essential tremor, are conditions that frequent the neuropsychiatric interface. Rates of depression in this population may approach 50%, and the rate of anxiety disorders is often higher due to the perceived social stigma and self-awareness of abnormal movements.[85,86] Not infrequently, these individuals present to the mental health clinician years prior to the onset of movement symptoms. For example, 30% to 40% of patients with Huntington's[87] disease or Wilson's[88] disease initially present with psychiatric symptoms, most commonly depression, but also anxiety, psychosis, or cognitive decline.[89] The onset of motor symptoms may be delayed for a decade or more. There is increasing recognition of the extensive burden of non-motor symptoms as well as efforts to identify subtypes of non-motor-predominant movement disorder.[90,91] For clinicians, the detection of depression is sometimes hampered by the affective and somatic changes that accompany movement disorders. For example, bradykinesia and flat affect may suggest depression but can be inconsistent with the internal mood state. Similarly, affective lability and disinhibition may not accurately reflect the underlying depressive emotions in someone with Huntington's.

Pharmacotherapy with SSRIs is often suggested for individuals with movement disorders, and several trials support their use.[92,93] Caution is needed in assessing the potential drug interactions with the medications used in treating movement disorders (e.g., L-dopa, ropinirole, selegiline). Dopaminergic medications may also escalate mood, libido, and reward-seeking behaviors that can suggest hypomania, especially if inadvertently overused.[94,95] Psychotherapy and movement-based therapies are often beneficial in this population as well.[96,97]

Depression following cerebrovascular accident is an important and treatable aspect of post-stroke rehabilitation. Approximately 30% of stroke survivors will experience depression in the following five years.[98] Post-stroke depression (PSD) has traditionally been associated with left frontal or left basal ganglia lesions,[99] although some studies refute this finding.[100] Greater impairment in activities of daily living, deficits in cognitive functioning, and a personal history and family history of depression are also prognostic factors in the development of PSD.[101,102] Recognition and treatment of depression in this population may improve rehabilitation and long-term outcome, although the impact of SSRIs on functional recovery has been inconsistent.[103,104] Treatment trials aimed at improving PSD support the use of SSRIs, although smaller studies have been done with non-SSRI medications.[106–107] Stimulants, such as methylphenidate, may also prove of benefit in addressing apathy and helping the patient to engage in physical rehabilitation.[108]

Approximately one-third of patients with epilepsy will meet criteria for depression at some point in their illness course.[109] The interplay between depression and seizures is complex, having multiple neurochemical and psychosocial determinants.[110,111] Seizure type, frequency, severity, and locus may affect the presentation of depression, with temporal lobe and drug-refractory epilepsies more closely associated with depression.[112] Concomitant anxiety disorders are also frequent in this population, with worsening symptoms sometimes occurring during the pre-ictal and post-ictal periods.[113] Episodic intense fear is characteristic of temporal lobe seizures and may be mistaken for panic.[114] Depression is one of the major determinants of quality of life in people with epilepsy, along with seizure frequency.[115]

Evidence supports the use of both psychotherapy and pharmacotherapy in the treatment of depression in the population with epilepsy.[116] Modern antidepressants, such as SSRIs and SNRIs, are thought to carry minimal risk of seizure exacerbation when used in therapeutic doses; however, tricyclic antidepressants and bupropion are not recommended due to their propensity to lower the seizure threshold.[117] Attention to drug–drug interactions is important when selecting and dosing the antidepressant.[118] For example, carbamazepine, phenytoin, and phenobarbital speed the metabolism of other medications being processed through the liver, effectively increasing the dose needed for many antidepressants. Valproic acid, in contrast, slows metabolism and may reduce the dose needed for antidepressants. Older agents like phenobarbital[119] and primidone,[120] along with the newer drug topiramate,[121] can lead to a feeling of depressed mood and cognitive dullness. Lamotrigine is generally well tolerated and appears to have a positive effect on mood.[122]

9.3.9. Cancer

Distinguishing depression from similar cancer-related somatic symptoms can be challenging.[123] The National Comprehensive Cancer Network and the American Society of Clinical Oncology have published comprehensive guidelines for the screening, assessment, and treatment of cancer patients with depressive symptoms, including the use of CBT and antidepressant medications with a careful consideration of risks and benefits for the individual patient.[124]

9.3.10. Pain

Comorbid depression and pain is one of the most common debilitating combinations in clinical practice to evaluate and manage. Depression coexists in almost 80% of pain patients, and the comorbidity is associated with impaired quality of life and treatment resistance to either the antidepressant or pain medication. Suggestive of heightened neuroplasticity, there are distinct changes in neural activation, neural circuitry, and molecular signaling pathways underlying the complex relationship between pain and depression and treatments for these comorbid conditions.[125]

SNRIs and tricyclic antidepressants are two classes of antidepressants that are have approval from the US Food and Drug Administration (FDA) for the treatment of depression and a variety of chronic pain conditions. Studies are ongoing to explore the efficacy of ketamine in sub-anesthetic doses, deep brain stimulation, transcranial magnetic stimulation, biofeedback, and CBT.

9.3.11. Infectious Disease

Human immunodeficiency virus[126] and syphilis[127] are classic examples of how infectious agents can have direct neuropsychiatric effects on the brain, particularly in white matter and deep structures. Depressed patients have higher rates of seropositivity than healthy controls for infections such as Borna disease virus, herpes simplex virus-1, varicella zoster virus, Epstein-Barr virus, and *Chlamydia trachomatis*.[128] Depression can be a sequela of the isolation and stigma associated with tuberculosis (TB) infection[129] and a significant contributor to nonadherence with anti-TB medications.[130] Fear, stigma, isolation, rurality, poverty, and limited access to and adherence to treatment are contributors to the interface of depression and many infectious illnesses.[131]

9. 3.12. Minerals and Bones

Serotonin's effects extend beyond the nervous system to include the GI tract, platelets, vascular endothelium, and osteoblasts. The impact of SSRIs on bone metabolism and osteoporosis has been under examination after several studies, but not all, found that fracture risk was increased and bone mineral density was decreased in SSRI users.[132] Confounding factors like ethnicity, body mass, nutritional status, smoking, and alcohol consumption, as well as the independent effects of depression on bone metabolism, are still unclear. Laboratory studies show that serotonin inhibits osteoblast proliferation, leading to bone loss.[133] The effects may be reversible, as one study found that risk of fracture was reduced after discontinuation of the SSRI medication.[134]

9.4. KEY ELEMENTS IN TREATMENT OF DEPRESSION AND MEDICAL ILLNESS

Systemic medical illnesses can mimic major depression. Conversely, patients with chronic medical conditions are at much higher risk for developing major depression. Untreated depression in patients with chronic medical conditions is both a marker and a risk factor for poorer outcomes. Recognizing depression early and conducting a careful differential diagnosis pays dividends in terms of improved function, better adherence to treatment regimens, and lower morbidity and mortality. Collaborative team approaches are essential in achieving the best outcome for depression due to or comorbid with general medical conditions.

REFERENCES

1. Katon WJ. Epidemiology and treatment of depression in patients with chronic medical illness. Dialog Clin Neurosci. 2011; 13(1):7–23.
2. Yates WR, Mitchell J, Rush AJ, et al. Clinical features of depressed outpatients with and without co-occurring general medical conditions in STAR*D. Gen Hosp Psychiatry. 2004; 26(6):421–429.
3. Cuijpers P, Vogelzangs N, Twisk J, et al. Differential mortality rates in major and subthreshold depression: a meta-analysis of studies that measured both. Br J Psychiatry. 2013; 202:22–27.
4. Warnke I, Nordt C, Kawohl W, et al. Age- and gender-specific mortality risk profiles for depressive outpatients with major chronic medical diseases. J Affect Disord. 2016; 193:295–304.
5. Katon W, Lin EH, Kroenke K. The association of depression and anxiety with medical symptom burden in patients with chronic medical illness. Gen Hosp Psychiatry. 2007; 29:147–155.
6. Kahl KG, Stapel B, Frieling H. Link between depression and cardiovascular diseases due to epigenomics and proteomics: focus on energy metabolism. Prog Neuropsychopharmacol Biol Psychiatry. 2019; 89:146–157.
7. Behan C, Doyle R, Masterson S, et al. A double-edged sword: review of the interplay between physical health and mental health. Ir J Med Sci. 2015; 184(1):107–112.
8. Uzun S, Kozumplik O, Topić R, Jakovljević M. Depressive disorders and comorbidity: somatic illness vs. side effect. Psychiatr Danub. 2009; 21(3):391–398.
9. Qato DM, Ozenbuerger K, Olfson M. Prevalence of prescription medications with depression as a potential adverse effect among adults in the United States. JAMA. 2018; 319(22):2289–2298.
10. Gan Y, Gong Y, Tong X, et al. Depression and the risk of coronary heart disease: a meta-analysis of prospective cohort studies. BMC Psychiatry. 2014; 14:371.
11. Cohen BE, Edmondson D, Kronish IM. State of the art review: depression, stress, anxiety, and cardiovascular disease. Am J Hypertens. 2015; 28(11):1295–1302.
12. Li Z, Li Y, Chen L, et al. Prevalence of depression in patients with hypertension: a systematic review and meta-analysis. Medicine. 2015; 94(31):e1317.
13. Lane D, Carroll D, Ring C, et al. The prevalence and persistence of depression and anxiety following myocardial infarction. Br J Health Psychol. 2002; 7:11–21.
14. Bartoli F, Lillia N, Lax A, et al. Depression after stroke and risk of mortality: a systematic review and meta-analysis. Stroke Res Treat 2013; 2013:862978.
15. Tully PJ. Psychological depression and cardiac surgery: a comprehensive review. J Extra Corpor Technol. 2012; 44(4):224–232.

16. Lichtman JH, Froelicher ES, Blumenthal JA, et al.; American Heart Association Statistics Committee of the Council on Epidemiology and Prevention and the Council on Cardiovascular and Stroke Nursing. Depression as a risk factor for poor prognosis among patients with acute coronary syndrome: systematic review and recommendations: a scientific statement from the American Heart Association. Circulation 2014; 129:1350–1369.

17. Vieweg WV, Hasnain M, Lesnefsky EJ, et al. Assessing the presence and severity of depression in subjects with comorbid coronary heart disease. Am J Med. 2010; 123(8):683–690.

18. Amare AT, Schubert KO, Klingler-Hoffmann M, et al. The genetic overlap between mood disorders and cardiometabolic diseases: a systematic review of genome wide and candidate gene studies. Transl Psychiatry. 2017; 7(1):e1007.

19. Berkman LF, Blumenthal J, Burg M, et al. Effects of treating depression and low perceived social support on clinical events after myocardial infarction: the Enhancing Recovery in Coronary Heart Disease Patients (ENRICHD) randomized trial. JAMA. 2003; 289:3106–3116.

20. Glassman AH, O'Connor CM, Califf RM, et al. Sertraline treatment of major depression in patients with acute MI or unstable angina. JAMA. 2002; 288:701–709.

21. Honig A, Kuyper AM, Schene AH, et al. Treatment of post-myocardial infarction depressive disorder: a randomized, placebo-controlled trial with mirtazapine. Psychosom Med. 2007; 69:606–613.

22. Freedland KE, Skala JA, Carney RM, et al. Treatment of depression after coronary artery bypass surgery: a randomized controlled trial. Arch Gen Psychiatry. 2009; 66:387–396.

23. Lesperance F, Frasure-Smith N, Koszycki D, et al. Effects of citalopram and interpersonal psychotherapy on depression in patients with coronary artery disease: the Canadian Cardiac Randomized Evaluation of Antidepressant and Psychotherapy Efficacy (CREATE) trial. JAMA. 2007; 297:367–379.

24. O'Connor CM, Jiang W, Kuchibhatla M, et al. Safety and efficacy of sertraline for depression in patients with heart failure: results of the SADHART-CHF (Sertraline Against Depression and Heart Disease in Chronic Heart Failure) trial. J Am Coll Cardiol. 2010; 56:692–699.

25. Matte DL, Pizzichini MM, Hoepers AT, et al. Prevalence of depression in COPD: a systematic review and meta-analysis of controlled studies. Respir Med. 2016; 117:154–161.

26. Blakemore A, Dickens C, Guthrie E, et al. Depression and anxiety predict health-related quality of life in chronic obstructive pulmonary disease: systematic review and meta-analysis. Int J Chron Obstruct Pulmon Dis. 2014; 9:501–512.

27. Sahin H, Varol Y, Naz I, Tuksavul F. Effectiveness of pulmonary rehabilitation in COPD patients receiving long-term oxygen therapy. Clin Respir J. 2018; 12(4):1439–1446.

28. Hedayati SS, Bosworth HB, Kuchibhatla M, et al. The predictive value of self-report scales compared with physician diagnosis of depression in hemodialysis patients. Kidney Int. 2006; 69(9):1662–1668.

29. Palmer S, Vecchio M, Craig JC, et al. Prevalence of depression in chronic kidney disease: systematic review and meta-analysis of observational studies. Kidney Int. 2013; 84(1):179–191.

30. Hedayati SS, Minhajuddin AT, Toto RD, et al. Validation of depression screening scales in patients with CKD. Am J Kidney Dis. 2009;54(3):433–439.

31. Farrokhi F, Abedi N, Beyene J, et al. Association between depression and mortality in patients receiving long-term dialysis: a systematic review and meta-analysis. Am J Kidney Dis. 2014; 63(4):623–635.

32. Uglešić B, Ljutić D, Lasić D, et al. Depression and serum interleukin-6 levels in patients on dialysis. Psychiatr Danub. 2015; 27(2):168–73.

33. Jaber BL, Lee Y, Collins AJ, et al.; FREEDOM Study Group. Effect of daily hemodialysis on depressive symptoms and postdialysis recovery time: interim report from the FREEDOM (Following Rehabilitation, Economics and Everyday-Dialysis Outcome Measurements) study. Am J Kidney Dis. 2010; 56(3):531–539.

34. Veater NL, East L. Exploring depression amongst kidney transplant recipients: a literature review. J Ren Care 2016; 42(3):172–184.

35. Palmer SC, Natale P, Ruospo M, et al. Antidepressants for treating depression in adults with end-stage kidney disease treated with dialysis. Cochrane Database Syst Rev. 2016; 5:CD004541.

36. Hedayati SS, Gregg LP, Carmody T, et al. Effect of sertraline on depressive symptoms in patients with chronic kidney disease without dialysis dependence: the CAST randomized clinical trial. JAMA. 2017; 318(19):1876–1890.

37. Friedli K, Guirguis A, Almond M, et al. Sertraline versus placebo in patients with major depressive disorder undergoing hemodialysis: a randomized, controlled feasibility trial. Clin J Am Soc Nephrol. 2017; 12(2):280–286.

38. Baghdady NT, Banik S, Swartz SA, McIntyre RS. Psychotropic drugs and renal failure: translating the evidence for clinical practice. Adv Ther. 2009; 26(4):404–424.

39. Mezuk B, Eaton W, Albrecht S, Golden S. Depression and type 2 diabetes over the lifespan: a meta-analysis. Diabetes Care. 2008; 31:2383–2390.

40. Ali S, Stone MA, Peters JL, et al. The prevalence of co-morbid depression in adults with type 2 diabetes: a systematic review and meta-analysis. Diabet Med. 2006; 23:1165–1173.

41. Lloyd CE, Nouwen A, Sartorius N, et al. Prevalence and correlates of depressive disorders in people with type 2 diabetes: results from the International Prevalence and Treatment of Diabetes and Depression (INTERPRET-DD) study, a collaborative study carried out in 14 countries. Diabet Med. 2018; 35(6):760–769.

42. Wong JJ, Hood KK, Breland JY. Correlates of health care use among White and minority men and women with diabetes: an NHANES study. Diabetes Res Clin Pract. 2019; 150: 122–128.

43. Lyra E, Silva NM, Lam MP, et al. Insulin resistance as a shared pathogenic mechanism between depression and type 2 diabetes. Front Psychiatry. 2019; 10:57.

44. Thase ME. Managing medical comorbidities in patients with depression to improve prognosis. J Clin Psychiatry. 2016; 77(S1):22–27.

45. Guo M, Mi J, Jiang QM, et al. Metformin may produce antidepressant effects through improvement of cognitive function among depressed patients with diabetes mellitus. Clin Exp Pharmacol Physiol. 2014; 41:650–656.

46. Sepanjnia K, Modabbernia A, Ashrafi M, et al. Pioglitazone adjunctive therapy for moderate-to-severe major depressive disorder: randomized double-blind placebo-controlled trial. Neuropsychopharmacology. 2012; 37:2093–100.

47. Wallace CJK, Milev R. The effects of probiotics on depressive symptoms in humans: a systematic review. Ann General Psychiatry. 2017; 16:14.

48. van der Feltz-Cornelis CM, Nuyen J, Stoop C, et al. Effect of interventions for major depressive disorder and significant depressive symptoms in patients with diabetes mellitus: a systematic review and meta-analysis. Gen Hosp Psychiatry. 2010; 32(4):380–395.

49. Roopan S, Larsen ER. Use of antidepressants in patients with depression and comorbid diabetes mellitus: a systematic review. Acta Neuropsychiatr. 2017; 29(3):127–139.

50. Semenkovich K, Brown ME, Svrakic DM, Lustman PJ. Depression in type 2 diabetes mellitus: prevalence, impact, and treatment. Drugs. 2015; 75(6):577–587.

51. Newby J, Robins L, Wilhelm K, et al. Web-based cognitive behavior therapy for depression in people with diabetes mellitus: a randomized controlled trial. J Med Internet Res. 2017; 19(5):e157.

52. Huang Y, Wei X, Wu T, et al. Collaborative care for patients with depression and diabetes mellitus: a systematic review and meta-analysis. BMC Psychiatry. 2013; 13:260.

53. Loh HH, Lim LL, Yee A, Loh HS. Association between subclinical hypothyroidism and depression: an updated systematic review and meta-analysis. BMC Psychiatry. 2019; 19(1):12.

54. Cohen BM, Sommer BR, Vuckovic A. Antidepressant-resistant depression in patients with comorbid subclinical hypothyroidism or high-normal TSH levels. Am J Psychiatry. 2018; 175(7):598–604.

55. Dinan TG, Cryan JF. The microbiome-gut-brain axis in health and disease. Gastroenterol Clin North Am. 2017; 46(1):77–89.

56. Laudisio A, Antonelli Incalzi R, Gemma A, et al. Use of proton-pump inhibitors is associated with depression: a population-based study. Int Psychogeriatr. 2018; 30(1):153–159.

57. Zhang AZ, Wang QC, Huang KM, et al. Prevalence of depression and anxiety in patients with chronic digestive system diseases: a multicenter epidemiological study. World J Gastroenterol. 2016; 22(42):9437–9444.

58. Parker G, Brotchie H. Pancreatic cancer and depression: a narrative review. J Nerv Ment Dis. 2017; 205(6):487–490.

59. Breitbart W, Rosenfeld B, Tobias K, et al. Depression, cytokines, and pancreatic cancer. J Psychooncology. 2014; 23(3):339–345.

60. Fond G, Loundou A, Hamdani N, et al. Anxiety and depression comorbidities in irritable bowel syndrome (IBS): a systematic review and meta-analysis. Eur Arch Psychiatry Clin Neurosci. 2014; 264(8):651–660.

61. Neuendorf R, Harding A, Stello N, et al. Depression and anxiety in patients with inflammatory bowel disease: a systematic review. J Psychosom Res. 2016; 87:70–80.

62. Mikocka-Walus A, Pittet V, Rossel JB, von Känel R; Swiss IBD Cohort Study Group. Symptoms of depression and anxiety are independently associated with clinical recurrence of inflammatory bowel disease. Clin Gastroenterol Hepatol. 2016; 14(6): 829–835.

63. Nigro G, Angelini G, Grosso SB, et al. Psychiatric predictors of noncompliance in inflammatory bowel disease: psychiatry and compliance. J Clin Gastroenterol. 2001; 32:66–68.

64. Ciriaco M, Ventrice P, Russo G, et al. Corticosteroid-related central nervous system side effects. J Pharmacol Pharmacother. 2013; 4(1):S94–S98.

65. Goodhand JR, Greig FI, Koodun Y, et al. Do antidepressants influence the disease course in inflammatory bowel disease? A retrospective case-matched observational study. Inflamm Bowel Dis. 2012; 18(7):1232–1239.

66. Wiles NJ, Thomas L, Turner N, et al. Long-term effectiveness and cost-effectiveness of cognitive behavioural therapy as an adjunct to pharmacotherapy for treatment-resistant depression in primary care: follow-up of the CoBalT randomised controlled trial. Lancet Psychiatry. 2016; 3(2):137–144.

67. Huang X, Liu X, Yu Y. Depression and chronic liver diseases: are there shared underlying mechanisms? Front Mol Neurosci. 2017; 10:134.

68. Baumeister H, Hutter N, Bengel J, Härter M. Quality of life in medically ill persons with comorbid mental disorders: a systematic review and meta-analysis. Psychother Psychosom. 2011; 80:275–86.

69. Leutscher PD, Lagging M, Buhl MR, et al. Evaluation of depression as a risk factor for treatment failure in chronic hepatitis C. Hepatology. 2010; 52: 430–435.

70. Singh N, Gayowski T, Wagener MM, Marino IR. Depression in patients with cirrhosis. Impact on outcome. Dig Dis Sci. 1997; 42:1421–1427.

71. Youssef NA, Abdelmalek MF, Binks M, et al. Associations of depression, anxiety and antidepressants with histological severity of nonalcoholic fatty liver disease. Liver Int 2013; 33:1062–70.

72. Rogal SS, Landsittel D, Surman O, et al. Pretransplant depression, antidepressant use, and outcomes of orthotopic liver transplantation. Liver Transpl. 2011; 17(3):251–260.

73. Choi JS, Kim W, Sohn BK, et al. Association of changes in mood status and psychosocial well-being with depression during interferon-based treatment for hepatitis C. Psychiatry Investig. 2017; 3:314–324.

74. Baranyi A, Meinitzer A, Stepan A, et al. A biopsychosocial model of interferon-alpha-induced depression in patients with chronic hepatitis C infection. Psychother Psychosom. 2013; 82(5):332–340.

75. Musselman DL, Lawson DH, Gumnick JF, et al. Paroxetine for the prevention of depression induced by high-dose interferon alfa. N Engl J Med. 2001; 344:961–966.

76. Tang LS, Masur J, Sims Z, et al. Safe and effective sofosbuvir-based therapy in patients with mental health disease on hepatitis C virus treatment. World J Hepatol. 2016; 8(31):1318–1326.

77. Takeda K, Noguchi R, Namisaki T, et al. Efficacy and tolerability of interferon-free regimen for patients with genotype-1 HCV infection. Exp Ther Med. 2018; 16(3):2743–2750.

78. Yarlott L, Heald E, Forton D. Hepatitis C virus infection, and neurological and psychiatric disorders: a review. J Adv Res. 2017; 8:139–148.

79. Zhang L, Fu T, Yin R, et al. Prevalence of depression and anxiety in systemic lupus erythematosus: a systematic review and meta-analysis. BMC Psychiatry. 2017; 17(1):70.

80. Dowlatshahi EA, Wakkee M, Arends LR, Nijsten T. The prevalence and odds of depressive symptoms and clinical depression in psoriasis patients: a systematic review and meta-analysis. J Invest Dermatol. 2014; 134(6):1542–1551.

81. Zhao S, Thong D, Miller N, et al. The prevalence of depression in axial spondyloarthritis and its association with disease activity: a systematic review and meta-analysis. Arthritis Res Ther. 2018; 20(1):140.

82. Pompili M, Innamorati M, Forte A, et al. Psychiatric comorbidity and suicidal ideation in psoriasis, melanoma and allergic disorders. Int J Psychiatry Clin Pract. 2017; 21(3):209–214.

83. Lafer B, Renshaw PF, Sachs GS. Major depression and the basal ganglia. Psychiatr Clin North Am. 1997; 20(4):885–896.

84. Marsh L. Depression and Parkinson's disease: current knowledge. Curr Neurol Neurosci Rep. 2013; 13(12):409.

85. Pontone GM1, Williams JR, Anderson KE, et al. Prevalence of anxiety disorders and anxiety subtypes in patients with Parkinson's disease. Mov Disord. 2009; 24(9):1333–1338.

86. Smeltere L, Kuzņecovs V, Erts R. Depression and social phobia in essential tremor and Parkinson's disease. Brain Behav. 2017; 7(9):e00781.

87. Paulsen JS, Miller AC, Hayes T, Shaw E. Cognitive and behavioral changes in Huntington disease before diagnosis. Handb Clin Neurol. 2017; 144:69–91.

88. Zimbrean PC, Schilsky ML. Psychiatric aspects of Wilson disease: a review. Gen Hosp Psychiatry. 2014; 36(1):53–62.

89. Poewe W. Non-motor symptoms in Parkinson's disease. Eur J Neurol. 2008; 15(Suppl 1):14–20.

90. Kim JI, Long JD, Mills JA, et al.; PREDICT-HD Investigators and Coordinators of the Huntington Study Group. Multivariate clustering of progression profiles reveals different depression patterns in prodromal Huntington disease. Neuropsychology. 2015; 29(6):949–960.

91. Sauerbier A, Jenner P, Todorova A, Chaudhuri KR. Non motor subtypes and Parkinson's disease. Parkinsonism Relat Disord. 2016; 22(Suppl 1):S41–S46.

92. Bomasang-Layno E, Fadlon I, Murray AN, Himelhoch S. Antidepressive treatments for Parkinson's disease: a systematic review and meta-analysis. Parkinsonism Relat Disord. 2015; 21(8):833–842.

93. Zhuo C, Xue R, Luo L, et al. Efficacy of antidepressive medication for depression in Parkinson disease: a network meta-analysis. Medicine. 2017; 96(22):e6698.

94. Voon V1, Thomsen T, Miyasaki JM, et al. Factors associated with dopaminergic drug-related pathological gambling in Parkinson disease. Arch Neurol. 2007; 64(2):212–216.

95. Maier F, Merkl J, Ellereit AL, et al. Hypomania and mania related to dopamine replacement therapy in Parkinson's disease. Parkinsonism Relat Disord. 2014; 20(4):421–427.

96. Sharp K, Hewitt J. Dance as an intervention for people with Parkinson's disease: a systematic review and meta-analysis. Neurosci Biobehav Rev. 2014; 47:445–456.

97. Xie CL, Wang XD, Chen J, et al. A systematic review and meta-analysis of cognitive behavioral and psychodynamic therapy for depression in Parkinson's disease patients. Neurol Sci. 2015; 36(6):833–843.

98. Robinson RG, Jorge RE. Post-stroke depression: a review. Am J Psychiatry. 2016; 173(3):221–231.

99. Robinson RG, Spalletta G. Poststroke depression: A review. Can J Psychiatry. 2010; 55:341–349.

100. Wei N1, Yong W, Li X, et al. Post-stroke depression and lesion location: a systematic review. J Neurol. 2015; 262(1):81–90.

101. Jørgensen TS, Wium-Andersen IK, Wium-Andersen MK, et al. Incidence of depression after stroke, and associated risk factors and mortality outcomes, in a large cohort of Danish patients. JAMA Psychiatry. 2016; 73:1032–1040.

102. Willey JZ, Disla N, Moon YP, et al. Early depressed mood after stroke predicts long-term disability: the Northern Manhattan Stroke Study (NOMASS). Stroke 2010; 41: 1896–1900.

103. Siepmann T, Penzlin A, Kepplinger J, et al. Selective serotonin reuptake inhibitors to improve outcome in acute ischemic stroke: possible mechanisms and clinical evidence. Brain Behav. 2015; 5(10):e003731.

104. FOCUS Trial Collaboration. Effects of fluoxetine on functional outcomes after acute stroke (FOCUS): a pragmatic, double-blind, randomised, controlled trial. Lancet. 2019; 393(10168):265–274.

105. Qin B, Chen H, Gao W, et al. Efficacy, acceptability, and tolerability of antidepressant treatments for patients with post-stroke depression: a network meta-analysis. Braz J Med Biol Res. 2018; 51(7):e7218.

106. Mead GE, Hsieh CF, Lee R, et al. Selective serotonin reuptake inhibitors (SSRIs) for stroke recovery. Cochrane Database Syst Rev. 2012; 11:CD009286.

107. Xu XM, Zou DZ, Shen LY, et al. Efficacy and feasibility of antidepressant treatment in patients with post-stroke depression. Medicine. 2016; 95(45):e5349.

108. Grade C, Redford B, Chrostowski J, et al. Methylphenidate in early poststroke recovery: a double-blind, placebo-controlled study. Arch Phys Med Rehabil. 1998; 79:1047–1050.

109. Fiest K, Dykeman J, Patten S, et al. Depression in epilepsy: a systematic review and meta-analysis Neurology. 2013; 80(6):590–599.

110. Blaszczyk B Czuczwar SJ. Epilepsy coexisting with depression. Pharmacol Rep. 2016; 68(5):1084–1092.

111. Jobe PC, Dailey JW, Wernicke JF. A noradrenergic and serotonergic hypothesis of the linkage between epilepsy and affective disorders. Crit Rev Neurobiol. 1999; 13(4): 317–356.

112. Gonçalves EB, de Oliveira Cardoso TAM, Yasuda CL, Cendes F. Depressive disorders in patients with pharmaco-resistant mesial temporal lobe epilepsy. J Int Med Res. 2017; 46(2):752–760.

113. Munger Clary HM. Anxiety and epilepsy: what neurologists and epileptologists should know. Curr Neurol Neurosci Rep. 2014; 14:445–449.

114. Boulogne S, Catenoix H, Ryvlin P, Rheims S. Long-lasting seizure-related anxiety in patients with temporal lobe epilepsy and comorbid psychiatric disorders. Epileptic Disord. 2015;17(3): 340–344.

115. Sajatovic M, Tatsuoka C, Welter E, et al. Correlates of quality of life among individuals with epilepsy enrolled in self-management research: from the US Centers for Disease Control and Prevention Managing Epilepsy Well Network. Epilepsy Behav. 2017; 69:177–180.

116. Mehndiratta P, Sajatovic M. Treatments for patients with comorbid epilepsy and depression: a systematic literature review. Epilepsy Behav. 2013; 28:36–40.

117. Koster M, Grohmann R, Engel RR, et al. Seizures during antidepressant treatment in psychiatric inpatients—results from the transnational pharmacovigilance project

"Arzneimittelsicherheit in der Psychatrie" (ASMP) 1993–2008. Psychopharmacology. 2013; 230(2):191–201.

118. Spina E, Perucca E. Clinical significant of pharmacokinetic interactions between antiepileptic and psychotropic drugs. Epilepsia 2002; 43(2):37–44.

119. Brent DA, Crumrine PK, Varma RR, et al. Phenobarbital treatment and major depressive disorder in children with epilepsy. Pediatrics. 1987; 80:909–917.

120. Lopez-Gomez M, Ramirez-Bermudez J, Campillo C, et al. Primidone is associated with interictal depression in patients with epilepsy. Epilepsy Behav. 2005; 6:413–416.

121. Fritz N, Glogau S, Hoffman J, et al. Efficacy and cognitive side effects of tiagabine and topriamate in patients with epilepsy. Epilepsy Behav 2005; 6:373–381.

122. Ettinger AB, Kustra RP, Hammer AE. Effect of lamotrigine on depressive symptoms in adult patients with epilepsy. Epilepsy Behav. 2007; 10:148–154.

123. Thompson LMA, Bobonis Babilonia M. Distinguishing depressive symptoms from similar cancer-related somatic symptoms: implications for assessment and management of major depression after breast cancer. South Med J. 2017; 110(10):667–672.

124. Ostuzzi G, Matcham F, Dauchy S, et al. Antidepressants for the treatment of depression in people with cancer. Cochrane Database Syst Rev. 2018; 4:CD011006.

125. Doan L, Manders T, Wang J. Neuroplasticity underlying the comorbidity of pain and depression. Neural Plast. 2015; 2015:504691.

126. Arseniou S, Arvaniti A, Smakouri M. HIV Infection and depression. Psychiatry Clin Neurosci. 2014; 68:96–109.

127. Costiniuk CT, MacPherson PA. Neurocognitive and psychiatric changes as the initial presentation of neurosyphilis. CMAJ. 2013; 185(6):499–503.

128. Wang X, Shang L, Lei Y, et al. Meta-analysis of infectious agents and depression. Sci Rep. 2014; 4:4530.

129. Gong Y, Yan S, Qiu L, et al. Prevalence of depressive symptoms and related risk factors among patients with tuberculosis in China: a multistage cross-sectional study. Am J Trop Med Hyg. 2018; 98(6):1624–1628.

130. Yan S, Zhang S, Tong Y, et al. Nonadherence to antituberculosis medications: the impact of stigma and depressive symptoms. Am J Trop Med Hyg. 2017; 98(1):262–265.

131. Pappas G, Kiriaze IJ, Giannakis P, Falagas ME. Psychosocial consequences of infectious diseases. Clin Microbiol Infection. 2009; 15(8):743–747.

132. Wadhwa R, Kumar M, Talegaonkar S, Vohora D. Serotonin reuptake inhibitors and bone health: a review of clinical studies and plausible mechanisms. Osteoporos Sarcopenia. 2017; 3(2):75–81.

133. Ducy P, Karsenty G. The two faces of serotonin in bone biology. J Cell Biol. 2010; 191:7–13.

134. van den Brand MW, Pouwels S, Samson MM, et al. Use of anti-depressants and the risk of fracture of the hip or femur. Osteoporos Int. 2009; 20:1705–1713.

/// 10 /// GENERAL MEDICAL CONDITIONS

Metabolic Disorders

SETH W. PERRY, MA-LI WONG, AND JULIO LICINIO

10.1. INTRODUCTION

Until relatively recently, the etiopathogeneses and thus treatment of seemingly dispa-
rate conditions such as depression and metabolic disorders were primarily considered
separately. Although efforts to understand depression in the context of metabolic
disorders date back at least half a century,[1,2] research interest in this field has grown
exponentially over the last 20 years, as evidenced by a PubMed default keyword
search for "metabolic," "disorder," and "depression." When defined most broadly,
there are a vast number of metabolic diseases or disorders—both inherited (genetic)
and acquired—and covering each and every one of them as they relate to depression would be a herculean task. Hence our discussions will be organized around
three major metabolic disease states to which depression has been most consistently
and strongly linked: obesity, type 2 diabetes mellitus (T2D), and cardiovascular disease (CVD). Closely intertwined with all of these diseases and also strongly linked
with depression is metabolic syndrome (MetS)—a collection of aberrant physiologic
parameters including obesity, unfavorable lipid profiles (e.g., high triglyceride and/
or low high-density lipoprotein [HDL] cholesterol levels), high blood pressure, and
high blood glucose (insulin resistance)—that, when present together or in combination, significantly increase one's risk for developing diabetes, CVD, and related
conditions. Because the pathogenic mechanisms of MetS are so closely intertwined
with obesity, T2D, and CVD, for simplicity we will discuss the connections between depression and MetS under the context of the most closely related disease. For

example, where it adds to the discussion, connections between altered lipid profiles and depression would be covered under the CVD section, and insulin resistance and depression would be covered under T2D.

Next, we will see that the pathophysiologic mechanisms shared between these very common metabolic conditions (obesity, T2D, CVD) and depression (i.e., inflammation, cytokine and hypothalamic–pituitary–adrenal [HPA] axis dysregulation, oxidative stress, neurotransmitter disruptions, neurogenesis and neuroplasticity, and the microbiome) are also likely relevant to the depression symptoms that accompany many of the rare but often devastating inherited metabolic disorders. Finally, we will make an argument for taking a more integrative approach toward understanding and treating depression as it presents comorbid with these and other metabolic disorders, and briefly discuss current and novel integrated therapeutic strategies for advancing treatment of these widespread and debilitating conditions.

10.2. OBESITY AND DEPRESSION

10.2.1. Molecules and Pathways

The arguments for bidirectional functional and mechanistic interactions between obesity and depression are many. Just some of the molecules and systems that have been shown to contribute to both depression and obesity in humans and/or animal models—and, in many cases, T2D and CVD too, discussed later in the chapter—include serotonin, norepinephrine, dopamine, leptin, neuropeptide Y (NPY), melanocortin-4 receptor (MC4), pro-opiomelanocortin (POMC), corticotropin releasing hormone (CRH), urocortin, melanin-concentrating hormone (MCH), galanin, leptin, adiponectin, ghrelin, cocaine- and amphetamine-regulated transcript (CART), orexins, cholecystokinin (CCK), bombesin, growth hormone (GH), glucagon-like peptide-1 (GLP-1), uncoupling proteins 2 and 3 (UCP2/UCP3), beta-adrenergic receptors, nuclear factor kappa B (NF-κB) and other transcription factors, glycogen synthase kinase-3 beta (GSK-3β), beta-catenin, tumor necrosis factor (TNF) (also known as TNF-alpha), interleukins, and brain derived neurotrophic factor (BDNF).[3] These molecules are involved in HPA-axis, neuroimmune, and endocrine regulation; central nervous system (CNS) and peripheral pro- and anti-inflammatory effects; synaptic transmission and function; appetite regulation; immune cell and system responses; gene transcription; and energy production, respiration, and protein packaging and transport. There is considerable cross-talk between these molecules and systems, and on the whole, self-amplifying feedback loops may develop at the molecular and behavioral levels whereby obesity leads to depression, which leads to greater obesity (or vice versa). For example, obesity often leads to low self-esteem and depressed mood and behavior. Depression in turn may cause increased food intake and decreased exercise, which together lead to increased body weight (body weight changes are a component of the official diagnostic criteria for depression) and elevated cortisol levels, which promote hunger (especially for unhealthy foods) and weight gain.[3] Accordingly, reciprocal meta-analyses of eight and nine longitudinal studies, respectively, showed that obesity at baseline was associated with a 1.55-fold increase in depression incidence at follow-up, and depression at baseline was associated with a 1.58 times increased risk of developing obesity.[4]

10.2.2. Shared Genetics: Functional Implications and Novel Targets

Compounding these molecular, physiologic, and behavioral effects, an individual's inherent genetic variation in these or other (known or unknown) molecular pathways likely plays a significant role in predetermining the risk for obesity and depression. The risk for both depression and obesity has heritable components, and evidence for a shared genetic architecture is rapidly growing. Using whole-exome sequencing of two family trios, each comprising the parents and an offspring with extreme morbid obesity, we recently identified sequence variants in the low-density lipoprotein (LDL) receptor-related protein 2 (*LRP2*) and *UCP2* genes, and overrepresentation of four pathways coded by the *UCP2* gene, with high likelihood of contributing to the extreme morbid obesity phenotype. The overrepresented pathways included peroxisome proliferator-activated receptor (PPAR) regulation of lipid metabolism; effects of insulin, insulin-like growth factor 1 (IGF-1), and TNF in brown adipocyte differentiation; mitochondrial dysfunction in neurodegenerative diseases; and roles of Sirtuin1 (SIRT1) and peroxisome proliferator-activated receptor gamma coactivator 1-alpha (PGC-1α) in oxidative stress.[5] Albeit a small study, these results have significant implications for identifying functional and mechanistic links between obesity and depression, since both genes and all the pathways have been linked with depression in humans or mouse models. UCP2, for example, is an inner mitochondrial membrane protein that participates in ATP (energy) production and regulation of oxidative stress, which has previously been strongly linked with obesity. One major theory of depression, the "network" theory, posits that reduced neurogenesis and/or neuroplasticity are significant contributors to depression, and that antidepressants' therapeutic action results from increasing monoamine levels, which in turn enhances neurogenesis and neuroplasticity to reduce depression.[6] The UCPs as a group play substantial roles in synaptic modulation and plasticity,[7,8] and more recently *Ucp2* knockout in particular was shown to induce depressive behaviors and impaired neurogenesis in a mouse model.[9] Similarly, there is significant cross-talk among the PPAR, insulin, IGF-1, TNF, and SIRT1 signaling pathways, and all of these molecules have been linked to depressive behaviors, neurogenesis, and/or neuroplasticity in humans or rodent models.[10–18] Finally, LRP2 (also known as megalin) levels were significantly higher in the amygdala and orbitofrontal cortex (Brodmann area 11) (BA11)— two brain regions that are central to depression pathology—of Alzheimer's disease patients with depression, compared to Alzheimer's patients without depression.[19] It would be useful to perform a similar study to see whether these findings can be replicated in major depressive disorder (MDD) patients versus controls, to help validate LRP2 as a potential novel therapeutic target for depression comorbid with obesity.

In a larger genomic study, we identified a substantial number of single nucleotide polymorphisms (SNPs) in 68 candidate genes for obesity, along with information on the expected functional effects of these SNPs.[20] Many of the 68 candidate genes have also been implicated in depression, including the UCPs, insulin, IGF, adrenergic receptors, dopamine receptor D2, leptin, and neuropeptide Y, among others. In genome-wide association studies (GWAS), Samaan et al. identified an SNP in the T-cell acute lymphocytic leukemia 1 gene (*TAL1* rs2984618) that is positively associated with risk of both obesity and MDD across multiethnic populations. In contrast, they found that another obesity risk allele, BDNF rs1401635, was ethnicity-specific: It contributed to MDD risk in Europeans but protected against MDD risk in non-Europeans.[4] This finding partially aligns with one of their previous studies in which they found that a polymorphic (rs9939609 A) variant in the "fat mass and obesity-associated" (*FTO*) gene, which is linked to obesity risk across multiethnic populations, was associated with lower risk of depression.[21] In contrast, Milaneschi et al. "found a positive association between the *FTO* rs9939609 A variant and MDD . . . [that] was completely driven by the atypical MDD subtype."[22] These results are especially intriguing because increased appetite and weight gain are principal diagnostic criteria of the "atypical" variant of MDD, whereas "melancholic" MDD is characterized by loss of appetite and weight.[23] Thus, one might expect the obesity risk *FTO* gene variants to be positively associated with atypical MDD but not melancholic MDD, as this study demonstrated. Together these findings show that stratifying depression into its various subgroups may be a key factor for genomic studies. Supporting this concept, a recent analysis of more than 25,000 samples[24] showed "a strong genetic correlation (0.53) between [body mass index] and MDD with increased appetite and/or weight gain."[25]

From a functional standpoint, most or all of the above-identified gene variants code for molecules that have been ascribed functional roles in obesity and depression. BDNF is a well-known regulator of neurogenesis and neuroplasticity that is implicated in regulation of food intake and obesity,[26] depression,[15] and depression comorbid with obesity.[27–29] Rivera et al. demonstrated that compared to psychiatrically healthy controls, individuals with depression showed a 2.2% increase in body mass index for each *FTO* rs9939609 A risk allele.[30] FTO is also expressed in adult neural stem cells and neurons and regulates adult neurogenesis in mice,[31] which presents an intriguing link to the neurogenesis theory of depression. Together these studies make FTO an attractive novel candidate therapeutic target for treating depression comorbid with obesity. TAL1 has identified roles in development and regulation of monoaminergic circuits[32] and is expressed in human cortical microglia[33] (brain microglia are increasingly appreciated as playing significant roles in normal and aberrant synaptic regulation, and in MDD and depression), making it another appealing candidate for further investigation.

Finally, analysis of multiple GWAS found that several genes linked to BMI and severe obesity—neuronal growth regulator 1 (*NEGR1*), olfactomedin 4 (*OLFM4*), and kinase suppressor of ras 2 (*KSR2*)—were also associated with depression phenotypes.[25] NEGR1 is a regulator of neuronal growth and development that modulates synaptic connectivity and activity in brain regions important to regulating appetite, behavior, and mood[25,34,35] and has thus far been investigated primarily in the context of obesity; its exact role in depression requires further elucidation. Similarly, KSR2 is a molecular scaffolding protein[36] that "regulates energy balance via control of feeding behavior and adaptive thermogenesis . . . [and] modulates sensitivity to leptin."[37] with still relatively unknown functional roles in depression. OLFM4 is involved in immune and inflammatory effects, with its best-identified roles in cancer.[38] Its role in the nervous system is still largely unknown, although intriguingly it is massively upregulated after axonal damage,[39] which may have novel implications for both obesity and depression. Recent methodologic advances in deciphering how genotype variations observed with GWAS may translate to mechanistic changes in protein expression and function and the observed disease phenotype[40] will enhance our understanding of the shared pathophysiologies of obesity and depression.

10.2.3. HPA Axis

The HPA axis is one of the four major neuroendocrine systems and, along with the sympathetic nervous system (SNS), one of two major neuroimmune interfaces that bidirectionally mediate the physiologic and functional responses to stress, along with many other bodily processes. A detailed overview of the HPA axis is beyond the scope of what we can cover here, but it has been expertly covered elsewhere,[41–43] as have the mechanistic and functional links between the HPA axis, depression, and obesity.[25,44-46] For our purposes in this chapter, the key take-home point is that even with the ever-growing list of molecules and systems thought to interact in the shared biology of obesity and depression, the vast majority of them will act, at least in part (and sometimes exclusively), via the HPA axis. We will briefly highlight just a couple of examples here and refer readers to the above and other reviews for more detailed discussions.

Hyperactivation of the HPA axis can occur through numerous mechanisms, including physical or emotional stressors, and leads to elevated cortisol levels, which in turn have been shown to promote both depression and obesity. Some of the earliest evidence that excess cortisol was related to obesity and depression comes from clinical observations of Cushing's syndrome, which is caused by a pathologic hypercortisolemia and typically accompanied by symptoms of obesity, depression, and other metabolic disruption, including glucose intolerance, dyslipidemia, and hypertension. While it is well established that HPA-axis activation and excess cortisol lead to metabolic syndrome and obesity, our understanding of the precise downstream mechanisms by which cortisol enacts these effects is growing yet remains incomplete—likely in large part because cortisol binds to the glucocorticoid receptor, and this complex then homodimerizes and translocates to the nucleus to enact a vast array of downstream effects by binding to glucocorticoid response elements and modulating transcription of numerous cortisol-responsive genes.[45,47] There are numerous pleiotropic and tightly intertwined downstream mediators in these effects, and we discuss a few of them briefly in Sections 10.2.3.1 and 10.2.3.2.

10.2.3.1. Adipose System, Glucocorticoids, Leptin, and Inflammation

Far from being a passive depot for fat storage, the adipose system is now understood to be a complex and dynamic array consisting of adipocytes (fat cells), immune cells, and blood vessels and other architectural components that act in concert to regulate metabolic and inflammatory processes as they impact health and disease.[48,49] Inflammatory mechanisms originating from adipose tissue and obesity phenotypes have earned newfound importance as likely contributors to diseases ranging from cancer to psychiatric disease, including depression. In the periphery, elevated cortisol levels are believed to contribute to obesity by glucocorticoid-mediated upregulation of pathways involved in adipogenesis and fat deposition.[50] In the brain, glucocorticoids stimulate food intake by interacting with several appetite-regulating targets in the arcuate nucleus of the hypothalamus: In this region, they increase adenosine monophosphate (AMP)-activated protein kinase signaling and upregulate expression of the orexigenic NPY and agouti-related peptide (AGRP).[51]

Glucocorticoids also help regulate leptin, the first identified "adipokine"—that is, cytokine-like hormones produced by adipose tissue that regulate physiologic processes such as food intake, energy metabolism, insulin sensitivity, reproduction, stress responses, bone growth, and inflammation.[52] Leptin released into the circulatory system by adipose tissue crosses the blood–brain barrier, whereupon it binds to leptin receptors in the hypothalamus, the primary brain center for regulating food intake and body weight.[53] Typically leptin acts as an anorexigenic adipokine, serving to decrease food intake (signal satiety and suppress appetite) and increase energy expenditure to maintain body fat stores at normal levels.[53] However, activated hypothalamic leptin receptors can either directly or indirectly induce downstream expression of various anorexigenic (e.g., POMC, CRH, BDNF) and orexigenic (e.g., NPY, AGRP, orexin) peptides,[53] so leptin may have pleiotropic effects that are ultimately dependent on the net result of all activated pathways. Glucocorticoids stimulate leptin release from adipocytes yet also promote leptin resistance in the brain,[51] so they too can also exert opposing effects on leptin pathways. The anorexigenic hormone ghrelin, secreted by the stomach and produced by some neurons in the brain, is one of the primary appetite-stimulatory signals and likely interplays bidirectionally with leptin pathways to regulate food intake and body fat.[53,54]

In 1997, Montague et al. discovered that congenital leptin deficiency in humans was associated with severe early-onset obesity,[55] and innate or acquired leptin resistance is associated with more common forms of obesity.[56] Obese individuals without congenital leptin deficiency (a rare condition) have high circulating leptin levels that are directly correlated with adiposity (fat mass) and develop leptin resistance (akin to the insulin resistance that develops in pre-T2D).[57] For this reason, leptin replacement therapy has been astonishingly effective at normalizing weight and metabolic profiles in those with congenital leptin deficiency, but less so in patients with common obesity.[56] We and others have also since discovered that leptin mediates or influences all components of MetS, including obesity, dyslipidemia, insulin sensitivity and glucose homeostasis, and blood pressure.[57–59] Leptin deficiency is linked to depression and antidepressant resistance in humans and animals, and leptin has antidepressant effects that have been shown to involve glucocorticoids, GSK-3β, β-catenin, synaptic plasticity, neurogenesis, glutamate, and dopamine.[60–66]

Beyond leptin, our understanding of how the HPA axis and these other molecular players also impact depression, as well as obesity, is expanding. Cortisol, glucocorticoids, leptin, ghrelin, NPY, AGRP, BDNF, and numerous pro- and anti-inflammatory cytokines, just to name a few, have all been implicated in the pathophysiology of MDD. Numerous studies have demonstrated that individuals with MetS have a higher prevalence of depression, and individuals with depression are more likely to have MetS.[67–69] Depression may lead to a vicious cycle of HPA-axis hyperactivation and consequent hypercortisolemia, leading to increased MetS, which further amplifies depression. Cortisol itself may promote depression directly via inhibitory actions on serotoninergic systems in the brain.[41] Obesity is characterized by a chronic, low-grade inflammatory state and release of pro-inflammatory cytokines and adipokines from adipose tissue, which can promote depression via stimulation of the HPA axis, or by direct molecular actions.[25,45] For example, pro-inflammatory cytokines such as interleukin-6 and TNF are known players in synaptic regulation, mediate sickness behavior, and are increasingly believed to contribute to depression pathology.[15] These and similar molecules are also implicated in neurodegeneration and neurodegenerative disorders, and thus may contribute to the hippocampal neurodegeneration found in depressed subjects.[6,15] There are far too many similar examples to cover each individually, but these kinds of functional and molecular interrelationships relevant to both obesity and depression have been well detailed elsewhere.[44,68,70–77]

10.2.3.2. Microbiome

Interestingly, HPA-axis–mediated effects of obesity on depression risk may even cross generations, as maternal obesity and HPA-axis dysregulation have been linked to an increased risk of obesity, depression, and other psychiatric disorders in offspring.[45,51,78–80] And the gut microbiome may be a potential mediator of this effect. Maternal high-fat diets or obesity prenatally or perinatally have been linked with changes in the offspring's synaptic and hippocampal function and behavior,[81–85] which in turn are believed to contribute to depression pathophysiology.[86] In another fascinating study, offspring from high-fat–fed mothers showed aberrant social behavior and synaptic deficits in the dopaminergic circuits of the ventral tegmental area

(VTA), accompanied by decreased abundance of several species of gut bacteria.[87] Interestingly, treatment with (i.e., microbial restoration of) only the single bacterial species that was most drastically reduced, *Lactobacillus reuteri*, ameliorated the behavioral and VTA synaptic deficits in the afflicted offspring by restoring oxytocin neurons in the paraventricular nucleus (PVN) of the hypothalamus (oxytocin-producing neurons in the PVN project to the VTA[88])—which the authors hypothesized was occurring via vagal nerve projections from the gut to the PVN.[87] The PVN is the central hypothalamic component of the HPA axis,[42] and the VTA (which projects to the hippocampus, among other areas) and oxytocin also have probable roles in depression, obesity, and T2D.[89-93]

The gut microbiome (i.e., the sum population of all bacterial species in the gut) is a chief component of the gut–brain axis, a bidirectional communication network consisting of the gut, microbiome, CNS (brain and spinal cord), autonomic and enteric nervous systems, and HPA axis, which serves to regulate metabolic and physiologic processes, and in recent years has become a significant topic of interest as a previously unappreciated mediator of both peripheral and CNS health and disease. A detailed appreciation of the microbiome and gut–brain axis is beyond the scope of what we can cover here (instead see references 94–98 and Chapter 24 in this volume for more complete coverage of this topic), but it involves all the same hormonal, immune, and neural molecular signals as we have described above. Figure 10.1 illustrates the various components of the microbiome–gut–brain axis and provides a top-level overview of many of the bidirectional signaling networks discussed in this chapter (Figure 10.1A), which when disrupted can lead to a variety of metabolic and psychiatric conditions (Figure 10.1B).

With these many shared effector pathways, the microbiome has recently been ascribed putative roles in obesity, T2D,[99] CVD, and depression, as well as numerous other neurologic, psychiatric, and peripheral diseases.[100-104] For example, we and colleagues recently reported that the gut microbiome mediates depressive-like behavior in a mouse model,[105] effects that may be regulated by inflammasome signaling via caspase-1.[106] Another mouse study demonstrated that consumption of *Lactobacillus rhamnosus* bacteria reduced anxiety- and depression-related behavior and stress-induced corticosterone levels, and altered gamma-aminobutyric acid (GABA) receptor expression (mRNA levels) in several brain regions relevant to depression.[107] And as the authors state very nicely:

> Moreover, the neurochemical and behavioral effects were not found in vagotomized mice, identifying the vagus as a major modulatory constitutive communication pathway between the bacteria exposed to the gut and the brain. Together, these findings highlight the important role of bacteria in the bidirectional communication of the gut–brain axis and suggest that certain organisms may prove to be useful therapeutic adjuncts in stress-related disorders such as anxiety and depression.[107]

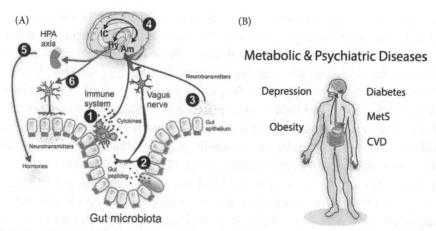

FIGURE 10.1. The microbiome–gut–brain axis in depression and metabolic disease. (A) Direct and indirect pathways make up the bidirectional interactions between the gut microbiota and the CNS, involving endocrine, immune, and neural signaling. Afferent pathways signaling to the brain (up arrows) include (1) peripheral lymphocytes or other immune cells that release pro- or anti-inflammatory cytokines, which can have endocrine or paracrine actions, (2) sensory nerve terminals, such as on the vagus nerve, may be activated by gut peptides released by enteroendocrine cells, and (3) neurotransmitters emanating from the gut, such as serotonin synthesized and released by enterochromaffin cells (an enteroendocrine cell subtype), also have endocrine and paracrine effects in both the CNS and periphery. (4) In the CNS, after the brainstem relays (e.g. the solitary nucleus), the amygdala (Am) and insular cortex (IC) integrate visceral inputs, and hypothalamic (Hy) activation initiates the efferent arm (down arrows), whereby (5) HPA-axis activation releases corticosteroids (e.g., cortisol), which effect many actions as described in this chapter, and can also modulate gut microbiota composition. (6) Activation of neuronal efferents releases neurotransmitters with a variety of effects on the periphery, including modulation of the gut microbiome. (B) Loss of homeostasis in one or more of these pathways is believed to contribute to numerous disease conditions, including but not limited to depression, obesity, MetS, T2D, and CVD, as we detail in this chapter. *The figure and legend are reprinted with modifications from reference 108 under the Creative Commons Attribution License (CC BY) (https://creativecommons.org/licenses/by/3.0/).*

This study illustrates one of many ways by which gut microbiota may contribute to the functional and synaptic pathophysiology of depression via these closely intertwined pathways. We are fortunate to be able to refer readers to our colleagues' Chapter 24 in this volume for complementary and much more comprehensive coverage of this complex topic.

10.2.4. Monoamines and Obesity

The monoaminergic neurotransmitters include the catecholamines dopamine, epinephrine (adrenaline), and norepinephrine (noradrenaline); the tryptamine serotonin; and histamine. Monoamines have long been understood to play key roles in MDD, and the vast majority of antidepressant drugs are believed to exert their therapeutic effect via one or more of these circuits. Moreover, at various points in the CNS, HPA axis, and microbiota–gut–brain axis, the monoaminergic circuits act either directly or in concert with many of the immune and endocrine molecules discussed in this section to regulate food intake, adiposity, metabolism, and body weight.[109–112] Hence it is not surprising that a frequently reported side effect of antidepressant medications is weight gain.[109] Indeed, a recent population study confirmed that individuals using antidepressants gained more weight than non-users. However, this effect was mostly due to selective serotonin reuptake inhibitor (SSRI) use (there was no association with tricyclic antidepressants [TCAs] or other antidepressant use and weight gain), and the link between SSRI use and weight gain was strongest in the context of unhealthy lifestyle factors such as high intake of a Western diet, sedentary habits, and smoking.[113] Other monoaminergic and neurotransmitter circuits have also been implicated in hunger, weight gain, and obesity.[110,112] Finally, obesity is associated with higher levels of circulating cytokines, which in turn play significant roles in modulating monoamine and other neurotransmitter signaling linked to both depression and obesity.[73]

10.3. T2D AND DEPRESSION

Obesity and MetS are known risk factors for developing insulin resistance and T2D; thus, unsurprisingly, the molecular links between depression and diabetes are similar to those discussed in Section 10.2.3. As with obesity, depressed individuals are more likely to have T2D,[114] and those with T2D are more likely to be depressed,[115] which may establish a similar self-amplifying feedback loop. T2D is also associated with a twofold increase in clinical depression risk, and depression comorbid with T2D is linked to poor glycemic control, higher mortality rates, and perhaps increased CVD risk (see reference 116 and references therein). In addition, insulin resistance and glucose dysregulation may have direct functional and metabolic consequences in the brain. Glucose is the key fuel for the brain and synaptic transmission, and either too little or too much of this key nutrient in the brain has been linked to depression, dementia, and a variety of neurodegenerative and peripheral diseases.[117,118] Similarly, insulin, the key molecule involved in systemic glucose homeostasis, regulates both brain function and systemic metabolism, and insulin resistance or dysregulation in the brain has likewise been linked to depression, cognitive dysfunction, and other neurologic disease.[119–132]

At the same time, common molecular mechanisms cannot entirely explain the links between T2D and depression, because versus the general population, depression prevalence is increased only in those with diagnosed diabetes, not in those with undiagnosed diabetes.[116,133] Moreover, diabetics with diabetic complications have a higher risk of depression than diabetics without complications.[134] Thus there appears to be an additional confounding element of psychological distress, or "diabetes distress" (i.e., "the concerns and worries about diabetes and its management"[116]) that contributes in significant yet still undefined ways to depression comorbid with diabetes. Greater understanding of how "diabetes distress" interacts with shared biologic mechanisms will be critical to preventing, identifying, and treating MDD together with T2D.

10.4. CVD AND DEPRESSION

10.4.1. Shared Genetics

In a familiar story, depression is associated with an increased risk of CVD, and vice versa, leading to increased morbidity and mortality when the conditions are comorbid, with many expected shared pathophysiologic mechanisms.[135–141] Here we will briefly discuss the epidemiologic and functional links between depression and specific aspects of CVD—for example, dyslipidemia and hypertension—to the extent not already covered in Sections 10.1 through 10.3.

Meta-analyses of numerous GWAS have associated depression or mood disorders with many genes linked to particular aspects of CVD, a few of which include the genes for methylenetetrahydrofolate reductase (MTHFR) (blood pressure); calcium voltage-gated channel subunit alpha1 D (CACNA1D) (blood pressure and hypertension); RE1-silencing transcription factor (REST) (coronary artery disease); FTO (HDL cholesterol or triglycerides); neurocan (NCAN) (total cholesterol, triglycerides, LDL cholesterol); GSK-3β (HDL cholesterol); apolipoprotein E (APOE) (HDL, LDL, total cholesterol). These and the other genes listed (see reference 142) provide attractive targets for identifying functional and mechanistic links between CVD and depression.

10.4.2. Cholesterol and Lipids

The associations between depression and genes related to lipid metabolism are especially interesting, in our view, because cholesterol and lipids have long been appreciated as central components of cellular and neuronal membranes, and hence critical regulators of neuronal and synaptic health and function.[143–148] Not surprisingly, then, there is solid evidence that dyslipidemia can, at minimum, be correlated with depression, suicidality, and other psychiatric disease.[149] However, the findings in this area are too nuanced to allow for simplistic conclusions such as "Any dyslipidemia associated with MetS (e.g., high total cholesterol, high triglycerides, low HDL/LDL or HDL/total cholesterol ratios) is positively correlated with depression." In fact, albeit with some exceptions that have reported positive or no associations between lipid levels and depression or suicide, the majority of reports have found that total and individual serum lipid levels (i.e., cholesterol, triglycerides, HDL, LDL) are negatively correlated with depression and suicidality—that is, lower across the board in depressed or suicidal patients versus controls.[149,150] This general finding is consistent with substantial other literature that has reported deficits in key synaptic lipids (e.g., multiple species of phosphatidylcholine and sphingomyelin in one example[151]) associated with depression and other psychiatric disease.[149,152,153] In other words, lower levels of various broad lipid types appear to correlate with deficits in key lipid subspecies that are critical to maintaining synaptic homeostasis.

At the same time, although low HDL ("good") cholesterol levels have consistently been linked to depression and suicidality (consistent with this model), the picture for LDL cholesterol and depression has been far more heterogeneous.[154] We expect, and there is some evidence[155] to suggest, that these inconsistencies likely result from the immune-inflammatory response seen in depression, which would tend to drive HDL levels down and LDL levels up.

Moving from correlative findings to potential causal mechanisms, many studies have linked deficits in key neuronal and synaptic lipid species to changes in neurotransmitter signaling.[149,152,153] In animal models, lower brain levels of polyunsaturated fatty acids (PUFAs) such as docosahexaenoic acid (DHA) correlate with lower serotonin (5-HT) and higher 5-HT_{2A} receptor levels, which is consistent with the reduced levels of 5-HT and increased 5-HT_{2A} found postmortem in brains of depressed patients and individuals dying by suicide.[152] Likewise, other human studies have consistently found lower DHA levels in depression- or suicide-relevant areas of the brains of depressed individuals.[152] In keeping with this model, HDL and 5-hydroxyindolacetic (5-HIAA) levels were both lower in suicide attempters versus controls[156] (5-HIAA is a 5-HT metabolite that correlates with 5-HT levels). Similar results have been found for multiple other types of lipid or fatty acid compounds, and other neurotransmitter systems involved in depression (reviewed in references 152 and 153). Overall, the data support the general principles that deficits of key neuronal and synaptic lipids may causally contribute to depression and other psychiatric disease, as one might anticipate given their critical roles in neuronal function.

10.4.3. Blood Pressure

As for the other aspects of CVD comorbid with depression, blood pressure control is influenced by the SNS, HPA axis, and immune-inflammatory molecules and mechanisms. Recent evidence also implicates the microbiome in hypertension[157,158] and hypertension comorbid with obesity.[159] Studies on the relationships between depression and blood pressure or hypertension have shown variable results. Some reports have found increased hypertension risk for MDD subjects, whereas others have found the opposite. Conversely, some longitudinal studies have reported that low blood pressure at baseline is predictive for later depressive symptoms, whereas other such studies concluded that high blood pressure at baseline predicts later depression. Hypertension is an important risk factor for CVD, and the studies of connections between depression and CVD have been less dichotomous. However, whether hypertension promotes depression, or vice versa, and whether similar mechanisms promote both independently remain open questions. Several observations may help explain these often conflicting findings. First, activation of the SNS is a hallmark of hypertension,[160] and Barton et al. reported a distinctly bimodal distribution of SNS activity in MDD patients, with one subset having lower SNS activity versus non-depressed normals and the other MDD subset having higher SNS activity versus normals.[161] This finding alone could explain the apparently variable associations between depression and hypertension. In addition, different types of antidepressants,[162] as well as antihypertensives, can have opposing effects on blood pressure, which makes medication status another key factor that likely contributes to this observed variability. While further research is needed to clarify exactly how blood pressure and hypertension relate to depression risk, the critical point is that, as for other elements of CVD, cross-talk between the same molecular pathways of the SNS, HPA axis, immune-inflammation, and the microbiome can be expected to influence both hypertension and depression morbidity, in ways that are likely reciprocal and may be causal.

10.4.4. Depression and Non-CVD Cardiac Risk

Depression also increases risk for several acute cardiac abnormalities not related to CVD or coronary artery disease—such as Takotsubo cardiomyopathy (aka "broken heart syndrome") and sudden cardiac death—likely through similar triggers, mechanisms, and pathways that include extreme (and often acute) emotional or physical stress or distress, SNS hyperactivity, and catecholamine overload.[163,164] Hence, similar mechanisms may link depression with non-CVD–related cardiac risk as well.

10.5. INHERITED METABOLIC DISEASES: TARGETING CELL STRESS

Inherited metabolic diseases (IMDs) are those "caused by defective activity in a single enzyme or transport protein" resulting from a defective gene (frequently autosomal recessive) and include "aminoacidopathies, creatine disorders, mitochondrial cytopathies, peroxisomal disorders and lysosomal storage disorders."[165] Although their affected genes and systems and thus symptomologies are too broad to link them all to depression, a large number of them include significant neurologic components, and often first manifest with psychiatric symptoms, including depression.[165–167] Very broad themes that emerge across all IMDs are that they may lead to neurologic or psychiatric symptoms, including depression, through their impact on neurodevelopmental processes and disruptions of neurotransmitter systems.[167] Significant for our discussion in this section, IMDs linked to mitochondrial or lysosomal storage dysfunctions often appear to have particularly strong links to depression. For example, depression incidence in Fabry disease, a lysosomal storage disorder, has been estimated at 15% to 62%,[168] with the largest study reporting a 42% prevalence.[169] Psychiatric illness can be the presenting symptom of mitochondrial disorders, with mood disorders being the most commonly associated psychiatric symptoms: In one analysis, 44% of patients with mitochondrial disorders presented with MDD, plus 4% with bipolar disorder (48% total with depression).[170]

While IMDs are relatively rare, they are relevant to our discussions because they as a whole,[167] and perhaps especially lysosomal storage and mitochondrial IMDs,[171] activate multiple pathogenic cascades significant to neuronal and synaptic function, including mitochondrial and oxidative stress, calcium homeostasis, endo/exocytosis and lipid trafficking, cell death pathways, endoplasmic reticulum (ER) stress, inflammation, and immune responses.[171] We have already covered the implications of many of these areas for depression pathophysiology in Sections 10.1 through 10.4 (e.g., inflammation, immune responses, and lipids), but in addition, mitochondrial, ER, and oxidative stress have become emerging therapeutic areas of interest for depression treatment. Thus these areas tie together the pathophysiologies of depression and IMDs and represent novel opportunities for integrated treatment of depression comorbid with IMDs.

10.6. ARE INTEGRATED THERAPIES THE FUTURE?

On the basis of existing knowledge, some have already suggested integrated therapeutic strategies for treating depression comorbid with various kinds of metabolic disease.[15,172] Here, we define "integrated therapies" as a single drug, or combination of drugs, expressly indicated to simultaneously benefit two or more conditions, such as depression comorbid with obesity (and/or T2D, CVD, etc.). For example, SSRIs may be an optimal pharmacologic treatment for depression in patients with CVD for their apparent beneficial (and fewer adverse) effects on myocardial infarction risk, ischemia–reperfusion injury, reduced platelet aggregation, and atherosclerosis compared to other antidepressants like TCAs.[15] More specifically, it has been suggested that "[d]ue to its low risk of drug–drug interactions, adverse effect profile and potential for beneficial antiplatelet activity, sertraline could be considered the choice antidepressant for patients with ischemic heart disease."[173] Similarly, SSRIs may be a good option for diabetes comorbid with depression for their favorable effects on glycemic control compared to other types of antidepressants.[15,174,175] On the other hand, these effects must be monitored closely, as in some cases SSRIs or other antidepressants may contribute to hypoglycemia in diabetics.[176,177]

SSRIs may also induce weight loss in the short term[109] but may lead to long-term weight gain, especially in conjunction with a sedentary lifestyle.[113] The 5-HT$_{2C}$ selective serotonin receptor agonist lorcaserin,[178] and the norepinephrine–dopamine reuptake inhibitor antidepressant bupropion in combination with the opioid receptor antagonist naltrexone,[179] are both believed to have anorexigenic actions in the hypothalamus and are two of the relatively few drugs that have been approved by the US Food and Drug Administration for weight loss.[180] Alternative emerging drug classes such as triple reuptake inhibitors may present new opportunities for simultaneously treating depression, eating disorders, obesity, and T2D,[181] but the need for development of additional novel integrated therapeutics remains. Throughout this chapter we have highlighted numerous genetic and molecular targets evidenced to be involved in the pathophysiology of both depression and comorbid conditions (e.g.,

LRP2 and FTO involvement in depression and obesity), thus making them attractive potential hits for future development of integrated drug therapies.

10.6.1. Side Effects and Contraindications: What Can They Teach Us?

While the 5-HT system is an attractive target for integrated therapies given its ability to influence the pathophysiology of MDD, T2D, and obesity, this allure is sobered by appreciation of the complexities of the serotonergic (and monoaminergic) networks and their sometimes contradictory effects—as we have highlighted throughout this chapter. For example, in the body there are separate CNS and peripheral serotonergic systems;[182] about 95% of the body's 5-HT is in the gut;[183] and weight loss may be triggered by (selectively?) increased 5-HT signaling in the CNS and/or by decreased 5-HT signaling in the periphery.[184] These contradictory signaling effects on weight loss may in part explain the acute versus chronic effects on weight sometimes observed with SSRIs.[109]

In addition to weight gain, another frequent side effect with SSRIs that is also common to and therefore may be further exacerbated by depression comorbidities such as T2D and CVD is sexual dysfunction. In such cases, the comorbidities themselves, and the side effects or exacerbations brought on by pharmacotherapies, may arise by common mechanisms and pathophysiology. For example, both male and female sexual dysfunction are common with obesity, CVD, metabolic syndrome, and T2D,[185] and nitric oxide is but one signaling mechanism common to all these disorders. Intriguingly, and perhaps not surprisingly in this context, while most drugs related to CVD (e.g., antihypertensives, diuretics, and beta-blockers) negatively impact sexual function, the beta-blocker nebivolol—which, like most erectile dysfunction drugs, increases nitric oxide availability and thus has favorable impacts on sexual function—has recently been demonstrated to protect against depressive-like behavior in rats.[186] Indeed, nitric oxide signaling is attracting increasing interest as a target for antidepressant therapies.[187] Similarly, the hypoglycemic drugs metformin, pioglitazone, and liraglutide have shown favorable results for erectile dysfunction,[185] and are all currently being evaluated as antidepressive therapies in humans and/or animal models.[188-190] These and similar studies highlight the growing need to harness and understand the complex interactions between depression, its many comorbidities, and the drugs that treat them, to develop novel integrated therapies for comorbid depression and metabolic disorders.

10.6.2. Drug–Drug Interactions in Depression Comorbidities

Serious adverse drug interactions with modern antidepressants such as SSRIs in clinically routine application are fairly uncommon, although greater potential for serious adverse interactions with older antidepressant classes such as monoamine oxidase inhibitors (MAOIs) and TCAs does exist.[191-193] Moreover, depression's long list of comorbidities means that many individuals are concomitantly taking numerous drugs.

This rise in polypharmacy has led to growing evidence for relevant and nontrivial drug interactions with antidepressants that may have been previously unappreciated, particularly with drugs for depression's major metabolic comorbidities.[173,176] In Section 10.6 we mentioned, for example, that SSRIs or other antidepressants may sometimes contribute to diabetic hypoglycemia.[176,177] Some antidepressants can increase the risk for or exacerbate several aspects of CVD.[173,176] For example, "[h]ypertension can be significant with serotonin norepinephrine reuptake inhibitors (SNRIs) and MAOIs" and "[t]he potential for QT prolongation is present with TCAs, certain selective serotonin reuptake inhibitors (SSRIs), certain SNRIs and mirtazapine."[173] These and similar findings (e.g., see references 173 and 176) highlight both the need for being acutely aware of potential drug interactions when prescribing other drugs concomitant with antidepressants, and the clear need for more deliberately tailored integrated therapies for depression and its comorbidities.

10.7. CONCLUSIONS

There is a tremendous need for novel therapies to treat depression comorbid with metabolic diseases. In this chapter we have highlighted multiple new and emerging potential target molecules and pathways common to depression and comorbid pathologies that are therefore ripe for further exploration, so that we may develop the most effective and comprehensive pharmacotherapies for treating depression in the context of metabolic disorders, to help reduce morbidity and mortality from these significant and growing global health burdens.

REFERENCES

1. Altschule MD. Metabolic disorders as causes of depressions. *Med Sci.* 1964;15:45.
2. Nordman LO. [Diabetes and depression]. *Nord Med.* 1951;46(38):1411–1412.
3. Licinio J, Wong ML. The interface of obesity and depression: risk factors for the metabolic syndrome. *Rev Bras Psiquiatr.* 2003;25(4):196–197.
4. Samaan Z, Lee YK, Gerstein HC, et al. Obesity genes and risk of major depressive disorder in a multiethnic population: a cross-sectional study. *J Clin Psychiatry.* 2015;76(12):e1611–1618.
5. Paz-Filho G, Boguszewski MC, Mastronardi CA, et al. Whole exome sequencing of extreme morbid obesity patients: translational implications for obesity and related disorders. *Genes (Basel).* 2014;5(3):709–725.
6. Dean J, Keshavan M. The neurobiology of depression: an integrated view. *Asian J Psychiatr.* 2017;27:101–111.
7. Cheng A, Hou Y, Mattson MP. Mitochondria and neuroplasticity. *ASN Neuro.* 2010;2(5):e00045.
8. Andrews ZB, Diano S, Horvath TL. Mitochondrial uncoupling proteins in the CNS: in support of function and survival. *Nat Rev Neurosci.* 2005;6(11):829–840.
9. Du RH, Wu FF, Lu M, et al. Uncoupling protein 2 modulation of the NLRP3 inflammasome in astrocytes and its implications in depression. *Redox Biol.* 2016;9:178–187.
10. Colle R, de Larminat D, Rotenberg S, et al. PPAR-gamma agonists for the treatment of major depression: a review. *Pharmacopsychiatry.* 2017;50(2):49–55.
11. Anderson MF, Aberg MA, Nilsson M, Eriksson PS. Insulin-like growth factor-I and neurogenesis in the adult mammalian brain. *Brain Res Dev Brain Res.* 2002;134(1–2):115–122.

12. Ji MJ, Yu XB, Mei ZL, et al. Hippocampal PPAR-delta overexpression or activation represses stress-induced depressive behaviors and enhances neurogenesis. *Int J Neuropsychopharmacol.* 2016;19(1):pyv083.

13. Sharma AN, da Costa e Silva BF, Soares JC, et al. Role of trophic factors GDNF, IGF-1 and VEGF in major depressive disorder: a comprehensive review of human studies. *J Affect Disord.* 2016;197:9–20.

14. Burgdorf J, Zhang XL, Colechio EM, et al. Insulin-like growth factor I produces an antidepressant-like effect and elicits N-methyl-D-aspartate receptor-independent long-term potentiation of synaptic transmission in medial prefrontal cortex and hippocampus. *Int J Neuropsychopharmacol.* 2015;19(2):pyv101.

15. Lang UE, Borgwardt S. Molecular mechanisms of depression: perspectives on new treatment strategies. *Cell Physiol Biochem.* 2013;31(6):761–777.

16. Eyre H, Baune BT. Neuroplastic changes in depression: a role for the immune system. *Psychoneuroendocrinology.* 2012;37(9):1397–1416.

17. Hashmi AM, Butt Z, Umair M. Is depression an inflammatory condition? A review of available evidence. *J Pak Med Assoc.* 2013;63(7):899–906.

18. Song J, Kim J. Role of sirtuins in linking metabolic syndrome with depression. *Front Cell Neurosci.* 2016;10:86.

19. Dekens DW, Naude PJ, Engelborghs S, et al. Neutrophil gelatinase-associated lipocalin and its receptors in Alzheimer's disease (AD) brain regions: differential findings in AD with and without depression. *J Alzheimers Dis.* 2017;55(2):763–776.

20. Irizarry K, Hu G, Wong ML, et al. Single nucleotide polymorphism identification in candidate gene systems of obesity. *Pharmacogenomics J.* 2001;1(3):193–203.

21. Samaan Z, Anand SS, Zhang X, et al. The protective effect of the obesity-associated rs9939609 A variant in fat mass- and obesity-associated gene on depression. *Mol Psychiatry.* 2013;18(12):1281–1286.

22. Milaneschi Y, Lamers F, Mbarek H, et al. The effect of FTO rs9939609 on major depression differs across MDD subtypes. *Mol Psychiatry.* 2014;19(9):960–962.

23. Woelfer M, Kasties V, Kahlfuss S, Walter M. The role of depressive subtypes within the neuroinflammation hypothesis of major depressive disorder. *Neuroscience.* 2019;403:93–110.

24. Milaneschi Y, Lamers F, Peyrot WJ, et al. Genetic association of major depression with atypical features and obesity-related immunometabolic dysregulations. *JAMA Psychiatry.* 2017;74(12):1214–1225.

25. Milaneschi Y, Simmons WK, van Rossum EFC, Penninx BW. Depression and obesity: evidence of shared biological mechanisms. *Mol Psychiatry.* 2019;24(1):18–33.

26. Rosas-Vargas H, Martinez-Ezquerro JD, Bienvenu T. Brain-derived neurotrophic factor, food intake regulation, and obesity. *Arch Med Res.* 2011;42(6):482–494.

27. Lee IT, Fu CP, Lee WJ, et al. Brain-derived neurotrophic factor, but not body weight, correlated with a reduction in depression scale scores in men with metabolic syndrome: a prospective weight-reduction study. *Diabetol Metab Syndr.* 2014;6(1):18.

28. Numakawa T, Richards M, Nakajima S, et al. The role of brain-derived neurotrophic factor in comorbid depression: possible linkage with steroid hormones, cytokines, and nutrition. *Front Psychiatry.* 2014;5:136.

29. Kurhe Y, Mahesh R. Mechanisms linking depression co-morbid with obesity: an approach for serotonergic type 3 receptor antagonist as novel therapeutic intervention. *Asian J Psychiatr.* 2015;17:3–9.

30. Rivera M, Locke AE, Corre T, et al. Interaction between the FTO gene, body mass index and depression: meta-analysis of 13701 individuals. *Br J Psychiatry.* 2017;211(2):70–76.

31. Li L, Zang L, Zhang F, et al. Fat mass and obesity-associated (FTO) protein regulates adult neurogenesis. *Hum Mol Genet.* 2017;26(13):2398–2411.

32. Lahti L, Haugas M, Tikker L, et al. Differentiation and molecular heterogeneity of inhibitory and excitatory neurons associated with midbrain dopaminergic nuclei. *Development.* 2016;143(3):516–529.

33. Galatro TF, Holtman IR, Lerario AM, et al. Transcriptomic analysis of purified human cortical microglia reveals age-associated changes. *Nat Neurosci.* 2017;20(8):1162–1171.

34. Singh K, Loreth D, Pottker B, et al. Neuronal growth and behavioral alterations in mice deficient for the psychiatric disease-associated Negr1 gene. *Front Mol Neurosci.* 2018;11:30.

35. Pischedda F, Szczurkowska J, Cirnaru MD, et al. A cell surface biotinylation assay to reveal membrane-associated neuronal cues: Negr1 regulates dendritic arborization. *Mol Cell Proteomics.* 2014;13(3):733–748.

36. Lim J, Ritt DA, Zhou M, Morrison DK. The CNK2 scaffold interacts with vilse and modulates Rac cycling during spine morphogenesis in hippocampal neurons. *Curr Biol.* 2014;24(7):786–792.

37. Guo L, Costanzo-Garvey DL, Smith DR, Neilsen BK, MacDonald RG, Lewis RE. Kinase suppressor of Ras 2 (KSR2) expression in the brain regulates energy balance and glucose homeostasis. *Mol Metab.* 2017;6(2):194–205.

38. Liu W, Rodgers GP. Olfactomedin 4 expression and functions in innate immunity, inflammation, and cancer. *Cancer Metastasis Rev.* 2016;35(2):201–212.

39. Saunders NR, Noor NM, Dziegielewska KM, et al. Age-dependent transcriptome and proteome following transection of neonatal spinal cord of *Monodelphis domestica* (South American grey short-tailed opossum). *PLoS One.* 2014;9(6):e99080.

40. Keller B, Martini S, Sedor J, Kretzler M. Linking variants from genome-wide association analysis to function via transcriptional network analysis. *Semin Nephrol.* 2010;30(2):177–184.

41. Haddad JJ, Saade NE, Safieh-Garabedian B. Cytokines and neuro-immune-endocrine interactions: a role for the hypothalamic-pituitary-adrenal revolving axis. *J Neuroimmunol.* 2002;133(1-2):1–19.

42. Smith SM, Vale WW. The role of the hypothalamic-pituitary-adrenal axis in neuroendocrine responses to stress. *Dialogues Clin Neurosci.* 2006;8(4):383–395.

43. Mitrovic I. Introduction to the hypothalamo-pituitary-adrenal (HPA) axis (Lecture). http://biochemistry2.ucsf.edu/programs/ptf/mn%20links/HPA%20Axis%20Physio.pdf.

44. Bornstein SR, Schuppenies A, Wong ML, Licinio J. Approaching the shared biology of obesity and depression: the stress axis as the locus of gene-environment interactions. *Mol Psychiatry.* 2006;11(10):892–902.

45. Bose M, Olivan B, Laferrere B. Stress and obesity: the role of the hypothalamic-pituitary-adrenal axis in metabolic disease. *Curr Opin Endocrinol Diabetes Obes.* 2009;16(5):340–346.

46. Lemche E, Chaban OS, Lemche AV. Neuroendorine and epigentic mechanisms subserving autonomic imbalance and HPA dysfunction in the metabolic syndrome. *Front Neurosci.* 2016;10:142.

47. Kyrou I, Chrousos GP, Tsigos C. Stress, visceral obesity, and metabolic complications. *Ann N Y Acad Sci.* 2006;1083:77–110.

48. Hotamisligil GS. Foundations of immunometabolism and implications for metabolic health and disease. *Immunity.* 2017;47(3):406–420.

49. Hotamisligil GS. Inflammation, metaflammation and immunometabolic disorders. *Nature.* 2017;542(7640):177–185.

50. Lee MJ, Pramyothin P, Karastergiou K, Fried SK. Deconstructing the roles of glucocorticoids in adipose tissue biology and the development of central obesity. *Biochim Biophys Acta.* 2014;1842(3):473–481.

51. Sominsky L, Spencer SJ. Eating behavior and stress: a pathway to obesity. *Front Psychol.* 2014;5:434.

52. Paz-Filho G, Wong ML, Licinio J. Ten years of leptin replacement therapy. *Obes Rev.* 2011;12(5):e315–323.

53. Klok MD, Jakobsdottir S, Drent ML. The role of leptin and ghrelin in the regulation of food intake and body weight in humans: a review. *Obes Rev.* 2007;8(1):21–34.

54. de Candia P, Matarese G. Leptin and ghrelin: sewing metabolism onto neurodegeneration. *Neuropharmacology.* 2018;136(Pt B):307–316.

55. Montague CT, Farooqi IS, Whitehead JP, et al. Congenital leptin deficiency is associated with severe early-onset obesity in humans. *Nature.* 1997;387(6636):903–908.

56. Paz-Filho G, Mastronardi CA, Licinio J. Leptin treatment: facts and expectations. *Metabolism.* 2015;64(1):146–156.

57. Paz-Filho G, Mastronardi C, Franco CB, et al. Leptin: molecular mechanisms, systemic pro-inflammatory effects, and clinical implications. *Arq Bras Endocrinol Metabol.* 2012;56(9):597–607.

58. Simonds SE, Pryor JT, Ravussin E, et al. Leptin mediates the increase in blood pressure associated with obesity. *Cell.* 2014;159(6):1404–1416.

59. Paz-Filho G, Mastronardi C, Wong ML, Licinio J. Leptin therapy, insulin sensitivity, and glucose homeostasis. *Indian J Endocrinol Metab.* 2012;16(Suppl 3):S549–S555.

60. Lu XY. The leptin hypothesis of depression: a potential link between mood disorders and obesity? *Curr Opin Pharmacol.* 2007;7(6):648–652.

61. Garza JC, Guo M, Zhang W, Lu XY. Leptin increases adult hippocampal neurogenesis in vivo and in vitro. *J Biol Chem.* 2008;283(26):18238–18247.

62. Guo M, Huang TY, Garza JC, et al. Selective deletion of leptin receptors in adult hippocampus induces depression-related behaviours. *Int J Neuropsychopharmacol.* 2013;16(4): 857–867.

63. Guo M, Lu XY. Leptin receptor deficiency confers resistance to behavioral effects of fluoxetine and desipramine via separable substrates. *Transl Psychiatry.* 2014;4:e486.

64. Guo M, Lu Y, Garza JC, et al. Forebrain glutamatergic neurons mediate leptin action on depression-like behaviors and synaptic depression. *Transl Psychiatry.* 2012;2:e83.

65. Liu J, Perez SM, Zhang W, et al. Selective deletion of the leptin receptor in dopamine neurons produces anxiogenic-like behavior and increases dopaminergic activity in amygdala. *Mol Psychiatry.* 2011;16(10):1024–1038.

66. Milaneschi Y, Lamers F, Bot M, et al. Leptin dysregulation is specifically associated with major depression with atypical features: evidence for a mechanism connecting obesity and depression. *Biol Psychiatry.* 2017;81(9):807–814.

67. Kucerova J, Babinska Z, Horska K, Kotolova H. The common pathophysiology underlying the metabolic syndrome, schizophrenia and depression. A review. *Biomed Pap Med Fac Univ Palacky Olomouc Czech Repub.* 2015;159(2):208–214.

68. Nousen EK, Franco JG, Sullivan EL. Unraveling the mechanisms responsible for the comorbidity between metabolic syndrome and mental health disorders. *Neuroendocrinology.* 2013;98(4):254–266.

69. Marazziti D, Rutigliano G, Baroni S, et al. Metabolic syndrome and major depression. *CNS Spectr.* 2014;19(4):293–304.

70. Wedrychowicz A, Zajac A, Pilecki M, et al. Peptides from adipose tissue in mental disorders. *World J Psychiatry.* 2014;4(4):103–111.

71. Doolin K, Farrell C, Tozzi L, et al. Diurnal hypothalamic-pituitary-adrenal axis measures and inflammatory marker correlates in major depressive disorder. *Int J Mol Sci.* 2017;18(10). doi:10.3390/ijms18102226.

72. Chesnokova V, Pechnick RN, Wawrowsky K. Chronic peripheral inflammation, hippocampal neurogenesis, and behavior. *Brain Behav Immun.* 2016;58:1–8.

73. Felger JC, Lotrich FE. Inflammatory cytokines in depression: neurobiological mechanisms and therapeutic implications. *Neuroscience.* 2013;246:199–229.

74. Shelton RC, Miller AH. Eating ourselves to death (and despair): the contribution of adiposity and inflammation to depression. *Prog Neurobiol.* 2010;91(4):275–299.

75. Choi AJ, Ryter SW. Inflammasomes: molecular regulation and implications for metabolic and cognitive diseases. *Mol Cells*. 2014;37(6):441–448.

76. McElroy SL, Keck PE, Jr. Metabolic syndrome in bipolar disorder: a review with a focus on bipolar depression. *J Clin Psychiatry*. 2014;75(1):46–61.

77. Singhal G, Jaehne EJ, Corrigan F, et al. Inflammasomes in neuroinflammation and changes in brain function: a focused review. *Front Neurosci*. 2014;8:315.

78. Goldstein JM, Holsen L, Huang G, et al. Prenatal stress-immune programming of sex differences in comorbidity of depression and obesity/metabolic syndrome. *Dialogues Clin Neurosci*. 2016;18(4):425–436.

79. Edlow AG. Maternal obesity and neurodevelopmental and psychiatric disorders in offspring. *Prenat Diagn*. 2017;37(1):95–110.

80. Rivera HM, Christiansen KJ, Sullivan EL. The role of maternal obesity in the risk of neuro-psychiatric disorders. *Front Neurosci*. 2015;9:194.

81. Walker CD, Naef L, d'Asti E, et al. Perinatal maternal fat intake affects metabolism and hippocampal function in the offspring: a potential role for leptin. *Ann N Y Acad Sci*. 2008;1144:189–202.

82. Sullivan EL, Nousen EK, Chamlou KA. Maternal high-fat diet consumption during the peri-natal period programs offspring behavior. *Physiol Behav*. 2014;123:236–242.

83. Sullivan EL, Riper KM, Lockard R, Valleau JC. Maternal high-fat diet programming of the neuroendocrine system and behavior. *Horm Behav*. 2015;76:153–161.

84. Sullivan EL, Nousen EK, Chamlou KA, Grove KL. The impact of maternal high-fat diet consumption on neural development and behavior of offspring. *Int J Obes Suppl*. 2012; 2:S7–S13.

85. Lin C, Shao B, Huang H, et al. Maternal high-fat diet programs stress-induced behavioral disorder in adult offspring. *Physiol Behav*. 2015;152(Pt A):119–127.

86. Marsden WN. Synaptic plasticity in depression: molecular, cellular and functional correlates. *Prog Neuropsychopharmacol Biol Psychiatry*. 2013;43:168–184.

87. Buffington SA, Di Prisco GV, Auchtung TA, et al. Microbial reconstitution reverses maternal diet-induced social and synaptic deficits in offspring. *Cell*. 2016;165(7): 1762–1775.

88. Hung LW, Neuner S, Polepalli JS, et al. Gating of social reward by oxytocin in the ventral tegmental area. *Science*. 2017;357(6358):1406–1411.

89. Maejima Y, Yokota S, Nishimori K, Shimomura K. The anorexigenic neural pathways of ox-ytocin and its clinical implication. *Neuroendocrinology*. 2018;107(1):91–104.

90. Zhang H, Wu C, Chen Q, et al. Treatment of obesity and diabetes using oxytocin or analogs in patients and mouse models. *PLoS One*. 2013;8(5):e61477.

91. Polter AM, Kauer JA. Stress and VTA synapses: implications for addiction and depression. *Eur J Neurosci*. 2014;39(7):1179–1188.

92. Naef L, Pitman KA, Borgland SL. Mesolimbic dopamine and its neuromodulators in obesity and binge eating. *CNS Spectr*. 2015;20(6):574–583.

93. Figlewicz DP. Expression of receptors for insulin and leptin in the ventral tegmental area/substantia nigra (VTA/SN) of the rat: historical perspective. *Brain Res*. 2016;1645: 68–70.

94. Agusti A, Garcia-Pardo MP, Lopez-Almela I, et al. Interplay between the gut-brain axis, obe-sity and cognitive function. *Front Neurosci*. 2018;12:155.

95. Carabotti M, Scirocco A, Maselli MA, Severi C. The gut-brain axis: interactions between en-teric microbiota, central and enteric nervous systems. *Ann Gastroenterol*. 2015;28(2):203–209.

96. Bonaz B, Bazin T, Pellissier S. The vagus nerve at the interface of the microbiota-gut-brain axis. *Front Neurosci*. 2018;12:49.

97. Bonaz B, Sinniger V, Pellissier S. The vagus nerve in the neuro-immune axis: implications in the pathology of the gastrointestinal tract. *Front Immunol*. 2017;8:1452.

98. Sherwin E, Sandhu KV, Dinan TG, Cryan JF. May the force be with you: the light and dark sides of the microbiota-gut-brain axis in neuropsychiatry. *CNS Drugs*. 2016;30(11):1019–1041.

99. Graessler J, Qin Y, Zhong H, et al. Metagenomic sequencing of the human gut microbiome before and after bariatric surgery in obese patients with type 2 diabetes: correlation with inflammatory and metabolic parameters. *Pharmacogenomics J*. 2013;13(6):514–522.

100. Rogers GB, Keating DJ, Young RL, et al. From gut dysbiosis to altered brain function and mental illness: mechanisms and pathways. *Mol Psychiatry*. 2016;21(6):738–748.

101. Gilbert JA, Blaser MJ, Caporaso JG, et al. Current understanding of the human microbiome. *Nat Med*. 2018;24(4):392–400.

102. Shreiner AB, Kao JY, Young VB. The gut microbiome in health and in disease. *Curr Opin Gastroenterol*. 2015;31(1):69–75.

103. Wiley NC, Dinan TG, Ross RP, et al. The microbiota-gut-brain axis as a key regulator of neural function and the stress response: implications for human and animal health. *J Anim Sci*. 2017;95(7):3225–3246.

104. Grenham S, Clarke G, Cryan JF, Dinan TG. Brain-gut-microbe communication in health and disease. *Front Physiol*. 2011;2:94.

105. Zheng P, Zeng B, Zhou C, et al. Gut microbiome remodeling induces depressive-like behaviors through a pathway mediated by the host's metabolism. *Mol Psychiatry*. 2016;21(6):786–796.

106. Wong ML, Inserra A, Lewis MD, et al. Inflammasome signaling affects anxiety- and depressive-like behavior and gut microbiome composition. *Mol Psychiatry*. 2016;21(6):797–805.

107. Bravo JA, Forsythe P, Chew MV, et al. Ingestion of Lactobacillus strain regulates emotional behavior and central GABA receptor expression in a mouse via the vagus nerve. *Proc Natl Acad Sci U S A*. 2011;108(38):16050–16055.

108. Montiel-Castro AJ, Gonzalez-Cervantes RM, Bravo-Ruiseco G, Pacheco-Lopez G. The microbiota-gut-brain axis: neurobehavioral correlates, health and sociality. *Front Integr Neurosci*. 2013;7:70.

109. Lee SH, Paz-Filho G, Mastronardi C, et al. Is increased antidepressant exposure a contributory factor to the obesity pandemic? *Transl Psychiatry*. 2016;6:e759.

110. Halford JC, Cooper GD, Dovey TM. The pharmacology of human appetite expression. *Curr Drug Targets*. 2004;5(3):221–240.

111. Harrold JA, Dovey TM, Blundell JE, Halford JC. CNS regulation of appetite. *Neuropharmacology*. 2012;63(1):3–17.

112. Halford JC, Harrold JA. Neuropharmacology of human appetite expression. *Dev Disabil Res Rev*. 2008;14(2):158–164.

113. Shi Z, Atlantis E, Taylor AW, et al. SSRI antidepressant use potentiates weight gain in the context of unhealthy lifestyles: results from a 4-year Australian follow-up study. *BMJ Open*. 2017;7(8):e016224.

114. Mezuk B, Eaton WW, Albrecht S, Golden SH. Depression and type 2 diabetes over the lifespan: a meta-analysis. *Diabetes Care*. 2008;31(12):2383–2390.

115. Nouwen A, Winkley K, Twisk J, et al. Type 2 diabetes mellitus as a risk factor for the onset of depression: a systematic review and meta-analysis. *Diabetologia*. 2010;53(12):2480–2486.

116. Nouwen A. Depression and diabetes distress. *Diabet Med*. 2015;32(10):1261–1263.

117. van Praag H, Fleshner M, Schwartz MW, Mattson MP. Exercise, energy intake, glucose homeostasis, and the brain. *J Neurosci*. 2014;34(46):15139–15149.

118. Mergenthaler P, Lindauer U, Dienel GA, Meisel A. Sugar for the brain: the role of glucose in physiological and pathological brain function. *Trends Neurosci*. 2013;36(10):587–597.

119. Banks WA, Owen JB, Erickson MA. Insulin in the brain: there and back again. *Pharmacol Ther*. 2012;136(1):82–93.

120. Moulton CD, Pickup JC, Ismail K. The link between depression and diabetes: the search for shared mechanisms. *Lancet Diabetes Endocrinol*. 2015;3(6):461–471.

121. Straub RH. Insulin resistance, selfish brain, and selfish immune system: an evolutionarily positively selected program used in chronic inflammatory diseases. *Arthritis Res Ther.* 2014;16(Suppl 2):S4.

122. Ghasemi R, Dargahi L, Haeri A, et al. Brain insulin dysregulation: implication for neurological and neuropsychiatric disorders. *Mol Neurobiol.* 2013;47(3):1045–1065.

123. Detka J, Kurek A, Basta-Kaim A, et al. Neuroendocrine link between stress, depression and diabetes. *Pharmacol Rep.* 2013;65(6):1591–1600.

124. Holden RJ. The role of brain insulin in the neurophysiology of serious mental disorders: review. *Med Hypotheses.* 1999;52(3):193–200.

125. Kullmann S, Heni M, Hallschmid M, et al. Brain insulin resistance at the crossroads of metabolic and cognitive disorders in humans. *Physiol Rev.* 2016;96(4):1169–1209.

126. Werner H, LeRoith D. Insulin and insulin-like growth factor receptors in the brain: physiological and pathological aspects. *Eur Neuropsychopharmacol.* 2014;24(12):1947–1953.

127. Kullmann S, Heni M, Fritsche A, Preissl H. Insulin action in the human brain: evidence from neuroimaging studies. *J Neuroendocrinol.* 2015;27(6):419–423.

128. Kleinridders A, Ferris HA, Cai W, Kahn CR. Insulin action in brain regulates systemic metabolism and brain function. *Diabetes.* 2014;63(7):2232–2243.

129. Gray SM, Meijer RI, Barrett EJ. Insulin regulates brain function, but how does it get there? *Diabetes.* 2014;63(12):3992–3997.

130. Cetinkalp S, Simsir IY, Ertek S. Insulin resistance in brain and possible therapeutic approaches. *Curr Vasc Pharmacol.* 2014;12(4):553–564.

131. Ghasemi R, Haeri A, Dargahi L, et al. Insulin in the brain: sources, localization and functions. *Mol Neurobiol.* 2013;47(1):145–171.

132. Derakhshan F, Toth C. Insulin and the brain. *Curr Diabetes Rev.* 2013;9(2):102–116.

133. Nouwen A, Nefs G, Caramlau I, et al. Prevalence of depression in individuals with impaired glucose metabolism or undiagnosed diabetes: a systematic review and meta-analysis of the European Depression in Diabetes (EDID) Research Consortium. *Diabetes Care.* 2011;34(3):752–762.

134. Pouwer F, Beekman AT, Nijpels G, et al. Rates and risks for co-morbid depression in patients with type 2 diabetes mellitus: results from a community-based study. *Diabetologia.* 2003;46(7):892–898.

135. Nemeroff CB, Goldschmidt-Clermont PJ. Heartache and heartbreak—the link between depression and cardiovascular disease. *Nat Rev Cardiol.* 2012;9(9):526–539.

136. Seligman F, Nemeroff CB. The interface of depression and cardiovascular disease: therapeutic implications. *Ann N Y Acad Sci.* 2015;1345:25–35.

137. Hare DL, Toukhsati SR, Johansson P, Jaarsma T. Depression and cardiovascular disease: a clinical review. *Eur Heart J.* 2014;35(21):1365–1372.

138. Halaris A. Co-morbidity between cardiovascular pathology and depression: role of inflammation. *Mod Trends Pharmacopsychiatry.* 2013;28:144–161.

139. Bradley SM, Rumsfeld JS. Depression and cardiovascular disease. *Trends Cardiovasc Med.* 2015;25(7):614–622.

140. Whooley MA, Wong JM. Depression and cardiovascular disorders. *Annu Rev Clin Psychol.* 2013;9:327–354.

141. Elderon L, Whooley MA. Depression and cardiovascular disease. *Prog Cardiovasc Dis.* 2013;55(6):511–523.

142. Amare AT, Schubert KO, Klingler-Hoffmann M, et al. The genetic overlap between mood disorders and cardiometabolic diseases: a systematic review of genome wide and candidate gene studies. *Transl Psychiatry.* 2017;7(1):e1007.

143. Aureli M, Grassi S, Prioni S, et al. Lipid membrane domains in the brain. *Biochim Biophys Acta.* 2015;1851(8):1006–1016.

144. Zhang J, Liu Q. Cholesterol metabolism and homeostasis in the brain. *Protein Cell.* 2015;6(4):254–264.

145. Borroni MV, Valles AS, Barrantes FJ. The lipid habitats of neurotransmitter receptors in brain. *Biochim Biophys Acta.* 2016;1858(11):2662–2670.

146. Davletov B, Montecucco C. Lipid function at synapses. *Curr Opin Neurobiol.* 2010;20(5):543–549.

147. Ueda Y. The role of phosphoinositides in synapse function. *Mol Neurobiol.* 2014;50(3):821–838.

148. Sebastiao AM, Colino-Oliveira M, Assaife-Lopes N, et al. Lipid rafts, synaptic transmission and plasticity: impact in age-related neurodegenerative diseases. *Neuropharmacology.* 2013;64:97–107.

149. Grela A, Rachel W, Cole M, et al. Application of fatty acid and lipid measurements in neuropsychiatry. *Clin Chem Lab Med.* 2016;54(2):197–206.

150. De Berardis D, Marini S, Piersanti M, et al. The relationships between cholesterol and suicide: an update. *ISRN Psychiatry.* 2012;2012:387901.

151. Demirkan A, Isaacs A, Ugocsai P, et al. Plasma phosphatidylcholine and sphingomyelin concentrations are associated with depression and anxiety symptoms in a Dutch family-based lipidomics study. *J Psychiatr Res.* 2013;47(3):357–362.

152. Schneider M, Levant B, Reichel M, et al. Lipids in psychiatric disorders and preventive medicine. *Neurosci Biobehav Rev.* 2017;76(Pt B):336–362.

153. Muller CP, Reichel M, Muhle C, et al. Brain membrane lipids in major depression and anxiety disorders. *Biochim Biophys Acta.* 2015;1851(8):1052–1065.

154. Persons JE, Fiedorowicz JG. Depression and serum low-density lipoprotein: a systematic review and meta-analysis. *J Affect Disord.* 2016;206:55–67.

155. Maes M, Smith R, Christophe A, et al. Lower serum high-density lipoprotein cholesterol (HDL-C) in major depression and in depressed men with serious suicidal attempts: relationship with immune-inflammatory markers. *Acta Psychiatr Scand.* 1997;95(3):212–221.

156. Jokinen J, Nordstrom AL, Nordstrom P. Cholesterol, CSF 5-HIAA, violence and intent in suicidal men. *Psychiatry Res.* 2010;178(1):217–219.

157. Jose PA, Raj D. Gut microbiota in hypertension. *Curr Opin Nephrol Hypertens.* 2015;24(5):403–409.

158. Yang T, Santisteban MM, Rodriguez V, et al. Gut dysbiosis is linked to hypertension. *Hypertension.* 2015;65(6):1331–1340.

159. DeMarco VG, Aroor AR, Sowers JR. The pathophysiology of hypertension in patients with obesity. *Nat Rev Endocrinol.* 2014;10(6):364–376.

160. Schlaich MP, Lambert E, Kaye DM, et al. Sympathetic augmentation in hypertension: role of nerve firing, norepinephrine reuptake, and angiotensin neuromodulation. *Hypertension.* 2004;43(2):169–175.

161. Barton DA, Dawood T, Lambert EA, et al. Sympathetic activity in major depressive disorder: identifying those at increased cardiac risk? *J Hypertens.* 2007;25(10):2117–2124.

162. Dawood T, Schlaich M, Brown A, Lambert G. Depression and blood pressure control: all antidepressants are not the same. *Hypertension.* 2009;54(1):e1; author reply e2.

163. Esler M. Mental stress and human cardiovascular disease. *Neurosci Biobehav Rev.* 2017;74(Pt B):269–276.

164. Nguyen SB, Cevik C, Otahbachi M, et al. Do comorbid psychiatric disorders contribute to the pathogenesis of Tako-tsubo syndrome? A review of pathogenesis. *Congest Heart Fail.* 2009;15(1):31–34.

165. Pierre G. Neurodegenerative disorders and metabolic disease. *Arch Dis Child.* 2013;98(8):618–624.

166. Nia S. Psychiatric signs and symptoms in treatable inborn errors of metabolism. *J Neurol.* 2014;261(Suppl 2):S559–S568.

167. Walterfang M, Bonnot O, Mocellin R, Velakoulis D. The neuropsychiatry of inborn errors of metabolism. *J Inherit Metab Dis*. 2013;36(4):687–702.

168. Ali N, Gillespie S, Laney D. Treatment of depression in adults with Fabry disease. *JIMD Rep*. 2018;38:13–21.

169. Bolsover FE, Murphy E, Cipolotti L, et al. Cognitive dysfunction and depression in Fabry disease: a systematic review. *J Inherit Metab Dis*. 2014;37(2):177–187.

170. Anglin RE, Garside SL, Tarnopolsky MA, et al. The psychiatric manifestations of mitochondrial disorders: a case and review of the literature. *J Clin Psychiatry*. 2012;73(4):506–512.

171. Vitner EB, Platt FM, Futerman AH. Common and uncommon pathogenic cascades in lysosomal storage diseases. *J Biol Chem*. 2010;285(27):20423–20427.

172. Gans RO. The metabolic syndrome, depression, and cardiovascular disease: interrelated conditions that share pathophysiologic mechanisms. *Med Clin North Am*. 2006;90(4):573–591.

173. Teply RM, Packard KA, White ND, et al. Treatment of depression in patients with concomitant cardiac disease. *Prog Cardiovasc Dis*. 2016;58(5):514–528.

174. Deuschle M. Effects of antidepressants on glucose metabolism and diabetes mellitus type 2 in adults. *Curr Opin Psychiatry*. 2013;26(1):60–65.

175. Roopan S, Larsen ER. Use of antidepressants in patients with depression and comorbid diabetes mellitus: a systematic review. *Acta Neuropsychiatr*. 2017;29(3):127–139.

176. Low Y, Setia S, Lima G. Drug-drug interactions involving antidepressants: focus on desvenlafaxine. *Neuropsychiatr Dis Treat*. 2018;14:567–580.

177. Derijks HJ, Heerdink ER, De Koning FH, et al. The association between antidepressant use and hypoglycaemia in diabetic patients: a nested case-control study. *Pharmacoepidemiol Drug Saf*. 2008;17(4):336–344.

178. Shukla AP, Kumar RB, Aronne LJ. Lorcaserin HCl for the treatment of obesity. *Expert Opin Pharmacother*. 2015;16(16):2531–2538.

179. Christou GA, Kiortsis DN. The efficacy and safety of the naltrexone/bupropion combination for the treatment of obesity: an update. *Hormones (Athens)*. 2015;14(3):370–375.

180. Dias S, Paredes S, Ribeiro L. Drugs involved in dyslipidemia and obesity treatment: focus on adipose tissue. *Int J Endocrinol*. 2018;2018:2637418.

181. Subbaiah MAM. Triple reuptake inhibitors as potential therapeutics for depression and other disorders: design paradigm and developmental challenges. *J Med Chem*. 2018;61(6):2133–2165.

182. Berger M, Gray JA, Roth BL. The expanded biology of serotonin. *Annu Rev Med*. 2009;60:355–366.

183. Gershon MD, Tack J. The serotonin signaling system: from basic understanding to drug development for functional GI disorders. *Gastroenterology*. 2007;132(1):397–414.

184. Oh CM, Park S, Kim H. Serotonin as a new therapeutic target for diabetes mellitus and obesity. *Diabetes Metab J*. 2016;40(2):89–98.

185. Imprialos KP, Stavropoulos K, Doumas M, et al. Sexual dysfunction, cardiovascular risk and effects of pharmacotherapy. *Curr Vasc Pharmacol*. 2018;16(2):130–142.

186. Abdelkader NF, Saad MA, Abdelsalam RM. Neuroprotective effect of nebivolol against cisplatin-associated depressive-like behavior in rats. *J Neurochem*. 2017;141(3):449–460.

187. Joca SRL, Sartim AG, Roncalho AL, Diniz CFA, Wegener G. Nitric oxide signalling and antidepressant action revisited. *Cell Tissue Res*. 2019;377(1):45–58.

188. Aftab A, Kemp DE, Ganocy SJ, et al. Double-blind, placebo-controlled trial of pioglitazone for bipolar depression. *J Affect Disord*. 2019;245:957–964.

189. Erensoy H, Niafar M, Ghafarzadeh S, et al. A pilot trial of metformin for insulin resistance and mood disturbances in adolescent and adult women with polycystic ovary syndrome. *Gynecol Endocrinol*. 2019;35(1):72–75.

190. Cuomo A, Bolognesi S, Goracci A, et al. Feasibility, adherence and efficacy of liraglutide treatment in a sample of individuals with mood disorders and obesity. *Front Psychiatry.* 2018;9:784.
191. Nieuwstraten C, Labiris NR, Holbrook A. Systematic overview of drug interactions with antidepressant medications. *Can J Psychiatry.* 2006;51(5):300–316.
192. Bleakley S. Antidepressant drug interactions: evidence and clinical significance. *Progr Neurol Psychiatry.* 2016;20(3):21–27.
193. Spina E, Trifiro G, Caraci F. Clinically significant drug interactions with newer antidepressants. *CNS Drugs.* 2012;26(1):39–67.

Pharmacotherapy for Depression

FIRST-LINE AND COMBINATION THERAPEUTICS FOR MAJOR DEPRESSIVE DISORDER

MANISH K. JHA

11.1. INTRODUCTION

Major depressive disorder (MDD) affects one in five adults during their lifetime and is the second leading cause of disability in the United States [1, 2]. Patients with MDD experience significant impairments in work and non-work-related productivity, quality of life, social and interpersonal relationships, and overall satisfaction with life [3, 4]. Despite the widespread prevalence, depression is often underrecognized and undertreated. In community settings, about 20% patients with MDD receive minimally adequate treatment [5], and only 6% attain remission of depressive symptoms [6]. Even among the patients who are diagnosed with depression, initiation of treatment is often delayed, with median duration of treatment initiation from onset of illness being 8 years [7]. Hence, current practice guidelines recommend universal screening for depression of adults who are seen in medical settings [8]. Combined with the efforts by payors to incentivize screening for depression and the initiatives by healthcare systems to implement large-scale screening for depression [9], the rates of undiagnosed depression will likely decrease and the identification of patients suffering from depression will improve. However, due to a shortage of mental health professionals, the burden of management of depression may fall on primary care providers or other healthcare providers [10]. Thus, the management approach after a positive screen for depression includes a diagnostic assessment, as outlined in Figure 11.1, to rule out other primary psychiatric conditions and to establish the presence of comorbid medical and psychiatric conditions that might affect

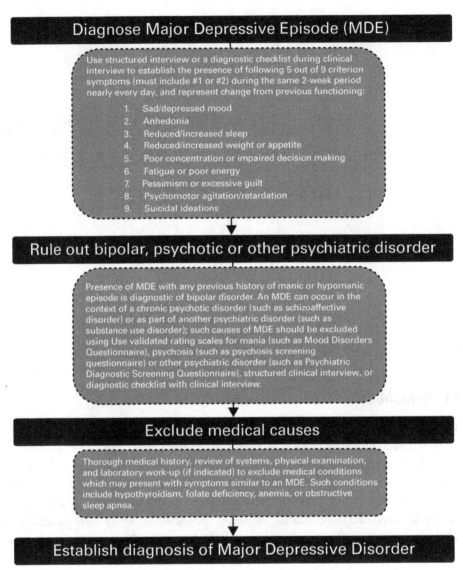

Diagnose Major Depressive Episode (MDE)

Use structured interview or a diagnostic checklist during clinical interview to establish the presence of following 5 out of 9 criterion symptoms (must include #1 or #2) during the same 2-week period nearly every day, and represent change from previous functioning:

1. Sad/depressed mood
2. Anhedonia
3. Reduced/increased sleep
4. Reduced/increased weight or appetite
5. Poor concentration or impaired decision making
6. Fatigue or poor energy
7. Pessimism or excessive guilt
8. Psychomotor agitation/retardation
9. Suicidal ideations

Rule out bipolar, psychotic or other psychiatric disorder

Presence of MDE with any previous history of manic or hypomanic episode is diagnostic of bipolar disorder. An MDE can occur in the context of a chronic psychotic disorder (such as schizoaffective disorder) or as part of another psychiatric disorder (such as substance use disorder); such causes of MDE should be excluded using Use validated rating scales for mania (such as Mood Disorders Questionnaire), psychosis (such as psychosis screening questionnaire) or other psychiatric disorder (such as Psychiatric Diagnostic Screening Questionnaire), structured clinical interview, or diagnostic checklist with clinical interview.

Exclude medical causes

Thorough medical history, review of systems, physical examination, and laboratory work-up (if indicated) to exclude medical conditions which may present with symptoms similar to an MDE. Such conditions include hypothyroidism, folate deficiency, anemia, or obstructive sleep apnea.

Establish diagnosis of Major Depressive Disorder

FIGURE 11.1. Diagnostic algorithm for MDD.

the outcomes of patients with MDD. Once the diagnosis of MDD is established, initiation of treatment should incorporate a measurement-based care approach.

11.2. MEASUREMENT-BASED CARE APPROACH

Systematic treatment of MDD includes assessment of symptom severity at baseline along with repeated measurements of symptom severity, treatment-emergent side effects, and adherence to treatment at follow-up visits. Such a measurement-based care (MBC) approach was operationalized by Trivedi et al. in the Sequenced Treatment Alternatives to Relive Depression (STAR*D) [11]. Patients with MDD, who were recruited from both primary care and psychiatric clinics, were started on citalopram, a selective serotonin reuptake inhibitor (SSRI), during level 1 of STAR*D and followed at regular intervals (every 2–3 weeks) with treatment changes made if side effects were tolerable, adherence to medication was good, and improvement in symptom severity was inadequate [11]. In a subsequent randomized controlled trial, the MBC approach was shown to have two times higher rates of remission and response versus treatment as usual [12]. The STAR*D study also demonstrated that treatment outcomes in primary care and psychiatric clinics were similar with the same antidepressant when a similar MBC approach was used [13]. More recent evidence suggests the utility of expanding the range of assessments for symptom severity in such an MBC approach [14]. For example, anxiety in patients with MDD is multidimensional and may not be adequately captured by any single scale [15]. Similarly, the presence of subthreshold hypomanic symptoms in patients with MDD is associated with poor response to most currently available antidepressants [16]. Advances in healthcare information technology may allow such multidimensional assessments to inform clinical decision making and should be considered when initiating antidepressant treatment [14].

11.3. FIRST-LINE TREATMENTS OF MDD

Recommendation for initial treatment of MDD is based on the severity of presenting symptoms and previous history, if any, of response to antidepressant treatment [17]. Thus, an MBC approach will also allow appropriate selection of antidepressant treatment. For those with mild depressive symptom severity, clinical trials have failed to establish a superiority of antidepressant medications over placebo [18]. Hence, to limit the potential for side effects, antidepressant medications should be avoided. Instead, first-line treatment recommendations for mild depressive symptom severity include psychotherapy, careful monitoring, or exercise [19]. For patients with moderate depressive symptom severity, practice guidelines recommend either pharmacotherapy or psychotherapy due to similar efficacy of both and no evidence for benefit with combination of the two modalities [17]. In patients with severe depression, first-line treatment may include a combination of pharmacotherapy and psychotherapy [17]. Using of invasive treatments, such as electroconvulsive treatment (ECT) or off-label use of ketamine, as first-line treatment may be considered for very severe depression associated with suicidality or catatonia (proven efficacy for ECT) [20]. Similarly, in patients with severe depression that is associated with psychotic symptoms, initial treatment may include a combination of antidepressants and antipsychotic medications [17]. These first-line treatments are discussed in greater detail later in the chapter.

11.3.1. Psychotherapy for MDD

Cognitive therapy (CT), behavioral activation (BA), and interpersonal therapy (IPT) are commonly used evidence-based psychotherapy modalities that have been shown to be efficacious in patients with MDD [19]. These therapies all share similar traits of being structured and being limited in duration for acute-phase treatment. While CT focuses on identification and modification of negative thoughts that influence mood and behavior, BA emphasizes scheduling activities that result in positive interactions. IPT is focused on modifying interpersonal relationships [19]. Less structured therapies such as psychodynamic psychotherapy and supportive counselling, while efficacious for some patients, are not as effective as CT, BA, and IPT [19]. Mindfulness-based cognitive therapy, often conducted as group therapy, can be used in patients with depression, especially after an acute episode, to disengage from thought patterns that mediate relapse or recurrence [21]. Most psychotherapy modalities involve weekly or twice-weekly visits during the acute phase, which may limit access for some patients. Technological advances are being used to reduce or eliminate barriers to psychotherapy. For example, a recent study reported on implementation of a video-conference system to conduct BA in patients with MDD who were receiving care at underserved clinics [22]. Similarly, CT delivered via the internet has been shown to be efficacious in patients with MDD. The choice of optimal psychotherapy modality often depends on the availability of trained therapists, the strength of the relationship between therapist and patient, and the presence of comorbid conditions [19]. For example, CT may be useful in patients with MDD who also have primary insomnia. Additionally, motivational therapy may be used in patients with MDD who have an active comorbid substance use disorder.

11.3.2. Exercise for MDD

Exercise is an effective treatment of MDD that is recommended in patients with mild to moderate symptom severity [23]. In a meta-analysis of 25 randomized controlled trials of exercise versus control, there was a significant and large effect of exercise on reduction in depressive symptom severity [24]. Exercise may also be considered as a first-line treatment in patients with cardiovascular disease. For example, in patients with congestive heart failure, while antidepressant medications have not been shown to be superior to placebo, exercise has been shown to reduce the self-reported depressive symptom severity and improve long-term survival [25, 26]. Exercise has also been shown to be an effective augmentation strategy after partial response to an antidepressant medication [27].

11.3.3. Pharmacotherapy for MDD

Antidepressants continue to be one of the most commonly prescribed classes of medications. However, about a third of prescriptions for antidepressants are considered inappropriate because they are being used without strong scientific evidence, such as no psychiatric diagnosis or lack of consideration for drug interactions [28]. Currently available and commonly used first-line antidepressant medications include selective serotonin reuptake inhibitor (SSRIs), serotonin norepinephrine reuptake inhibitors

(SNRIs), and other agents with miscellaneous mechanisms of action (Table 11.1). As this report is focused on first-line treatment, older antidepressants such as tricyclic and tetracyclic antidepressants and monoamine oxidase inhibitors will not be discussed. All antidepressant medications have a US Food and Drug Administration (FDA) black-box warning that their use may be associated with an increased risk of suicidal thoughts and behaviors in children, adolescents, and young adults; thus, their use should be accompanied by monitoring for worsening and emergence of suicidal thoughts and behaviors. The classes of antidepressant medications differ slightly in their anticipated side-effect profiles (see Table 11.1). They also differ in the rates of discontinuation symptoms; thus, patients should be advised about these symptoms if discontinuation is planned [29]. Head-to-head comparisons of the medications have failed to find a significant pattern of superiority of any one medication (or class of medication) over others [17]. Hence, practice guidelines recommend basing the choice of antidepressant medications on subjective factors such as matching existing symptoms to anticipated side-effect profiles, patient or provider preference, and cost [17]. For example, in a patient with insomnia as a severe symptom of depression, treatment with mirtazapine may be preferred due to its sedating side effects and bupropion may be avoided as it is associated with insomnia. However, in a prospective study of patients in the Combining Medication to Enhance Depression Outcomes (CO-MED) trial, there was no significant difference in remission between patients who received bupropion (plus escitalopram) or mirtazapine (plus venlafaxine) [30], suggesting a limited utility of selecting treatments based on anticipated side-effect profiles. Several other reports have failed to find utility of baseline clinical features (such as anxious, atypical, melancholic, or anhedonic), symptom severity, or chronicity of illness in predicting response to one antidepressant medication versus another [9, 31–33]. Emerging literature suggests that inflammation-related markers may assist in the selection of one antidepressant versus another [34–37]. Body mass index (BMI) is such a marker that can be used in clinical practice to guide antidepressant treatment selection [38, 39].

11.4. PREDICTION OF CLINICAL OUTCOMES OF PHARMACOTHERAPY

All currently available first-line pharmacotherapy medications take two to three months at an adequate dose to be maximally effective. Early improvement in depressive symptoms is a strong predictor of subsequent response. For example, in the CO-MED trial, outpatients with MDD who attained remission at 6 weeks were 14.4 times more likely to be in remission after 12 weeks of treatment versus those who did not attain remission at 6 weeks [40]. Greater severity of depressive symptoms prior to treatment initiation has been consistently shown to reduce the likelihood of attaining remission [40]. Other predictors of poor response to antidepressant medications include greater burden of comorbid psychiatric and medical conditions, previous history of nonresponse to antidepressant treatments, and higher levels of inflammatory markers [41, 42]. However, the prediction of outcomes using baseline

TABLE 11.1. First-Step Pharmacotherapy for MDD

Drug	Common Side Effects	Clinical Considerations and Drug Interactions
SSRIs (dose)		
Fluoxetine (initial: 20 mg; target: 20–80 mg)	GI (anorexia, dry mouth, diarrhea, dyspepsia, nausea), general (flu syndrome, pharyngitis, rash, sinusitis, increased sweating, tremor), sexual dysfunction (abnormal ejaculation, impotence, decreased libido), psychiatric (abnormal dreams, anxiety, insomnia, nervousness, somnolence)	Longest half-life among SSRIs, lowest risk of discontinuation symptoms among all antidepressants. Drug interactions include reduced metabolism of beta-blockers and certain anti-arrhythmic agents. Increased risk of hyponatremia and bleeding (esp. in patients on aspirin or anticoagulants).
Citalopram (initial: 20 mg; target: 20–40 mg)	GI (dry mouth, nausea), sleep (somnolence), sexual dysfunction (abnormal ejaculation, decreased libido, orgasmic disturbance), cardiovascular (tachycardia, hypotension, postural hypotension)	Increased risk of QTc prolongation especially at doses >40 mg. Drug interactions include reduced metabolism of beta-blockers and certain anti-arrhythmic agents. Increased risk of hyponatremia and bleeding (esp. in patients on aspirin or anticoagulants).
Escitalopram (initial: 10 mg; target: 10–20 mg)	Sleep (insomnia, somnolence), general (increased sweating, fatigue), GI (nausea), sexual dysfunction (abnormal ejaculation, decreased libido, orgasmic disturbance), cardiovascular (hypertension and palpitation)	Drug interactions include reduced metabolism of beta-blockers and certain anti-arrhythmic agents. Increased risk of hyponatremia and bleeding (esp. in patients on aspirin or anticoagulants).
Paroxetine (initial: 20 mg IR, 25 mg CR; target: 20–50 mg IR, 25–62.5 mg CR)	GI (nausea, diarrhea, constipation), sleep (somnolence, insomnia), sexual dysfunction (decreased libido, abnormal ejaculation, orgasmic disturbance); highest potential for weight gain among SSRIs	Reduced metabolism of CYP 1A2. Increased risk of hyponatremia and bleeding (esp. in patients on aspirin or anticoagulants). Highest risk of discontinuation symptoms among all SSRIs, higher with IR than CR.

TABLE 11.1. Continued

Drug	Common Side Effects	Clinical Considerations and Drug Interactions
Sertraline (initial: 50 mg; target: 50–200 mg)	GI (nausea, diarrhea, dyspepsia, decreased appetite), general (tremor, increased sweating), sexual dysfunction (abnormal ejaculation, decreased libido)	Reduced metabolism of CYP 2D6 substrates at higher doses. Increased risk of hyponatremia and bleeding (esp. in patients on aspirin or anticoagulants).
SNRIs (dose)		
Venlafaxine (initial: 75 mg; target: 150–375 mg)	Sleep (insomnia, abnormal dreams), GI (weight loss, nausea), general (increased sweating, nervousness), cardiovascular (tachycardia, sustained hypertension at doses >300 mg/day), sexual (abnormal ejaculation)	Risk of discontinuation symptoms, higher with the IR than ER formulation. Increased risk of hyponatremia and bleeding (esp. in patients on aspirin or anticoagulants).
Desvenlafaxine (initial: 50 mg; target: 50 mg)	GI (nausea, constipation, reduced appetite), sleep (insomnia, somnolence), general (dizziness, increased sweating, anxiety), sexual dysfunction, cardiovascular (cholesterol and triglyceride elevation, and orthostatic hypotension in patients ≥65 years of age)	Dose adjustment needed in patients with renal insufficiency. Risk of discontinuation symptoms similar to venlafaxine, of which this is the main active metabolite. Increased risk of hyponatremia and bleeding (esp. in patients on aspirin or anticoagulants).
Duloxetine (initial: 40–60 mg; target: 60–120 mg)	GI (nausea, dry mouth, constipation, reduced appetite), general (fatigue, increased sweating), somnolence, orthostatic hypotension	Lower risk of hyponatremia than SSRIs, may be preferred for patients with pain disorders. Drug interactions include reduced metabolism of beta-blockers and certain anti-arrhythmic agents.
Others (dose)		
Levomilnacipram (initial: 20 mg; target: 40–120 mg)	GI (nausea, vomiting, constipation), increased sweating, erectile dysfunction, palpitations	Better tolerability, including lower weight gain and sexual dysfunction, than SSRIs. Increased risk of hyponatremia and bleeding (esp. in patients on aspirin or anticoagulants).

(*continued*)

TABLE 11.1. Continued

Drug	Common Side Effects	Clinical Considerations and Drug Interactions
Bupropion (initial: 150 mg; target: 300–450 mg)	GI (dry mouth, nausea), insomnia, dizziness, increased sweating, palpitations	Decreased plasma concentration of digoxin. Slight increase in risk of seizures; higher doses have higher risk of seizures. Preferred for patients with sexual dysfunction on SSRIs or SNRIs. Contraindicated in presence of eating disorder or seizure disorder, or in presence of alcohol or benzodiazepine withdrawal.
Mirtazapine (initial: 15 mg; target: 15–45 mg)	Sleep (somnolence), weight gain, dizziness, cardiovascular (orthostatic hypotension, hypertension)	Lower risk of hyponatremia than SSRIs, increased risk of bleeding; bedtime dosing preferred due to sedating side effects
Trazodone (initial: 150 mg; target: 150–375 mg ER, 300–600 mg IR)	Somnolence, dizziness, blurred vision, constipation, priapism, cardiovascular (orthostatic hypotension, QTc prolongation)	Increased risk of bleeding (esp. in patients on aspirin or anticoagulants), increased level of digoxin
Vilazodone (initial: 10 mg; target: 40 mg)	GI (diarrhea, nausea, vomiting), insomnia	Increased risk of bleeding (esp. in patients on aspirin or anticoagulants). Should be taken with food.
Vortioxetine (initial: 10 mg; target: 10–20 mg)	GI (nausea, vomiting, constipation)	May help with cognitive symptoms of depression. Increased risk of hyponatremia and bleeding (esp. in patients on aspirin or anticoagulants).

CR = controlled release; ER = extended release; GI = gastrointestinal; IR = immediate release.

features is highly variable and not significant after controlling for early changes in depression severity. Adding measurements of functional improvement, such as work- or non-work-related productivity, can improve the precision in estimating the clinical outcomes [33, 43].

11.5. COMBINATION THERAPEUTICS FOR MDD

11.5.1. As First-Line Treatment

As outlined earlier in the chapter, combination therapeutics across different modalities (pharmacotherapy plus psychotherapy, antidepressant plus antipsychotic, antidepressant plus ECT) are typically indicated in patients with severe depression or in case of imminent threat to the safety of patients. However, a combination of antidepressant medications as first-line treatment has not been shown to be more efficacious or to lead to faster remission. In the large-scale CO-MED trial, which compared escitalopram monotherapy with combinations of bupropion plus escitalopram and venlafaxine plus mirtazapine, there was no significant difference in treatment outcomes among the three treatment arms [44]. However, the combination of venlafaxine and mirtazapine was associated with higher rates of burdensome side effects [44]. Thus, a combination of antidepressant medications should be avoided as first-line treatment. Based on patient presentation, short courses of other treatments may need to be initiated concomitantly to address comorbid psychiatric conditions such as anxiety disorder or insomnia [17].

11.5.2. After Inadequate Response to First-Line Treatment

Level 2 of the STAR*D trial tested the utility of adding another medication to ongoing antidepressant therapy in the augmentation arm. In this study of 565 patients, augmentation of citalopram with bupropion had similar remission rates compared with augmentation with buspirone [45]. However, augmentation with bupropion was better tolerated and was associated with lower dropout rates due to intolerance. Since the publication of these STAR*D findings, several second-generation antipsychotic medications have been approved by the FDA to augment the effect of ongoing antidepressant treatment (Table 11.2). A recent study compared the effectiveness of switch to bupropion versus augmentation with bupropion or augmentation with aripiprazole in patients with MDD who had failed to respond to at least one adequate antidepressant trial. In this study, response rates with aripiprazole augmentation were superior to the other two treatment arms [46]. Thus, augmentation with second-generation antipsychotics may be considered in patients with MDD who have failed to improve adequately with a first-line pharmacotherapy agent. Among the second-generation antipsychotics currently approved for augmentation, there is no evidence for superiority of one medication over another. However, their use may be guided by the side-effect profile of these medications. Olanzapine and quetiapine are both sedating and associated with significant metabolic burden. Thus, their prolonged use warrants monitoring of weight, lipid levels, hemoglobin A1C, and waist circumference. Aripiprazole has significantly lower weight-gain potential but is associated with akathisia in about one in four patients with MDD, which may be a dose-limiting side effect of the medication.

TABLE 11.2. Second-Generation Antipsychotics for Augmentation After Inadequate Response to First-Line Pharmacotherapy

Drug	Dose	Common Side Effects
Olanzapine	Initial: 5 mg Target: 5–20 mg	GI (constipation, dry mouth), metabolic (increased appetite, weight gain, hyperglycemia, hyperlipidemia), sleep (somnolence), general (dizziness), cardiovascular (QTc prolongation, orthostatic hypotension, tachycardia, hypertension, enhanced effect of antihypertensive drugs)
Quetiapine	Initial: 50 mg Target: 150–300 mg	Sleep (somnolence), general (dizziness, fatigue, dysarthria, nasal congestion), GI (dry mouth, constipation, dyspepsia), metabolic (increased appetite, weight gain, hyperglycemia, hyperlipidemia), cardiovascular (orthostatic hypotension, tachycardia, hypertension, enhanced effect of antihypertensive drugs)
Aripiprazole	Initial: 2.5 mg Target: 5–15 mg	Extrapyramidal (akathisia, restlessness), sleep (insomnia), general (fatigue, blurred vision), GI (constipation), metabolic (dyslipidemia), cardiovascular (orthostatic hypotension, bradycardia, palpitations, enhanced effect of antihypertensive drugs by alpha adrenergic antagonism)
Brexipiprazole	Initial: 0.5–1 mg Target: 2–3 mg	Extrapyramidal (akathisia, restlessness), metabolic (weight gain, increased cortisol, dyslipidemia), cardiovascular (orthostatic hypotension)

GI = gastrointestinal.

11.6. CONTINUATION-PHASE TREATMENT

Patients who improve with the acute-phase treatment may require ongoing treatment to prevent relapse/recurrence. In the STAR*D study, patients who improved with one or more treatments entered a naturalistic follow-up phase where they were encouraged to stay on the treatment that worked for them as well as make any changes based on the clinician judgments. Relapse among these patients was very common [11]. Lowest relapse rates (about 40%) were seen in patients who had remitted with the first-level treatment, while highest relapse rates (>80%) were seen in patients who took more than two medication trials to improve [11]. To assess the durability of improvement with CT, Jarrett et al. conducted a three-stage study where 523 patients were treated with acute-phase CT [47]. Those who met criteria for stable remission (operationalized as 17-item Hamilton Depression Rating Scale score of <7 for last seven assessments during the acute phase) were followed without any treatment for 32 months [47]. The remaining responders (labeled as high-risk responders) were randomized to treatment with either continuation-phase CT (C-CT), fluoxetine, or placebo for 8 months followed by 24 months of follow-up [47]. In this study, continuation-phase treatment with either C-CT or fluoxetine attenuated the risk of relapse in high-risk responders versus those who had attained a stable remission. Over the next 24 months of follow-up, the benefit with active-continuation phase improvement did not persist. Relapse rates among those with stable remission and high-risk responders treated with an eight-month course of C-CT, fluoxetine, or placebo were similar [47, 48]. Taken together, these findings suggest that for most patients with MDD, continued treatment is often necessary to sustain the improvement seen with acute-phase treatments.

11.7. CONCLUSIONS

There are multiple treatment options available for patients with MDD. Nonpharmacologic treatments may be considered for those with mild symptom severity. Pharmacologic treatments or psychotherapy should be considered in those with moderate to severe symptom severity. The combination of antidepressant medications and psychotherapy should be considered in those with severe or very severe symptom severity. Presence of psychotic symptoms, catatonia, and/or imminent risk of harm may necessitate combination treatments as well as interventional treatments such as ECT. There currently are no recommended objective markers to guide selection of one antidepressant medication over another in clinical practice. However, exciting new research promises to utilize an array of clinical and biologic markers to personalize treatment selection. After the failure of first-line antidepressant medication, augmentation strategies may be considered if the first antidepressant was well tolerated. However, future research is needed to compare the effectiveness of augmentation versus switch to another antidepressant medication.

REFERENCES

1. Hasin, D.S., et al., Epidemiology of adult DSM-5 major depressive disorder and its specifiers in the United States. JAMA Psychiatry, 2018. **75**(4): pp. 336–346.
2. Vos, T., et al., Global, regional, and national incidence, prevalence, and years lived with disability for 328 diseases and injuries for 195 countries, 1990–2016: a systematic analysis for the Global Burden of Disease Study 2016. Lancet, 2017. **390**(10100): pp. 1211–1259.
3. Jha, M.K., et al., Improvement in self-reported quality of life with cognitive therapy for recurrent major depressive disorder. J Affect Disord, 2014. **167**: pp. 37–43.
4. Greer, T.L., et al., Improvements in psychosocial functioning and health-related quality of life following exercise augmentation in patients with treatment response but nonremitted major depressive disorder: results from the TREAD study. Depress Anxiety, 2016. **33**(9): pp. 870–881.

5. Kessler, R.C., et al., The epidemiology of major depressive disorder: results from the national comorbidity survey replication (NCS-R). JAMA, 2003. **289**(23): pp. 3095–3105.

6. Pence, B.W., et al. The depression treatment cascade in primary care: a public health perspective. Curr Psychiatry Rep, 2012. **14**(4): pp. 328–335.

7. Wang, P.S., et al., Failure and delay in initial treatment contact after first onset of mental disorders in the National Comorbidity Survey Replication. Arch Gen Psychiatry, 2005. **62**(6): pp. 603–613.

8. Siu, A.L., and U.S. Preventive Services Task Force, Screening for depression in adults. JAMA, 2016. **315**(4): pp. 380–387.

9. Sung, S.C., et al., The impact of chronic depression on acute and long-term outcomes in a randomized trial comparing selective serotonin reuptake inhibitor monotherapy versus each of 2 different antidepressant medication combinations. J Clin Psychiatry, 2012. **73**(7): pp. 967–976.

10. Jha, M., et al., A structured approach for universal screening of depression and measurement-based treatment of major depressive disorder in primary care clinics. Ann Fam Med, 2019 Jul. **17**(4): pp. 326–335. doi: 10.1370/afm.2418.

11. Trivedi, M.H., et al., Evaluation of outcomes with citalopram for depression using measurement-based care in STAR*D: implications for clinical practice. Am J Psychiatry, 2006. **163**(1): pp. 28–40.

12. Guo, T., et al., Measurement-based care versus standard care for major depression: a randomized controlled trial with blind raters. Am J Psychiatry, 2015. **172**(10): pp. 1004–1013.

13. Gaynes, B.N., et al., Primary versus specialty care outcomes for depressed outpatients managed with measurement-based care: results from STAR*D. J Gen Intern Med, 2008. **23**(5): pp. 551–560.

14. Jha, M., et al., Irritability and its clinical utility in major depressive disorder: prediction of individual-level acute-phase outcomes using early changes in irritability and depression severity. Am J Psychiatry, 2019. **176**(5): pp. 358–366.

15. Trombello, J.M., et al., Characterizing anxiety subtypes and the relationship to behavioral phenotyping in major depression: results from the EMBARC study. J Psychiatr Res, 2018. **102**: pp. 207–215.

16. Jha, M.K., et al., Do baseline sub-threshold hypomanic symptoms affect acute-phase antidepressant outcome in outpatients with major depressive disorder? Preliminary findings from the randomized CO-MED trial. Neuropsychopharmacology, 2018. **43**(11): pp. 2197–2203.

17. Gelenberg, A.J., et al., Practice guideline for the treatment of patients with major depressive disorder third edition. Am J Psychiatry, 2010. **167**(10): p. 1.

18. Fournier, J.C., et al., Antidepressant drug effects and depression severity: a patient-level meta-analysis. JAMA, 2010. **303**(1): pp. 47–53.

19. Park, L.T., and C.A. Zarate Jr, Depression in the primary care setting. N Engl J Med, 2019. **380**(6): pp. 559–568.

20. Fava, M., et al., Double-blind, placebo-controlled, dose-ranging trial of intravenous ketamine as adjunctive therapy in treatment-resistant depression (TRD). Mol Psychiatry, 2018. doi: 10.1038/s41380-018-0256-5.

21. Kuyken, W., et al., Mindfulness-based cognitive therapy to prevent relapse in recurrent depression. J Consult Clin Psychol, 2008. **76**(6): p. 966.

22. Trombello, J.M., et al., Efficacy of a behavioral activation teletherapy intervention to treat depression and anxiety in primary care VitalSign6 program. Prim Care Companion CNS Disord, 2017. **19**(5). doi: 10.4088/PCC.17m02146.

23. Cleare, A., et al., Evidence-based guidelines for treating depressive disorders with antidepressants: a revision of the 2008 British Association for Psychopharmacology guidelines. J Psychopharmacol, 2015. **29**(5): pp. 459–525.

24. Schuch, F.B., et al., Exercise as a treatment for depression: a meta-analysis adjusting for publication bias. J Psychiatr Res, 2016. **77**: pp. 42–51.
25. Blumenthal, J.A., et al., Exercise, depression, and mortality after myocardial infarction in the ENRICHD trial. Med Scie Sports Exercise, 2004. **36**(5): pp. 746–755.
26. Blumenthal, J.A., et al., Effects of exercise training on depressive symptoms in patients with chronic heart failure: The HF-action randomized trial. JAMA, 2012. **308**(5): pp. 465–474.
27. Greer, T.L., et al., Evaluation of the benefits of exercise on cognition in major depressive disorder. Gen Hosp Psychiatry, 2017. **49**:19–25.
28. Cruickshank, G., et al., Cross-sectional survey of patients in receipt of long-term repeat prescriptions for antidepressant drugs in primary care. Ment Health Fam Med, 2008. **5**(2): pp. 105–109.
29. Jha, M.K., et al., When discontinuing SSRI antidepressants is a challenge: management tips. Am J Psychiatry, 2018. **175**(12): pp. 1176–1184.
30. Sung, S.C., et al., Pre-treatment insomnia as a predictor of single and combination antidepressant outcomes: a CO-MED report. J Affect Disord, 2015. **174**: pp. 157–164.
31. Friedman, E.S., et al., Baseline depression severity as a predictor of single and combination antidepressant treatment outcome: results from the CO-MED trial. Eur Neuropsychopharmacol, 2012. **22**(3): pp. 183–199.
32. Arnow, B.A., et al., Depression subtypes in predicting antidepressant response: a report from the iSPOT-D trial. Am J Psychiatry, 2015. **172**(8): pp. 743–750.
33. Chan, H.N., et al., Correlates and outcomes of depressed out-patients with greater and fewer anxious symptoms: a CO-MED report. Int J Neuropsychopharmacol, 2012. **15**(10): pp. 1387–1399.
34. Jha, M.K., et al., Platelet-derived growth factor as an antidepressant treatment selection biomarker: higher levels selectively predict better outcomes with bupropion-SSRI combination. Int J Neuropsychopharmacol, 2017. **20**(11): pp. 919–927.
35. Jha, M.K., et al., Interleukin 17 selectively predicts better outcomes with bupropion-SSRI combination: novel T cell biomarker for antidepressant medication selection. Brain Behav Immun, 2017. **66**: pp. 103–110.
36. Gadad, B.S., et al., Proteomics profiling reveals inflammatory biomarkers of antidepressant treatment response: findings from the CO-MED trial. J Psychiatr Res, 2017. **94**: pp. 1–6.
37. Jha, M.K., et al., Can C-reactive protein inform antidepressant medication selection in depressed outpatients? Findings from the CO-MED trial. Psychoneuroendocrinology, 2017. **78**: pp. 105–113.
38. Jha, M.K., et al., Validating pre-treatment body mass index as moderator of antidepressant treatment outcomes: findings from CO-MED trial. J Affect Disord, 2018. **234**: pp. 34–37.
39. Green, E., et al., Personalizing antidepressant choice by sex, body mass index, and symptom profile: an iSPOT-D report. Personal Med Psychiatry, 2017. **1**: pp. 65–73.
40. Jha, M.K., et al., Early improvement in work productivity predicts future clinical course in depressed outpatients: findings from the CO-MED trial. Am J Psychiatry, 2016. **173**(12): pp. 1196–1204.
41. Kuk, A.Y., et al., Recursive subsetting to identify patients in the STAR*D: a method to enhance the accuracy of early prediction of treatment outcome and to inform personalized care. J Clin Psychiatry, 2010. **71**(11): pp. 1502–1508.
42. Haroon, E., et al., Antidepressant treatment resistance is associated with increased inflammatory markers in patients with major depressive disorder. Psychoneuroendocrinology, 2018. **95**: pp. 43–49.
43. Jha, M.K., et al., Daily activity level improvement with antidepressant medications predicts long-term clinical outcomes in outpatients with major depressive disorder. Neuropsychiatr Dis Treat, 2017. **13**: pp. 803–813.

44. Rush, A.J., et al., Combining medications to enhance depression outcomes (CO-MED): acute and long-term outcomes of a single-blind randomized study. Am J Psychiatry, 2011. **168**(7): pp. 689–701.

45. Trivedi, M.H., et al., Medication augmentation after the failure of SSRIs for depression. N Engl J Med, 2006. **354**(12): pp. 1243–1252.

46. Mohamed, S., et al., Effect of antidepressant switching vs augmentation on remission among patients with major depressive disorder unresponsive to antidepressant treatment: the VAST-D randomized clinical trial. JAMA, 2017. **318**(2): pp. 132–145.

47. Jarrett, R.B., et al., Preventing depressive relapse and recurrence in higher-risk cognitive therapy responders: a randomized trial of continuation phase cognitive therapy, fluoxetine, or matched pill placebo. JAMA Psychiatry, 2013. **70**(11): pp. 1152–1160.

48. Jarrett, R.B., et al., Quantifying and qualifying the preventive effects of acute-phase cognitive therapy: pathways to personalizing care. J Consult Clin Psychol, 2016. **84**(4): pp. 365–376.

/// 12 /// PRIMER ON DEPRESSION

Augmentation Strategies

NAJI C. SALLOUM AND
GEORGE I. PAPAKOSTAS

12.1. INTRODUCTION

Although there are many available first-line treatments today for major depressive disorder (MDD), around two-thirds of patients fail to remit after an initial trial and may benefit from other treatment strategies (1). Augmentation therapy refers to the addition of a treatment to an existing treatment regimen in order to enhance response in patients who have not, or have only partially, responded to an initial antidepressant trial. Augmentation strategies can therefore help improve an initial partial response, and possibly enhance outcome faster than switching from one antidepressant to another. In this chapter, we will discuss the augmentation options, highlighting their pharmacologic profile, empirical evidence supporting their role as augmentation agents, and adverse effects that the prescriber should be mindful of. Table 12.1 outlines dosing recommendations.

12.2. ATYPICAL ANTIPSYCHOTICS

Atypical antipsychotics (AAPs) started gaining attention as adjunctive treatment for patients with MDD after a case series in 1999 demonstrated the sustained efficacy of risperidone as an augmentation therapy in MDD patients who were unresponsive to monotherapy with a selective serotonin reuptake inhibitor (SSRI) (2). Since then, AAPs have become the most studied class of drugs for adjunctive therapy in MDD, and three (aripiprazole, brexpiprazole, and quetiapine) compounds have gained approval from the US Food and Drug Administration (FDA) for that indication in the past decade (the olanzapine–fluoxetine combination therapy is FDA approved as a

TABLE 12.1. Dosing Recommendations of Augmenting Marketed Agents

	Starting Dose Daily (mg)	Dose Escalation	Recommended Daily Dose (mg)
Aripiprazole	2–5	5-mg increments/week	5–10
Brexpiprazole	0.5–1	0.5- to 1-mg increments/week	2
Olanzapine	5*	2.5- to 5-mg increments every 1–2 weeks	5–20
Quetiapine	50	Increase to 150 mg on day 3	150–300
Risperidone	0.5–1	0.5-mg increments/week	0.5–3
Ziprasidone	40**	40-mg increments/week	80–160**
Cariprazine	0.5	1.5-mg increments/week	2–4.5
Lithium	300–600	150–300 mg increments with lithium levels monitoring	Trough lithium level of 0.6–0.9 mEq/L
Triiodothyronine	25 mcg+	12- to 25-mcg increments/week	25–50
Methylphenidate	5++	2.5–5 mg every 1–2 days	5–30
Modafinil	100	100-mg increments every 3 days	200
Pramipexole	0.5#	1 mg after 1 week, 1.5 mg after 2 weeks, 2 mg after 3 weeks#	0.5–2
L-methylfolate	15	N/A	15
SAMe	800	1,600 mg after 2 weeks	800–1,600

*2.5 mg in the elderly or patients with risk of hypotension;

**Recommend bid dosing and taken with food;

+12.5 mcg in frail and elderly individuals;

++2.5 mg in frail individuals or with a history of cardiovascular disease;

#recommend bid dosing.

"switch" therapy in treatment-resistant depression [TRD]). From a pharmacologic standpoint, AAP receptor binding profiles offer a compelling scientific rationale for their utility in the treatment of depression, owing to their role in the modulation of the serotonergic system.

12.2.1. Aripiprazole

12.2.1.1. Pharmacologic Profile

Aripiprazole, similarly to other AAPs, acts as a serotonin-2($5HT_2$) receptor antagonist. It also acts as an agonist at the serotonin-1A($5HT_{1a}$) receptor. In addition, aripiprazole is a dopamine-2 (D_2) receptor partial agonist (3).

12.2.1.2. Empirical Evidence

Aripiprazole was approved by the FDA in 2007, the first drug to receive such approval. An earlier study done on a small cohort of patients with MDD who had an inadequate trial of an SSRI yielded a response rate of 58% after augmenting with aripiprazole (4). Subsequently, two identically designed randomized placebo-controlled trials (RPCTs) were conducted, in which augmentation with aripiprazole resulted in significantly higher remission rates than augmentation with placebo in patients who had previously not experienced sufficient symptom improvement after one to three antidepressant trials (5, 6). Evidence from these trials resulted in the FDA approval of aripiprazole in 2007 as an adjunctive agent for the treatment of MDD. Since then, other RPCTs have replicated these results, including in patients older than 60 (7–9). In addition, a small ($n = 101$), preliminary, open-label, rater-blinded randomized comparative trial of aripiprazole augmentation versus antidepressant switching in Korean and Taiwanese outpatients resulted in a greater Montgomery–Asberg Depression Rating Scale (MADRS) score mean change (score difference between groups: -8.7; $p < .0001$) for patients in the augmentation arm (10). However, a recent, large trial of 1,522 patients at 35 US Veterans Health Administration medical centers who were diagnosed with nonpsychotic MDD, unresponsive to at least one antidepressant course, meeting minimal standards for treatment dose and duration showed no statistically significant difference on the study's primary outcome measure (remission) between aripiprazole and bupropion augmentation groups (11). However, a statistically significant greater response to aripiprazole augmentation (74.3%) compared to either bupropion augmentation (65.6%) or switch (62.4%) was reported (respective numbers needed to treat of, approximately, 12 and 8) (11). Thus, the relative efficacy of these three strategies remains unclear.

12.2.1.3. Notable Adverse Effects

Aripiprazole may lead to weight gain and metabolic syndrome, although to a much lesser extent than olanzapine, making it a more favorable choice than other agents in the same class for overweight patients or those with diabetes mellitus and/or hyperlipidemia. Multiple studies have shown a significantly increased rate of akathisia with aripiprazole compared to placebo, warranting periodic assessment and dose adjustment or discontinuation when necessary.

12.2.2. Brexpiprazole

12.2.2.1. Pharmacologic Profile

Similar to aripiprazole, brexpiprazole acts as a D_2-receptor partial agonist, a partial agonist at 5-HT_{1a}, and an antagonist at 5-HT_{2a} receptors, however with much higher affinity to serotonin receptors than aripiprazole (12).

12.2.2.2. Empirical Evidence

In 2015, brexpiprazole was approved by the FDA as an adjunctive therapy for the treatment of MDD. Supporting its approval were two phase III RPCTs demonstrating its efficacy over placebo, with both 2- and 3-mg doses but not a 1-mg dose, as adjunctive treatment to standard antidepressant therapy in patients who failed to respond to one to three antidepressant trials (13, 14). A post-hoc pooled analysis from both studies resulted in brexpiprazole showing greater improvement than placebo in both patients with and without anxious distress (15). A recent RPCT also demonstrated the superiority of adjunct brexpiprazole (2–3 mg) over placebo in MDD patients who had failed to respond to one to three antidepressant trials and were currently on an antidepressant regimen. However, in this study, adjunct quetiapine extended release (XR; 150–300 mg/day), which was used as a measure of clinical trial "assay sensitivity," did not separate from placebo (16).

12.2.2.3. Notable Adverse Effects

The most common adverse effects observed with 2 and 3 mg of brexpiprazole daily were weight gain, somnolence, headache, and akathisia (13, 14, 16).

12.2.3. Olanzapine

12.2.3.1. Pharmacologic Profile

Olanzapine antagonizes the D_2-receptor as well as several serotonin receptors, including 5-$HT_{2A/2C}$, with high affinity. It also blocks adrenergic, muscarinic, and histamininergic receptors, the latter two with very strong affinity (17).

12.2.3.2. Empirical Evidence

Olanzapine was the first AAP to be tested as adjunctive therapy for MDD in a controlled trial comparing the olanzapine and fluoxetine combination (OFC) to either one alone. The study demonstrated a significantly superior efficacy of OFC over either monotherapy (18). In 2009, the FDA approved the use of OFC for TRD following the results from two large-scale studies with similar designs published in the same articler (19), comparing OFC to either drug in monotherapy. In the first study ($n = 638$), the combination did not separate in efficacy from either monotherapy. However, one factor that might explain this is the robust effect of fluoxetine monotherapy seen by the study's end. The second study ($n = 675$) did show superiority in efficacy of OFC over either monotherapy (MADRS change in OFC [−14.5] vs. fluoxetine [−8.6, $p < .001$] and olanzapine [−7.0, $p < .001$]). Furthermore, these results were replicated with pooled analyses from both studies. To note, two earlier clinical trials testing OFC did not yield positive results (20, 21). A more recent study demonstrated longer time to relapse ($p < .001$) and lower relapse rates (15.8% vs. 31.8%, $p < .001$) with OFC versus fluoxetine, respectively (22).

12.2.3.3. Notable Adverse Effects

Owing to the spectrum of receptors it targets, several notable adverse effects should be considered with olanzapine, including weight gain, metabolic syndrome, and sedation. The risk for extrapyramidal symptoms is relatively lower than with aripiprazole, risperidone, and brexpiprazole.

12.2.4. Quetiapine

12.2.4.1. Pharmacologic Profile

Quetiapine acts as an antagonist primarily to 5-HT$_2$ receptors, in addition to D$_1$ and D$_2$ receptors and, albeit with low potency, alpha-adrenergic and histamine receptors (23). This pharmacodynamics profile makes quetiapine more favorable than other APPs in terms of extrapyramidal symptoms (EPS).

12.2.4.2. Empirical Evidence

Quetiapine ER was approved by the FDA as an adjunctive therapy in MDD in 2009. Supportive evidence of efficacy was extracted from two large six-week RPCTs ($n = 936$) (24, 25), in which quetiapine ER (150 and 300 mg/day) augmentation to antidepressant therapy in patients who already failed to respond to at least one antidepressant trial resulted in a significantly greater reduction in MARDS score compared to placebo, in both trials for the 300-mg/day dose and only one trial for the 150-mg/day dose. Quetiapine's efficacy was also demonstrated as augmentation therapy to venlafaxine (26) and cognitive–behavioral therapy (CBT) (27), and in different clinical phenotypes, including psychotic depression (26) and depression with comorbid anxiety (28). A large open-label trial found that add-on quetiapine XR 300 mg/day ($n = 231$) was non-inferior to add-on lithium ($n = 229$) in patients with TRD (29). One RPCT did not demonstrate a significant difference between quetiapine and placebo as adjunct therapy to fluoxetine in MDD (30); however, the mean quetiapine dose (47 mg/day) administered was significantly lower than what was used in other trials.

12.2.4.3. Notable Adverse Effects

Somnolence, dry mouth, constipation, dizziness, and weight gain are common side effects with quetiapine, although weight gain appears to be notably less than with olanzapine. Patients should be regularly monitored for metabolic syndrome. EPS are seen with lower frequency compared to aripiprazole, risperidone, and brexpiprazole, but tardive dyskinesia and neuroleptic malignant syndrome can still occur.

12.2.5. Risperidone

12.2.5.1. Pharmacologic Profile

Risperidone is a strong and one of the most potent D$_2$ receptor antagonists among the AAPs, as well as a 5-HT$_2$ receptor antagonist (31).

12.2.5.2. Empirical Evidence

Results from two RPCTs comparing the effect of risperidone versus placebo augmentation therapy on time to relapse in TRD did not find statistically significant differences (32, 33). It is worth noting, though, that numerically in both studies, the median time to relapse for subjects on risperidone was greater (102–105 days) than for subjects on placebo (57–85 days). Further, two other RPCTs (total $n = 365$) demonstrated superior efficacy of risperidone over placebo as adjunct therapy in TRD on both response and remission rates (34, 35). Of note, risperidone is not FDA approved for the treatment of MDD.

12.2.5.3. Notable Adverse Effects

Due to its high potency on D_2 receptors, risperidone leads to an increased risk of EPS, especially at higher doses, as well as hyperprolactinemia and galactorrhea. As with other AAPs, it can also cause weight gain and metabolic syndrome.

12.2.6. Ziprasidone

12.2.6.1. Pharmacologic Profile

Ziprasidone, like risperidone, is a potent D_2 and 5-HT_2 receptor antagonist (31). In addition, it inhibits serotonin and norepinephrine reuptake similarly to imipramine (36).

12.2.6.2. Empirical Evidence

The first evidence for ziprasidone's efficacy as augmentation therapy in MDD came from an open-label trial of 20 subjects with TRD who had an incomplete response to an SSRI and were subsequently treated with ziprasidone. Fifty percent of the subjects were responders (37). These preliminary results were not supported, however, by a later randomized, open-label trial of MDD subjects who prospectively failed to respond to a trial of sertraline and were then randomized to receive sertraline alone, sertraline with ziprasidone 80 mg/day (mean dose 78 mg/day), or sertraline with ziprasidone 160 mg/day (mean dose 130 mg/day). The groups did not differ statistically on the mean change from baseline in the MADRS score, although a trend was observed with the highest score change in the ziprasidone 160 mg/day augmentation group (−8.27), followed by the ziprasidone 80 mg/d group (−5.98) and the sertraline monotherapy groups (−4.45) (38). A more recent RPCT testing the effect of ziprasidone versus placebo adjunctive therapy to escitalopram in subjects with MDD found significantly higher rates of clinical response and mean improvement in Hamilton Depression Rating Scale (HAM-D)-17 scores to adjunctive ziprasidone than adjunctive placebo (39). Of note, ziprasidone is not FDA approved for the treatment of MDD.

12.2.6.3. Notable Adverse Effects

Patients on ziprasidone should be monitored for EPS, akathisia, and QT prolongation. The drug can also cause somnolence, dizziness, headache, and nausea. Of note, there is a much lower risk of weight gain than with olanzapine.

12.2.7. Cariprazine

12.2.7.1. Pharmacologic Profile

Cariprazine is a partial agonist at D_2 and D_3 receptors, with 10-fold higher affinity to D_3, a receptor predominantly found in brain regions associated with motivation reward-related behavior, hence offering a rationale for its investigation as an augmentation agent in depression (40, 41). Cariprazine is also a partial agonist at 5-HT_{1A} and an antagonist at 5-HT_{2A} and 5-HT_7.

12.2.7.2. Empirical Evidence

Cariprazine is a new AAP approved by the FDA in 2015 for the treatment of schizophrenia and bipolar type 1 disorder. One large RPCT ($n = 819$) has so far been published to investigate its efficacy as an adjunctive agent to antidepressants in MDD patients who have a history of inadequate response to antidepressants. A cariprazine dose of 2 to 4.5 mg/day, but not 1 to 2 mg/day, was shown to significantly reduce the MADRS score at week 8 to a greater extent than adjunctive placebo (42). Of note, cariprazine is not FDA approved for the treatment of MDD.

12.2.7.3. Notable Adverse Effects

Adverse effects seen most commonly ($\geq$ %) with cariprazine include akathisia, EPS, insomnia, and nausea.

12.3. LITHIUM

12.3.1 Pharmacologic Profile

The mechanism of action by which lithium exerts its antidepressant augmentation properties is still not well understood. Lithium modulates and increases serotonin neurotransmission, possibly explaining its antidepressant potentiation effect (43, 44). It decreases oxidative stress by targeting second-messenger pathways; it also has neuroprotective effects by increasing the concentration of protective proteins such as brain-derived neurotrophic factor (BDNF) and inhibiting glycogen synthase kinase 3 (GSK-3β), therefore reducing apoptosis (45).

12.3.2. Empirical Evidence

Lithium augmentation to tricyclic antidepressants was first described in 1981, and 10 RPCTs were subsequently conducted in the following 20 years, offering strong support for its efficacy in depressed nonresponders (46). This is reflected by the fact that lithium is a commonly recommended augmentation strategy by treatment guidelines. A meta-analysis pooling results from all 10 trials and 231 depressed patients found that lithium augmentation was significantly more effective than placebo, with an odds ratio (OR) of 3.11 and a number needed to treat of 5 (47).

12.3.3. Notable Adverse Effects

To receive optimal efficacy and decrease the risk of serious adverse events, lithium levels should be checked five to seven days after any dose changes, and target trough levels should be between 0.6 and 0.9 mEq/L. For patients on steady doses of lithium, a lithium level should be checked every 6 to 12 months. Nevertheless, lithium can cause side effects even within the therapeutic range. It can lead to decreased glomerular filtration rate and renal dysfunction, as well as hypothyroidism and hyperparathyroidism. Therefore, levels of creatinine, thyroid hormones, and calcium should be monitored periodically. Other side effects include weight gain, tremor, diarrhea, drowsiness, polyuria, and polydipsia.

12.4. TRIIODOTHYRONINE

12.4.1. Pharmacologic Profile

Triiodothyronine (T_3) is a thyroid hormone produced naturally by the thyroid gland in response to the thyroid-stimulating hormone (TSH). The use of T_3 as an augmentation strategy is based on supporting evidence of a relationship between thyroid function and depression, although it is still not well understood.

12.4.2. Empirical Evidence

T_3 augmentation therapy in depression is still recommended by most treatment guidelines, but evidence for its efficacy is mixed. An RPCT of T_3 and lithium augmentation in depressed patients who failed to respond to tricyclic antidepressants found superior efficacy of both augmentation strategies over placebo but no significant difference between the two (48). Moreover, results from a STAR*D report, where unipolar depressed subjects who had already failed to respond to two treatment trials were randomized to either lithium or T_3, showed remission rates of 15.9% and 24.7%, respectively, although the difference did not reach statistical significance (49). However, a meta-analysis of four clinical trials ($n = 444$) did not find a significance difference in efficacy between the co-initiation of an SSRI and T_3 on one hand and SSRI monotherapy on the other hand, in the treatment of MDD (50).

12.4.3. Notable Adverse Effects

T_3 is generally well tolerated, with a favorable side-effect profile compared to other augmentation strategies. T_3 may cause hyperthyroidism-like symptoms, including tremor, sweating, palpitations, shortness of breath, and increased frequency of bowel movements. Long-term use may lead to osteoporosis and a higher risk of fracture.

12.5. COMBINATION ANTIDEPRESSANTS

Combination antidepressant therapy, a commonly used strategy in patients who fail to respond to antidepressant monotherapy, refers to using a combination of antidepressants from different classes. The rationale behind this strategy is to combine antidepressants with different mechanisms of action, leading to a synergistic effect. However, using combination strategy as the initial treatment is generally not recommended due to the lack of evidence showing any benefit over a monotherapy trial (51). It is also important to note that certain antidepressant combinations should be avoided due to the high risk of drug–drug interactions leading to serious adverse events (e.g., using a monoamine oxidase inhibitor with an antidepressant that increases serotonin reuptake leads to a significant increase in the risk of serotonin syndrome). Likewise, it is not recommended to use antidepressants with pharmacokinetics interactions, such as the blockade by the first antidepressant of one or more CYP450 enzymes that have a primary role in metabolism of the second antidepressant. A detailed description of the different antidepressants used in combination therapy is given in other chapters.

12.6. NUTRACEUTICALS

12.6.1. Pharmacologic Profile

Omega-3 modulates serotonin, norepinephrine, and dopamine neurotransmission and increases glutathione antioxidant capacity, potentially underpinning its antidepressant properties. L-methylfolate and S-adenosyl methionine (SAMe) are involved in monoamines' methylation, potentially explaining their utility in depression treatment.

12.6.2. Empirical Evidence

Several RPCTs have demonstrated efficacy of omega-3 fatty acids as an augmentation strategy in MDD. A meta-analysis of eight double-blind randomized controlled trials ($n = 448$) found that depressed patients on adjunctive omega-3 (primarily eicosapentaenoic acid [EPA]) for a period of 4 to 12 weeks improved significantly compared to patients on adjunctive placebo, with a moderate to large effect size (Hedges' g) of 0.61 ($p = .009$) (52).

An L-methylfolate dose of 15 mg/day was compared to placebo as adjunctive therapy for 75 patients with SSRI-resistant depression in an RPCT. The L-methylfolate arm had a significantly higher response rate (32.3% vs. 14.6%; $p = .04$) and decrease in HAM-D score (-5.58 vs. -3.04; $p = .05$) compared to placebo, with a number needed to treat of 6 to achieve response with adjunct L-methylfolate (53).

An RPCT of 73 serotonin reuptake inhibitor nonresponders with a diagnosis of MDD comparing adjunctive SAMe (target dose 1,600 mg/day) to placebo resulted in statistically significantly higher response (36.1% vs. 17.6%) and re-mission rates (25.8% vs. 11.7%) with SAMe versus placebo, respectively (54). Also, the side-effect profile was comparable between the SAMe and placebo arms. Of note, there was no significant reduction in the HAM-D score between the two groups. Other open-label trials have showed consistent results in favor of the efficacy of SAMe as an augmenting agent in TRD, at doses of both 800 and 1,600 mg/day (55, 56).

12.6.3. Notable Adverse Effects

All the nutraceuticals are generally well tolerated, with very low rates of dropouts due to side effects in clinical trials. The most commonly observed adverse effects are gastrointestinal symptoms. SAMe, especially when administered intramuscularly or intravenously, has also been reported to induce hypomania/mania in depressed patients, particularly bipolar patients.

12.7. INVESTIGATIONAL DRUGS

12.7.1. Ketamine

Ketamine is an N-methyl-D-aspartate (NMDA) receptor antagonist, although the exact mechanism of action underlying its antidepressant properties is still poorly understood. Ketamine is used as an anesthetic but has garnered great interest for its rapid and robust antidepressant effects in uncontrolled studies (For a more detailed description of the efficacy of ketamine in MDD, including ketamine monotherapy trials, see Chapter 13 in this volume). An RPCT of adjunctive single-dose intrave-nous ketamine (0.5 mg/kg) plus escitalopram versus placebo plus escitalopram in 30 patients with severe MDD showed that the former group had significantly higher response (92.3% v. 57.1%, $p = .04$) and remission rates (76.9% v. 14.3%, $p = .001$), as well as shorter time to response and remission (57). Another RPCT ($n = 67$) tested the efficacy of intravenous ketamine augmentation (two or three times a week for up to four weeks) versus placebo while the antidepressant regimen remained unchanged (58). Ketamine performed significantly better than placebo in both the twice-weekly (-18.4 vs. -5.7; $p < .001$) and thrice-weekly (-17.7 vs. -3.1; $p < .001$) groups over 15 days. Despite these positive results, it is still recommended to limit the off-label use of ketamine to situations where benefits clearly outweigh risks, and until more is known about the long-term maintenance of its antidepressant properties, its adverse-effects profile, and its potential for abuse. A consensus statement from the American Psychiatric Association Council of Research Task Force on Novel Biomarkers and Treatments has been published to offer guidance on the proper use of ketamine in MDD (59).

12.7.2. Esketamine

Esketamine, the S(+) enantiomer of ketamine and a more potent NMDA receptor antagonist than its stereoisomer, is a compound that was recently approved by the FDA for patients who failed to respond to two or more treatment trials and as a combination with a newly started antidepressant, but not as an add-on to a previously existing one (60). An RPCT ($n = 67$ TRD patients) investigated the efficacy of intranasal esketamine (28, 56, 84 mg twice weekly) augmentation to the existing antidepressant regimen, compared to placebo augmentation (61). A dose–response relationship on the MADRS score change was observed, with the maximum improvement notable in the group receiving esketamine 84 mg (esketamine 28 mg: −4.2 [2.09], $p = .02$; 56 mg: −6.3 [2.07], $p = .001$; 84 mg: −9.0 [2.13], $p < .001$). The antidepressant effect was further maintained in an open-label extension phase of 74 days where the esketamine dosing frequency was gradually tapered to once every two weeks. Another recent RPCT (n = 68 hospitalized patients with severe MDD and imminent risk of suicide) also found significant improvement in MADRS score change over 4 and 24 hours, but not 25 days, in patients receiving augmentation with intranasal esketamine 84 mg versus placebo twice weekly (62). More recently, three phase 3 trials comparing esketamine to placebo over four weeks were completed, with one demonstrating a significantly superior response to esketamine vs. placebo (63), and two others not meeting the primary efficacy endpoint (64, 65). Another long-term maintenance trial showed a significantly longer time to relapse in responders who were continued on esketamine plus an oral antidepressant versus ones on placebo and an oral antidepressant (66). Side effects observed with esketamine include dizziness, headache, nausea, dissociation, and unpleasant taste.

12.7.3. ALKS 5461

ALKS 5461 is a combination of buprenorphine, a μ partial agonist and weak κ antagonist, and samidorphan, a μ antagonist. The resulting combination therefore acts as a selective κ-opoid receptor (KOR) antagonist. ALKS 5461 is currently under development for the indication of adjunctive therapy in TRD. A two-stage sequential parallel comparison design (SPCD) RPCT ($n = 98$ patients with TRD) demonstrated significant improvement on all primary outcomes measures for the adjunctive treatment with 2 mg/2 mg of buprenorphine/samidorphan (HAM-D: −2.8, 95% confidence interval [CI] = −5.1, −0.6; MADRS: −4.9, 95% CI = −8.2, −1.6; Clinical Global Impression—Severity [CGI-S]: −0.5, 95% CI = −0.9, −0.1) but not for the group receiving the 8 mg/8 mg combination (67). Three phase 3 trials have also been conducted and published: (1) One trial did not meet its primary endpoint (68), (2) another one trended toward efficacy with the 2 mg/2 mg dose on the primary endpoint and showed significant treatment differences on other regulatory-accepted endpoints, such as the MADRS; and (3) the third SPCD trial met its primary endpoint on 2 mg/2 mg dose (69). One other RCT is pending.

12.8. PSYCHOTHERAPY

Psychotherapy, covered more thoroughly in other chapters, can be a valuable treatment option for augmentation, especially in patients with comorbidities and higher risk from polypharmacy. In the STAR*D trial, patients not responding to citalopram monotherapy received augmentation with either CBT or medication (bupropion or buspirone) in a nonrandomized fashion (70). Although the medication augmentation group remitted faster than the CBT augmentation group (55 vs. 40 days), no significant difference was seen in terms of remission rates between the two groups. A more recent RCT examining adjunct CBT to pharmacotherapy in 469 patients with TRD found that 46% in the CBT + usual care group responded versus only 22% in the usual care group (OR = 3.26, $p < .001$) (71).

12.9. AUGMENTATION TREATMENTS WITH LITTLE EVIDENCE

12.9.1. Buspirone

Buspirone was compared to bupropion as an augmenting agent to citalopram in the STAR*D randomized, open-label trial comprising 565 patients with unipolar depression. No statistically significant differences in response (26.9% vs. 31.8%) or remission rates (30.1% vs. 29.7%) were seen between the two agents, respectively (72). However, results from two RPCTs ($n = 119$ and 102) failed to show a significant difference between buspirone and placebo augmentation in SSRI-resistant patients with unipolar depression (73, 74).

12.9.2. Pindolol

In a meta-analysis of 12 RPCTs ($n = 889$) comparing augmentation with pindolol versus placebo in MDD, patients on pindolol and citalopram showed higher rates of accelerated response than those taking placebo and citalopram in the first two weeks (relative risk [RR] = 1.68; 95% CI, 1.18–2.39; $p = .004$) and at four to six weeks (RR = 1.11; 95% CI, 1.02–1.20; $p = .02$). However, no statistically significant advantage to pindolol augmentation was seen at end-of-study response outcomes (75).

12.9.3. Methylphenidate

Methylphenidate is pharmacologically related to amphetamine and is thought to block norepinephrine and dopamine reuptake and rapidly increase the release of monoamines in the synaptic cleft. Two RPCTs testing the augmentation of methylphenidate in adults with TRD did not show any statistically significant difference from placebo outcomes (76, 77). However, methylphenidate's augmentation in TRD has been more beneficial in late-life depression. A small RPCT ($n = 16$) showed a significantly better response to adjunctive methylphenidate than placebo in older patients (mean age 74 years) with TRD treated with citalopram (78). Subsequently, the same group published a larger RPCT where 143 patients (mean age 70 years) with MDD (41% with TRD) were treated with citalopram plus methylphenidate, citalopram plus placebo, and methylphenidate plus placebo. The combination treatment outperformed the other two monotherapy arms (79). Potential benefits of adjunctive methylphenidate in older adults should be weighed against adverse effects such as anxiety, insomnia, decreased appetite, nausea, headache, and adverse cardiac effects.

12.9.4. Modafinil

Modafinil, a psychostimulant-like drug, has been investigated as an adjunct to ongoing antidepressant treatment in two major RPCTs, both of which failed to demonstrate superior efficacy against placebo on primary outcomes (80, 81). In a meta-analysis of three RPCTs ($n = 522$) comparing adjunctive modafinil to placebo in unipolar major depression, modafinil was a more efficacious augmenting agent than placebo, although the effect was small (Hedges' g = -0.18; 95% CI, -0.35, -0.01; $p = .04$) (82). A sub-analysis of six studies including patients with both unipolar and bipolar depression showed that modafinil is particularly effective for treating fatigue symptoms.

12.9.5. Pramipexole

Evidence for pramipexole, a dopamine-receptor agonist, is still limited, with only one RPCT ($n = 60$) to date investigating its augmenting effect versus placebo in TRD (83). Pramipexole was shown to have a small but significant ($p = .038$) augmenting effect over adjunctive placebo on depressive symptoms after eight weeks of treatment. Another RPCT published negative results in the same year; however, it was testing a combination treatment of pramipexole and escitalopram (started simultaneously) rather than the former as an augmenting agent, compared to pramipexole or escitalopram monotherapy (84). The study also suffered from a high dropout rate in the combination arm due to subjects not being able to tolerate the dose titration schedule of pramipexole.

12.9.6. Testosterone

Testosterone has also been investigated as an add-on for the treatment of MDD, but several RPCTs have provided conflicting results. One study of 100 hypogonadal men with MDD using add-on testosterone gel and another one with 32 hypogonadal men using add-on intramuscular testosterone did not find significant differences between testosterone and placebo (85, 86). In contrast, 22 hypogonadal men with MDD were randomized to 1% testosterone gel 10 g/day or matching placebo, with results pointing to the superiority of testosterone over placebo in reducing depressive symptoms after eight weeks (87). In two other RPCTs of hypogonadal ($n = 18$; testosterone gel) (88) and eugonadal ($n = 26$; intramuscular testosterone) (89) depressed men, testosterone was found numerically superior to placebo in terms of reduction of depressive symptoms and treatment response, respectively. However, these results were not statistically significant. In sum, adjunct testosterone may be helpful in depressed men with low testosterone level, but larger studies are warranted.

12.10. SUMMARY AND RECOMMENDATIONS

The pathophysiology of MDD is complex and potentially involves multiple neurotransmitter circuits. Therefore patients who have had a partial response and who are able to tolerate first-line antidepressant monotherapy often benefit from an augmenting agent with a different mechanism of action. Therefore, it is recommended to use an augmenting agent and/or psychotherapy for patients who partially respond to initial treatment. Perhaps the most important lesson from STAR*D is that monotherapies become progressively more futile after second-line treatment (1, 90, 91). Therefore, augmentation should be equally considered for partial responders as well as frank nonresponders to antidepressant monotherapy after two failed trials. AAPs and lithium remain the most evidence-based and widely used augmenting agents. Intranasal esketamine is approved for use for patients who fail to respond to more than two treatments, but only in combination with a newly initiated antidepressant (as opposed to adjunctive use with a preexisting one).

AUTHOR NOTE

Funding Support: None.
Acknowledgments: None.
Conflict of Interest: NCS has no conflict of interest to report. As part of his current fellowship training, he also works in the digital medicine group at Pfizer Inc.; however, this work has no relevance or conflict of interest with the subject of this chapter. GIP has served as a consultant for Abbott Laboratories, Acadia Pharmaceuticals, Inc.,* Alkermes, Inc., AstraZeneca PLC, Avanir Pharmaceuticals, Axsome Therapeutics,* Boston Pharmaceuticals, Inc., Brainsway Ltd., Bristol-Myers Squibb Company, Cephalon Inc., Dey Pharma, L.P., Eli Lilly Co., Genentech, Inc.,* Genomind, Inc.,* GlaxoSmithKline, Evotec AG, H. Lundbeck A/S, Inflabloc Pharmaceuticals, Janssen Global Services LLC,* Jazz Pharmaceuticals, Johnson & Johnson Companies,* Methylation Sciences Inc., Mylan Inc.,* Novartis Pharma AG, One Carbon Therapeutics, Inc.,* Osmotica Pharmaceutical Corp.,* Otsuka Pharmaceuticals, PAMLAB LLC, Pfizer Inc., Pierre Fabre Laboratories, Ridge Diagnostics (formerly known as Precision Human Biolaboratories), Shire Pharmaceuticals, Sunovion Pharmaceuticals, Taisho Pharmaceutical Co, Ltd., Takeda Pharmaceutical Company LTD, Theracos, Inc., and Wyeth, Inc. GIP has received honoraria (for lectures or consultancy) from Abbott Laboratories, Acadia Pharmaceuticals Inc., Alkermes Inc.,

Asopharma America Central y Caribe, Astra Zeneca PLC, Avanir Pharmaceuticals, Bristol-Myers Squibb Company, Brainsway Ltd., Cephalon Inc., Dey Pharma, L.P., Eli Lilly Co., Evotec AG, Forest Pharmaceuticals, GlaxoSmithKline, Inflabloc Pharmaceuticals, Grunbiotics Pty LTD, Jazz Pharmaceuticals, H. Lundbeck A/S, Medichem Pharmaceuticals, Inc., Meiji Seika Pharma Co. Ltd., Novartis Pharma AG, Otsuka Pharmaceuticals, PAMLAB LLC, Pfizer, Pharma Trade SAS, Pierre Fabre Laboratories, Ridge Diagnostics, Shire Pharmaceuticals, Sunovion Pharmaceuticals, Takeda Pharmaceutical Company LTD, Theracos, Inc., Titan Pharmaceuticals, and Wyeth Inc. GIP has received research support (paid to hospital) from AstraZeneca PLC, Bristol-Myers Squibb Company, Forest Pharmaceuticals, the National Institute of Mental Health, Neuralstem, Inc.,* PAMLAB LLC, Pfizer Inc., Ridge Diagnostics (formerly known as Precision Human Biolaboratories), Sunovion Pharmaceuticals, Tal Medical, and Theracos, Inc. GIP has served (not currently) on the speaker's bureau for BristolMyersSquibb Co and Pfizer, Inc. * Asterisk denotes activity undertaken on behalf of Massachusetts General Hospital.

REFERENCES

1. Rush AJ, Trivedi MH, Wisniewski SR, Nierenberg AA, Stewart JW, Warden D, et al. Acute and longer-term outcomes in depressed outpatients requiring one or several treatment steps: a STAR*D report. Am J Psychiatry. 2006;163(11):1905–1917.
2. Ostroff RB, Nelson JC. Risperidone augmentation of selective serotonin reuptake inhibitors in major depression. J Clin Psychiatry. 1999;60(4):256–259.
3. Lawler CP, Prioleau C, Lewis MM, Mak C, Jiang D, Schetz JA, et al. Interactions of the novel antipsychotic aripiprazole (OPC-14597) with dopamine and serotonin receptor subtypes. Neuropsychopharmacology. 1999;20(6):612–627.
4. Papakostas GI, Petersen TJ, Kinrys G, Burns AM, Worthington JJ, Alpert JE, et al. Aripiprazole augmentation of selective serotonin reuptake inhibitors for treatment-resistant major depressive disorder. J Clin Psychiatry. 2005;66(10):1326–1330.
5. Berman RM, Marcus RN, Swanink R, McQuade RD, Carson WH, Corey-Lisle PK, et al. The efficacy and safety of aripiprazole as adjunctive therapy in major depressive disorder: a multicenter, randomized, double-blind, placebo-controlled study. J Clin Psychiatry. 2007;68(6):843–853.
6. Marcus RN, McQuade RD, Carson WH, Hennicken D, Fava M, Simon JS, et al. The efficacy and safety of aripiprazole as adjunctive therapy in major depressive disorder: a second multicenter, randomized, double-blind, placebo-controlled study. J Clin Psychopharmacol. 2008;28(2):156–165.
7. Lenze EJ, Mulsant BH, Blumberger DM, Karp JF, Newcomer JW, Anderson SJ, et al. Efficacy, safety, and tolerability of augmentation pharmacotherapy with aripiprazole for treatment-resistant depression in late life: a randomised, double-blind, placebo-controlled trial. Lancet. 2015;386(10011):2404–12.
8. Kamijima K, Higuchi T, Ishigooka J, Ohmori T, Ozaki N, Kanba S, et al. Aripiprazole augmentation to antidepressant therapy in Japanese patients with major depressive disorder: a randomized, double-blind, placebo-controlled study (ADMIRE study). J Affect Disord. 2013;151(3):899–905.
9. Berman RM, Fava M, Thase ME, Trivedi MH, Swanink R, McQuade RD, et al. Aripiprazole augmentation in major depressive disorder: a double-blind, placebo-controlled study in patients with inadequate response to antidepressants. CNS Spectr. 2009;14(4):197–206.

10. Han C, Wang SM, Kwak KP, Won WY, Lee H, Chang CM, et al. Aripiprazole augmentation versus antidepressant switching for patients with major depressive disorder: a 6-week, randomized, rater-blinded, prospective study. J Psychiatr Res. 2015;66–67:84–94.

11. Mohamed S, Johnson GR, Chen P, Hicks PB, Davis LL, Yoon J, et al. Effect of antidepressant switching vs augmentation on remission among patients with major depressive disorder unresponsive to antidepressant treatment: the VAST-D randomized clinical trial. JAMA. 2017;318(2):132–145.

12. Maeda K, Lerdrup L, Sugino H, Akazawa H, Amada N, McQuade RD, et al. Brexpiprazole II: antipsychotic-like and procognitive effects of a novel serotonin-dopamine activity modulator. J Pharmacol Exp Ther. 2014;350(3):605–614.

13. Thase ME, Youakim JM, Skuban A, Hobart M, Zhang P, McQuade RD, et al. Adjunctive brexpiprazole 1 and 3 mg for patients with major depressive disorder following inadequate response to antidepressants: a phase 3, randomized, double-blind study. J Clin Psychiatry. 2015;76(9):1232–1240.

14. Thase ME, Youakim JM, Skuban A, Hobart M, Augustine C, Zhang P, et al. Efficacy and safety of adjunctive brexpiprazole 2 mg in major depressive disorder: a phase 3, randomized, placebo-controlled study in patients with inadequate response to antidepressants. J Clin Psychiatry. 2015;76(9):1224–1231.

15. McIntyre RS, Weiller E, Zhang P, Weiss C. Brexpiprazole as adjunctive treatment of major depressive disorder with anxious distress: results from a post-hoc analysis of two randomised controlled trials. J Affect Disord. 2016;201:116–123.

16. Hobart M, Skuban A, Zhang P, Josiassen MK, Hefting N, Augustine C, et al. Efficacy and safety of flexibly dosed brexpiprazole for the adjunctive treatment of major depressive disorder: a randomized, active-referenced, placebo-controlled study. Curr Med Res Opin. 2018;34(4):633–642.

17. Mauri MC, Paletta S, Maffini M, Colasanti A, Dragogna F, Di Pace C, et al. Clinical pharmacology of atypical antipsychotics: an update. EXCLI J. 2014;13:1163–1191.

18. Shelton RC, Tollefson GD, Tohen M, Stahl S, Gannon KS, Jacobs TG, et al. A novel augmentation strategy for treating resistant major depression. Am J Psychiatry. 2001;158(1):131–134.

19. Thase ME, Corya SA, Osuntokun O, Case M, Henley DB, Sanger TM, et al. A randomized, double-blind comparison of olanzapine/fluoxetine combination, olanzapine, and fluoxetine in treatment-resistant major depressive disorder. J Clin Psychiatry. 2007;68(2):224–236.

20. Shelton RC, Williamson DJ, Corya SA, Sanger TM, Van Campen LE, Case M, et al. Olanzapine/fluoxetine combination for treatment-resistant depression: a controlled study of SSRI and nortriptyline resistance. J Clin Psychiatry. 2005;66(10):1289–1297.

21. Corya SA, Williamson D, Sanger TM, Briggs SD, Case M, Tollefson G. A randomized, double-blind comparison of olanzapine/fluoxetine combination, olanzapine, fluoxetine, and venlafaxine in treatment-resistant depression. Depress Anxiety. 2006;23(6):364–372.

22. Brunner E, Tohen M, Osuntokun O, Landry J, Thase ME. Efficacy and safety of olanzapine/fluoxetine combination vs fluoxetine monotherapy following successful combination therapy of treatment-resistant major depressive disorder. Neuropsychopharmacology. 2014;39(11):2549–2559.

23. Saller CF, Salama AI. Seroquel: biochemical profile of a potential atypical antipsychotic. Psychopharmacology (Berl). 1993;112(2–3):285–292.

24. Bauer M, Pretorius HW, Constant EL, Earley WR, Szamosi J, Brecher M. Extended-release quetiapine as adjunct to an antidepressant in patients with major depressive disorder: results of a randomized, placebo-controlled, double-blind study. J Clin Psychiatry. 2009;70(4):540–549.

25. El-Khalili N, Joyce M, Atkinson S, Buynak RJ, Datto C, Lindgren P, et al. Extended-release quetiapine fumarate (quetiapine XR) as adjunctive therapy in major depressive disorder (MDD) in patients with an inadequate response to ongoing antidepressant treatment: a multicentre,

randomized, double-blind, placebo-controlled study. Int J Neuropsychopharmacol. 2010;13(7):917–932.

26. Wijkstra J, Burger H, van den Broek WW, Birkenhäger TK, Janzing JG, Boks MP, et al. Treatment of unipolar psychotic depression: a randomized, double-blind study comparing imipramine, venlafaxine, and venlafaxine plus quetiapine. Acta Psychiatr Scand. 2010;121(3):190–200.

27. Chaput Y, Magnan A, Gendron A. The co-administration of quetiapine or placebo to cognitive-behavior therapy in treatment refractory depression: a preliminary trial. BMC Psychiatry. 2008;8:73.

28. McIntyre A, Gendron A. Quetiapine adjunct to selective serotonin reuptake inhibitors or venlafaxine in patients with major depression, comorbid anxiety, and residual depressive symptoms: a randomized, placebo-controlled pilot study. Depress Anxiety. 2007;24(7):487–494.

29. Bauer M, Dell'osso L, Kasper S, Pitchot W, Dencker Vansvik E, Köhler J, et al. Extended-release quetiapine fumarate (quetiapine XR) monotherapy and quetiapine XR or lithium as add-on to antidepressants in patients with treatment-resistant major depressive disorder. J Affect Disord. 2013;151(1):209–219.

30. Garakani A, Martinez JM, Marcus S, Weaver J, Rickels K, Fava M, et al. A randomized, double-blind, and placebo-controlled trial of quetiapine augmentation of fluoxetine in major depressive disorder. Int Clin Psychopharmacol. 2008;23(5):269–275.

31. Richelson E, Souder T. Binding of antipsychotic drugs to human brain receptors focus on newer generation compounds. Life Sci. 2000;68(1):29–39.

32. Rapaport MH, Gharabawi GM, Canuso CM, Mahmoud RA, Keller MB, Bossie CA, et al. Effects of risperidone augmentation in patients with treatment-resistant depression: results of open-label treatment followed by double-blind continuation. Neuropsychopharmacology. 2006;31(11):2505–2513.

33. Alexopoulos GS, Canuso CM, Gharabawi GM, Bossie CA, Greenspan A, Turkoz I, et al. Placebo-controlled study of relapse prevention with risperidone augmentation in older patients with resistant depression. Am J Geriatr Psychiatry. 2008;16(1):21–30.

34. Mahmoud RA, Pandina GJ, Turkoz I, Kosik-Gonzalez C, Canuso CM, Kujawa MJ, et al. Risperidone for treatment-refractory major depressive disorder: a randomized trial. Ann Intern Med. 2007;147(9):593–602.

35. Keitner GI, Garlow SJ, Ryan CE, Ninan PT, Solomon DA, Nemeroff CB, et al. A randomized, placebo-controlled trial of risperidone augmentation for patients with difficult-to-treat unipolar, non-psychotic major depression. J Psychiatr Res. 2009;43(3):205–214.

36. Schmidt AW, Lebel LA, Howard HR, Zorn SH. Ziprasidone: a novel antipsychotic agent with a unique human receptor binding profile. Eur J Pharmacol. 2001;425(3):197–201.

37. Papakostas GI, Petersen TJ, Nierenberg AA, Murakami JL, Alpert JE, Rosenbaum JF, et al. Ziprasidone augmentation of selective serotonin reuptake inhibitors (SSRIs) for SSRI-resistant major depressive disorder. J Clin Psychiatry. 2004;65(2):217–221.

38. Dunner DL, Amsterdam JD, Shelton RC, Loebel A, Romano SJ. Efficacy and tolerability of adjunctive ziprasidone in treatment-resistant depression: a randomized, open-label, pilot study. J Clin Psychiatry. 2007;68(7):1071–1077.

39. Papakostas GI, Fava M, Baer L, Swee MB, Jaeger A, Bobo WV, et al. Ziprasidone augmentation of escitalopram for major depressive disorder: efficacy results from a randomized, double-blind, placebo-controlled study. Am J Psychiatry. 2015;172(12):1251–1258.

40. Kiss B, Horváth A, Némethy Z, Schmidt E, Laszlovszky I, Bugovics G, et al. Cariprazine (RGH-188), a dopamine D(3) receptor-preferring, D(3)/D(2) dopamine receptor antagonist-partial agonist antipsychotic candidate: in vitro and neurochemical profile. J Pharmacol Exp Ther. 2010;333(1):328–340.

41. Leggio GM, Salomone S, Bucolo C, Platania C, Micale V, Caraci F, et al. Dopamine D(3) receptor as a new pharmacological target for the treatment of depression. Eur J Pharmacol. 2013;719(1-3):25–33.

42. Durgam S, Earley W, Guo H, Li D, Németh G, Laszlovszky I, et al. Efficacy and safety of adjunctive cariprazine in inadequate responders to antidepressants: a randomized, double-blind, placebo-controlled study in adult patients with major depressive disorder. J Clin Psychiatry. 2016;77(3):371–378.

43. Wegener G, Bandpey Z, Heiberg IL, Mørk A, Rosenberg R. Increased extracellular serotonin level in rat hippocampus induced by chronic citalopram is augmented by subchronic lithium: neurochemical and behavioural studies in the rat. Psychopharmacology (Berl). 2003;166(2):188–194.

44. Okamoto Y, Motohasi N, Hayakawa H, Muraoka M, Yamawaki S. Addition of lithium to chronic antidepressant treatment potentiates presynaptic serotonergic function without changes in serotonergic receptors in the rat cerebral cortex. Neuropsychobiology. 1996;33(1): 17–20.

45. Malhi GS, Tanious M, Das P, Coulston CM, Berk M. Potential mechanisms of action of lithium in bipolar disorder. Current understanding. CNS Drugs. 2013;27(2):135–153.

46. Bauer M, Adli M, Bschor T, Pilhatsch M, Pfennig A, Sasse J, et al. Lithium's emerging role in the treatment of refractory major depressive episodes: augmentation of antidepressants. Neuropsychobiology. 2010;62(1):36–42.

47. Crossley NA, Bauer M. Acceleration and augmentation of antidepressants with lithium for depressive disorders: two meta-analyses of randomized, placebo-controlled trials. J Clin Psychiatry. 2007;68(6):935–940.

48. Joffe RT, Singer W, Levitt AJ, MacDonald C. A placebo-controlled comparison of lithium and triiodothyronine augmentation of tricyclic antidepressants in unipolar refractory depression. Arch Gen Psychiatry. 1993;50(5):387–393.

49. Nierenberg AA, Fava M, Trivedi MH, Wisniewski SR, Thase ME, McGrath PJ, et al. A comparison of lithium and T(3) augmentation following two failed medication treatments for depression: a STAR*D report. Am J Psychiatry. 2006;163(9):1519–1530.

50. Papakostas GI, Cooper-Kazaz R, Appelhof BC, Posternak MA, Johnson DP, Klibanski A, et al. Simultaneous initiation (coinitiation) of pharmacotherapy with triiodothyronine and a selective serotonin reuptake inhibitor for major depressive disorder: a quantitative synthesis of double-blind studies. Int Clin Psychopharmacol. 2009;24(1):19–25.

51. Rush AJ, Trivedi MH, Stewart JW, Nierenberg AA, Fava M, Kurian BT, et al. Combining medications to enhance depression outcomes (CO-MED): acute and long-term outcomes of a single-blind randomized study. Am J Psychiatry. 2011;168(7):689–701.

52. Sarris J, Murphy J, Mischoulon D, Papakostas GI, Fava M, Berk M, et al. Adjunctive nutraceuticals for depression: a systematic review and meta-analyses. Am J Psychiatry. 2016;173(6):575–587.

53. Papakostas GI, Shelton RC, Zajecka JM, Etemad B, Rickels K, Clain A, et al. L-methylfolate as adjunctive therapy for SSRI-resistant major depression: results of two randomized, double-blind, parallel-sequential trials. Am J Psychiatry. 2012;169(12):1267–1274.

54. Papakostas GI, Mischoulon D, Shyu I, Alpert JE, Fava M. S-adenosyl methionine (SAMe) augmentation of serotonin reuptake inhibitors for antidepressant nonresponders with major depressive disorder: a double-blind, randomized clinical trial. Am J Psychiatry. 2010;167(8):942–948.

55. De Berardis D, Marini S, Serroni N, Rapini G, Iasevoli F, Valchera A, et al. S-adenosyl-L-methionine augmentation in patients with stage II treatment-resistant major depressive disorder: an open label, fixed dose, single-blind study. Scientific World Journal. 2013;2013:204649.

56. Alpert JE, Papakostas G, Mischoulon D, Worthington JJ, Petersen T, Mahal Y, et al. S-adenosyl-L-methionine (SAMe) as an adjunct for resistant major depressive disorder: an open trial following partial or nonresponse to selective serotonin reuptake inhibitors or venlafaxine. J Clin Psychopharmacol. 2004;24(6):661–664.

57. Hu YD, Xiang YT, Fang JX, Zu S, Sha S, Shi H, et al. Single i.v. ketamine augmentation of newly initiated escitalopram for major depression: results from a randomized, placebo-controlled 4-week study. Psychol Med. 2016;46(3):623–635.

58. Singh JB, Fedgchin M, Daly EJ, De Boer P, Cooper K, Lim P, et al. A double-blind, randomized, placebo-controlled, dose-frequency study of intravenous ketamine in patients with treatment-resistant depression. Am J Psychiatry. 2016;173(8):816–826.

59. Sanacora G, Frye MA, McDonald W, Mathew SJ, Turner MS, Schatzberg AF, et al. A consensus statement on the use of ketamine in the treatment of mood disorders. JAMA Psychiatry. 2017;74(4):399–405.

60. FDA approves new nasal spray medication for treatment-resistant depression; available only at a certified doctor's office or clinic. [press release]. U.S. Food & Drug Administration. 2019.

61. Daly EJ, Singh JB, Fedgchin M, Cooper K, Lim P, Shelton RC, et al. Efficacy and safety of intranasal esketamine adjunctive to oral antidepressant therapy in treatment-resistant depression: a randomized clinical trial. JAMA Psychiatry. 2018;75(2):139–148.

62. Canuso CM, Singh JB, Fedgchin M, Alphs L, Lane R, Lim P, et al. Efficacy and safety of intranasal esketamine for the rapid reduction of symptoms of depression and suicidality in patients at imminent risk for suicide: results of a double-blind, randomized, placebo-controlled study. Am J Psychiatry. 2018;175(7):620–630.

63. Janssen R&D. Randomized, double-blind study of flexibly-dosed intranasal esketamine plus oral antidepressant vs. active control in treatment-resistant depression. Poster presented at the 2018 Annual Meeting of the American Society of Clinical Psychopharmacology, May 30, 2018, Miami, FL. Poster W30.

64. Janssen R&D. Randomized, double-blind study of fixed-dosed intranasal esketamine plus oral antidepressant vs. active control in treatment-resistant depression. Poster presented at the 9th Biennial Conference of the International Society for Affective Disorders (ISAD), September 20–22, 2018, Houston, TX.

65. Janssen R&D. Efficacy and safety of esketamine nasal spray plus an oral antidepressant in elderly patients with treatment-resistant depression. Poster presented at the 2018 Annual Meeting of the American Society of Clinical Psychopharmacology, May 29–June 1, 2018. Poster W27.

66. Janssen R&D. A randomized withdrawal, double-blind, multicenter study of esketamine nasal spray plus an oral antidepressant for relapse prevention in treatment-resistant depression. Poster presented at the 2018 Annual Meeting of American Society of Clinical Psychopharmacology, May 30, 2018, Miami, FL. Poster W68.

67. Fava M, Memisoglu A, Thase ME, Bodkin JA, Trivedi MH, de Somer M, et al. Opioid modulation with buprenorphine/samidorphan as adjunctive treatment for inadequate response to antidepressants: a randomized double-blind placebo-controlled trial. Am J Psychiatry. 2016;173(5):499–508.

68. Zajecka JM, Stanford AD, Memisoglu A, Martin WF, Pathak S. Buprenorphine/samidorphan combination for the adjunctive treatment of major depressive disorder: results of a phase III clinical trial (FORWARD-3). Neuropsychiatr Dis Treat. 2019;15:795–808.

69. Fava M, Thase ME, Trivedi MH, Ehrich E, Martin WF, Memisoglu A, et al. Opioid system modulation with buprenorphine/samidorphan combination for major depressive disorder: two randomized controlled studies. Mol Psychiatry. 2018. doi: 10.1038/s41380-018-0284-1.

70. Thase ME, Friedman ES, Biggs MM, Wisniewski SR, Trivedi MH, Luther JF, et al. Cognitive therapy versus medication in augmentation and switch strategies as second-step treatments: a STAR*D report. Am J Psychiatry. 2007;164(5):739–752.

71. Wiles N, Thomas L, Abel A, Ridgway N, Turner N, Campbell J, et al. Cognitive behavioural therapy as an adjunct to pharmacotherapy for primary care based patients with treatment resistant depression: results of the CoBalT randomised controlled trial. Lancet. 2013;381(9864):375–384.

72. Trivedi MH, Fava M, Wisniewski SR, Thase ME, Quitkin F, Warden D, et al. Medication augmentation after the failure of SSRIs for depression. N Engl J Med. 2006;354(12):1243–1252.

73. Appelberg BG, Syvälahti EK, Koskinen TE, Mehtonen OP, Muhonen TT, Naukkarinen HH. Patients with severe depression may benefit from buspirone augmentation of selective serotonin reuptake inhibitors: results from a placebo-controlled, randomized, double-blind, placebo wash-in study. J Clin Psychiatry. 2001;62(6):448–452.

74. Landén M, Björling G, Agren H, Fahlén T. A randomized, double-blind, placebo-controlled trial of buspirone in combination with an SSRI in patients with treatment-refractory depression. J Clin Psychiatry. 1998;59(12):664–668.

75. Portella MJ, de Diego-Adeliño J, Ballesteros J, Puigdemont D, Oller S, Santos B, et al. Can we really accelerate and enhance the selective serotonin reuptake inhibitor antidepressant effect? A randomized clinical trial and a meta-analysis of pindolol in nonresistant depression. J Clin Psychiatry. 2011;72(7):962–969.

76. Ravindran AV, Kennedy SH, O'Donovan MC, Fallu A, Camacho F, Binder CE. Osmotic-release oral system methylphenidate augmentation of antidepressant monotherapy in major depressive disorder: results of a double-blind, randomized, placebo-controlled trial. J Clin Psychiatry. 2008;69(1):87–94.

77. Patkar AA, Masand PS, Pae CU, Peindl K, Hooper-Wood C, Mannelli P, et al. A randomized, double-blind, placebo-controlled trial of augmentation with an extended release formulation of methylphenidate in outpatients with treatment-resistant depression. J Clin Psychopharmacol. 2006;26(6):653–656.

78. Lavretsky H, Park S, Siddarth P, Kumar A, Reynolds CF. Methylphenidate-enhanced antidepressant response to citalopram in the elderly: a double-blind, placebo-controlled pilot trial. Am J Geriatr Psychiatry. 2006;14(2):181–185.

79. Lavretsky H, Reinlieb M, St Cyr N, Siddarth P, Ercoli LM, Senturk D. Citalopram, methylphenidate, or their combination in geriatric depression: a randomized, double-blind, placebo-controlled trial. Am J Psychiatry. 2015;172(6):561–569.

80. DeBattista C, Doghramji K, Menza MA, Rosenthal MH, Fieve RR, Group MiDS. Adjunct modafinil for the short-term treatment of fatigue and sleepiness in patients with major depressive disorder: a preliminary double-blind, placebo-controlled study. J Clin Psychiatry. 2003;64(9):1057–1064.

81. Fava M, Thase ME, DeBattista C. A multicenter, placebo-controlled study of modafinil augmentation in partial responders to selective serotonin reuptake inhibitors with persistent fatigue and sleepiness. J Clin Psychiatry. 2005;66(1):85–93.

82. Goss AJ, Kaser M, Costafreda SG, Sahakian BJ, Fu CH. Modafinil augmentation therapy in unipolar and bipolar depression: a systematic review and meta-analysis of randomized controlled trials. J Clin Psychiatry. 2013;74(11):1101–1107.

83. Cusin C, Iovieno N, Iosifescu DV, Nierenberg AA, Fava M, Rush AJ, et al. A randomized, double-blind, placebo-controlled trial of pramipexole augmentation in treatment-resistant major depressive disorder. J Clin Psychiatry. 2013;74(7):e636–641.

84. Franco-Chaves JA, Mateus CF, Luckenbaugh DA, Martinez PE, Mallinger AG, Zarate CA. Combining a dopamine agonist and selective serotonin reuptake inhibitor for the treatment of depression: a double-blind, randomized pilot study. J Affect Disord. 2013;149(1–3):319–325.

85. Pope HG, Amiaz R, Brennan BP, Orr G, Weiser M, Kelly JF, et al. Parallel-group placebo-controlled trial of testosterone gel in men with major depressive disorder displaying an incomplete response to standard antidepressant treatment. J Clin Psychopharmacol. 2010;30(2):126–134.

86. Seidman SN, Spatz E, Rizzo C, Roose SP. Testosterone replacement therapy for hypogonadal men with major depressive disorder: a randomized, placebo-controlled clinical trial. J Clin Psychiatry. 2001;62(6):406–412.

87. Pope HG, Cohane GH, Kanayama G, Siegel AJ, Hudson JI. Testosterone gel supplementation for men with refractory depression: a randomized, placebo-controlled trial. Am J Psychiatry. 2003;160(1):105–111.

88. Orengo CA, Fullerton L, Kunik ME. Safety and efficacy of testosterone gel 1% augmentation in depressed men with partial response to antidepressant therapy. J Geriatr Psychiatry Neurol. 2005;18(1):20–24.

89. Seidman SN, Miyazaki M, Roose SP. Intramuscular testosterone supplementation to selective serotonin reuptake inhibitor in treatment-resistant depressed men: randomized placebo-controlled clinical trial. J Clin Psychopharmacol. 2005;25(6):584–588.

90. Fava M, Rush AJ, Wisniewski SR, Nierenberg AA, Alpert JE, McGrath PJ, et al. A comparison of mirtazapine and nortriptyline following two consecutive failed medication treatments for depressed outpatients: a STAR*D report. Am J Psychiatry. 2006;163(7):1161–1172.

91. McGrath PJ, Stewart JW, Fava M, Trivedi MH, Wisniewski SR, Nierenberg AA, et al. Tranylcypromine versus venlafaxine plus mirtazapine following three failed antidepressant medication trials for depression: a STAR*D report. Am J Psychiatry. 2006;163(9):1531–1541.

/// 13 /// RAPID-ACTING ANTIDEPRESSANTS

BASHKIM KADRIU, SUBHA SUBRAMANIAN,
ZHI-DE DENG, IOLINE D. HENTER,
LAWRENCE T. PARK, AND
CARLOS A. ZARATE JR.

13.1. INTRODUCTION

Major depressive disorder (MDD) is a highly prevalent condition that affects nearly 20% of the population at some point during their lives. MDD is currently the second leading cause of disability worldwide,[1] and the World Health Organization (WHO) has predicted that, by 2020, it will be the number one cause of disability.[2] MDD is also the *Diagnostic and Statistical Manual of Mental Disorders* diagnosis most strongly associated with suicide attempt (53.8%),[3] a phenomenon whose rates have sharply increased over the past two decades in the United States.[4]

Current first-line treatment options for MDD include pharmacological agents primarily directed at monoaminergic targets (mostly based on serotonin or norepinephrine) as well as cognitive-based therapies. However, despite the critical role that pharmacological and cognitive therapies play in the treatment of MDD, a large proportion of patients remain inadequately treated.[5,6] Indeed, the large Sequenced Treatment Alternatives to Relieve Depression (STAR*D) study of approximately 4,000 outpatients with MDD, funded by the National Institute of Mental Health, found that standard pharmacological monotherapy was effective in ameliorating depressive symptoms in only one-third of these individuals.[6] Another third of patients failed to achieve remission even after four attempts to change therapeutics, augment medications, or use cognitive–behavioral therapy,[6] with each attempt lasting 12 to 14 weeks. These data suggest that a large proportion of individuals with MDD face poor outcomes even with standard treatment. This lack of immediate response—or no response in the case of individuals with treatment-resistant depression (TRD)— coupled with the prolonged period needed to achieve remission even in those who do respond to currently available medications exposes patients to polypharmacy; this trend further underscores the notion that currently available antidepressant treatments are inadequate for many MDD patients.

MDD is a complex, heterogeneous condition associated with a multifaceted constellation of symptoms that likely represent divergent biological mechanisms, which complicates treatment algorithms. As we have noted, monoaminergic-based treatments such as selective serotonin reuptake inhibitors (SSRIs), serotonin–norepinephrine reuptake inhibitors (SNRIs), tricyclic antidepressants (TCAs), and monoamine oxidase inhibitors (MAOIs) take weeks to months to exert their full antidepressant effects; this lag time often leads to patients discontinuing their treatment early or relapsing after initial response. Finally, even effective therapeutics used to treat severe TRD, such as MAOIs, are not target-specific and are thus associated with metabolic or cardiac side effects, further decreasing patient compliance and increasing comorbidities.

The recent discovery that glutamatergic-based drugs are uniquely capable of rapidly and robustly treating mood disorders has ushered in a new therapeutic era in the quest to develop novel and efficacious antidepressant treatments.[7,8] This chapter highlights pivotal research into these novel fast-acting pharmacological agents, as well as novel and existing neuromodulatory interventions associated with the rapid alleviation of depressive symptoms. Recent research into the mechanistic underpinnings of these treatment modalities is also described, as these data continue to help the scientific community understand the etiology of MDD and TRD.

13.2. KETAMINE

13.2.1. Mechanism of Action

Ketamine is a prototypic glutamatergic modulator that acts as a noncompetitive, high-affinity, N-methyl-D-aspartate receptor (NMDAR) blocker. Ketamine rapidly increases the number and function of spine synapses[9] and has high lipid solubility and limited protein binding, which allows the brain to rapidly absorb and redistribute the compound, with a plasma distribution half-life of four to 10 minutes and a terminal half-life of two hours.[10,11] Over the past two decades, ketamine's well-documented rapid antidepressant effects have galvanized efforts to understand its underlying mechanism of antidepressant action. Several broad classifications of this hypothesized mechanism have emerged, including both NMDAR-dependent and -independent mechanisms. NMDAR-dependent mechanisms include, among others, (1) disinhibition of gamma-aminobutyric acid (GABA)-ergic intraneurons driven by presynaptic NMDAR blockade;[12] (2) direct inhibition of extrasynaptic GluN2B-containing NMDARs;[13] and (3) inhibition of NMDAR burst activity coming from the lateral habenula.[14] NMDAR-independent mechanisms include, among others, (1) conversion of ketamine to its plasma metabolite hydroxynorketamine (HNK), which induces rapid-onset and sustained activation of α-amino-3-hydroxy-5-methyl-4-isoxazolepropionic acid (AMPA) throughput coupled with downstream signaling changes;[15] and (2) the regulation of glutamate release via the stabilization of excitatory and inhibitory interactions.[9,16]

One model hypothesized that ketamine blocks NMDARs on interneurons in the prefrontal cortex (PFC), which disinhibits pyramidal neurons and leads to a glutamate surge and to AMPA receptor (AMPAR) activation.[17] AMPAR activation then triggers the translation and release of brain-derived neurotrophic factor (BDNF). BDNF, in turn, binds to and activates the tropomyosin receptor kinase B (TrkB) receptor, triggering the activation of the mechanistic target of rapamycin (mTOR)1 pathway and protein synthesis.[18] Another model proposed that ketamine blocks NMDARs at rest, which disinhibits eukaryotic elongation factor 2 (eEF2), promotes BDNF translation, and increases protein synthesis and synaptogenesis.[19] The result is a net increase in BDNF, protein synthesis, and synaptogenesis that reverses chronic stress and neuronal atrophy (Figure 13.1).

BDNF is a key regulator of synaptic plasticity and has been implicated in the neurobiology of depression.[20] Loosely defined, synaptic plasticity is an adaptive process by which local or global neural circuits adjust to changes in the environment (e.g., aging, stress, learning); either the number of synapses or the strength of connectivity can increase. One theory of MDD posits that environmental triggers such as stress increase extracellular glutamate, leading to neuronal toxicity, the retraction of dendritic spines, and decreased spine density.[9,21,22] This synaptic downregulation then culminates in gray matter changes in the PFC and hippocampus.[23,24] Molecular evidence suggests that inhibition of mTOR (an upstream regulator of BDNF) or a decrease in BDNF levels leads to synaptic deregulation in the PFC. One study found that individuals with the BDNF *Val66Met* polymorphism were more vulnerable to depression if exposed to early life stress.[25] Intriguingly, cellular signaling studies suggest that BDNF is necessary for ketamine's antidepressant effects. For instance, ketamine's effects were abolished in mice with a knock-in of the BDNF *Val66Met* allele, which blocks the processing- and activity-dependent release of BDNF.[26] Further evidence that activity-dependent BDNF release is key to ketamine's antidepressant effects is drawn from studies demonstrating that infusion of a function-blocking antibody into the medial prefrontal cortex (mPFC) blocks ketamine's antidepressant actions.[27]

From a global mechanistic perspective, neuroimaging and electrophysiological studies have been used to determine the key brain areas involved in pre- and postdepressive states (i.e., before and after ketamine infusion). Positron emission tomography (PET) imaging studies have found increased glucose metabolism in the PFC of individuals with MDD after ketamine infusion.[28] In addition, studies in animals[29,30] and humans[31] found that ketamine infusion may increase gamma power oscillations by increasing glutamate release and silencing GABAergic interneurons;

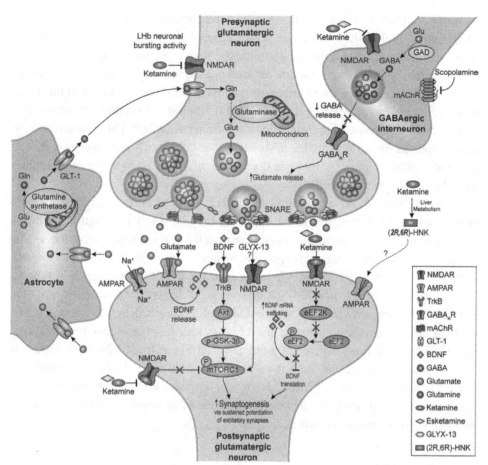

FIGURE 13.1. Proposed mechanisms of action of glutamatergic modulators and other putative rapid-acting antidepressant treatments.

Disinhibition hypothesis: Ketamine and esketamine selectively block NMDARs, and scopolamine selectively blocks mAChRs. These are expressed on GABA-ergic inhibitory interneurons, and their blockade decreases interneuron activity, which leads to a disinhibition of pyramidal neurons and enhances glutamatergic firing. Glutamate then binds to and activates postsynaptic AMPARs.

The role of ketamine metabolites: HNK exerts NMDAR inhibition-independent antidepressant actions by activating AMPAR-mediated synaptic potentiation.

Other glutamatergic modulators: GLYX-13, which has partial agonist properties at NMDARs, is hypothesized to activate mTORC and subsequently induce protein synthesis. GLYX-13 requires AMPA and activity-dependent BDNF release but, unlike ketamine, does not produce glutamate bursts. AMPAR activation enhances BDNF release, activates the TrkB receptor, and subsequently promotes protein synthesis by activating the mTORC complex.

Inhibition of extrasynaptic NMDARs: Ketamine selectively blocks extra-synaptic GluN2B-containing NMDARs, which are tonically activated by low levels of ambient glutamate regulated by the glutamate transporter 1 (EAAT2) located on astrocytes. Inhibition of the extrasynaptic GluN2B-NMDARs desuppresses mTORC1 function, which in turn induces protein synthesis. Finally, blockade of spontaneous NMDAR activation inhibits eukaryotic elongation factor 2 kinase (eEF2K) activity, thus preventing phosphorylation of its eEF2 substrate. This effect subsequently enhances BDNF translation and, ultimately, protein synthesis. *Reproduced with permission from reference 137.*

this, in turn, leads to the activation of AMPA receptors at the synapse.[32] One study of 20 healthy male volunteers assessed the neuronal effects of a 0.5 mg/kg ketamine infusion by measuring task-induced gamma oscillations in motor and visual cortices. The researchers found that ketamine reduced peak gamma frequency to full contrast stimuli in the visual cortex and increased gamma oscillation amplitudes in the motor and visual cortices, suggesting that NMDAR inhibition via ketamine increases cortical excitability, possibly by disinhibiting pyramidal cells.[33] This phenomenon is also supported by animal studies postulating that ketamine's antidepressant effects are mediated by its ability to increase the number of AMPARs in synapses and spines in cell layer V pyramidal cells.[18]

Notably, several novel preclinical studies have recently energized this already exciting field and, if clinically proven, may be a key paradigm shift in the development of novel antidepressants. Specifically, a preclinical study found that ketamine's antidepressant effects appear to be due to one of its metabolites, (2R,6R)-hydroxynorketamine (HNK), an effect mediated via an NMDAR-independent mechanism that seems to enhance AMPAR activation.[15,34] In rodent models of depression (the 24-hour forced swim test, suppressed feeding, learned helplessness, chronic corticosterone-induced anhedonia, and chronic social defeat stress models), (2R, 6R)-HNK exerted dose-dependent antidepressant-like effects.[15] Nevertheless, it is important to emphasize that these results were found in mice. Additional research is needed to ascertain whether (2R,6R)-HNK will have similar antidepressant effects in humans; toward this end, this metabolite is currently in development as a treatment and will soon be tested in humans.

13.2.2. Clinical Evidence

Ketamine is administered via various routes; bioavailability for the intravenous, intramuscular, and intranasal routes is 100%, 93%, and 8% to 45% respectively.[35] Intravenous ketamine is generally composed of an equal mixture of R- and S-ketamine enantiomers and is by far the most extensively studied route of administration.

In 2000, Berman and colleagues published the first double-blind clinical trial demonstrating that a sub-anesthetic dose of intravenous ketamine (0.5 mg/kg administered over 40 minutes) had antidepressant effects. Intravenous ketamine improved Hamilton Depression Rating Scale (HAM-D) scores in seven participants (one with bipolar depression and six with MDD).[36] Since then, numerous larger-scale, randomized control trials of individuals with MDD[37–39] as well as bipolar depression[40,41]—both with and without TRD—have confirmed that ketamine infusion at this dose (1) rapidly improves depressive symptoms (within hours); (2) has robust antidepressant effects that reach peak improvement within 24 hours (with effect sizes ranging from ~60–71%); and (3) maintains antidepressant efficacy for up to a week or more in 30% to 50% of patients.[42] What is particularly striking is that the rapid and sustained response to a single ketamine infusion is comparable or superior to that seen after roughly eight weeks of treatment with currently available monoaminergic-based antidepressants. Indeed, ketamine's ability to induce remission in roughly one-third of TRD patients, as well as the magnitude of their treatment response, differs sharply from the effectiveness of currently available monoaminergic-based antidepressants, which traditionally require 10 to 14 weeks of chronic administration before similar remission rates are observed.[6] As we noted earlier in the chapter, ketamine, used adjunctively with therapeutic doses of either lithium or valproate, has also been found to produce similarly rapid, robust, and sustained antidepressant effects in individuals with treatment-resistant bipolar depression.[40,41,43,44] These effects were not accompanied by increased risk of inducing mania or hypomania.[45]

Of particular interest from a public health perspective, ketamine has also been found to have rapid antisuicidal effects in patients with mood and anxiety spectrum disorders[38,46-48] as well as those with bipolar depression.[38,46-49] A recent meta-analysis of 167 patients with a range of mood disorder diagnoses found that ketamine reduced suicidal thoughts compared to placebo as rapidly as within a few hours and lasting up to seven days.[50] Another study found that these reductions in active suicidal ideation in response to ketamine were present even when compared to a midazolam control.[51] Another study used the implicit association test (IAT) to measure differences in suicidal behavior before and 24 hours after ketamine or midazolam infusions. Fifty-four percent of those who received ketamine had IAT scores of zero versus 24% percent of those who received midazolam ($p = .03$)[47]. Notably, some studies suggest that ketamine's ability to reduce suicidal ideation may occur independently of its antidepressant effects.[49,50] Although the biological mechanisms underlying ketamine's antisuicidal effects remain unknown, one study found that MDD patients who experienced an antisuicidal response to ketamine showed reduced nocturnal wakefulness,[52] a finding that is particularly important given that self-reported sleep disturbances may confer elevated risk for suicidal ideation, suicide attempts, or suicide deaths.[53-55]

Taken together, the evidence suggests that ketamine possesses considerable antidepressant effects. Indeed, a systematic review and meta-analysis of placebo-controlled, double-blind, randomized clinical ketamine studies (encompassing 147 participants drawn from seven trials) found that the cumulative odds ratio of ketamine response within 24 hours was 9.87 (95% confidence interval [CI] 4.37–22.29) and that the cumulative odds ratio for transient remission was 14.47 (95% CI 2.67–78.49).[56] Another meta-analysis pooled nine studies that tested single-dose intravenous ketamine ($n = 234$) and reported a reduction in depressive symptoms as early as 40 to 60 minutes, which peaked at day 1, and with effects lasting until days 5 through 8.[57]

While the clinical pan-therapeutic effects of ketamine are being tested across various clinical settings, optimal dose efficacy studies are also ongoing. Toward this end, a recent multicenter trial of 99 TRD patients tested four different intravenous ketamine doses (0.1, 0.2, 0.5, and 1.0 mg/kg).[58] In an attempt to decrease perception bias of symptom improvement, ketamine was compared with an active placebo—a drug that, like ketamine, induces side effects. The study found that single intravenous doses of 0.5 and 1.0 mg/kg were superior to active placebo in reducing depressive symptoms over a three-day period. The two lower doses (0.1 and 0.2 mg/kg) did not provide significant symptom relief, although some improvement was noted with the lowest dose (0.1 mg/kg).[58]

Repeated or chronic ketamine infusions have also been investigated in an effort to prolong ketamine's rapid but transient antidepressant effects. To date, preliminary data suggest that up to two or three 0.5 mg/kg intravenous infusions per week for two weeks are well-tolerated and effective.[59–61] A recent, randomized, multicenter, double-blind study assessed change in Montgomery–Asberg Depression Rating Scale (MADRS) score in 67 MDD patients who received ketamine and found that mean MADRS scores improved from baseline to day 15 in both groups receiving ketamine compared to their placebo counterparts.[62] Change in MADRS score for those receiving ketamine twice per week for two weeks was −18.4 (standard deviation [SD] = 12.0) for the ketamine group versus −5.7 (SD = 10.2) ($p < .001$) for the placebo group. In those receiving ketamine three times per week for two weeks, change in MADRS score was −17.7 (SD = 7.3) for the ketamine group versus −3.1 (SD = 5.7) ($p < .001$) for the placebo group. There was no difference in MADRS score between the two frequencies and no difference in the number of treatment-based adverse effects reported. In addition, transient dissociative symptoms appeared to lessen with repeated dosing.[62] Another study reported similar decreases in MADRS scores of 18.9 (SD = 6.6, $p < .001$) when assessing the effects of an open-label ketamine infusion six times over 12 days in a group of 24 individuals with TRD.[63] These results suggest that ketamine may not only ameliorate depressive symptoms within hours of administration but that its effects may be sustained when administered over multiple sessions.

Given these promising findings, considerable research efforts have been made to identify putative biomarkers of treatment response to ketamine.[64,65] One study found that a family history of alcoholism was associated with a better antidepressant response to ketamine.[66] Another study of 126 subjects with either MDD or bipolar depression found that ketamine-induced dissociative effects (such as depersonalization and derealization) were also associated with antidepressant response.[67] Another randomized, placebo-controlled study investigating ketamine's mechanism of action in 35 unmedicated TRD subjects and 25 healthy volunteers found that gamma power was increased in subjects six to nine hours after ketamine infusion and, furthermore, that baseline gamma levels moderated the relationship between increased gamma power after ketamine administration and antidepressant response.[68] This suggests that resting gamma oscillations may provide a measure of inhibition–excitation balance and homeostasis[68] and further adds to the growing literature characterizing depression as a disorder of homeostatic regulation. Interestingly, the MDD subjects in that study had a robust antidepressant response to ketamine until day 11 and reported significant symptom improvement across a wide variety of relevant psychiatric domains, including, among others, anhedonia, anxiety, post-traumatic stress disorder, atypical depressive symptoms, suicidal ideation, and quality of life.[68] This finding suggests that the breadth of therapeutic response to ketamine occurs trans-diagnostically across a number of relevant domains of psychiatric disorders.

Finally, preclinical studies of ketamine and its metabolite (2R,6R)-HNK suggest that this metabolite may have greater antidepressant effects in females versus males,[15] although this has not been reported to occur in humans.[69,70] Interestingly, serum- and brain-level increases in (2R,6R)-HNK have been observed after ketamine administration in both mice and humans, suggesting that (2R,6R)-HNK could be used as a biomarker to evaluate ketamine response; however, to date, no association between increased (2R,6R)-HNK levels and antidepressant response has been observed in humans.[15,69]

13.2.3. Adverse Effects

Despite ketamine's unparalleled antidepressant effects, long-term safety guidelines for its use in depression are lacking, in part because many repeat-dose studies remain ongoing. Ketamine is associated with a number of side effects, including dissociative and psychotomimetic symptoms as well as drowsiness, dizziness, poor coordination, floating, and feelings of strangeness or unreality.[71] In addition, transient cardiovascular symptoms such as elevations in heart rate and blood pressure have been reported in patients during intravenous ketamine infusion.[71,72] Although typically mild and transient in nature, these side effects should be taken seriously, especially in the absence of well-controlled longitudinal studies of this issue. Additional side effects related to acute dosing include, among others, neurological symptoms (sedation, faintness, unsteadiness), cognitive symptoms (memory loss, cognitive impairment), and urological symptoms (interstitial cystitis) (for a comprehensive review, see reference 71). Finally, ketamine is a street drug with recreational abuse potential and is known to induce cravings and tolerance in repeat uncontrolled users.[73] Thus, extreme caution is needed when regulating its use to treat depression.

13.3. ESKETAMINE

Esketamine, the S-enantiomer of ketamine, binds with three- to four-fold higher affinity to the NMDAR than racemic R-ketamine. Esketamine is currently available in intravenous and intranasal formulations. From a clinical perspective, intranasal esketamine is particularly appealing because it offers an opportunity for outpatient administration. In 2013 and 2016, the US Food and Drug Administration (FDA) granted "breakthrough therapy designation" for intravenous and intranasal esketamine, respectively—the first rapid-acting antidepressant to receive this designation. In March 2019, the FDA approved intranasal esketamine (Spravato) for adults with TRD.[74]

In a multicenter, randomized, proof-of-concept trial, 30 individuals with TRD received either an intravenous esketamine infusion (either 0.20 or 0.40 mg/kg) or placebo over 40 minutes.[75] Those who did not respond to placebo then received 0.20 mg/kg esketamine. The esketamine infusion significantly improved MADRS scores within two hours, with a response rate of 67% for the 0.20 mg/kg dose and 64% for the 0.40 mg/kg dose of esketamine.[75] Interestingly, there was no statistical difference between treatment effects at either esketamine dose, suggesting that the lower dose could be equally beneficial. Transient adverse effects included dissociative symptoms within one hour of the 0.40 mg/kg dose, and common side effects included nausea and headache.

A recent, phase 2, double-blind study randomized 67 individuals with TRD to receive intranasal esketamine (28, 56, or 84 mg twice weekly) or placebo adjunctive to their oral antidepressant treatment.[76] It should be noted that 56 and 84 mg are pharmacokinetically equivalent to 0.2 and 0.5 mg/kg of intravenous ketamine, respectively. Those who received intranasal esketamine in all three groups had improved MADRS scores one week after receiving two doses. Furthermore, improvement in depressive symptoms was maintained with reduced dosing frequency for up to nine weeks in the open-label phase of the trial. Only 5% of the participants discontinued treatment due to adverse effects, which included dizziness, headache, and transient dissociative symptoms.[76]

Another double-blind, multicenter, inpatient and outpatient study found reduced MADRS scores in a group of TRD patients receiving 84 mg intranasal esketamine twice weekly for four weeks. Compared to placebo, the response rate for the treatment group was 61% at four hours and 65% at 24 hours; approximately 35% of subjects maintained an antidepressant response until day 25.[77] The same investigators also used the MADRS suicidal thoughts item, the Suicide Ideation and Behavior Assessment Tool, and the Beck Scale for Suicide Ideation to assess intranasal esketamine's possible antisuicidal effects. Intranasal esketamine significantly reduced depressive symptoms as well as suicidal ideation at four hours. However, esketamine's effects did not differentiate from placebo at 24 hours or day 25.[77]

Taken together, the data indicate that esketamine rapidly improves depressive symptoms as well as measures of suicidal ideation, underscoring its potential effectiveness in treating depressed patients with acute suicidal risk. In light of these results, and as noted earlier in the chapter, in March 2019 the FDA approved Spravato for adults with TRD; this agent is the first mechanistically distinct drug approved to treat depression in over three decades.[74]

As with ketamine, caution is warranted with esketamine due to its dissociative symptoms and potential abuse liability.[78] According to recently published data, most of the adverse effects associated with esketamine were of mild to moderate severity and typically resolved within the same day of dosing. The most common treatment-emergent adverse effects (affecting <10% of subjects) were observed during the induction double-blind phase and were primarily associated with the highest intranasal dose tested (84 mg) plus oral antidepressant. The symptoms included nausea, dissociation, dizziness, headache, vertigo, sleepiness, dysgeusia (taste disturbance), hypoesthesia (diminished sense of touch or sensation), and vomiting.[76,79] Like ketamine, esketamine has been observed to transiently elevate systemic blood pressure (systolic ~20 mmHg; diastolic, ~11 mmHg), with a peak effect observed 10 to 40 minutes after dosing.[76]

13.4. NITROUS OXIDE

Nitrous oxide, originally known as "laughing gas" for its euphoric effects, is an inhaled anesthetic that has been used for its analgesic and anxiolytic properties since its discovery in 1772. Nitrous oxide has multiple targets in the central nervous system, including glutamate, GABA, and calcium channel blocking pathways. Like ketamine, the effects of nitrous oxide are largely confined to postsynaptic targets as well as to the AMPA-kainate subtype of the glutamate receptor.[80] While nitrous oxide largely mimics the histological effects of ketamine,[81] high concentrations of nitrous oxide may only partially block NMDARs.[82] Nitrous oxide produces nitric oxide (NO), a metabolite associated with antidepressant and anxiolytic effects. NO is neurotoxic at high concentrations but may be neuroprotective at physiological concentrations. Interestingly, individuals with MDD appear to have lower levels of nitric oxide synthase activity in platelets and fewer NO metabolites than control subjects.[83] Nitric oxide synthase has also been implicated in the regulation of key neurotransmitters that are altered in mood disorders, such as serotonin, noradrenaline, and GABA.[84] Furthermore, the mood stabilizer lithium has been found to increase NO levels in individuals with mood disorders.[85]

In a randomized, placebo-controlled, crossover pilot study, 20 individuals with TRD received an hour of inhaled nitrous oxide (50% nitrous oxide and 50% oxygen) or placebo (50% nitrogen and 50% oxygen) during two treatment sessions separated by one week.[86] Within two hours, depressive symptoms improved in response to nitrous oxide versus placebo, and this effect remained for 24 hours; a median reduction of 5.5 points was observed on the HAM-D, the primary outcome measure. Nausea, vomiting, headache, numbness, and paresthesia were the top mild to moderate adverse outcomes, and all were transient, suggesting that nitrous oxide was generally well tolerated in this study population.[86]

While other phase 1 and 2 double-blind clinical trials are actively assessing the efficacy, dose optimization, and safety of nitrous oxide in TRD and bipolar depression, its feasibility as a rapid-acting antidepressant requires further exploration. In particular, studies have yet to determine the safety and efficacy of repeated doses of nitrous oxide. Two studies are currently investigating nitrous oxide's effects in TRD and its relationship to neural connectivity via magnetic resonance imaging (MRI) assessments.

While studies assessing the safety of nitrous oxide in depression are limited, the original study by Nagele and colleagues showed that an acute, one-time administration of nitrous oxide was relatively safe.[86] However, previous studies that sought to characterize the sub-anesthetic properties of nitrous oxide reported psychedelic effects, with symptoms ranging from perceptual disturbances, detachment, and euphoric effects to altered body awareness and image.[87] Another key issue is nitrous oxide's abuse potential, as well as its inactivation of vitamin B12, which could potentially lead to megaloblastic anemia, myelopathy, and the interruption of folate metabolism, all of which have also been noted in clinical studies.[88–90]

13.5. SCOPOLAMINE

Scopolamine is a nonselective muscarinic acetylcholine receptor (mAChR) antagonist with potentially selective inhibitory actions on muscarinic subtypes 1 and 2 (M1 and M2). Unlike ketamine, esketamine, and nitrous oxide, scopolamine directly affects the cholinergic pathway but does not directly modulate the glutamatergic pathway. The cholinergic–adrenergic balance hypothesis of MDD, first proposed in 1972,[91] posits that depression is due to the relative predominance of central cholinergic versus adrenergic tone. Evidence that cholinergic overdrive and cholinergic receptor upregulation occurred after withdrawal from antidepressant medications lent further support to this theory.[92]

Another theory postulates that the antidepressant actions of scopolamine occur by acutely inhibiting muscarinic mAChRs on GABAergic interneurons, leading to glutamate disinhibition, which in turn may induce a rapid glutamate burst in the mPFC, increased mechanistic target of rapamycin complex (mTORC) signaling, and increased synapse formation. For antidepressant effects and synapse formation to occur, it appears that both BDNF and mTORC are necessary[93–95] (see Figure 13.1).

In the first human trial of scopolamine for depression, 0.4 mg intramuscular scopolamine was administered for three consecutive nights to 10 individuals with MDD and 10 healthy controls; mild antidepressant effects were found on the second day of scopolamine administration.[96] These preliminary findings were expanded in several double-blind, placebo-controlled scopolamine trials. In the first study, the investigators explored scopolamine's cognitive effects in eight individuals with MDD or bipolar depression; scopolamine infusions were provided over 15 minutes and separated by three to five days. The investigators found that MADRS score—their secondary outcome measure—was lower after the fourth administration of scopolamine compared to placebo, especially at a higher scopolamine dose of 4.0 ug/kg.[97] These findings were replicated in 22 patients with MDD who received six scopolamine infusions (4.0 ug/kg); reductions in MADRS scores of 32% and 53% were observed after the first three and second three sets of infusions, respectively.[98] Individuals who received scopolamine and then placebo had lower MADRS scores than those who received placebo and then scopolamine. Despite these promising results, a recent study found that scopolamine had no antidepressant effects in a group of 23 MDD subjects and, furthermore, that scopolamine administration did not alter BDNF levels or MEG gamma power, both of which have previously been associated with antidepressant response to ketamine.[99] The authors hypothesized that the lack of clinical and physiological response may have been due to the fact that the subject sample was more treatment-resistant than in previous studies.

Further investigation is needed to determine the extent of scopolamine's antidepressant effects and whether specific subpopulations of individuals with MDD might respond preferentially to this agent. In addition, studies are needed to better understand the mechanism of action underlying antidepressant response to scopolamine, particularly whether scopolamine shares a mechanism of action with other rapid-acting antidepressants such as ketamine. Ongoing clinical trials are currently investigating the effects of intravenous scopolamine augmentation during electroconvulsive therapy (ECT) as well as escitalopram and naltrexone treatment.

In placebo-controlled trials, the side effects of scopolamine included drowsiness, blurred vision, dry mouth, and light-headedness.[100] Scopolamine administration also decreased heart rate and blood pressure, likely due to its effects on cholinergic parasympathetic autonomic function, although no subject developed symptoms of hypotension or evidence of cardiovascular insufficiency.[100] These transient side effects were associated with scopolamine administration and resolved within a two- to four-hour window.

13.6. GLYX-13 (RAPASTINEL)

GLYX-13 (rapastinel) is a synthetic peptide with functional partial agonist properties at the NMDAR.[101,102] GLYX-13 has glycine-like enhancing properties, although it binds to an allosteric site on the complex.[103] In preclinical studies, GLYX-13 was found to increase BDNF levels and synaptic connectivity in the PFC and exert rapid antidepressant effects, all of which depend on postsynaptic glutamate activation as well as on the manipulation of AMPARs and voltage-gated calcium channels.[104] Unlike ketamine, GLYX-13 does not produce a glutamate burst and thus is not associated with underlying dissociative symptoms.[105] These findings lend further credence to the theory that NMDAR inhibition is primarily linked to ketamine's side effects but that NMDAR activation occurring via either enhanced synaptic glutamatergic neurotransmission (as is the case for ketamine) or via direct activation of the receptor (as is the case for GLYX-13) results in the antidepressant actions of these drugs.[101,103]

In a large phase 2b trial, 116 unmedicated TRD inpatients were randomized to receive either intravenous GLYX-13 (1 mg/kg [$n = 25$], 5 mg/kg [$n = 20$], 10 mg/kg [$n = 17$], or 30 mg/kg [$n = 21$]) or a single saline placebo ($n = 33$) over 3 to 15 minutes.[102] One week after administration, subjects who had received either 5 or 10 mg/kg GLYX-13 had significantly improved depressive symptom scores compared to those who had received saline placebo.

In another double-blind, randomized clinical trial, investigators explored adjunctive GLYX-13 use in 116 TRD patients who were concurrently maintained on a psychotropic medication regimen.[106] Subjects were randomized to receive weekly intravenous GLYX-13 infusions (either 1, 5, or 10 mg/kg) or placebo. Follow-up occurred on days 3, 7, and 14. After an interim safety and efficacy analysis, an additional group of subjects was added to the study. These received intravenous GLYX-13 (30 mg/kg) or placebo, with follow-up at days 3, 7, 14, 21, and 28. As assessed via the Bech-6 subscale of the HAM-D, onset of action occurred within two hours. Subjects who received 5 or 10 mg/kg of intravenous GLYX-13 had significantly lower HAM-D scores on days 1 through 7 versus placebo, though no antidepressant effects were observed after day 7. It is possible that the U-shaped dose–response curve observed for GLYX-13 may be due to this agent's unique molecular interactions as a partial agonist on the glycine site of the NMDAR.

Because of these promising preliminary findings, GLYX-13 received breakthrough therapy designation from the FDA for adjunctive treatment of MDD in January 2016.[107] Several clinical trials are currently investigating the safety and efficacy of this agent as monotherapy or as adjunctive treatment in MDD and suicidality. However, a recent press release highlighted three acute studies in MDD (RAP-MD-01, -02, -03) indicating that rapastinel treatment arms did not differentiate from placebo on the primary and key secondary endpoints. In all three acute studies rapastinel was well tolerated without any sign of psychotomimetic side effects.[108] Future development of this compound is unknown at this time.

Unlike ketamine, GLYX-13 does not induce sensory dissociation or psychotomimetic properties and does not display abuse liability properties in rodents.[101] Studies found that only a small percentage (~5%) of subjects reported side effects, which included dizziness, headache, somnolence, fatigue, and dysgeusia. In addition, no differences in vital signs, cardiovascular effects, oxygen saturation, or laboratory and hematological data were observed between the placebo and active treatment groups.[102,103] In the clinical trials that we noted earlier, GLYX-13 infusion at any dose was not associated with serious adverse events and caused no psychotomimetic symptoms;[106,108] dizziness was the most common side effect (10%).[102]

13.7. BUPRENORPHINE

Opiate receptors are densely expressed in cortical and subcortical areas linked to stress response and emotional regulation.[109] Depression is thought to be at least partly associated with dysregulation of mu and kappa opioid receptor tone. There is evidence that endogenous opioids play an important role in human mood, as mu receptor agonists release serotonin and dopamine in the CNS, and lower levels of endorphins have been found in the postmortem brains of depressed and suicidal patients .[110,111]

Interestingly, opium was the primary treatment for melancholia until the 1950s, when MAOIs and TCAs were introduced. Use of antidepressants led to a decrease in opium-based treatments, in part because of their known risk of abuse and addiction. Nevertheless, given the high rates of TRD and the imperfect response of most individuals to available antidepressants, the scientific community has reevaluated previous evidence over the past decade and conducted rigorous human and animal studies to further understand the role that endogenous opioids play in depression.

Buprenorphine is a synthetic opiate with partial mu receptor agonist and kappa receptor antagonist properties. This latter property is beneficial because withdrawal symptoms in opioid addiction are thought to be related to kappa receptor overactivity.[112] Buprenorphine is used to treat opioid use and is clinically useful in reducing withdrawal symptoms and cravings. It also decreases symptoms such as anxiety, depression, dysphoria, non-suicidal self-injury, and myalgia via kappa receptor antagonism.[113] Rodent studies suggest that kappa receptor antagonism has antidepressant effects[114] and that buprenorphine is implicated in the hypothalamic–pituitary–adrenal (HPA) axis and serotonergic pathway.[115]

A recent combination of buprenorphine and the mu receptor antagonist samidorphan was developed in an effort to lessen endogenous opioid tone in areas with high mu and kappa activity and to improve opioid tone in brain regions where ligand activity was altered. Investigators tested the combination drug (known as ALKS 5461) in a pilot trial in depression and found that a 1:1 ratio of 8 mg buprenorphine and 8 mg samidorphan blocked measures of mu receptor opioid activity, as assessed via pupillometry, visual analog scale assessments, and questionnaires related to drug liking and euphoria.[116] HAM-D scores were improved after one week ($p = .032$), and the combination was found to be well tolerated among participants. The same research group then conducted a multicenter, randomized, double-blind, placebo-controlled study in 142 MDD subjects. Patients received either a 2 mg/2 mg combination, an 8 mg/8 mg combination, or placebo. Compared to placebo, HAM-D and MADRS scores improved significantly in the 2 mg/2 mg group but not in the 8 mg/8 mg group.[117] Another randomized, double-blind, placebo-controlled trial of low-dose adjunctive sublingual buprenorphine (0.1 mg administered once or twice daily) examined the effects of this agent on suicidal ideation in 40 suicidal individuals and found significantly lower Beck Suicide Ideation Scale scores two and four weeks after administration.[118] In addition, results from two recent phase 3 clinical trials (FORWARD-4 and FORWARD-5) further support the safety and efficacy of adjunctive ALKS-5461 in decreasing depressive symptoms in TRD patients.[119] In both studies, TRD patients were randomized to receive a combination of buprenorphine and samidorphan (either adjunctive 2 mg/2 mg, adjunctive 1 mg/1 mg, or adjunctive 0.5 mg/0.5 mg) or placebo for five weeks. In the FORWARD-5 study, the combination of adjunctive 2 mg buprenorphine and 2 mg samidorphan reduced depressive symptoms (as measured via MADRS scores) across multiple time points compared to placebo, and met its primary endpoint by reducing depression scores. However, FORWARD-4 did not reach its primary endpoint, as change in MADRS score from baseline to the end of the treatment period was not significantly different at any dose.[119]

This series of studies was not designed to examine rapid onset of antidepressant action; for instance, in the study by Fava and colleagues[117] the earliest time point examining response was one week, and there was no evidence at this time point for superiority in response or remission over placebo. Future studies designed to specifically assess early response are needed to address this question. It should be noted, however, that the FDA recently turned down Alkermes's bid to win approval for ALKS 5461 in MDD and requested additional clinical data.[120]

A recently completed, longitudinal (52 weeks), open-label, adjunct-medication study of ALKS 5461 (given as 2 mg buprenorphine/2 mg samidorphan) found that adverse effects were mostly reported at study onset but resolved during treatment. The most frequent side effects, observed in about 5% of patients, included headache, constipation, dizziness, nausea, and vomiting.[119] However, significant caution is warranted with buprenorphine because it is a Schedule III controlled substance, underscoring its potential for low to moderate physical and psychological dependence. However, in the aforementioned trial the authors observed no withdrawal, suicidal, or behavioral disturbances on discontinuation of the drug.[119]

13.8. SLEEP DEPRIVATION

It has been hypothesized that a subset of patients with severe MDD who experience circadian rhythm abnormalities—including in mood, sleep, hormonal levels, and/or temperature regulation—have a state-related defect in clock gene machinery. This hypothesis is supported by the findings that chronotherapeutic treatments that alter clock gene processes, such as sleep deprivation (SD) and sleep phase advance, can rapidly and dramatically improve symptoms in MDD subjects.[121] The circadian mechanism hypothesis posits that SD activates *CLOCK* gene transcription, which then leads to *PER2* expression in the cortex.[122] Another possible mechanism involves the monoaminergic system, as SD increases levels of serotonin, norepinephrine, and dopamine.[123,124] A BOLD functional MRI study found that activation of the dorsolateral PFC and dorsal anterior cingulate cortex in subjects with bipolar depression correlated with antidepressant response to SD in homozygous carriers of the serotonin transporter gene (*5-HTTLPR*),[125] suggesting that acute changes in serotonin levels are associated with ameliorations in mood due to SD. A third possible mechanism involves the synaptic plasticity model, which posits that therapeutic SD strengthens synapses and shifts the deficient long-term potentiation in patients with MDD to a favorable range of plasticity.[126] Like many of the rapid-acting antidepressants we have discussed, SD regulates neuroplasticity and increases dendritic spine density in the hippocampus.[127] SD also increases phosphorylation of glycogen synthase kinase 3B (GSK3β), which has been shown to contribute to synaptic potentiation in ketamine studies.[128] In particular, individuals who have the rs334558 SNP, located on the *GSK3β* gene, have a mood response to SD.[128]

SD can include both total and partial therapy. In the former, individuals are deprived of sleep for an average of 36 hours; in the latter, patients sleep for up to three to four hours and sustain 20 to 21 hours of wakefulness. Over two centuries ago, Heinroth successfully experimented with SD as a treatment for melancholia, presenting anecdotal evidence from three depressed individuals who self-treated themselves; the first modern studies in this area drew on that work.[129,130] Since then, a large number of studies have confirmed the antidepressant effects of SD.

A comprehensive analysis of these investigations reported an average antidepressant response to SD of 59%.[131] A more recent meta-analysis of 66 studies ranging from 1974 to 2016 found a response rate to SD of 45% in studies with randomized control groups.[132] The investigators also found that partial SD was as effective as total SD, and that concurrent use of antidepressant medications did not significantly influence response to SD.[132] Despite these successes, adoption of SD in clinical settings has lagged because symptom improvements are short-lived, typically disappearing after a night of sleep. Indeed, up to 80% of those who initially responded to SD relapsed after a night of sleep.[133,134] Augmentation therapies may improve these rates, as both chronobiological treatments and use of the mood stabilizer lithium have been shown to prevent depression relapse and sustain the antidepressant effects of SD over time.[135,136]

13.9. CONCLUSIONS

This chapter provides an overview of rapid-acting agents and procedures that are shifting the current paradigm of treatment for MDD. These therapies act rapidly—within hours to days instead of weeks to months. In particular, ketamine and esketamine are currently being adapted in non-experimental clinical settings to treat acute depressive symptoms and TRD. However, given the complexity of mood disorders, many questions remain. What populations are these agents best suited for? Can ideal candidates for novel treatments be identified by genotype, serum markers, or neuroimaging modalities? What neural perturbations are specific to those who are ketamine (or esketamine, etc.) responders versus nonresponders? Do different treatment modalities share common underlying mechanisms? How can we reduce the high relapse rates associated with these rapid-acting treatments? To identify and create patient-specific treatments, exploring these fundamental mechanistic questions will allow us to not only investigate the molecular mechanisms underlying depression but also understand individual variability in treatment response.

AUTHOR NOTE

Funding for this work was supported by the Intramural Research Program at the National Institute of Mental Health, National Institutes of Health (IRP-NIMH-NIH), by a NARSAD Independent Investigator Award to Dr. Zarate, and by a Brain and Behavior Mood Disorders Research Award to Dr. Zarate. Dr. Zarate is listed as a co-inventor on a patent for the use of ketamine in major depression and suicidal ideation; as a co-inventor on a patent for the use of (2R,6R)-hydroxynorketamine, (S)-dehydronorketamine, and other stereoisomeric dehydro and hydroxylated metabolites of (R,S)-ketamine metabolites in the treatment of depression and neuropathic pain; and as a co-inventor on a patent application for the use of (2R,6R)-hydroxynorketamine and (2S,6S)-hydroxynorketamine in the treatment of depression, anxiety, anhedonia, suicidal ideation, and post-traumatic stress disorders. He has assigned his patent rights to the U.S. government but will share a percentage of any royalties that may be received by the government. All other authors have no conflict of interest to disclose, financial or otherwise.

REFERENCES

1. Ferrari AJ, Charlson FJ, Norman RE, et al. Burden of depressive disorders by country, sex, age, and year: findings from the global burden of disease study 2010. *PLoS Med* 2013; 10: e1001547.
2. World Health Organization. Depression. 2018. http://www.who.int/en/news-room/fact-sheets/detail/depression.
3. Nock MK, Kessler RC. Prevalence of and risk factors for suicide attempts versus suicide gestures: analysis of the National Comorbidity Survey. *J Abnorm Psychol* 2006; 115: 616–623.
4. Stone DM, Simon TR, Fowler KA, et al. Vital signs: trends in state suicide rates—United States, 1999–2016 and circumstances contributing to suicide—27 states, 2015. *MMWR Morb Mortal Wkly Rep* 2018; 67: 617–624.
5. Rush AJ, Trivedi MH, Wisniewski SR, et al. Acute and longer-term outcomes in depressed outpatients requiring one or several treatment steps: a STAR*D report. *Am J Psychiatry* 2006; 163: 1905–1917.
6. Trivedi MH, Rush AJ, Wisniewski SR, et al. Evaluation of outcomes with citalopram for depression using measurement-based care in STAR*D: implications for clinical practice. *Am J Psychiatry* 2006; 163: 28–40.
7. Henter ID, de Sousa RT, Zarate CA, Jr. Glutamatergic modulators in depression. *Harv Rev Psychiatry* 2018; 26: 307–319.
8. Ionescu DF, Papakostas GI. Current trends in identifying rapidly acting treatments for depression. *Curr Behav Neurosci Rep* 2016; 3: 185–191.
9. Duman RS, Aghajanian GK, Sanacora G, et al. Synaptic plasticity and depression: new insights from stress and rapid-acting antidepressants. *Nat Med* 2016; 22: 238–249.
10. Clements JA, Nimmo WS, Grant IS. Bioavailability, pharmacokinetics, and analgesic activity of ketamine in humans. *J Pharm Sci* 1982; 71: 539–542.
11. Zhao X, Venkata SL, Moaddel R, et al. Simultaneous population pharmacokinetic modelling of ketamine and three major metabolites in patients with treatment-resistant bipolar depression. *Br J Clin Pharmacol* 2012; 74: 304–314.
12. Moghaddam B, Adams B, Verma A, et al. Activation of glutamatergic neurotransmission by ketamine: a novel step in the pathway from NMDA receptor blockade to dopaminergic and cognitive disruptions associated with the prefrontal cortex. *J Neurosci* 1997; 17: 2921–2927.
13. Miller OH, Yang L, Wang CC, et al. GluN2B-containing NMDA receptors regulate depression-like behavior and are critical for the rapid antidepressant actions of ketamine. *Elife* 2014; 3: e03581.
14. Yang Y, Cui Y, Sang K, et al. Ketamine blocks bursting in the lateral habenula to rapidly relieve depression. *Nature* 2018; 554: 317–322.
15. Zanos P, Moaddel R, Morris PJ, et al. NMDAR inhibition-independent antidepressant actions of ketamine metabolites. *Nature* 2016; 533: 481–486.
16. Musazzi L, Tornese P, Sala N, et al. Acute or chronic? A stressful question. *Trends Neurosci* 2017; 40: 525–535.
17. Widman AJ, McMahon LL. Disinhibition of CA1 pyramidal cells by low-dose ketamine and other antagonists with rapid antidepressant efficacy. *Proc Natl Acad Sci USA* 2018; 115: E3007–E3016.
18. Li N, Lee B, Liu RJ, et al. mTOR-dependent synapse formation underlies the rapid antidepressant effects of NMDA antagonists. *Science* 2010; 329: 959–964.

19. Autry AE, Adachi M, Nosyreva E, et al. NMDA receptor blockade at rest triggers rapid behavioural antidepressant responses. *Nature* 2011; 475: 91–95.

20. Bjorkholm C, Monteggia LM. BDNF: a key transducer of antidepressant effects. *Neuropharmacology* 2016; 102: 72–79.

21. Kang HJ, Voleti B, Hajszan T, et al. Decreased expression of synapse-related genes and loss of synapses in major depressive disorder. *Nat Med* 2012; 18: 1413–1417.

22. Duman RS, Aghajanian GK. Neurobiology of rapid acting antidepressants: role of BDNF and GSK-3beta. *Neuropsychopharmacology* 2014; 39: 233.

23. Kempton MJ, Salvador Z, Munafo MR, et al. Structural neuroimaging studies in major depressive disorder: meta-analysis and comparison with bipolar disorder. *Arch Gen Psychiatry* 2011; 68: 675–690.

24. Kassem MS, Lagopoulos J, Stait-Gardner T, et al. Stress-induced grey matter loss determined by MRI is primarily due to loss of dendrites and their synapses. *Mol Neurobiol* 2013; 47: 645–661.

25. Gatt JM, Nemeroff CB, Dobson-Stone C, et al. Interactions between BDNF Val66Met polymorphism and early life stress predict brain and arousal pathways to syndromal depression and anxiety. *Mol Psychiatry* 2009; 14: 681–695.

26. Liu R, Lee F, Li X, et al. Brain-derived neurotrophic factor Val66Met allele impairs basal and ketamine-stimulated synaptogenesis in prefrontal cortex. *Biol Psychiatry* 2012; 71: 996–1005.

27. Lepack AE, Fuchikami M, Dwyer JM, et al. BDNF release is required for the behavioral actions of ketamine. *Int J Neuropsychopharmacol* 2014; 18: pii:pyu033.

28. Lally N, Nugent AC, Luckenbaugh DA, et al. Neural correlates of change in major depressive disorder anhedonia following open-label ketamine. *J Psychopharmacol* 2015; 29: 596–607.

29. Zhang Y, Yoshida T, Katz DB, et al. NMDAR antagonist action in thalamus imposes δ oscillations on the hippocampus. *J Neurophysiol* 2012; 107: 3181–3189.

30. Pinault D. N-methyl-D-aspartate receptor antagonists ketamine and MK-801 induce wake-related aberrant gamma oscillations in the rat neocortex. *Biol Psychiatry* 2008; 63: 730–735.

31. Rivolta D, Heidegger T, Scheller B, et al. Ketamine dysregulates the amplitude and connectivity of high-frequency oscillations in cortical-subcortical networks in humans: evidence from resting-state magnetoencephalography-recordings. *Schizophr Bull* 2015; 41: 1105–1114.

32. Ren Z, Pribiag H, Jefferson SJ, et al. Bidirectional homeostatic regulation of a depression-related brain state by gamma-aminobutyric acidergic deficits and ketamine treatment. *Biol Psychiatry* 2016; 80: 457–468.

33. Shaw AD, Saxena N, L EJ, et al. Ketamine amplifies induced gamma frequency oscillations in the human cerebral cortex. *Eur Neuropsychopharmacol* 2015; 25: 1136–1146.

34. Lumsden EW, Troppoli TA, Myers SJ, et al. Antidepressant-relevant concentrations of the ketamine metabolite (2R,6R)-hydroxynorketamine do not block NMDA receptor function. *Proc Natl Acad Sci USA* 2019; 116(11): 5160–5169.

35. Li L, Vlisides PE. Ketamine: 50 years of modulating the mind. *Front Hum Neurosci* 2016; 10: 612.

36. Berman RM, Cappiello A, Anand A, et al. Antidepressant effects of ketamine in depressed patients. *Biol Psychiatry* 2000; 47: 351–354.

37. Ibrahim L, Diazgranados N, Luckenbaugh DA, et al. Rapid decrease in depressive symptoms with an N-methyl-D-aspartate antagonist in ECT-resistant major depression. *Prog Neuropsychopharmacol Biol Psychiatry* 2011; 35: 1155–1159.

38. Diazgranados N, Ibrahim L, Brutsche NE, et al. Rapid resolution of suicidal ideation after a single infusion of an N-methyl-D-aspartate antagonist in patients with treatment-resistant major depressive disorder. *J Clin Psychiatry* 2010; 71: 1605–1611.

39. Zarate CA, Jr., Singh JB, Carlson PJ, et al. A randomized trial of an N-methyl-D-aspartate antagonist in treatment-resistant major depression. *Arch Gen Psychiatry* 2006; 63: 856–864.

40. Zarate CA, Brutsche N, Ibrahim L, et al. Replication of ketamine's antidepressant efficacy in bipolar depression: a randomized controlled add-on trial. *Biol Psychiatry* 2012; 71: 939–946.

41. Diazgranados N, Ibrahim L, Brutsche NE, et al. A randomized add-on trial of an N-methyl-D-aspartate antagonist in treatment-resistant bipolar depression. *Arch Gen Psychiatry* 2010; 67: 793–802.

42. Iadarola ND, Niciu MJ, Richards EM, et al. Ketamine and other N-methyl-D-aspartate receptor antagonists in the treatment of depression: a perspective review. *Ther Adv Chronic Dis* 2015; 6: 97–114.

43. Permoda-Osip A, Kisielewski J, Bartkowska-Sniatkowska A, et al. Single ketamine infusion and neurocognitive performance in bipolar depression. *Pharmacopsychiatry* 2015; 48: 78–79.

44. Kantrowitz JT, Halberstam B, Gangwisch J. Single-dose ketamine followed by daily D-cycloserine in treatment-resistant bipolar depression. *J Clin Psychiatry* 2015; 76: 737–738.

45. Niciu MJ, Luckenbaugh DA, Ionescu DF, et al. Subanesthetic dose ketamine does not induce an affective switch in three independent samples of treatment-resistant major depression. *Biol Psychiatry* 2013; 74: e23–e24.

46. Price RB, Nock MK, Charney DS, et al. Effects of intravenous ketamine on explicit and implicit measures of suicidality in treatment-resistant depression. *Biol Psychiatry* 2009; 66: 522–526.

47. Price RB, Iosifescu DV, Murrough JW, et al. Effects of ketamine on explicit and implicit suicidal cognition: a randomized controlled trial in treatment-resistant depression. *Depress Anxiety* 2014; 31: 335–343.

48. Murrough JW, Soleimani L, DeWilde KE, et al. Ketamine for rapid reduction of suicidal ideation: a randomized controlled trial. *Psychol Med* 2015; 45: 3571–3580.

49. Ballard ED, Ionescu DF, Vande Voort JL, et al. Improvement in suicidal ideation after ketamine infusion: relationship to reductions in depression and anxiety. *J Psychiatr Res* 2014; 58: 161–166.

50. Wilkinson ST, Ballard ED, Bloch MH, et al. The effect of a single dose of intravenous ketamine on suicidal ideation: a systematic review and individual participant data meta-analysis. *Am J Psychiatry* 2017; 175: 150–158.

51. Grunebaum MF, Galfalvy HC, Choo TH, et al. Ketamine for rapid reduction of suicidal thoughts in major depression: a midazolam-controlled randomized clinical trial. *Am J Psychiatry* 2017; 175: 327–335.

52. Vande Voort JL, Ballard ED, Luckenbaugh D, et al. Antisuicidal response following ketamine infusion is associated with decreased nighttime wakefulness in major depressive disorder and bipolar disorder. *J Clin Psychiatry* 2017; 78: 1068–1074.

53. McCall WV, Black CG. The link between suicide and insomnia: theoretical mechanisms. *Curr Psychiatry Rep* 2013; 15: 389.

54. Bernert RA, Turvey CL, Conwell Y, et al. Association of poor subjective sleep quality with risk for death by suicide during a 10-year period: a longitudinal, population-based study of late life. *JAMA Psychiatry* 2014; 71: 1129–1137.

55. Pigeon WR, Pinquart M, Conner K. Meta-analysis of sleep disturbance and suicidal thoughts and behaviors. *J Clin Psychiatry* 2012; 73: e1160–e1167.

56. Newport DJ, Carpenter LL, McDonald WM, et al. Ketamine and other NMDA antagonists: early clinical trials and possible mechanisms in depression. *Am J Psychiatry* 2015; 172: 950–966.

57. Kishimoto T, Chawla JM, Hagi K, et al. Single-dose infusion ketamine and non-ketamine N-methyl-D-aspartate receptor antagonists for unipolar and bipolar depression: a meta-analysis of efficacy, safety and time trajectories. *Psychol Med* 2016; 46: 1459–1472.

58. Fava M, Freeman MP, Flynn M, et al. Double-blind, placebo-controlled, dose-ranging trial of intravenous ketamine as adjunctive therapy in treatment-resistant depression (TRD). *Mol Psychiatry* 2018 [Epub ahead of print]. doi:10.1038/s41380-018-0256-5.

59. Diamond PR, Farmery AD, Atkinson S, et al. Ketamine infusions for treatment resistant depression: a series of 28 patients treated weekly or twice weekly in an ECT clinic. *J Psychopharmacol* 2014; 28: 536–544.

60. aan het Rot M, Collins KA, Murrough JW, et al. Safety and efficacy of repeated-dose intravenous ketamine for treatment-resistant depression. *Biol Psychiatry* 2010; 67: 139–145.

61. Rasmussen KG, Lineberry TW, Galardy CW, et al. Serial infusions of low-dose ketamine for major depression. *J Psychopharmacol* 2013; 27: 444–450.

62. Singh JB, Fedgchin M, Daly EJ, et al. A double-blind, randomized, placebo-controlled, dose-frequency study of intravenous ketamine in patients with treatment-resistant depression. *Am J Psychiatry* 2016; 173: 816–826.

63. Murrough JW, Iosifescu DV, Chang LC, et al. Antidepressant efficacy of ketamine in treatment-resistant major depression: a two-site randomized controlled trial. *Am J Psychiatry* 2013; 170: 1134–1142.

64. Zarate CA, Jr., Mathews DC, Furey ML. Human biomarkers of rapid antidepressant effects. *Biol Psychiatry* 2013; 73: 1142–1155.

65. Niciu MJ, Mathews DC, Ionescu DF, et al. Biomarkers in mood disorders research: developing new and improved therapeutics. *Rev Psiquiatr Clin* 2014; 41: 131–134.

66. Phelps LE, Brutsche N, Moral JR, et al. Family history of alcohol dependence and initial antidepressant response to an N-methyl-D-aspartate antagonist. *Biol Psychiatry* 2009; 65: 181–184.

67. Niciu MJ, Shovestul BJ, Jaso BA, et al. Features of dissociation differentially predict antidepressant response to ketamine in treatment-resistant depression. *J Affect Disord* 2018; 232: 310–315.

68. Nugent AC, Ballard ED, Gould TD, et al. Ketamine has distinct electrophysiological and behavioral effects in depressed and healthy subjects. *Mol Psychiatry* 2018 [Epub ahead of print]. doi: 10.1038/s41380-018-0028-2.

69. Zarate CA, Jr., Brutsche N, Laje G, et al. Relationship of ketamine's plasma metabolites with response, diagnosis, and side effects in major depression. *Biol Psychiatry* 2012; 72: 331–338.

70. Freeman MP, Papakostas GI, Hoeppner BB, et al. Sex differences in response to ketamine as a rapidly acting intervention for treatment resistant depression. *J Psychiatr Res* 2019; 110: 166–171.

71. Short B, Fong J, Galvez V, et al. Side-effects associated with ketamine use in depression: a systematic review. *Lancet Psychiatry* 2018; 5: 65–78.

72. Andrade C. Ketamine for depression, 1: Clinical summary of issues related to efficacy, adverse effects, and mechanism of action. *J Clin Psychiatry* 2017; 78: e415–e419.

73. Liu Y, Lin D, Wu B, et al. Ketamine abuse potential and use disorder. *Brain Res Bull* 2016; 126 (Pt 1): 68–73.

74. U.S. Food & Drug Administration. FDA approves new nasal spray medication for treatment-resistant depression. 2019.

75. Singh JB, Fedgchin M, Daly E, et al. Intravenous esketamine in adult treatment-resistant depression: a double-blind, double-randomization, placebo-controlled study. *Biol Psychiatry* 2016; 80: 424–431.

76. Daly EJ, Singh JB, Fedgchin M, et al. Efficacy and safety of intranasal esketamine adjunctive to oral antidepressant therapy in treatment-resistant depression: a randomized clinical trial. *JAMA Psychiatry* 2018; 75: 139–148.

77. Canuso CM, Singh JB, Fedgchin M, et al. Efficacy and safety of intranasal esketamine for the rapid reduction of symptoms of depression and suicidality in patients at imminent risk for suicide: results of a double-blind, randomized, placebo-controlled study. *Am J Psychiatry* 2018; 175: 620–630.

78. Freedman R, Brown AS, Cannon TD, et al. Can a framework be established for the safe use of ketamine? *Am J Psychiatry* 2018; 175: 587–589.

79. Popova V, Daly EJ, Trivedi MH, et al. Randomized, double-blind study of flexibly dosed intranasal esketamine plus oral antidepressant versus active control in treatment-resistant depression. Annual Meeting of the American Psychiatric Association, 2018, New York.

80. Lew V, McKay E, Maze M. Past, present, and future of nitrous oxide. *Br Med Bull* 2018; 125: 103–119.

81. Jevtovic-Todorovic V, Todorovic SM, Mennerick S, et al. Nitrous oxide (laughing gas) is an NMDA antagonist, neuroprotectant and neurotoxin. *Nat Med* 1998; 4: 460–463.

82. Mennerick S, Jevtovic-Todorovic V, Todorovic SM, et al. Effect of nitrous oxide on excitatory and inhibitory synaptic transmission in hippocampal cultures. *J Neurosci* 1998; 18: 9716–9726.

83. Chrapko WE, Jurasz P, Radomski MW, et al. Decreased platelet nitric oxide synthase activity and plasma nitric oxide metabolites in major depressive disorder. *Biol Psychiatry* 2004; 56: 129–134.

84. Dhir A, Kulkarni SK. Nitric oxide and major depression. *Nitric Oxide* 2011; 24: 125–131.

85. de Sousa RT, Zanetti MV, Busatto GF, et al. Lithium increases nitric oxide levels in subjects with bipolar disorder during depressive episodes. *J Psychiatr Res* 2014; 55: 96–100.

86. Nagele P, Duma A, Kopec M, et al. Nitrous oxide for treatment-resistant major depression: a proof-of-concept trial. *Biol Psychiatry* 2015; 78: 10–18.

87. Block RI, Ghoneim MM, Kumar V, et al. Psychedelic effects of a subanesthetic concentration of nitrous oxide. *Anesth Prog* 1990; 37: 271–276.

88. Nunn JF, Sharer NM, Bottiglieri T, et al. Effect of short-term administration of nitrous oxide on plasma concentrations of methionine, tryptophan, phenylalanine and S-adenosyl methionine in man. *Br J Anaesth* 1986; 58: 1–10.

89. Layzer RB, Fishman RA, Schafer JA. Neuropathy following abuse of nitrous oxide. *Neurology* 1978; 28: 504–506.

90. Kinsella LJ, Green R. "Anesthesia paresthetica": nitrous oxide-induced cobalamin deficiency. *Neurology* 1995; 45: 1608–1610.

91. Janowsky D, el-Yousef MK, Davis JM, et al. A cholinergic-adrenergic hypothesis of mania and depression. *Lancet* 1972; 2: 632–635.

92. Dilsaver SC, Greden JF, Snider RM. Antidepressant withdrawal syndromes: phenomenology and pathophysiology. *Int Clin Psychopharmacol* 1987; 2: 1–19.

93. Wohleb ES, Gerhard D, Thomas A, et al. Molecular and cellular mechanisms of rapid-acting antidepressants ketamine and scopolamine. *Curr Neuropharmacol* 2017; 15: 11–20.

94. Wohleb ES, Wu M, Gerhard DM, et al. GABA interneurons mediate the rapid antidepressant-like effects of scopolamine. *J Clin Invest* 2016; 126: 2482–2494.

95. Ghosal S, Bang E, Yue W, et al. Activity-dependent brain-derived neurotrophic factor release is required for the rapid antidepressant actions of scopolamine. *Biol Psychiatry* 2018; 83: 29–37.

96. Gillin JC, Sutton L, Ruiz C, et al. The effects of scopolamine on sleep and mood in depressed patients with a history of alcoholism and a normal comparison group. *Biol Psychiatry* 1991; 30: 157–169.

97. Furey ML, Drevets WC. Antidepressant efficacy of the antimuscarinic drug scopolamine: a randomized, placebo-controlled clinical trial. *Arch Gen Psychiatry* 2006; 63: 1121–1129.

98. Drevets WC, Furey ML. Replication of scopolamine's antidepressant efficacy in major depressive disorder: a randomized, placebo-controlled clinical trial. *Biol Psychiatry* 2010; 67: 432–438.

99. Park LT, Furey ML, Nugent AC, et al. Neurophysiological changes associated with antidepressant response to ketamine not observed in a negative trial of scopolamine in major depressive disorder. *Int J Neuropsychopharmacol* 2019; 22: 10–18.

100. Drevets WC, Zarate CA, Jr., Furey ML. Antidepressant effects of the muscarinic cholinergic receptor antagonist scopolamine: a review. *Biol Psychiatry* 2013; 73: 1156–1163.
101. Burgdorf J, Zhang XL, Weiss C, et al. The long-lasting antidepressant effects of rapastinel (GLYX-13) are associated with a metaplasticity process in the medial prefrontal cortex and hippocampus. *Neuroscience* 2015; 308: 202–211.
102. Moskal JR, Burch R, Burgdorf JS, et al. GLYX-13, an NMDA receptor glycine site functional partial agonist enhances cognition and produces antidepressant effects without the psychotomimetic side effects of NMDA receptor antagonists. *Expert Opin Investig Drugs* 2014; 23: 243–254.
103. Moskal JR, Burgdorf JS, Stanton PK, et al. The development of rapastinel (formerly GLYX-13); a rapid acting and long lasting antidepressant. *Curr Neuropharmacol* 2017; 15: 47–56.
104. Liu RJ, Duman C, Kato T, et al. GLYX-13 produces rapid antidepressant responses with key synaptic and behavioral effects distinct from ketamine. *Neuropsychopharmacology* 2017; 42: 1231–1242.
105. Kato T, Fogaca MV, Deyama S, et al. BDNF release and signaling are required for the antidepressant actions of GLYX-13. *Mol Psychiatry* 2018; 23: 2007–2017.
106. Preskorn S, Macaluso M, Mehra DO, et al. Randomized proof of concept trial of GLYX-13, an N-methyl-D-aspartate receptor glycine site partial agonist, in major depressive disorder nonresponsive to a previous antidepressant agent. *J Psychiatr Pract* 2015; 21: 140–149.
107. Allergan. Allergan's rapastinel receives FDA breakthrough therapy designation for adjunctive treatment of major depressive disorder (MDD). March 8, 2017. https://www.allergan.com/news/news/thomson-reuters/allergan-s-rapastinel-receives-fda-breakthrough-th.
108. Allergan. Allergan announces Phase 3 results for rapastinel as an adjunctive treatment of major depressive disorder (MDD). 2019.
109. Kennedy SE, Koeppe RA, Young EA, et al. Dysregulation of endogenous opioid emotion regulation circuitry in major depression in women. *Arch Gen Psychiatry* 2006; 63: 1199–1208.
110. Scarone S, Gambini O, Calabrese G, et al. Asymmetrical distribution of beta-endorphin in cerebral hemispheres of suicides: preliminary data. *Psychiatry Res* 1990; 32: 159–166.
111. Gross-Isseroff R, Dillon KA, Israeli M, et al. Regionally selective increases in mu opioid receptor density in the brains of suicide victims. *Brain Res* 1990; 530: 312–316.
112. Woody GE. Advances in the treatment of opioid use disorders. *F1000Res* 2017; 6: 87.
113. Sher L. Buprenorphine and the treatment of depression, anxiety, non-suicidal self-injury, and suicidality. *Acta Psychiatr Scand* 2016; 134: 84–85.
114. Mague SD, Pliakas AM, Todtenkopf MS, et al. Antidepressant-like effects of kappa-opioid receptor antagonists in the forced swim test in rats. *J Pharmacol Exp Ther* 2003; 305: 323–330.
115. Sbrenna S, Marti M, Morari M, et al. Modulation of 5-hydroxytryptamine efflux from rat cortical synaptosomes by opioids and nociceptin. *Br J Pharmacol* 2000; 130: 425–433.
116. Ehrich E, Turncliff R, Du Y, et al. Evaluation of opioid modulation in major depressive disorder. *Neuropsychopharmacology* 2015; 40: 1448–1455.
117. Fava M, Memisoglu A, Thase ME, et al. Opioid modulation with buprenorphine/samidorphan as adjunctive treatment for inadequate response to antidepressants: a randomized double-blind placebo-controlled trial. *Am J Psychiatry* 2016; 173: 499–508.
118. Yovell Y, Bar G, Mashiah M, et al. Ultra-low-dose buprenorphine as a time-limited treatment for severe suicidal ideation: a randomized controlled trial. *Am J Psychiatry* 2016; 173: 491–498.
119. Fava M, Thase ME, Trivedi MH, et al. Opioid system modulation with buprenorphine/samidorphan combination for major depressive disorder: two randomized controlled studies. *Mol Psychiatry* 2018.
120. FierceBiotech. FDA rejects Alkermes' depression drug ALKS 5461. 2019.

121. Bunney BG, Bunney WE. Mechanisms of rapid antidepressant effects of sleep deprivation therapy: clock genes and circadian rhythms. *Biol Psychiatry* 2013; 73: 1164–1171.

122. Mongrain V, La Spada F, Curie T, et al. Sleep loss reduces the DNA-binding of BMAL1, CLOCK, and NPAS2 to specific clock genes in the mouse cerebral cortex. *PLoS One* 2011; 6: e26622.

123. Stern WC, Miller FP, Cox RH, et al. Brain norepinephrine and serotonin levels following REM sleep deprivation in the rat. *Psychopharmacologia* 1971; 22: 50–55.

124. Volkow ND, Wang GJ, Telang F, et al. Sleep deprivation decreases binding of [11C]raclopride to dopamine D2/D3 receptors in the human brain. *J Neurosci* 2008; 28: 8454–8461.

125. Benedetti F, Bernasconi A, Blasi V, et al. Neural and genetic correlates of antidepressant response to sleep deprivation: a functional magnetic resonance imaging study of moral valence decision in bipolar depression. *Arch Gen Psychiatry* 2007; 64: 179–187.

126. Wolf E, Kuhn M, Normann C, et al. Synaptic plasticity model of therapeutic sleep deprivation in major depression. *Sleep Med Rev* 2016; 30: 53–62.

127. Vyazovskiy VV, Cirelli C, Pfister-Genskow M, et al. Molecular and electrophysiological evidence for net synaptic potentiation in wake and depression in sleep. *Nat Neurosci* 2008; 11: 200–208.

128. Benedetti F, Serretti A, Colombo C, et al. A glycogen synthase kinase 3-beta promoter gene single nucleotide polymorphism is associated with age at onset and response to total sleep deprivation in bipolar depression. *Neurosci Lett* 2004; 368: 123–126.

129. Pflug B, Tolle R. Disturbance of the 24-hour rhythm in endogenous depression and the treatment of endogenous depression by sleep deprivation. *Int Pharmacopsychiatry* 1971; 6: 187–196.

130. Schulte W. [Clinical experiences with the getting out of a melancholic phase]. *Arztl Forsch* 1968; 22: 145–148.

131. Wu JC, Bunney WE. The biological basis of an antidepressant response to sleep deprivation and relapse: review and hypothesis. *Am J Psychiatry* 1990; 147: 14–21.

132. Boland EM, Rao H, Dinges DF, et al. Meta-analysis of the antidepressant effects of acute sleep deprivation. *J Clin Psychiatry* 2017; 78: e1020–e1034.

133. Hemmeter UM, Hemmeter-Spernal J, Krieg JC. Sleep deprivation in depression. *Expert Rev Neurother* 2010; 10: 1101–1115.

134. Giedke H, Schwarzler F. Therapeutic use of sleep deprivation in depression. *Sleep Med Rev* 2002; 6: 361–377.

135. Benedetti F, Barbini B, Bernasconi A, et al. Acute antidepressant response to sleep deprivation combined with light therapy is influenced by the catechol-O-methyltransferase Val(108/158)Met polymorphism. *J Affect Disord* 2010; 121: 68–72.

136. Benedetti F, Riccaboni R, Locatelli C, et al. Rapid treatment response of suicidal symptoms to lithium, sleep deprivation, and light therapy (chronotherapeutics) in drug-resistant bipolar depression. *J Clin Psychiatry* 2014; 75: 133–140.

137. Kadriu B, Musazzi L, Henter ID, et al. Glutamatergic neurotransmission: pathway to developing novel rapid-acting antidepressant treatments. *Int J Neuropsychopharmacol* 2019; 22: 119–135.

/// 14 /// MANAGEMENT OF SIDE EFFECTS OF ANTIDEPRESSANT MEDICATIONS

RAJNISH MAGO

14.1. WHY ARE SIDE EFFECTS SO IMPORTANT?

Depressive disorders are among the most prevalent of mental disorders (Kessler et al., 2003; 2005) and are associated with considerable suffering, disability, and mortality (Murray et al., 2012). Antidepressant medications have a central role in the management of many patients with major depressive disorder, especially those with more severe and recurrent depression. The use of antidepressants has increased manifold since the introduction of the selective serotonin reuptake inhibitors (SSRIs) in 1998 (Paulose-Ram et al., 2007; Kantor et al., 2015). So why have the prevalence of depressive disorders, the disability associated with them, and the rates of suicide not decreased? There are probably many reasons for this, but one important one is that it is shockingly common for patients to prematurely stop taking their antidepressant medication. In one study, 28% of patients completely stopped taking any antidepressant within the first three months after starting an antidepressant, and more stopped it later on (Bull et al., 2002b). While nonadherence to antidepressant medications is undoubtedly multifactorial, one of the most important reasons for it is the side effects associated with these medications (Bull et al., 2002a; Crawford et al., 2014).

We must understand and appreciate that to patients the suffering caused by the side effects of antidepressants is distressing just as the symptoms of depression are. Patients should not have to choose between the depression and the side effects of medication for it. Patients report that they consider the side effects of antidepressants to be as important as improvement in the symptoms of depression and reduction in the risk of relapse (Wouters et al., 2014). Consistent with this, the most frequent reason given by psychiatrists for prescribing a particular antidepressant was its potential side effects (Zimmerman et al., 2004). Also, occasionally, side effects of antidepressant medications can be "medically serious," such as hyponatremia, seizures, abnormal bleeding, etc. (Mago et al., 2008).

14.2. HOW COMMON AND BOTHERSOME ARE THESE SIDE EFFECTS?

It is often thought that side effects of antidepressants occur in a minority of patients and are mild in most cases. This is far from the truth. We can look at adverse events that were spontaneously reported in placebo-controlled clinical trials (as described in the Prescribing Information for each medication) and that occurred at least twice as often as on placebo, suggesting that they were probably associated with the medication. For commonly used antidepressants, the drug–placebo difference for such adverse events ranged from 5% to 36% (Mago, 2016). And even these estimates are probably on the lower side given that patients are rarely specifically questioned about any adverse events they may have had. Also, in one fairly large survey of patients who were prescribed an SSRI, 52% reported having had three or more side effects that they attributed to the SSRI (Bull et al., 2002a; Hu et al., 2004). Also, 55% of them reported having had one or more side effects that were "a lot" or "extremely" bothersome.

14.3. WHAT CAN WE DO?

While some clinicians may consider side effects to be "unfortunate, unwanted, and perhaps inevitable accompaniments of the benefits of these medications" (Mago, 2016), in fact, there *are* things we can do. We can talk to patients about side effects before starting the medication and on an ongoing basis—but how should this be done in a way that helps patients to deal appropriately with any side effects that may occur? We can take measures from a "menu of options" to, if possible, reduce the incidence of side effects when possible and to manage them when they occur.

I classify these measures into *first-line, second-line, or third-line*, depending on how important it is that the medication not be stopped. First-line measures include simple actions with little downside. Second-line measures include those that are more active, including adding some treatment, but carry little risk. Third-line measures include more active, energetic measures, including those that may carry risks of their own. Third-line measures are, therefore, used only when it is very important that the patient continue the medication that is causing the side effect. For example, if a person with severe major depressive disorder failed to respond to numerous antidepressants but is doing very well on another antidepressant, it may be very important to treat any persistent and troubling side effects from this antidepressant.

14.4. TWO IMPORTANT ISSUES TO DISCUSS WITH PATIENTS

I believe that it is important for us to distinguish between "nuisance side effects" and "medically serious side effects" and to convey this distinction to patients. Nuisance side effects like headache, nausea, tremors, and jitteriness are definitely quite bothersome to patients but in almost all cases do not suggest there is any significant or lasting harm to any organ of the body. This is in contrast to "medical serious side effects" like hepatotoxicity, seizures, and so on.

Unfortunately, the side effects that most frequently cause patients to discontinue their medications tend to be nuisance side effects, in many cases those that would probably have soon subsided if the patient could have been helped to stay on the medication. For example, in one study, the side effects that most frequently led to patients stopping treatment with an SSRI were drowsiness/fatigue, anxiety, headache, and nausea (Bull et al., 2002b).

So, before starting the medication and on an ongoing basis, we should educate our patients on the difference between "nuisance" and "medically serious" side effects. We should also tell them that the great majority of side effects from antidepressant medications are nuisance side effects. We should acknowledge that these nuisance side effects are bothersome and assure patients that we will try our best to manage them. Nevertheless, they need to be kept in context.

The other issue that we should talk to patients about is that many side effects tend to occur early on and to gradually subside. In general, the-side effect burden associated with antidepressants tends to be worst in the first 30 days. If we can support the person in getting through the first 30 days, many side effects will subside or, at least, decrease in intensity. This is, unfortunately, not true for some other side effects, including sexual dysfunction, weight gain, excessive sweating, and so on, that may become more apparent later on and generally tend to persist as long as the antidepressant is taken.

14.5. WILL DISCUSSING SIDE EFFECTS LEAD TO MORE PROBLEMS?

Let's bring these concerns out into the open and discuss them. It is a widespread belief among clinicians that discussing potential side effects or those that the patient is experiencing will lead patients, through the power of suggestion, to report more side effects—and that discussing potential or actual side effects with patients will cause patients to either refuse to take the antidepressant or to stop taking it.

But in one study done in "real world" settings, while patients who said that they had been told by their physicians about potential adverse effects of the antidepressant being prescribed did report mild to moderate adverse effects more often, they did not prematurely discontinue taking the antidepressant more often (Bull et al., 2002b). Patients who reported that they had discussed side effects with their physicians were much more likely to have the antidepressant changed, but, importantly, their risk of stopping antidepressant treatment was reduced by half (Bull et al., 2002a). A discussion of side effects may lead to the antidepressant being changed, allowing the patient to continue treatment with an antidepressant rather than discontinuing treatment altogether. To the best of my knowledge, there are no data to support the idea that educating patients about potential side effects may increase the risk of their stopping the antidepressant altogether.

14.6. WHICH SIDE EFFECTS SHOULD WE TELL PATIENTS ABOUT?

Before starting an antidepressant (or other medication), we must tell the patient about potential side effects. Researchers have largely neglected the issue of how adequately this is being done in clinical practice or suggested ways of doing this effectively within the constraints of a busy clinical practice.

Somewhat surprisingly, we do not agree about what the potential side effects of a medication are. I have proposed a simple strategy that may be a good starting point (Mago, 2014). I suggest that patients should be told about all "adverse events" that occurred in placebo-controlled clinical trials at least twice as often as on placebo *and* occurred in at least 5% more patients on the drug than on placebo (Mago, 2016). The rationale for this is as follows. It is likely that adverse events that occurred at least twice as often as on placebo were, in fact, related to the drug. Focusing on adverse events that occurred in 5% or more patients on the drug than on placebo allows us to give patients a relatively limited list of "common side effects" for each medication rather than an exhaustive list of potential side effects, which may be difficult for patients to process. Clinicians can obtain (at no cost) patient handouts with such lists of common potential side effects at https://simpleandpractical.com/aehandouts.

In addition to telling patients about common side effects in this manner, we should also tell them about any potentially serious or life-threatening side effects. Within the time constraints of clinical practice, this is a challenging task. We have to customize this information for individual patients.

It is not possible, in this chapter, to discuss the large number of strategies that can be used to mitigate the dozens of potential adverse effects of antidepressant medications. Some of the strategies are discussed later in the chapter. For a more comprehensive discussion (without the space constraint of this chapter) of how to prevent and manage various antidepressant side effects, the reader is referred to https://simpleandpractical.com/side-effects or to my book *Side Effects of Psychiatric Medications: Prevention, Assessment, and Management.*

14.6.1. Bleeding, Excessive

The reason serotonergic antidepressants increase the risk of bleeding is that they inhibit the aggregation of platelets by inhibiting the serotonin transporter that is present on platelets as well as neurons.

BOX 14.1.

RISK FACTORS FOR EXCESSIVE BLEEDING ASSOCIATED WITH SEROTONERGIC ANTIDEPRESSANTS

DEMOGRAPHIC FACTORS
Older adults

COMORBID MEDICAL CONDITIONS
Hepatitis C[1]
Cirrhosis of liver/portal hypertension[2]

CONCOMITANT MEDICATIONS
Aspirin
NSAIDs
Antiplatelet agents (e.g., heparin, clopidogrel)[3]
Vitamin E
Fish oil

---

[1] *Patients with hepatitis C may be given a serotonergic antidepressant for the treatment of major depression or for the prophylaxis or treatment of interferon-induced depression. Excessive bleeding, sometimes very serious, can occur (e.g., Weinrieb et al., 2003).*
[2] *Presence of cirrhosis/portal hypertension increases the risk of gastrointestinal bleeding, but only a small percentage of these patients actually experience such bleeding (Martin et al., 2007).*
[3] *E.g., Labos et al. (2011).*

14.6.1.1. Evaluation

The most important thing with regard to the risk of excessive bleeding is to understand who is at greater risk (Box 14.1). In particular, patients who have more than one risk factor are at a significantly increased risk of bleeding.

Patients should be asked about all medications they are taking, including over-the-counter supplements. They should also be monitored for early signs of increased bleeding tendency. Here are some examples (Mago, 2014):

- Easy bruising (e.g., after a minor bump)
- Bleeding for longer than expected after getting blood drawn for laboratory tests
- Bleeding for longer than expected after a cut while shaving (or any other injury)
- New onset of bleeding after flossing.

14.6.1.2. Management

If the patient has one or more risk factors for increased bleeding, we should try to avoid prescribing SSRIs if possible. Alternatives include a non-serotonergic antidepressant (e.g., bupropion, agomelatine, reboxetine) or an antidepressant that increases serotonergic activity through a mechanism other than serotonin reuptake inhibition (e.g., mirtazapine, a monoamine oxidase inhibitor).

As discussed in Section 14.6.1.1., patients who are taking an SSRI and frequently or daily also take aspirin or a nonsteroidal anti-inflammatory are at increased risk of bleeding from the stomach. These may include patients with a rheumatologic condition (e.g., rheumatoid arthritis) or a painful musculoskeletal condition. In such cases, the addition of a proton-pump inhibitor should be strongly considered because this may reduce the risk of gastrointestinal bleeding.

14.6.2. Bruxism

Bruxism refers to involuntary clenching, grinding of the teeth, or both, that can occur during the day, during sleep, or both. Sleep bruxism is actually a form of parasomnia that occurs during non-REM sleep when muscle tone is intact and movement can occur. Serotonergic antidepressants are a common cause of bruxism. As many as 14% of patients taking an antidepressant may have bruxism (Uca et al., 2015). Bruxism can cause pain, headache, serious damage to the enamel of the teeth, inflammation of the temporomandibular joint, and so on. Management is as follows:

1. Waiting and watching: Antidepressant-induced bruxism may subside on its own (e.g., Iskander et al., 2012).
2. Reduction in the dose of the antidepressant, if possible, because bruxism is dose-related (Ranjan et al., 2006).
3. Switching the antidepressant: The bruxism may (e.g., Jaffee and Bostwick, 2000; Kuloglu et al., 2010) or may not (e.g., Chang et al., 2011) occur with the other antidepressant.
4. Wearing a night guard: To prevent damage to the teeth, a night guard should be worn in the mouth while sleeping.
5. Smoking cessation, if applicable, because smoking makes bruxism worse.
6. Regular monitoring by a dentist.
7. Adding an "antidote": The antidote most frequently used to treat antidepressant-induced bruxism is buspirone (Ellison and Stanziani, 1993: Romanelli et al., 1996; Bostwick and Jaffe, 1999; Jaffe and Bostwick, 2000; Wise, 2001; Pavlovic, 2004; Sabuncuoglu et al., 2009; Kuloglu et al., 2010; Çolak Sivri et al., 2016). For sleep bruxism, the buspirone may be given only at bedtime.

14.6.3. Dry Mouth

Dry mouth is a common and important side effect not only of tricyclic antidepressants (TCAs) but also of second-generation antidepressants. For example, up to a third of patients on SSRIs may have dry mouth. It is important not only because it is uncomfortable for the patient but also because saliva has antibacterial, buffering, and remineralization effects and, therefore, protects the teeth, tongue, and mouth. Patients who have dry mouth are more prone to develop dental caries and can even develop an infection of the tongue or mouth. Dry mouth may also lead to other problems like impairment in taste, halitosis, dry lips, and impaired fitting of dentures. Since patients may not spontaneously report it, we should ask patients whether they have dry mouth. We can also examine the mouth and tongue to see if they are dry.

Management of dry mouth includes the following:

1. Avoid things that may worsen the dry mouth, such as alcohol-based mouthwashes, tobacco, and caffeine.
2. Improve oral hygiene: Persons with depressive disorders may be more likely than others to neglect their oral hygiene, but if dry mouth is present, greater than usual attention to oral hygiene should be recommended.
3. Eat foods that stimulate the production of saliva, such as carrots, apples, and celery.
4. Use sugarless chewing gum or candy to stimulate saliva production.
5. Sip water while eating, which can be helpful in swallowing food and may improve the taste of food.
6. Suck on ice chips for symptomatic relief.
7. Use a cool mist humidifier, especially in the winter.
8. Use over-the-counter saliva substitutes.
9. Use xylitol-containing chewing gum. Xylitol is a sweetener that can reduce dental caries and help to remineralize the enamel.
10. Use a pilocarpine mouthwash (e.g., Tanigawa et al., 2015).
11. If applicable, consider changing to an antidepressant with less anticholinergic activity.

14.6.4. Glaucoma

Angle-closure glaucoma is a medical emergency because it can lead to loss of vision. Antidepressant medications that may cause this include bupropion, SSRIs (especially paroxetine), mirtazapine, venlafaxine, and TCAs. They do this by making the pupils dilate, which can precipitate this kind of glaucoma in persons who are predisposed. The single most important thing we can do to anticipate this adverse effect is to ask whether the patient or any family member has ever had glaucoma or increased pressure in the eye. Persons with a family history of acute angle-closure glaucoma are 10 times more likely to develop acute angle-closure glaucoma.

14.6.5. Hypersensitivity Reaction

In rare cases, a hypersensitivity syndrome occurs about one to six weeks after starting the antidepressant. It presents with fever and rash. If this is suspected, a blood count (to look for eosinophilia) and hepatic function tests should be urgently obtained.

14.6.6. Hypertension

While SSRIs have not convincingly been shown to increase blood pressure, serotonin–norepinephrine reuptake inhibitors (SNRIs) have been associated with at least some risk of doing so (Zhong et al., 2017). In the case of venlafaxine, this may be clinically significant only at doses greater than 300 mg/day (Thase, 1998). However, it should be noted that in clinical trials, patients with poorly controlled hypertension are generally excluded. In such patients, it may be best to avoid SNRIs if possible.

Bupropion has been associated with elevated blood pressure (e.g., Kiev et al., 2004). The Prescribing Information includes a warning that extended-release bupropion "can increase blood pressure. Monitor blood pressure before initiating treatment and periodically during treatment." The increase in blood pressure may be more likely in persons taking bupropion along with a nicotine patch for smoking cessation (Thase et al., 2008). However, in clinical trials in seasonal affective disorder, increased blood pressure was found in 2% of patients on bupropion and none on placebo (Prescribing Information). In a systematic study of bupropion that included ambulatory monitoring, no elevation of blood pressure was found (Thase et al., 2008). Thus, the question of how often bupropion is associated with increased blood pressure is not fully resolved.

14.6.7. Hyponatremia

Serotonergic antidepressants may be associated with hyponatremia (Mago et al., 2008), especially in persons with one or more of the risk factors (Box 14.2). It is critical that we understand that the hyponatremia is not due to a deficiency of salt, a misconception that is surprisingly common among clinicians and patients alike. It is due to a syndrome of inappropriate antidiuretic hormone secretion (SIADH), which leads to retention of water, leading, in turn, to a reduction in the serum sodium concentration.

BOX 14.2.

RISK FACTORS FOR ANTIDEPRESSANT-INDUCED HYPONATREMIA

Older adult
Female gender
Underweight
Concomitant use of a diuretic
Low baseline serum sodium
History of hyponatremia in the past

14.6.7.1. Identification

1. Be aware of persons who have one or more risk factors.
2. The early symptoms of hyponatremia are nonspecific (e.g., fatigue, cognitive impairment, malaise, and so on). These may easily be attributed to other causes, including the depressive disorder itself. In persons with risk factors for hyponatremia, however, we should be vigilant for them.
3. It is useful to know that hyponatremia typically occurs early on—within a few days of starting the antidepressant. Thus, in a person with risk factors for hyponatremia or with symptoms that may suggest hyponatremia, checking the serum sodium once or twice in the first two to three weeks should be considered. Without keeping a high index of suspicion, it is likely that we will miss many cases of antidepressant-induced hyponatremia.
4. Early detection. If hyponatremia is identified while it is still mild, it might be much easier to manage than if it has progressed and is severe.
5. To differentiate between SIADH and psychogenic polydipsia, both of which can lead to hyponatremia, we can check the plasma osmolality and the urine osmolality at the same time. In polydipsia, the urine will be dilute. In SIADH, the urine will be concentrated even though the plasma is dilute.

14.6.7.2. Management

Do not encourage these patients to drink rehydration drinks like Gatorade or give them intravenous normal saline; the last thing they need is more fluids. Instead, ask the patient to actively restrict fluid intake. If the person is taking a diuretic, try to stop the diuretic, if at all possible. Change to another antihypertensive if needed. In some cases, it may become essential to stop the antidepressant that is believed to be causing the hyponatremia. If continued antidepressant treatment is essential, it may be better to switch to an antidepressant with lower or no risk of causing hyponatremia, such as, bupropion, mirtazapine. If that is not possible, we should consider switching to a different serotonergic antidepressant, though hyponatremia may occur with the second antidepressant as well.

Can we rechallenge the patient by starting the same serotonergic antidepressant after the hyponatremia resolves? If the risk/benefit analysis supports this, yes, we can. The hyponatremia may or may not recur.

14.6.8. Liver Injury

While the exact prevalence is not known, milder liver injury is estimated to occur in between 0.5% and 3% of those taking an antidepressant. Typically, antidepressant-induced liver injury is mild and asymptomatic, with only slight elevation of liver enzymes. But, in rare cases, fulminant liver disease and even death have been associated with use of an antidepressant.

Liver injury is generally unrelated to the dose of the antidepressant. It may occur within a few days of starting the antidepressant or up to six months later. All antidepressants can be associated with liver injury, but some of them may be associated with an increased risk (Voican et al., 2014). These include (alphabetically) agomelatine, amitriptyline, bupropion, duloxetine, imipramine, nefazodone, phenelzine, tianeptine, and trazodone.

Evaluation and management is as follows:

1. The patient must be evaluated for other potential causes of liver injury.
2. Since antidepressant-induced liver injury is idiosyncratic and may occur rapidly, routinely ordering hepatic function tests after starting an antidepressant is not recommended.
3. If liver injury is suspected, hepatic function tests should be obtained. In antidepressant-induced liver injury, the ALT will typically be elevated more than the AST. Note that an increase in AST, ALT, or both to up to five times the upper limit of normal (i.e., to about 200 IU/L) is considered "mild." An increase in AST and/or ALT to between 5 and 10 times the upper limit of normal (i.e., from about 200–400 IU/L) is considered "moderate."
4. If AST or ALT is elevated to at least three times the upper limit of normal and bilirubin is increased to at least twice the upper limit of normal ("Hy's law"), this is very serious and the antidepressant must be stopped immediately (Voican et al., 2014). The patient should be referred for urgent evaluation and possible hospitalization.
5. If the abnormal hepatic function tests clearly appeared within the first six months after an antidepressant was started *and* there is no other apparent cause of liver injury, the antidepressant should usually be stopped.
6. In any of the following situations, a consultation with a liver specialist or other appropriate physician should be obtained right away: (1) the elevation of liver enzymes is severe, (2) serum bilirubin is elevated to twice the upper limit of normal or more, or (3) the abnormalities in the hepatic function tests are progressing.
9. If, after evaluation, the liver injury is believed to have been due to the antidepressant, the person should be clearly told to never in his or her life take that antidepressant again because severe liver failure can occur if the person is rechallenged with the same antidepressant (Voican et al., 2014).

14.6.9. Nausea

Nausea is one of the most common side effects of many antidepressants. This is true not only of the SSRIs and SNRIs but of bupropion as well. Also, nausea is one of the most common reasons why patients discontinue an antidepressant. Tips for prevention and management are as follows:

1. All antidepressants except mirtazapine should generally be taken after a substantial amount of food is eaten.
2. A simple strategy to reduce the incidence of nausea is to always start it at half the dose recommended in the Prescribing Information and then increase the dose after a few days. For example, starting duloxetine at 30 mg/day for one week before increasing it to 60 mg/day reduced the incidence of nausea to 16% compared to 33% when the duloxetine was started directly at 60 mg/day (Dunner et al., 2006).
3. If a sustained-release preparation of the medication is available and the patient is not already taking it (e.g., bupropion, paroxetine), changing to a sustained-release preparation may reduce the nausea.
4. Ginger has been shown in placebo-controlled clinical trials to treat postoperative nausea/vomiting (Chaiyakunapruk et al., 2006), nausea associated with pregnancy (Bryer, 2005), and other conditions that may be associated with nausea. This is a relatively but not completely benign intervention that, while not systematically studied specifically for antidepressant-induced nausea, has been successfully used in clinical practice by many psychopharmacologists.
5. Since the nausea associated with SSRIs and SNRIs is believed to be mediated in large part through postsynaptic 5-HT3 receptors, use of ondansetron, which is a 5-HT3 antagonist, is a simple and effective strategy to treat nausea associated with these medications.
6. Since it is itself an antagonist of 5-HT3 receptors, vortioxetine is an exception to the recommendation above to use 5-HT3 receptor antagonists to treat nausea associated with serotonergic antidepressants.

14.6.10. Seizures

Some antidepressants have been convincingly shown to increase the risk of seizures (Mago et al., 2008). The risk of a seizure associated with taking a TCA may be as high as 1%. The risk of a new-onset seizure associated with sustained-release bupropion up to 300 mg/day in persons who do not have any risk factors for seizures is about 0.1%, which is about the same as the risk with SSRIs. However, at its highest recommended dose, 400 mg/day, sustained-release bupropion is associated with a 0.4% risk of a seizure, or about four times more than at lower doses. At doses above the range approved by the US Food and Drug Administration (FDA), which are not recommended, the risk of a seizure associated with bupropion climbs steeply to about 4%. Patients with risk factors for seizures should generally not be prescribed TCAs or bupropion.

14.6.11. Sexual Dysfunction

Antidepressant-induced sexual dysfunction is both common and tends to persist for as long as the antidepressant is taken. It is distressing to patients and a common cause of nonadherence to antidepressants. Serotonergic antidepressants can cause sexual dysfunction related to any of the phases of the sexual response cycle—desire, arousal, and orgasm—but especially affect orgasm. How common is it? This depends on the antidepressant, with the incidence varying widely between antidepressants and how the sexual dysfunction was identified. But a rough estimate is that sexual dysfunction that can be attributed to the antidepressant occurs in about a quarter of patients overall (Clayton et al., 2002).

Management is as follows:

1. Wait and watch: Antidepressant-induced sexual dysfunction subsides, even in follow-up for up to 38 months, in only about 10% of cases (Ashton and Rosen, 1998).
2. Reduce the dose of the antidepressant, if possible.
3. Change to an antidepressant that is less likely to cause sexual dysfunction, such as (alphabetically) agomelatine, bupropion, mirtazapine, or moclobemide.
4. Drug holidays: Drug holidays for two days a week may temporarily reduce sexual dysfunction in a high proportion of patients, though this has been demonstrated only in an uncontrolled clinical trial (Rothschild, 1995). Drug holidays are not suitable for antidepressants that have a long half-life (e.g., fluoxetine, vortioxetine), those that are associated with a higher risk of discontinuation symptoms (e.g., venlafaxine), in patients whose depression is not well controlled, etc.
5. Contrary to popular practice, adding bupropion is unlikely to reverse antidepressant-induced sexual dysfunction. All three randomized, placebo-controlled trials of this strategy conducted in the United States (Masand et al., 2001; Clayton et al., 2004; DeBattista et al., 2005) did *not* find it to be effective. More recently, two large single-center studies from outside the United States reported addition of bupropion to a serotonergic antidepressant to be efficacious, but one of these studies has been withdrawn due to concerns about its methodology.
6. Add a phosphodiesterase inhibitor: Phosphodiesterase inhibitors have been shown in placebo-controlled clinical trials to reverse antidepressant-induced erectile dysfunction in a high proportion of patients (Nurnberg et al., 2003; Fava et al., 2006).
7. Refer the patient for possible treatment with testosterone gel: Testosterone gel has been found in randomized, placebo-controlled clinical trials to be effective for antidepressant-induced sexual dysfunction in both men (Amiaz et al., 2011) and women (Fooladi et al., 2014) with low or low-normal testosterone levels.

14.6.12. Sweating, Excessive (Hyperhidrosis)

Antidepressant-induced excessive sweating (ADIES) can occur with all or almost all antidepressants. These include TCAs, SSRIs, SNRIs, and bupropion. When looking at adverse events that occurred in clinical trials at least twice as often as on placebo, excessive sweating has been reported in between 5% and 14% of patients taking an SSRI or SNRI. ADIES is, thus, common, and it may cause significant distress and functional impairment in some patients. The first clinical trial ever for the treatment of ADIES (Mago et al., 2013) also systematically explored for the first time the clinical features of ADIES. In contrast to environmental or emotional sweating, ADIES had a distinct and consistent pattern of being prominent in the scalp, face, neck, and upper chest.

Management is as follows:

1. Wait and watch: This strategy may be inappropriate after the first few weeks because ADIES may persist for as long as the antidepressant is taken.
2. Reduce the dose, if possible.
3. Switch from bupropion or an SNRI to an SSRI since bupropion and SNRIs seem to be associated with higher rates of excessive sweating.
4. If the ADIES is due to an SSRI, a trial of changing to another SSRI may be considered, though ADIES may occur with the other SSRI as well.
5. In our uncontrolled clinical trial, terazosin (an alpha-1 blocker), 1 to 6 mg/day, was shown to be effective for ADIES in almost all patients.
6. Although not supported by any clinical trial thus far, glycopyrrolate (an anticholinergic medication that does not substantially cross the blood–brain barrier) 2 to 6 mg/day (Mago, 2013) is currently what I use first-line for ADIES in my patients.

14.7. CONCLUSIONS

The success of antidepressant treatment depends greatly on adherence, which in turn depends greatly on managing side effects. Side effects are common, distressing, and impairing. I hope that this chapter, while not comprehensive, has given readers an indication that many strategies can potentially be used to mitigate the adverse effects of antidepressants. My hope is that this active approach to managing side effects will benefit many of your patients.

REFERENCES

Amiaz R, Pope HG Jr, Mahne T, Kelly JF, Brennan BP, Kanayama G, Weiser M, Hudson JI, Seidman SN. Testosterone gel replacement improves sexual function in depressed men taking serotonergic antidepressants: a randomized, placebo-controlled clinical trial. J Sex Marital Ther. 2011;37(4):243–54.

Ashton AK, Rosen RC. Accommodation to serotonin reuptake inhibitor-induced sexual dysfunction. J Sex Marital Ther. 1998;24(3):191–2.

Bostwick JM, Jaffee MS. Buspirone as an antidote to SSRI-induced bruxism in 4 cases. J Clin Psychiatry. 1999;60(12):857–60.

Bryer E. A literature review of the effectiveness of ginger in alleviating mild-to-moderate nausea and vomiting of pregnancy. J Midwifery Womens Health. 2005;50(1):e1–3.

Bull SA, Hu XH, Hunkeler EM, Lee JY, Ming EE, Markson LE, Fireman B. Discontinuation of use and switching of antidepressants: influence of patient-physician communication. JAMA. 2002a;288(11):1403–9.

Bull SA, Hunkeler EM, Lee JY, Rowland CR, Williamson TE, Schwab JR, Hurt SW. Discontinuing or switching selective serotonin-reuptake inhibitors. Ann Pharmacother. 2002b;36(4): 578–84.

Chang JP, Wu CC, Su KP. A case of venlafaxine-induced bruxism alleviated by duloxetine substitution. Prog Neuropsychopharmacol Biol Psychiatry. 2011 Jan 15;35(1):307. doi: 10.1016/j.pnpbp.2010.11.025. Epub 2010 Nov 24. PubMed PMID:21111016.

Chaiyakunapruk N, Kitikannakorn N, Nathisuwan S, Leeprakobboon K, Leelasettagool C. The efficacy of ginger for the prevention of postoperative nausea and vomiting: a meta-analysis. Am J Obstet Gynecol. 2006;194(1):95–9.

Clayton AH, Pradko JF, Croft HA, Montano CB, Leadbetter RA, Bolden-Watson C, Bass KI, Donahue RM, Jamerson BD, Metz A. Prevalence of sexual dysfunction among newer antidepressants. J Clin Psychiatry. 2002;63(4):357–66.

Clayton AH, Warnock JK, Kornstein SG, Pinkerton R, Sheldon-Keller A, McGarvey EL. A placebo-controlled trial of bupropion SR as an antidote for selective serotonin reuptake inhibitor-induced sexual dysfunction. J Clin Psychiatry. 2004;65(1):62–7.

Çolak Sivri R, Akça ÖF. Buspirone in the treatment of fluoxetine-induced sleep bruxism. J Child Adolesc Psychopharmacol. 2016;26(8):762–3.

Crawford AA, Lewis S, Nutt D, Peters TJ, Cowen P, O'Donovan MC, Wiles N, Lewis G. Adverse effects from antidepressant treatment: randomised controlled trial of 601 depressed individuals. Psychopharmacology (Berl). 2014;231(15):2921–31.

DeBattista C, Solvason B, Poirier J, Kendrick E, Loraas E. A placebo-controlled, randomized, double-blind study of adjunctive bupropion sustained release in the treatment of SSRI-induced sexual dysfunction. J Clin Psychiatry. 2005;66(7):844–8.

Dunner DL, Wohlreich MM, Mallinckrodt CH, Watkin JG, Fava M. Clinical consequences of initial duloxetine dosing strategies: comparison of 30 and 60 mg QD starting doses. Curr Ther Res Clin Exp. 2005;66(6):522–40.

Ellison JM, Stanziani P. SSRI-associated nocturnal bruxism in four patients. J Clin Psychiatry. 1993;54(11):432–4.

Fava M, Nurnberg HG, Seidman SN, Holloway W, Nicholas S, Tseng LJ, Stecher VJ. Efficacy and safety of sildenafil in men with serotonergic antidepressant-associated erectile dysfunction: results from a randomized, double-blind, placebo-controlled trial. J Clin Psychiatry. 2006;67(2):240–6.

Fooladi E, Bell RJ, Jane F, Robinson PJ, Kulkarni J, Davis SR. Testosterone improves antidepressant-emergent loss of libido in women: findings from a randomized, double-blind, placebo-controlled trial. J Sex Med. 2014;11(3):831–9.

Hu XH, Bull SA, Hunkeler EM, Ming E, Lee JY, Fireman B, Markson LE. Incidence and duration of side effects and those rated as bothersome with selective serotonin reuptake inhibitor treatment for depression: patient report versus physician estimate. J Clin Psychiatry. 2004;65(7):959–65.

Iskandar JW, Wood B, Ali R, Wood R. Successful monitoring of fluoxetine-induced nocturnal bruxism. J Clin Psychiatry. 2012;73(3):366.

Jaffee MS, Bostwick JM. Buspirone as an antidote to venlafaxine-induced bruxism. Psychosomatics. 2000;41(6):535–6.

Kantor ED, Rehm CD, Haas JS, Chan AT, Giovannucci EL. Trends in prescription drug use among adults in the United States from 1999–2012. JAMA. 2015;314(17):1818–31.

Kessler RC, Berglund P, Demler O, Jin R, Koretz D, Merikangas KR, Rush AJ, Walters EE, Wang PS. The epidemiology of major depressive disorder: results from the National Comorbidity Survey Replication (NCS-R). JAMA. 2003;289(23):3095–105.

Kessler RC, Berglund P, Demler O, Jin R, Merikangas KR, Walters EE. Lifetime prevalence and age-of-onset distributions of DSM-IV disorders in the National Comorbidity Survey Replication. Arch Gen Psychiatry. 2005;62(6):593–602.

Kiev A, Masco HL, Wenger TL, Johnston JA, Batey SR, Holloman LC. The cardiovascular effects of bupropion and nortriptyline in depressed outpatients. Ann Clin Psychiatry. 1994;6(2):107–15.

Kuloglu M, Ekinci O, Caykoylu A. Venlafaxine-associated nocturnal bruxism in a depressive patient successfully treated with buspirone. J Psychopharmacol. 2010;24(4):627–8.

Labos C, Dasgupta K, Nedjar H, Turecki G, Rahme E. Risk of bleeding associated with combined use of selective serotonin reuptake inhibitors and antiplatelet therapy following acute myocardial infarction. CMAJ. 2011;183(16):1835–43.

Mago R. Glycopyrrolate for antidepressant-associated excessive sweating. J Clin Psychopharmacol. 2013;33(2):279–80.

Mago R. *Side Effects of Psychiatric Medications: Prevention, Assessment, and Management.* Seattle, WA: Amazon Digital Services, Inc; 2014.

Mago R. Adverse effects of psychotropic medications: a call to action. Psychiatr Clin North Am. 2016;39(3):361–73.

Mago R, Mahajan R, Borra D. Antidepressant-induced sexual dysfunction: an updated review. Curr Sex Health Rep. 2014;6(3):177–83.

Mago R, Mahajan R, Thase M. Medically serious adverse effects of newer antidepressants. Curr Psychiatry Rep. 2008;10(3):249–57.

Mago R, Thase ME, Rovner BW. Antidepressant-induced excessive sweating: clinical features and treatment with, 2013). Ann Clin Psychiatry. 2013;25(2):E1–E7.

Mago R, Tripathi N, Andrade C. Cardiovascular adverse effects of newer antidepressants. Expert Rev Neurother. 2014;14(5):539–51.

Martin KA, Krahn LE, Balan V, Rosati MJ. Selective serotonin reuptake inhibitors in the context of hepatitis C infection: reexamining the risks of bleeding. J Clin Psychiatry. 2007;68(7):1024–6.

Masand PS, Ashton AK, Gupta S, Frank B. Sustained-release bupropion for selective serotonin reuptake inhibitor-induced sexual dysfunction: a randomized, double-blind, placebo-controlled, parallel-group study. Am J Psychiatry. 2001;158(5):805–7.

Murray CJ, Vos T, Lozano R, Naghavi M, Flaxman AD, Michaud C, et al. Disability-adjusted life years (DALYs) for 291 diseases and injuries in 21 regions, 1990–2010: a systematic analysis for the Global Burden of Disease Study 2010. Lancet. 2012;380(9859):2197–223.

Nurnberg HG, Hensley PL, Gelenberg AJ, Fava M, Lauriello J, Paine S. Treatment of antidepressant-associated sexual dysfunction with sildenafil: a randomized controlled trial. JAMA. 2003;289(1):56–64.

Paulose-Ram R, Safran MA, Jonas BS, Gu Q, Orwig D. Trends in psychotropic medication use among U.S. adults. Pharmacoepidemiol Drug Saf. 2007;16(5):560–70.

Pavlovic ZM. Buspirone to improve compliance in venlafaxine-induced movement disorder. Int J Neuropsychopharmacol. 2004;7(4):523–4.

Ranjan S, S Chandra P, Prabhu S. Antidepressant-induced bruxism: need for buspirone? Int J Neuropsychopharmacol. 2006;9(4):485–7.

Romanelli F, Adler DA, Bungay KM. Possible paroxetine-induced bruxism. Ann Pharmacother. 1996;30(11):1246–8.

Rothschild AJ. Selective serotonin reuptake inhibitor-induced sexual dysfunction: efficacy of a drug holiday. Am J Psychiatry. 1995;152(10):1514–6.

Sabuncuoglu O, Ekinci O, Berkem M. Fluoxetine-induced sleep bruxism in an adolescent treated with buspirone: a case report. Spec Care Dentist. 2009;29(5):215–7.

Tanigawa T, Yamashita J, Sato T, Shinohara A, Shibata R, Ueda H, Sasaki H. Efficacy and safety of pilocarpine mouthwash in elderly patients with xerostomia. Spec Care Dentist. 2015;35(4):164–9.

Thase ME. Effects of venlafaxine on blood pressure: a meta-analysis of original data from 3744 depressed patients. J Clin Psychiatry. 1998;59(10):502–8.

Thase ME, Haight BR, Johnson MC, Hunt T, Krishen A, Fleck RJ, Modell JG. A randomized, double-blind, placebo-controlled study of the effect of sustained-release bupropion on blood pressure in individuals with mild untreated hypertension. J Clin Psychopharmacol. 2008;28(3):302–7.

Uca AU, Uğuz F, Kozak HH, Gümüş H, Aksoy F, Seyithanoğlu A, Kurt HG. Antidepressant-induced sleep bruxism: prevalence, incidence, and related factors. Clin Neuropharmacol. 2015;38(6):227–30.

Voican CS, Corruble E, Naveau S, Perlemuter G. Antidepressant-induced liver injury: a review for clinicians. Am J Psychiatry. 2014;171(4):404–15.

Weinrieb RM, Auriacombe M, Lynch KG, Chang KM, Lewis JD. A critical review of selective serotonin reuptake inhibitor-associated bleeding: balancing the risk of treating hepatitis C-infected patients. J Clin Psychiatry. 2003;64(12):1502–10.

Wise M. Citalopram-induced bruxism. Br J Psychiatry. 2001;178:182.

Wouters H, Van Dijk L, Van Geffen EC, Gardarsdottir H, Stiggelbout AM, Bouvy ML. Primary-care patients' trade-off preferences with regard to antidepressants. Psychol Med. 2014;44(11):2301–8.

Zhong Z, Wang L, Wen X, Liu Y, Fan Y, Liu Z. A meta-analysis of effects of selective serotonin reuptake inhibitors on blood pressure in depression treatment: outcomes from placebo and serotonin and noradrenaline reuptake inhibitor controlled trials. Neuropsychiatr Dis Treat. 2017;13:2781–96.

Zimmerman M, Posternak M, Friedman M, Attiullah N, Baymiller S, Boland R, Berlowitz S, Rahman S, Uy K, Singer S. Which factors influence psychiatrists' selection of antidepressants? Am J Psychiatry. 2004;161(7):1285–9.

/// 15 /// PHARMACOLOGICAL STRATEGIES FOR TARGETING RESIDUAL SYMPTOMS IN DEPRESSION

MAURIZIO FAVA

15.1. INTRODUCTION

Antidepressant monotherapies have shown to have limited efficacy in the treatment of major depressive disorder (MDD) (Rush et al., 2006), as evidenced by the relatively high rate of residual symptoms even among responders to antidepressant treatments (Fava and Davidson, 1996; Nierenberg et al., 2010). Effective treatment of residual symptoms is essential, since their persistence correlates with a greater risk of MDD recurrence (Paykel et al., 1995; Flint and Rifat, 1997; Judd et al., 1997) and relapse (Thase et al., 1992; Paykel et al., 1995). A study of a predominantly inpatient population with MDD ($n = 70$) found that subjects with residual symptoms at the time of remission had a relapse rate of 76%, compared with 25% among subjects without such symptoms (Paykel et al., 1995).

In some cases, it may be unclear whether the symptoms reported are truly residual or instead are side effects of the antidepressant therapy (Freeman et al., 2017). A systematic assessment of symptoms prior to beginning pharmacological treatment can help distinguish between residual symptoms and treatment side effects. Either way, there is a clear need to completely treat the acute symptoms of MDD and to sustain those benefits over time in order to prevent relapse (Nierenberg et al., 2010). In addition, many patients with MDD who are treated with antidepressants achieve only partial treatment responses and may suffer from residual symptoms, contributing to a poorer outcome (Nierenberg et al., 2010). A longitudinal study of patients with MDD found that residual symptoms were generally mild manifestations of typical depressive symptoms and included anxiety, insomnia, depressed mood, and work impairment, among other symptoms (Paykel et al., 1995). In an open study of 215 outpatients treated with fluoxetine, we found that the most common residual symptoms were sleep disturbances (44% of nonresponders and partial responders), fatigue (38%), and lack of interest (27%) (Nierenberg et al., 1999). Partial treatment responders may suffer from persistent psychological, behavioral, and somatic symptoms, including sadness, anhedonia, guilt, fatigue, insomnia, decreased appetite, decreased motivation, cognitive deficits, and even pain (Fava and Rush, 2006; Freeman et al., 2017). Therefore, achieving full symptom remission should be the ultimate objective in the treatment of depressed patients. In order to obtain this, it is common practice to use augmentation or combination strategies. In this chapter, we will review how to best assess residual symptoms and some of the preferred pharmacological strategies to address them.

15.2. ASSESSMENT OF RESIDUAL SYMPTOMS IN MDD

Clinicians and clinical researchers typically define treatment response in depression as a 50% or greater reduction in depressive symptoms from baseline, regardless of whatever instrument they use to measure outcome. However, there is great variability in both number and nature of symptoms tracked across rating scales. The standard scales used to assess depressive symptoms, such as the 17-item Hamilton Rating Scale for Depression (HAM-D; Hamilton, 1960) and the 10-item Montgomery–Asberg Depression Rating Scale (MADRS; Montgomery and Asberg, 1979) focus on symptoms that are characteristic of severe and/or melancholic depression and fail to measure a large number of symptoms that are characteristic of the various subtypes of depression. The 44-item Symptoms of Depression Questionnaire (SDQ) is a validated self-rating instrument that assesses an extremely broad range of symptoms, including cognitive impairment, irritability, anger attacks, and anxiety symptoms, together with the more commonly considered symptoms of depression (Pedrelli et al., 2014). Analysis of the factor structure of the SDQ identified five subscales with adequate internal consistency and concurrent validity. We have found the SDQ to be a valuable new tool to better characterize residual symptoms of depression (Pedrelli et al., 2014).

15.3. PHARMACOLOGICAL STRATEGIES TO TREAT RESIDUAL SYMPTOMS

The first step in dealing with the presence of residual symptoms is to optimize the antidepressant therapy. It is critical to encourage treatment adherence at adequate doses for an adequate duration (at least 8–12 weeks) and, in some cases where the treatment is tolerated, to increase the dose significantly to maximize its benefits. The usefulness of dose increases to increase the odds of full remission has been well demonstrated (Fava et al., 1994, 2002). It is also important to diagnose and treat any comorbid psychiatric or medical disorders, such as substance abuse, since these conditions may contribute to the presence of residual symptoms. When optimization of antidepressant therapy is unsuccessful, many clinicians are using augmentation or combination pharmacotherapy to address residual symptoms. Augmentation treatment involves adding a medication that is not considered a standard antidepressant drug, like thyroid supplementation, to a typically used antidepressant. Alternatively, combination treatments involve the use of two known antidepressants simultaneously. It is important to emphasize that all of these approaches, with few exceptions, are off-label strategies because they have not been approved by the US Food and Drug Administration (FDA).

15.3.1. Residual Anxiety

Both somatic and psychological anxiety are common residual symptoms in MDD (Opdyke et al., 1996) and predict a shorter time to relapse or recurrence (Flint and Rifat, 1997). In a two-year study of patients with unipolar depression who had responded to treatment of the index episode, the probability of remaining well without relapse or recurrence was much greater for the patients without anxiety at the time of remission (0.768 vs. 0.375) (Flint and Rifat, 1997). Anxiety and nervousness are also common side effects of antidepressant treatment (Fava et al., 2002). Augmentation with benzodiazepines can substantially improve residual anxiety (Fava, 2006). We have also reported the benefit of adding pregabalin to ongoing antidepressant therapy in MDD patients with residual anxiety (Vitali et al., 2013). Similarly, atypical antipsychotic drugs such as brexpiprazole (Davis et al., 2016; Thase et al., 2018), quetiapine (McIntyre et al., 2007), and aripiprazole (Trivedi et al., 2008) have been found to be helpful adjuncts in the treatment of MDD with anxiety. Other drugs that can be used as adjunctive treatment for anxiety include anticonvulsants and buspirone (Table 15.1).

15.3.2. Residual Irritability

In a large epidemiological study excluding bipolar spectrum disorders, irritability during depressive episodes was reported by roughly half of respondents with lifetime MDD based on criteria in the fourth edition of the American Psychiatric Association's *Diagnostic and Statistical Manual of Mental Disorders* (DSM-IV; Fava et al., 2010). Irritability in MDD was associated with early age of onset, lifetime persistence, comorbidity with anxiety and impulse-control disorders, fatigue and self-reproach during episodes, and disability (Fava et al., 2010). Irritability is also a common residual symptom in MDD in both pediatric and adult populations (Tao et al., 2010; Nierenberg et al., 2015). Atypical antipsychotic drugs such as brexpiprazole (Fava et al., 2016, 2017) have been found to be helpful adjuncts in the treatment of MDD with irritability. Anticonvulsants have also been shown to be

TABLE 15.1. Commonly Used Pharmacological Treatments
for Anxiety as Residual Symptom in MDD

Generic Name	Suggested Dosage
Lorazepam	0.5–2.0 mg BID or TID
Alprazolam	0.25–1.0 mg BID or TID
Clonazepam	0.25–1.0 mg BID
Gabapentin	300–1,200 mg BID or TID
Pregabalin	25–100 mg BID or TID
Buspirone	10–30 mg BID or TID
Quetiapine	25–200 mg QD or BID
Aripiprazole	2–15 mg QD
Brexpiprazole	1–3 mg QD
Quetiapine	50–200 mg QD or BID
Cariprazine	1.5–6 mg QD
Lurasidone	20–120 mg QD

effective in the treatment of MDD with irritability (Vigo and Baldessarini, 2009). Other drugs that can be used as adjunctive treatment for irritability include lithium and buspirone (Table 15.2).

15.3.3. Residual Insomnia

Sleep disturbance is common in MDD patients and can cause significant impairment (Mendlewicz, 2009). Insomnia may persist after remission in MDD and is a common residual symptom (Nierenberg et al., 1999) that has been found be associated with an increased risk for relapse (Mendlewicz et al., 2009). In a group of subjects with persistent insomnia, despite effective treatment with a selective serotonin reuptake inhibitor (SSRI), sleep symptoms included prolonged sleep latency (1 hour), total sleep time of less than 6.5 hours, multiple awakenings during the night, and clinically significant daytime impairment (Asnis et al., 1999). Among patients with residual symptoms in a naturalistic study, a significant proportion had early insomnia of moderate or greater severity (Paykel et al., 1995). Insomnia can also be a side effect of antidepressant treatment and is thought to reflect the activating effects of numerous antidepressant agents (Winokur and Reynolds, 1994). In an open study of 215 MDD patients treated with fluoxetine, insomnia was an important residual symptom (Nierenberg et al., 1999). A number of different agents can be used as augmentation therapy to reduce residual insomnia (Table 15.3). A double-blind, placebo-controlled trial of MDD patients treated with a tricyclic antidepressant and either a benzodiazepine hypnotic or placebo demonstrated significant improvement in sleep disturbance with the addition of the hypnotic (Nolen et al., 1993). After four weeks of co-therapy, the

TABLE 15.2. Commonly Used Pharmacological Treatments
for Irritability as Residual Symptom in MDD

Generic Name	Suggested Dosage
Lithium	600–1,200 mg/day
Carbamazepine	200–1,200 mg/day
Oxcarbazepine	300–900 mg QD
Valproic acid	500–1,500 mg/day
Gabapentin	300–1200 mg BID or TID
Pregabalin	25–100 mg BID or TID
Buspirone	10–30 mg BID or TID
Quetiapine	25–200 mg QD or BID
Aripiprazole	2–15 mg QD
Brexpiprazole	1–3 mg QD
Quetiapine	50–200 mg BID
Cariprazine	1.5–6 mg QD
Lurasidone	20 to 120 mg QD

HAM-D insomnia subscore decreased significantly more in patients treated with the benzodiazepine hypnotic than in those who received placebo (Nolen et al., 1993). In a randomized, placebo-controlled study of 190 patients with persistent insomnia after treatment with an SSRI, zolpidem augmentation was associated

TABLE 15.3. Commonly Used Pharmacological Treatments
for Insomnia as Residual Symptom in MDD

Generic Name	Suggested Dosage
Lorazepam	0.5–3.0 mg QHS
Alprazolam	0.5–2.0 mg QHS
Clonazepam	0.25–1.0 mg QHS
Zolpidem	10–20 mg QHS
Eszopiclone	1–3 mg QHS
Melatonin	3–10 mg QHS
Trazodone	50–200 mg QHS
Mirtazapine	15–30 mg QHS
Doxepin	10–25 mg QHS
Amitriptyline	10–25 mg QHS
Trimipramine	10–30 mg QHS
Gabapentin	300–1,200 mg QHS
Pregabalin	50–200 mg QHS
Suvorexant	10–20 mg QHS

with significant improvement compared with placebo in a number of sleep parameters, including sleep quality and duration (Asnis et al., 1999). In a study of patients with DSM-IV criteria for both MDD and insomnia ($n = 545$) receiving morning fluoxetine and randomized to nightly eszopiclone 3 mg or placebo for eight weeks, patients in the eszopiclone-plus-fluoxetine group had significantly decreased sleep latency, wake time after sleep onset, increased total sleep time, sleep quality, and depth of sleep at all double-blind time points (all $p < .05$) compared to the placebo-plus-fluoxetine group (Fava et al., 2006). Given the fact that the hypnotic orexin antagonists have been shown to possess antidepressant-like properties in some animal models of MDD (Shariq et al., 2018), there has been in interest among clinicians in the use of these compounds for the treatment of residual insomnia in MDD, although there are no published placebo-controlled studies yet.

15.3.4. Residual Somnolence/Fatigue

Fatigue is a frequently reported symptom in MDD, occurring in over 90% of patients, and presents with physical, cognitive, and emotional aspects (Ghanean et al., 2018). Somnolence or excessive daytime sleepiness is also relatively common in MDD and is associated with higher body mass index (Hein et al., 2019). Both somnolence and fatigue are important residual symptoms among MDD patients treated with antidepressants, with fatigue occurring in almost 40% of responders in one study (Nierenberg et al., 1999). These symptoms can also be side effects of antidepressant treatment, with SSRIs having been associated with fatigue and excessive daytime sleepiness as well (Fava et al., 2002a). Somnolence was reported in 14.7% of patients at week 4 in an open-label fluoxetine study (Zajecka et al., 1999). In MDD patients suffering from residual somnolence or fatigue in MDD, it is critical to consider whether the symptoms reflect an underlying sleep disturbance that requires further evaluation and treatment, such as obstructive sleep apnea or restless leg syndrome. If poor sleep quality exists in the absence of a primary sleep disorder, an agent with hypnotic effects can be added. If a sleep disturbance is not present, a number of agents can be used as augmentation therapy for patients with somnolence or fatigue (Table 15.4). For example, a retrospective analysis pooling the data of 348 patients (aged 18–65 years) participating in two randomized, double-blind, placebo-controlled studies of modafinil (six-week, flexible-dose study of 100–400 mg/day or eight-week, fixed-dose study of 200 mg/day) plus SSRI therapy and meeting criteria for several residual symptoms (Epworth Sleepiness Scale [ESS] score of at least 10; 17-item HAM-D score between 4 and 25; and Fatigue Severity Scale [FSS] score of at least 4) showed that, compared to placebo, modafinil augmentation rapidly (within one week) and significantly improved overall clinical condition (Clinical Global Impression–Improvement), wakefulness (ESS), depressive symptoms (17-item HAM-D), and fatigue (FSS) ($p < .01$ for all) (Fava et al., 2007).

TABLE 15.4. Commonly Used Pharmacological Treatments
for Fatigue/Somnolence as Residual Symptom in MDD

Generic Name	Suggested Dosage
Methylphenidate	20–80 mg QD
Dextroamphetamine	10–40 mg QD
Modafinil	100–400 mg QD
Armodafinil	150–300 mg QD
Bupropion	100–300 mg QD
Reboxetine	2–4 mg QD
Atomoxetine	40–80 mg QD
Protriptyline	10–20 mg QD
SAMe	400–800 mg BID
Solriamfetol	75–150 mg QD
Pitolisant	17.8–35.6 mg QD

15.3.5. Residual Apathy

Apathy is a relatively common symptom of depression, particularly in geriatric populations (Marin et al., 2003). Apathy has also been reported both as a residual symptom of MDD and as a side effect of antidepressant treatment (Paykel et al., 1995; Bolling and Kohlenberg, 2004; Fava et al., 2006a). Among a convenience sample of 161 adults who had completed a course of MDD treatment with an SSRI, 18.6% of respondents experienced apathy as a side effect of treatment (Bolling and Kohlenberg, 2004). A number of agents can be used to combat apathy, whether it is a residual symptom of MDD or a side effect of treatment, including psychostimulants, modafinil, bupropion, norepinephrine reuptake inhibitors (NRIs), and dopamine agonists (Table 15.5).

TABLE 15.5. Commonly Used Pharmacological Treatments
for Apathy as Residual Symptom in MDD

Generic Name	Suggested Dosage
Methylphenidate	20–80 mg QD
Dextroamphetamine	10–40 mg QD
Modafinil	100–400 mg QD
Armodafinil	150–300 mg QD
Bupropion	100–300 mg QD
Reboxetine	2–4 mg QD
Atomoxetine	40–80 mg QD
Pramipexole	0.125–1.0 mg BID or TID
Ropinirole	0.125–1.0 mg BID or TID
SAMe	400–800 BID

TABLE 15.6. Commonly used Pharmacological Treatments for Cognitive Impairment and Executive Dysfunction as Residual Symptoms in MDD

Generic Name	Suggested Dosage
Donepezil	5–10 mg QD
Memantine	10–20 mg QD
Galantamine	8–24 mg QD
Methylphenidate	20–80 mg QD
Dextroamphetamine	10–40 mg QD
Modafinil	100–400 mg QD
Armodafinil	150–300 mg QD
Bupropion	100–300 mg QD
Vortioxetine	5–20 mg QD
Reboxetine	2–4 mg QD
Atomoxetine	40–80 mg QD
Pramipexole	0.125–1.0 mg BID or TID
Ropinirole	0.125–1.0 mg BID or TID
SAMe	400–800 mg BID

15.3.6. Residual Cognitive Impairment and Executive Dysfunction

Cognitive impairments, such as memory deficits and executive impairment, are common among patients with MDD and can be captured with objective or subjective assessments (Fava et al., 2018). Investigators have found that depressed patients perform worse on a neuropsychological test battery than nondepressed subjects (Rush and Weissenburger, 1983). Cognitive symptoms generally improve with antidepressant treatment but may persist despite response (Fava et al., 2006a; Freeman et al., 2017). Cognitive dysfunction, such as reduced performance on immediate recall testing, can also present as a side effect of antidepressant treatment, especially with highly anticholinergic antidepressants (Meyers et al., 1991; Freeman et al., 2017). A number of agents can be used to combat cognitive impairment and executive dysfunction, whether a residual symptom of MDD or a side effect of treatment, including psychostimulants, modafinil, bupropion, vortioxetine, NRIs, and dopamine agonists (Table 15.6).

15.4. CONCLUSION

Residual symptoms are common among individuals treated for MDD. These symptoms, which include anxiety, irritability, insomnia, somnolence/fatigue, apathy, and cognitive and executive dysfunction, are associated with an increased risk of relapse and poor psychosocial functioning. Comprehensive clinical data are not yet available to guide management of symptoms—whether residual or drug-related—in patients treated pharmacologically for depressive disorders. Suggested approaches to the management of residual symptoms include addressing treatment-emergent side effects and comorbid conditions, optimizing antidepressant dosing, and using augmentation therapies.

REFERENCES

Asnis GM, Chakraburtty A, DuBoff EA, Krystal A, Londborg PD, Rosenberg R, Roth-Schechter B, Scharf MB, Walsh JK. Zolpidem for persistent insomnia in SSRI-treated depressed patients. J Clin Psychiatry. 1999;60:668–676.

Bolling MY, Kohlenberg RJ. Reasons for quitting serotonin reuptake inhibitor therapy: paradoxical psychological side effects and patient satisfaction. Psychother Psychosom. 2004;73: 380–385.

Davis LL, Ota A, Perry P, Tsuneyoshi K, Weiller E, Baker RA. Adjunctive brexpiprazole in patients with major depressive disorder and anxiety symptoms: an exploratory study. Brain Behav. 2016;6(10):e00520.

Fava M. Pharmacological approaches to the treatment of residual symptoms. J Psychopharmacol. 2006;20(3 Suppl):29–34.

Fava M, Alpert J, Nierenberg A, Lagomasino I, Sonawalla S, Tedlow J, Worthington J, Baer L, Rosenbaum JF. Double-blind study of high-dose fluoxetine versus lithium or desipramine augmentation of fluoxetine in partial responders and nonresponders to fluoxetine. J Clin Psychopharmacol. 2002;22(4):379–387.

Fava M, Davidson KG. Definition and epidemiology of treatment resistant depression. Psychiatr Clin North Am. 1996;19:179–200.

Fava M, Graves LM, Benazzi F, Scalia MJ, Iosifescu DV, Alpert JE, Papakostas GI. A cross-sectional study of the prevalence of cognitive and physical symptoms during long-term antidepressant treatment. J Clin Psychiatry. 2006a;67(11):1754–1759.

Fava M, Hoog SL, Judge RA, Kopp JB, Nilsson ME, Gonzales JS. Acute efficacy of fluoxetine versus sertraline and paroxetine in major depressive disorder including effects of baseline insomnia. J Clin Psychopharmacol. 2002a;22:137–147.

Fava M, Hwang I, Rush AJ, Sampson N, Walters EE, Kessler RC. The importance of irritability as a symptom of major depressive disorder: results from the National Comorbidity Survey Replication. Mol Psychiatry. 2010;15(8):856–867.

Fava M, Mahableshwarkar AR, Jacobson W, Zhong W, Keefe RS, Olsen CK, Jaeger J. What is the overlap between subjective and objective cognitive impairments in MDD? Ann Clin Psychiatry. 2018;30(3):176–184.

Fava M, McCall WV, Krystal A, Wessel T, Rubens R, Caron J, Amato D, Roth T. Eszopiclone co-administered with fluoxetine in patients with insomnia coexisting with major depressive disorder. Biol Psychiatry. 2006;59(11):1052–1060.

Fava M, Ménard F, Davidsen CK, Baker RA. Adjunctive brexpiprazole in patients with major depressive disorder and irritability: an exploratory study. J Clin Psychiatry. 2016;77(12): 1695–1701.

Fava M, Rosenbaum JF, McGrath PJ, Stewart JW, Amsterdam JD, Quitkin FM. Lithium and tricyclic augmentation of fluoxetine treatment for resistant major depression: a double-blind, controlled study. Am J Psychiatry. 1994;151(9):1372–1374.

Fava M, Rush AJ. Current status of augmentation and combination treatments for major depressive disorder: a literature review and a proposal for a novel approach to improve practice. Psychother Psychosom. 2006;75:139–153.

Fava M, Thase ME, DeBattista C, Doghramji K, Arora S, Hughes RJ. Modafinil augmentation of selective serotonin reuptake inhibitor therapy in MDD partial responders with persistent fatigue and sleepiness. Ann Clin Psychiatry. 2007;19(3):153–159.

Fava M, Weiller E, Zhang P, Weiss C. Efficacy of brexpiprazole as adjunctive treatment in major depressive disorder with irritability: post hoc analysis of 2 pivotal clinical studies. J Clin Psychopharmacol. 2017;37(2):276–278.

Flint AJ, Rifat SL. Two-year outcome of elderly patients with anxious depression. Psychiatry Res. 1997;66:23–31.

Freeman MP, Fisher L, Clain A, Rabbitt R, Pooley J, Baer L, Fava M. Differentiating residual symptoms of depression from adverse events among patients initiating treatment with an antidepressant. Ann Clin Psychiatry. 2017;29(1):28–34.

Ghanean H, Ceniti AK, Kennedy SH. Fatigue in patients with major depressive disorder: prevalence, burden and pharmacological approaches to management. CNS Drugs. 2018;32(1):65–74.

Hamilton M: A rating scale for depression. J Neurol Neurosurg Psychiatry. 1960;23:56–62.

Hein M, Lanquart JP, Loas G, Hubain P, Linkowski P. Prevalence and risk factors of excessive daytime sleepiness in major depression: a study with 703 individuals referred for polysomnography. J Affect Disord. 2019;243:23–32.

Judd LL, Akiskal HS, Paulus MP. The role and clinical significance of subsyndromal depressive symptoms (SSD) in unipolar major depressive disorder. J Affect Disord. 1997;45:5–17.

Marin RS, Butters MA, Mulsant BH, Pollock BG, Reynolds CF 3rd. Apathy and executive function in depressed elderly. J Geriatr Psychiatry Neurol. 2003;16(2):112–116.

McIntyre A, Gendron A, McIntyre A. Quetiapine adjunct to selective serotonin reuptake inhibitors or venlafaxine in patients with major depression, comorbid anxiety, and residual depressive symptoms: a randomized, placebo-controlled pilot study. Depress Anxiety. 2007;24(7):487–494.

Mendlewicz J. Sleep disturbances: core symptoms of major depressive disorder rather than associated or comorbid disorders. World J Biol Psychiatry. 2009;10(4):269–275.

Meyers BS, Mattis S, Gabriele M, Kakuma T. Effects of nortriptyline on memory self-assessment and performance in recovered elderly depressives. Psychopharmacol Bull. 1991;27:295–299.

Montgomery SA, Asberg M. A new depression scale designed to be sensitive to change. Br J Psychiatry. 1979;134:382–389.

Nierenberg AA. Residual symptoms in depression: prevalence and impact. J Clin Psychiatry. 2015;76(11):e1480.

Nierenberg AA, Husain MM, Trivedi MH, Fava M, Warden D, Wisniewski SR, Miyahara S, Rush AJ. Residual symptoms after remission of major depressive disorder with citalopram and risk of relapse: a STAR*D report. Psychol Med. 2010;40(1):41–50.

Nierenberg AA, Keefe BR, Leslie VC, Alpert JE, Pava JA, Worthington JJIII, Rosenbaum JF, Fava M. Residual symptoms in depressed patients who respond acutely to fluoxetine. J Clin Psychiatry. 1999;60:221–225.

Nolen WA, Haffmans PM, Bouvy PF, Duivenvoorden HJ. Hypnotics as concurrent medication in depression. A placebo-controlled, double-blind comparison of flunitrazepam and lormetazepam in patients with major depression, treated with a (tri)cyclic antidepressant. J Affect Disord. 1993;28:179–188.

Opdyke KS, Reynolds CFIII, Frank E, Begley AE, Buysse DJ, Dew MA, Mulsant BH, Shear MK, Mazumdar S, Kupfer DJ. Effect of continuation treatment on residual symptoms in late-life depression: how well is 'well'? Depress Anxiety. 1996;4:312–319.

Paykel ES, Ramana R, Cooper Z, Hayhurst H, Kerr J, Barocka A. Residual symptoms after partial remission: an important outcome in depression. Psychol Med. 1995;25:1171–1180.

Pedrelli P, Blais MA, Alpert JE, Shelton RC, Walker RS, Fava M. Reliability and validity of the Symptoms of Depression Questionnaire (SDQ). CNS Spectr. 2014;19(6):535–546.

Rush AJ, Trivedi MH, Wisniewski SR, Nierenberg AA, Stewart JW, Warden D, Niederehe G, Thase ME, Lavori PW, Lebowitz BD, McGrath PJ, Rosenbaum JF, Sackeim HA, Kupfer DJ, Luther J, Fava M. Acute and longer-term outcomes in depressed outpatients requiring one or several treatment steps: a STAR*D report. Am J Psychiatry. 2006;163(11):1905–1917.

Rush AJ, Weissenburger J, Vinson DB, Giles DE. Neuropsychological dysfunctions in unipolar nonpsychotic major depressions. J Affect Disord. 1983;5:281–287.

Shariq AS, Rosenblat JD, Alageel A, Mansur RB, Rong C, Ho RC, Ragguett RM, Pan Z, Brietzke E, McIntyre RS. Evaluating the role of orexins in the pathophysiology and treatment of depression: a comprehensive review. Prog Neuropsychopharmacol Biol Psychiatry. 2018;92:1–7.

Tao R, Emslie GJ, Mayes TL, Nakonezny PA, Kennard BD. Symptom improvement and residual symptoms during acute antidepressant treatment in pediatric major depressive disorder. J Child Adolesc Psychopharmacol. 2010;20(5):423–430.

Thase ME, Simons AD, McGeary J, Cahalane JF, Hughes C, Harden T, Friedman E. Relapse after cognitive behavior therapy of depression: potential implications for longer courses of treatment. Am J Psychiatry. 1992;149:1046–1052.

Thase ME, Weiller E, Zhang P, Weiss C, McIntyre RS. Adjunctive brexpiprazole in patients with major depressive disorder and anxiety symptoms: post hoc analyses of three placebo-controlled studies. Neuropsychiatr Dis Treat. 2018;15:37–45.

Trivedi MH, Thase ME, Fava M, Nelson CJ, Yang H, Qi Y, Tran QV, Pikalov A, Carlson BX, Marcus RN, Berman RM. Adjunctive aripiprazole in major depressive disorder: analysis of efficacy and safety in patients with anxious and atypical features. J Clin Psychiatry. 2008;69(12):1928–1936.

Vigo DV, Baldessarini RJ. Anticonvulsants in the treatment of major depressive disorder: an overview. Harv Rev Psychiatry. 2009;17(4):231–241.

Vitali M, Tedeschini E, Mistretta M, Fehling K, Aceti F, Ceccanti M, Fava M. Adjunctive pregabalin in partial responders with major depressive disorder and residual anxiety. J Clin Psychopharmacol. 2013;33(1):95–98.

Winokur A, Reynolds CF. The effects of antidepressants and sleep physiology. Prim Psychiatry. 1994;1:22–27.

Zajecka J, Amsterdam JD, Quitkin FM, Reimherr FW, Rosenbaum JF, Tamura RN, Sundell KL, Michelson D, Beasley CMJr. Changes in adverse events reported by patients during 6 months of fluoxetine therapy. J Clin Psychiatry. 1999;60:389–394.

Psychotherapy and Modalities of Delivery for Depression

/// 16 /// COGNITIVE BEHAVIOR THERAPY

STEVEN D. HOLLON

16.1. INTRODUCTION

Cognitive behavior therapy (CBT) was the first of the psychosocial interventions to hold its own with antidepressant medications (ADM) and has an enduring effect that lasts beyond the end of treatment. There are several different variants of CBT, but cognitive therapy, the version developed by Aaron Beck at the University of Pennsylvania, was the first and most widely practiced.[1] Throughout the chapter I will use the more generic term CBT to refer to that approach and will indicate when I am referring to another variant.

16.2. EMPIRICAL STATUS

16.2.1. Acute Treatment

In 1977, when Rush and colleagues reported that CBT was superior to ADM, it created quite a stir because up until that time, no psychosocial intervention had even held its own with medications.[2] When Blackburn and colleagues followed in 1981 with a similar finding out of Edinburgh, the empirical status of CBT seemed secure.[3] As it turned out, both studies did a less-than-adequate job of implementing ADM and subsequent trials typically found the two to be of comparable efficacy.[4,5] That verdict held until the publication of the NIMH Treatment of Depression Collaborative Research Program (TDCRP) in 1989, in which CBT was found to be less efficacious than ADM and no better than pill-placebo (PLA) among patients with more severe depressions.[6] However, there were problems with the implementation of CBT in that trial (the reverse of what happened in Rush and Blackburn),[7] and DeRubeis and colleagues were able to pool the data from the five trials just cited to conduct an individual patient data meta-analysis (IPDMA) that showed that across all the studies CBT was comparable to ADM even in the treatment of patients with more severe depressions.[8]

Nonetheless, the perception held that CBT (as well as other psychosocial interventions) was not as efficacious as ADM in the treatment of more severe depressions, so my colleague Robert DeRubeis and I initiated a two-site trial at the University of Pennsylvania and Vanderbilt University that focused solely on such patients. In that trial, CBT was as efficacious as ADM, and both beat PLA.[9] Jarrett and colleagues also found that CBT was comparable to ADM with monoamine oxidase inhibitors and each was better than placebo in a trial with patients who met criteria for atypical depression.[10] Although an occasional trial finds CBT less efficacious than ADM (or the converse), that typically is because one or the other was implemented less than adequately.[11] A recent IPDMA pooling data from 1,700 patients over 16 trials (the other 8 relevant trials were mostly older and had not retained their data) found a very modest advantage for ADM overall, but no evidence of any severity-by-treatment interaction.[12] In essence, CBT and ADM are about comparably efficacious when each is adequately implemented.

16.2.2. Enduring Effects

As efficacious as ADMs can be, they stop working when you stop taking them. CBT, however, appears to have an enduring effect that protects against subsequent relapse or recurrence even after treatment is over. This enduring effect was first detected in the aftermath of the original trial by Rush and colleagues and has been evident in almost every subsequent CBT-versus-ADM comparison.[13–19] The sole exception was the small pilot study published by Jarrett and colleagues in the follow-up to her atypical depression trial.[20] Two of those trials randomized patients who remitted on ADM to either stay on study medications for a year or be withdrawn onto PLA.[18,19] In both studies, patients who had been treated with CBT did just as well as patients who continued on ADM and were less likely to experience recurrence during the second year of follow-up when ADM patients were withdrawn from medications. Cuijpers and colleagues conducted a meta-analyses of the follow-up data from those eight studies and found that prior CBT cut risk for relapse by more than half relative to ADM withdrawal and by a quarter relative to ADM continuation.[21]

16.2.3. Combined Treatment

Combined treatment with CBT plus ADM typically outperforms either monotherapy alone with respect to acute response, but with a couple of caveats.[22] First, this advantage is heavily moderated. In a recent three-site trial (adding Rush Medical Center in Chicago to Penn and Vanderbilt), we found that virtually all of the 10% increment from adding CBT to ADM was clustered in the third of the sample that was more severely depressed but not chronic, for whom the increment was 30%.[23] If you were less severely depressed but not chronic, you did not need to add CBT; alternatively, if you were chronic (regardless of severity), you did not benefit from adding CBT.

The second caveat is that adding ADM appeared to wipe out CBT's enduring effect. We did not expect this to happen and were somewhat puzzled by it, since two of the three sites (and many of the therapists) were the same as those we used in the earlier Penn/Vanderbilt project. Three of the earlier trials also included a combined treatment condition; one found no enduring effect for CBT plus ADM,[15] whereas another did,[16] and a third pooled the conditions, so it was largely uninterpretable.[14] It would be premature to conclude that ADM interferes with CBT's enduring effect, but the field needs to be alert to the possibility.

16.2.4. Moderation

Prognostic information tells you which patients are likely to do better than others in a given treatment (you hold treatment constant and let patients vary), whereas prescriptive information tells you which treatment is likely to work better for a given patient (you hold patient characteristics constant and let treatments vary). Prognostic information can help you anticipate how well someone is likely to do in treatment and how much of it he or she is likely to need, whereas prescriptive information helps you select the best treatment for that patient. In the Penn/Vanderbilt project we found that patients with chronic depression did more poorly than nonchronic patients regardless of modality (prognostic), whereas patients who were married or unemployed or who had more prior precipitants did better in CBT than in ADM (prescriptive).[24] We also found that number of prior exposures to medication predicted poorer response to ADM but not to CBT (prescriptive).[25] All these latter indices were ordinal; patients with that characteristic did better in one modality or the other, whereas those without that characteristic did not show a differential response. We did find one that was disordinal: Patients with personality disorders did better in ADM (although they were particularly likely to relapse when discontinued), whereas those without personality disorders did better in CBT.[26]

My colleague Robert DeRubeis and his students combined these indices to form what he calls a personalized advantage index (PAI).[27] In his original approach he used multiple regressions to generate two prediction equations for each patient, one estimating how that patient would have done in CBT and the other in ADM, with any differential indicating the patient's optimal assignment. Critically, each equation was generated using only the data from the other patients so as to reduce the risk of capitalizing on chance. They then compared patients who were randomized to their optimal treatment to those who were not and found a difference between the two sets of patients that was as large as the drug–placebo difference. This means we could improve the efficiency of the mental health system by getting the optimal treatment to each patient even without improving either treatment. DeRubeis and his students are now using machine learning to generate their selection algorithms. This promises to revolutionize mental health service delivery.[28]

16.2.5. Mediation

It is easier to detect an effect than it is to explain it, but to the extent we can identify the active ingredients that make treatments work (processes) and the causal mechanisms they mobilize in the patient, the more we can hone our treatments to maximize their impact.[29] Cognitive theory holds that it is not just what happens to you that determines how you feel and what you do, but rather how you interpret those events. With respect to treatment process, DeRubeis and students have shown that adherence to specific cognitive and behavioral strategies leads to early symptom change in CBT that in turns drives the rated quality of the therapeutic alliance.[30] This is the converse of the conventional wisdom regarding the role of nonspecific factors.

Early tests of mechanism often failed because ADM produced as much change in cognition as CBT, and investigators misinterpreted nonspecificity for noncausality.[31] DeRubeis and colleagues found that in CBT, cognitive change predicted subsequent change in depression, whereas in ADM, change in depression predicted subsequent change in cognition, an early instance of moderated mediation.[32] Strunk and colleagues found that patients who could best perform the skills taught in CBT in later therapy sessions or who best enacted those skills when asked to respond to hypothetical stressors were the ones least likely to relapse following the end of treatment.[33] Tang and colleagues found that patients who showed "sudden gains" in treatment, sharp drops in symptom scores preceded by insight into the cognitive model, also were less likely to relapse than patients who showed a comparable amount of change in a more gradual fashion.[34] These findings suggest that CBT works through cognitive mechanisms to produce its enduring effect.[35]

16.3. CLINICAL IMPLEMENTATION

16.3.1. Basics of CBT

CBT is based on a cognitive model that posits that it is not just what happens to you that determines how you feel and respond, but the way that you interpret the event. It was developed as a brief, structured intervention that teaches the patient to examine the accuracy of beliefs (often with behavioral experiments) to reduce emotional distress and increase coping. In its original 1970s version, it was intended to be an intensive short-term (for those days) intervention but was subsequently extended to deal with chronic depressions and those superimposed on underlying personality disorders.[36]

The essence of that modification was the introduction of something called the "three-legged stool," as described in the rest of this paragraph. The original 1970s version of CBT focused almost exclusively on current life problems; exploration of childhood antecedents was rare and largely confined to later sessions, and the therapeutic relationship was discussed only if problems arose. In its modified 1990s version, sometimes referred to as "schema therapy," the therapist interweaves a focus on current life issues with consideration of childhood antecedents and attention to the therapeutic relationship. Patients with chronic depression or depressions superimposed on personality disorders have no other way to think about themselves and can process their interactions only through that problematic schema.

Two patients will be used to highlight this distinction. The first was a forty-something college art professor (a sculptor) who had lost his teaching job when his small liberal arts university got into financial trouble and had to jettison his small department. He had spent the last three years working as a handyman in a condominium complex and hated every minute of it because he thought it far beneath his talent and skills. He saw his depression as "reality based" and could not imagine how he could get over it until he got a teaching job again. Although his depression was severe, it was not complicated.

The second patient was a woman in her late twenties who maneuvered her way into the Penn/Vanderbilt study with a touch of deceit. She had just returned to Nashville from New York where she had run off to meet a man she had met only through the internet, leaving her husband in another city to do so. The new relationship lasted less than a week, and she returned to Nashville to take a job as a kindergarten teacher where she had done her student teaching.

She heard about the study from a friend and went to ClinicalTrials.gov to look up its inclusion criteria. On learning that patients with borderline personality were screened out, she borrowed a copy of the American Psychiatric Association's *Diagnostic and Statistical Manual of Mental Disorders* (DSM) to see what she had to deny to get into the trial. At the first session she informed the therapist (me) that protocol treatment (24 sessions over 16 weeks) was simply not enough and she wanted what Woody Allen got, up to five sessions a week for the rest of her life. She further informed me that she would not be that much of a burden because she did not intend to turn 30 (six months off). Finally, she noted she was a compulsive liar and that I could not believe a word she said. Like the sculptor, her depression was severe but she was considerably more complex.

16.3.2. Setting Rationale

There are several things that I want to accomplish in the first treatment session. I want to find out what the patient thinks is going wrong and what accounts for it. My patients are always depressed (although, like the kindergarten teacher, some are more than that) and almost all have a characterological explanation for what is going wrong in their lives. The sculptor saw himself as "incompetent" whereas the kindergarten teacher saw herself as "unlovable." People who are prone to depression tend to treat life as a test of character and assume that they have failed, rather than a test of strategy. In most instances the underlying theme is to help patients focus more on what they do (strategy) than on what they are (character). Some strategies just work better than others.

I also want to give patients a preview of what CBT is about so as to see if it fits for them (rather than if they fit the therapy), and I try to do so in an experiential fashion. I ask patients to recall a recent experience in which they experienced a distressing negative affect or were not happy with how they behaved and walk me through the instance in a detailed and specific fashion, filling in the nodes on the Greenberger and Padesky circular cognitive model.[37] I first ask them to describe the situation in some detail, like a reporter (who, what, where, when, and how), then move directly to their affect (how did you feel when that was happening?), then bounce to their physiological reaction (usually either aroused if anxiety or angry or deflated if sad or guilty). I then ask what they did behaviorally, and especially if they had the impulse to do something that they did not act on. Then and only then do I ask what was going on inside their head (cognition). The reason for holding the cognition for last is that I want the patient to be fully immersed in the immediacy of the situation and because I want to end with the cognition. If they respond with thoughts when I ask for a description of the situation or their feelings or physiology, I put it in the cognition space and note the distinction ("When you think you are defeated, how do you feel?") and then get back to filling out the circle diagram in the order described above (situation, affect, physiology, behavior, cognition).

I want to do several things with this exercise. First I want to introduce the notion that thoughts, feelings, physiology, and behavior are separate components of a coherent whole. I want patients to look for each of those components in any given situation, but I also want them to recognize that they will always form a coherent whole. Sadness comes from a sense of loss or an inability to anticipate future gain and is usually associated with a physiological sense of being deflated and behavioral inertia; anxiety comes from the perception of threat and is associated with physiological arousal and a desire to escape or avoid behaviorally (flight); anger comes from a sense of moral injustice (the violation of a "should") and is also arousing but with a propensity to approach in a hostile fashion (fight); and guilt also comes from a sense of moral injustice (another "should") but this time on the part of the patient with physiological deflation and behavioral inertia. Even patients in the midst of a psychosis will always exhibit coherence: Their affect and physiology and behavioral impulses will be consistent with their ideation; it is just that their ideation is divorced from reality ("Space aliens are beaming thoughts into my head"). This coherence is why when the kindergarten teacher asked whether her being an incorrigible liar would interfere with therapy, I was able to reply without any hesitation that it would not. Even if she told me fabricated stories, they would be coherent with respect to thoughts, feelings, physiology, and behavior that I needed to teach her the relevant CBT skills. She was quite surprised and not a little bemused.

When the English talk about "Theory A and Theory B," what they mean is that patients come to therapy with the assumption that they are deeply flawed, usually "incompetent" or "unlovable" (Theory A) and that therapy proceeds best if you can lay out an alternative explanation: "You may be neither incompetent nor unlovable but simply using the wrong strategies" (Theory B). The sculptor was so sure that he was incompetent that he did not send out job applications, and the kindergarten teacher was so sure that she was unlovable that she sabotaged relationships before her partner could reject her. Both engaged in "self-fulfilling prophecies"; they behaved in ways consistent with their beliefs so as to produce the very outcomes they feared and then took those outcomes as evidence for the accuracy of those beliefs. The sculptor was simply depressed; the actions he did not take simply kept him stuck in his misery (although that did annoy his wife), whereas the actions that the kindergarten teacher took were provocative and distressing to others, especially those with whom she was in an intimate relationship (that latter is the essence of a personality disorder). I did not bother with the "three-legged stool" with the sculptor. He did not need it because he did not have a personality disorder; but with the kindergarten teacher I invoked it from the first session on, in anticipation that she would be as provocative and demanding with me as she was with everyone else because she would process our relationship through the same distorted lens.

16.3.3. Training in Self-Monitoring

The first homework that I ask my patients to do is some systematic self-monitoring. The reason is that depression lives in the recollection and the expectation. For patients who are depressed, their actual experience is rarely as negative as they anticipate or as they recall; monitoring their affect on a systematic basis greatly facilitates testing their beliefs. It also highlights excesses and deficits in the patient's life; does the patient's mood rise and fall on a diurnal basis or in response to others or specific situations?

I ask patients to rate four things about once an hour:

1. Rate your mood at the moment on a scale of zero to 100 ("If zero is the worst that you have ever felt and 100 is the best, where would you put yourself right now?")
2. Write a couple of words about what you have been doing over the last hour.
3. Note whether anything pleasurable happened in the last hour (P).
4. Note whether you did anything masterful (M).

When we reviewed the sculptor's self-monitoring in session two, it was evident that his mood was much worse when he was home in the evenings and weekends thinking about his "dead-end" job than it was when he was at work, which he actually found pleasurable. It became apparent to both him and to me that the problem was not the job itself (he got to make things "pretty" with his hands), but rather with the way he thought about his job. He could not have told me that (and did not do so in the first session), but his systematic ratings made it clear.

16.3.4. Behavioral Activation

It is not that depressed patients cannot do, it is that they do not start. Response initiation deficit is the sine qua non of depression, and anything you can do to help them get started is likely to improve their situation.[38] The problem is not that they do not value, but rather that they do not expect. Motivation is a product of value by expectation. Whereas dynamic theories posit that the root cause of depression lies in unconscious desires, CBT focuses on unduly negative expectations. A variety of behavioral strategies are used to help the patient overcome this behavioral inertia, including scheduling and breaking big tasks down into a number of smaller steps ("chunking") in order to help the patient get started. In many instances, the problem is just one of passive noncompliance (the sculptor did not apply for other jobs because he did not expect it to work), whereas in others there is active resistance so as to not make things worse (the kindergarten teacher lied and manipulated so as not to be rejected).

The weekends were so much worse for the sculptor than when he was at work that we decided to devise an experiment to see if could do something interesting just for fun. There was a Picasso exhibit touring the country at the time that he would have gone to see had he not been so depressed, but every time he thought of going he got overwhelmed and never started. I simply asked him to list the steps that anyone would have to go through to get to the exhibit (check to see if it is still in town and if he still could get tickets and so forth) and encouraged him to take the first step or two while he was still in session (it was and he could) and cross each off the list as it was accomplished. He found that this simple strategy of breaking a big task into smaller steps helped him get over his inertia, and he and his wife went to the exhibit that weekend. He did not enjoy it as much as he would if he had not been depressed, but he enjoyed it more than he did the previous weekend. We then used the same strategy (breaking a big task into smaller steps) to put his portfolio together in a matter of weeks and he started applying again for jobs.

The thing that makes CBT different from more purely behavioral interventions that do not address cognition is that we use behavioral strategies not just to get the patient moving but also to test the accuracy of their beliefs by pitting Theory A versus Theory B. For the sculptor, the fact that he got to the exhibit and put his portfolio together suggested that the problem was the strategies he chose and not some basic character defect in him.

16.3.5. Identifying Thoughts

Most of the automatic negative thoughts that patients have occur on the edge of the sensorium, the kinds of things people think to themselves but rarely want to say in public. We use this metaphor to teach patients how to recognize the "hot" thoughts that are driving their affect. A second major cue occurs when patients use the verb "feel" to describe a belief. That is perfectly acceptable English, since the dictionary defines "feel" either as an affective state or a loosely held belief that is hard to defend logically. We ask patients to refrain from using the term "feel" to refer to their beliefs since we want to highlight the distinction between thoughts and feelings. The essential difference is that beliefs can be examined with respect to accuracy, whereas feelings cannot; they simply are. While it is important not to "invalidate" a patient's affective experience, the central premise of CBT is that correcting inaccurate beliefs can influence affect and behavior.

The single most effective way to find out how someone thinks about a situation is to put him or her in it, either in real life or in imagination. That is why I ask patients to describe the recent problematic situation in such detail when I work through the example in the first session. I want the exercise to be as immersive as it can be to facilitate recall of the thoughts. An even more powerful technique is to ask the patient to enter the situation.

We train patients to use the dysfunctional thought record (DTR) to capture automatic negative thoughts and the affects that they generate. Patients record the situation in the first column, their emotions in the second (it is usually easier to access the affect than the belief), and the problematic automatic negative thoughts ("hot" cognitions) in the third, rating the strength of both feelings and thoughts. We also ask patients to draw arrows connecting thoughts to feelings. If there is a "hot" thought without a feeling, we are curious as to why (some people are trained not to express strong feelings), and a feeling without a thought is an indication that we do not understand what it means to the patient. In instances when the thoughts identified do not fully account for the affect reported, we play "downward arrow," asking patients what that situation means about them or the other persons involved or their future (Beck's negative cognitive triad). We have a saying in CBT that affects are the royal road to the conscious.

16.3.6. Examining Beliefs

Once you identify beliefs, you can proceed to examine their accuracy. This is the heart of CBT. Staying with the DTR, one of the most effective things to do is to ask three questions":

1. What is the **evidence** for that belief?
2. Is there an **alternative explanation** for that event?
3. Even if true, what are its real **implications**?

These questions can be asked any time in therapy, and I do so from the first session on. But they lend themselves nicely to the DTR, and we want them to become habit for our patients.

Another thing that the sculptor had not done since he lost his teaching job was to pay his income taxes. Several weeks into therapy, as he was starting to feel better, he decided to get this financial affairs in order (he was getting paid in cash but had kept records) and headed down into his basement on a Sunday morning with a hot cup of coffee to do so. He got as far as the bottom step, looked across the room at the box in which he kept his receipts, and sank down on the bottom step ruminating furiously about what happens to long-haired artistic types when they get sent to a federal penitentiary. After a couple of minutes he went back upstairs, poured himself another hot cup of coffee, and worked through the top row in the DTR (see Figure 16.1). He first asked himself what **evidence** he had that he never got his work done and reminded himself of recent instances when he got to the Picasso exhibit and put his portfolio together. Nonetheless, he was not getting his taxes done that morning, so he asked himself if there was an **alternative explanation** other than that he was "a failure again" and "no good." When he did, he was able to remind himself that when he did get things done, it was in smaller bits and not all at once. He then went back downstairs, grabbed a handful of records, and brought them upstairs to sort through them. He did that several more times over the next several Sunday mornings and was able to finish the task in a couple of weeks. This was yet another instance of a bad strategy being misinterpreted as a character flaw.

That still left the question of what to do about the Internal Revenue Service (IRS). He very much did not want to be sent to prison, but he did want to bring things to closure. Although it does not show up on his DTR, he used the **implications** question in a manner that did not increase his risk of incarceration by calling the IRS from a pay phone (we had them in those days) to inquire about their policies. What the IRS told him was that it would not send him to jail if he came in voluntarily, although he would have to pay a fine; if he waited until the IRS caught up to him, he might well be sent to jail. After making a second call from a different pay phone using a different pseudonym and getting the same response, he went to the IRS and negotiated a schedule to pay off his back taxes.

16.3.7. Core Beliefs and Underlying Schema

Core beliefs and underlying schema represent "deep structures" at the core of an individual's meaning system and have implications for how a person processes incoming information. The sculptor was a tall gangly kid with a speech impediment and a younger brother who did everything right and was favored by their father. It is not hard to see where his core beliefs about "incompetence" and "not being good enough" originated.

The kindergarten teacher was close to her mother but not her father, who had a drinking problem and a dissolute lifestyle. Things took a turn for the worse when her mother died from cancer when she was 15. Her father moved his mistress into the house and commenced a series of drunken parties that culminated in the patient getting gang-raped in her own bedroom by her father's drinking buddies. The rape was bad enough, but what really got her was the total lack of concern that her father showed for her welfare. In essence, she learned that "I am nothing" and "someone no one could love."

THOUGHT RECORD

Directions: When you notice your mood getting worse, ask yourself, "What' s going throught my mind right now?" and as soon as possible jot down the throught or mental image in the Automatic Thoughts column. Then consider how realistic those thoughts are.

Date	Situation	Emotions	Automatic Thoughts	Alternative Responses	Outcome
	Where are you –and what was going on –when you got upset?	What emotions did you feel (sad, anxious, angry, etc.)? Rate intensity (0-100%).	What thoughts and/or images went through your mind? Rate your belief in each (0-100%).	Use the questions at the bottom to compose responses to the automatic thoughts. Rate your belief in each (0-100%). Also, consult the list of possible distortions.	Rerate belief in your automatic thoughts (0-100%) and in the intensity of your emotions (0-100%).
2/5	Not getting filing and lots of other stuff done	Anxious – sad –angry 85%	A failure again, I can never get my work done, I'm no good 85%	I have gotten filing and other work done in the past, but usually in smaller bites not all at once 80%	1. 45% 2. Anxious –sad –angry 50%
2/7	Sitting and idly looking thru some old books –6:30 am	Anxious 75%	Feeling guilty because I'm not doing work, I'm going to slip back into funk if I am not careful 70%	After twele hours of high energy work yesterday (phone work, filing, building, letter, therapy, driving) I think it is ok to relax from 5:30 am to 6:30 am the following day 95%	1. 10% 2. Joyful, exuberant 95%
	*********	*********	***************	******************	*********
1/29	I can't handle it anymore –too much in the past to undo –misuse of time	Depressed 80%	No options –either direct job in my speciality or nothing at all 90%	The present does not predict the future 20%	1. 95% 2. Depressed 95%

(1) What is the evidence that the automatic thought is true? What is the evidence that it is not true?

(2) Are there alternative explanations for that event, or alternative ways to view the situation?

(3) What are the implications if the thought is true? What' s most upsetting about it? What' s the most realistic? What can I do about it?

(4) What would I tell a good friend in the same situation?

Possible Distortions: All-or-none Thinking; Overgeneralizing; Discounting the Positives; Jumping to Conclusions; Mind-reading; Fortune-telling; Magnifying/Minimizing; Emotional Reasoning; Making "Should" Statements; Labelling; Inappropriate Blaming

FIGURE 16.1. Sample Thought Record illustrating application of "three questions" to deal with negative automatic thoughts and core beliefs relative to difficulty pulling together his tax records (first row).

It took about three months to persuade her to relive the story in therapy (she had alluded to something bad that had happened to her as a teen but did not want to talk about it), and when she did, two clusters of beliefs came out: (1) "I am worthless and unlovable and anyone I would be interested in would reject me if they knew what happened" and (2) it was so frightening to think that something so unfair could happen to someone who did not deserve it, that it was more comfortable to think of herself as a bad person who manipulated to get what she wanted. Her behaviors fell in line with her beliefs, and she engaged in a series of compensatory strategies (safety behaviors) that protected her from being rejected by others at the expense of rejecting them first.

We formulated a cognitive conceptualization diagram (CCD) that started with specific instances from her thought records to identify the core beliefs ("I am un-lovable") that lead to her underlying assumptions ("if I let someone get to know the real me, they will reject me") that led in turn to her compensatory strategies (lie, cheat, and manipulate to get what you want) that were understandably hard on her relationships. The hallmark of patients with a personality disorder is that they do not recognize that it is their own behaviors that annoy and frustrate others and keep them from getting what they want.

Armed with the CCD (we kept a copy on the desk between us at every session), we then set about testing her core beliefs. Marsha Linehan has a principle that she calls "opposite action" that she uses with her borderline patients: Whatever your inclination is to do under strong states of affect, do the opposite.[39] That is what we did with the kindergarten teacher. She had a new boyfriend whom she liked, but the last thing she could imagine doing was to tell him what had happened to her. She had already described the event to me, but I did not count because therapists are sup-posed to be nonjudgmental. She agreed to tell a childhood friend about the event, and when she did, the friend was nothing but supportive and consoling. Her friend was sorry that it happened to her but that fact did nothing to change how her girl-friend thought about her. The patient still was not willing to talk with her boyfriend yet, so we devised a plan to have me tape interviews with a number of young male soccer coaches from overseas (my son was playing indoor soccer at the time) for which she wrote out a description of what had happened to her and questions for me to ask. I conducted the survey over a tournament weekend, and although a couple of the young men indicated that they would stay away from someone who might be "damaged" as a consequence of the trauma, most had no concern. They were sorry about what happened to her, but they only thing that would matter to them was how she treated them. Armed with that information, she talked with her new boyfriend, who was nothing but sympathetic and consoling and then asked if she wanted get something to eat.

It took several more months of taking chances, asking for what she wanted in an assertive fashion instead of manipulating to get it and letting other people know the "real" person inside, before it became second nature, but it did. The key to dealing with core beliefs is not to talk them to death, but instead look for specific ways to test their accuracy, which usually means doing the opposite of your initial impulse. Judy Beck describes other helpful strategies in her treatise, but encouraging patients to drop their compensatory strategies to test their beliefs heads the list.[40] It was not until the kindergarten teacher stopped whistling that she learned there were no tigers to keep away.

16.3.8. Termination and Relapse Prevention

I start preparing the patients for termination in the first session by making it clear that CBT is a skills-based approach and that they can learn to do anything for themselves that I can do for them (that is when the kindergarten teacher informed me that she was so deeply damaged that she needed therapy for the rest of her life). The rationale for doing work between sessions is so that patients come to master those skills. Any reduction in session frequency is treated as a "dry run" for termination. Near the end of therapy, it is helpful to ask patients to imagine what they would do if the worst were to happen; fire drills do not increase the likelihood of fires but they do increase the odds of survival if a fire occurs.

The sculptor got over his depression within a couple of months without getting another teaching job. He did start dropping by a nursing home in his neighborhood one evening a week to teach art to the residents. He loved it and they loved him. He called about six months after treatment ended to indicate that he had changed jobs. He had been sitting reading the paper one morning before work in a coffee shop when another patron asked to borrow his sports section. They struck up a conversation, and when the sculptor indicated that he was an artist temporarily working as a handyman, the other patron suggested he stop by Tonka Toys, since they hired sculptors in their design department. The sculptor did, and he got hired and would never consider going back to teaching.

The kindergarten teacher got less depressed over the course of the year (and well over a hundred sessions) and we continued working in a less intensive fashion over the following year. She got quite skilled at asking for what she wanted without demanding that she get it (we spent considerable time role playing around assertion). She reached out to her by then ex-husband through her former in-laws (whom she continued to call "Mom" and "Pop") and agreed to meet him in New York to debrief about their marriage. He stood her up, which she handled with aplomb ("he missed an opportunity for me to take the blame"). She went to her brother's wedding knowing that her father would be there and felt more sorrow for him than anger when he was unable to respond (he "could have had a daughter"). She lived for several years very much in love with the next big star in country music but put an end to the relationship when he turned to drink and became abusive after the expected recording contract failed to materialize (as she put it, "better no relationship than a bad one"). She had clearly moved beyond the core beliefs and compensatory strategies that led her to sabotage her earlier relationships.

16.4. CONCLUSIONS

CBT can be as efficacious as ADM when adequately implemented and has an enduring effect not found for medications. Studies indicate that it can reduce risk for future episodes by half, and in a chronically recurrent disorder, that is a real boon. Likely that enduring effect comes from teaching patients how to be their own therapist. It is suitable and relatively brief for patients with uncomplicated depressions (regardless of severity) but can also be adapted for patients with chronic depressions or depressions superimposed on longstanding personality disorders. It does not work for everyone, but it works for many, and for those for whom it does work, it provides lasting benefits.

REFERENCES

1. Beck AT, Rush AJ, Shaw BF, Emery G. *Cognitive Therapy of Depression*. New York: Guilford Press; 1979.
2. Rush AJ, Beck AT, Kovacs M, Hollon SD. Comparative efficacy of cognitive therapy and pharmacotherapy in the treatment of depressed outpatients. *Cognit Ther Res*. 1977; 1: 17–37.
3. Blackburn IM, Bishop S, Glen AI, et al. The efficacy of cognitive therapy in depression: a treatment trial using cognitive therapy and pharmacotherapy, each alone and in combination. *Br J Psychiatry*. 1981; 139: 181–189.
4. Murphy GE, Simons AD, Wetzel RD, Lustman PJ. Cognitive therapy and pharmacotherapy: singly and together in the treatment of depression. *Arch Gen Psychiatry*. 1984; 41: 33–41.
5. Hollon SD, DeRubeis RJ, Evans MD, et al. Cognitive therapy and pharmacotherapy for depression: singly and in combination. *Arch Gen Psychiatry*. 1992; 49: 774–781.
6. Elkin I, Shea MT, Watkins JT, et al. National Institute of Mental Health Treatment of Depression Collaborative Research Program: general effectiveness of treatments. *Arch Gen Psychiatry*. 1989; 46: 971–982.
7. Jacobson NS, Hollon SD. Prospects for future comparisons between drugs and psychotherapy: lessons from the CBT vs. pharmacotherapy exchange. *J Consult Clin Psychol*. 1996; 64: 104–108.
8. DeRubeis RJ, Gelfand LA, Tang TZ, Simons A. Medications versus cognitive behavioral therapy for severely depressed outpatients: mega-analysis of four randomized comparisons. *Am J Psychiatry*. 1999; 156: 1007–1013.
9. DeRubeis RJ, Hollon SD, Amsterdam JD, et al. Cognitive therapy vs. medications in the treatment of moderate to severe depression. *Arch Gen Psychiatry*. 2005; 62: 409–416.
10. Jarrett RB, Schaffer M, McIntire D, et al. Treatment of atypical depression with cognitive therapy or phenelzine: a double-blind, placebo-controlled trial. *Arch Gen Psychiatry*. 1999; 56: 431–437.
11. Dimidjian S, Hollon SD, Dobson KS, et al. Behavioral activation, cognitive therapy, and antidepressant medication in the acute treatment of major depression. *J Consult Clin Psychol*. 2006; 74: 658–670.
12. Weitz ES, Hollon SD, Twisk J, et al. Baseline depression severity as moderator of depression outcomes between CBT versus pharmacotherapy: an individual patient data meta-analysis. *JAMA Psychiatry*. 2015; 72: 1102–1109.
13. Kovacs M, Rush AJ, Beck AT, Hollon SD. Depressed outpatients treated with cognitive therapy or pharmacotherapy: a one-year follow-up. *Arch Gen Psychiatry*. 1981; 38: 33–39.

14. Blackburn IM, Eunson KM, Bishop S. A two-year naturalistic follow-up of depressed patients treated with cognitive therapy, pharmacotherapy and a combination of both. *J Affect Disord.* 1986; 10: 67–75.

15. Simons AD, Murphy GE, Levine JL, Wetzel RD. Cognitive therapy and pharmacotherapy for depression: sustained improvement over one year. *Arch Gen Psychiatry.* 1986; 43: 43–48.

16. Evans MD, Hollon SD, DeRubeis RJ, et al. Differential relapse following cognitive therapy and pharmacotherapy for depression. *Arch Gen Psychiatry.* 1992; 49: 802–808.

17. Shea MT, Elkin I, Imber SD, et al. Course of depressive symptoms over followup: findings from the National Institute of Mental Health Treatment of Depression Collaborative Research Program. *Arch Gen Psychiatry.* 1992; 49: 782–787.

18. Hollon SD, DeRubeis RJ, Shelton RC, et al. Prevention of relapse following cognitive therapy vs. medications in moderate to severe depression. *Arch Gen Psychiatry.* 2005; 62: 417–422.

19. Dobson KS, Hollon SD, Dimidjian S, et al. Randomized trial of behavioral activation, cognitive therapy, and antidepressant medication in the prevention of relapse and recurrence in major depression. *J Consult Clin Psychol.* 2008; 76: 468–477.

20. Jarrett RB, Kraft D, Schaffer M, et al. Reducing relapse in depressed outpatients with atypical features: a pilot study. *Psychother Psychosomat.* 2000; 69: 232–239.

21. Cuijpers P, Hollon SD, van Straten A, et al. Does cognitive behaviour therapy have an enduring effect that is superior to keeping patients on continuation pharmacotherapy? A meta-analysis. *BMJ Open.* 2013; 3(4): e002542.

22. Hollon SD, Jarrett RB, Nierenberg AA, et al. Psychotherapy and medication in the treatment of adult and geriatric depression: which monotherapy or combined treatment? *J Clin Psychiatry.* 2005; 66: 455–468.

23. Hollon SD, DeRubeis RJ, Fawcett J, et al. Effect of cognitive therapy with antidepressant medications vs. antidepressants alone on the rate of recovery in major depressive disorder: a randomized clinical trial. *JAMA Psychiatry.* 2014; 71: 1157–1164.

24. Fournier JC, DeRubeis RJ, Shelton RC, et al. Prediction of response to medication and cognitive therapy in the treatment of moderate to severe depression. *J Consult Clin Psychol.* 2009; 77: 775–787.

25. Leykin Y, Amsterdam JD, DeRubeis RJ, et al. Progressive resistance to selective serotonin reuptake inhibitor but not to cognitive therapy in the treatment of major depression. *J Consult Clin Psychol.* 2007; 75: 267–276.

26. Fournier JC, DeRubeis RJ, Shelton RC, et al. Antidepressant medications versus cognitive therapy in people with depression with or without personality disorder. *Br J Psychiatry.* 2008; 192: 124–129.

27. DeRubeis RJ, Cohen ZD, Forand NR, et al. The Personalized Advantage Index: translating research on prediction into individualized treatment recommendations. A demonstration. *PLoS One.* 2014; 9(1): e83875.

28. Cohen ZD, DeRubeis RJ. Treatment selection in depression. *Annu Rev Clin Psychol.* 2018; 14: 15.1–15.28.

29. Kazdin AE. Mediators and mechanisms of change in psychotherapy research. *Annu Rev Clin Psychol.* 2007; 3: 1–27.

30. Feeley M, DeRubeis RJ, Gelfand LA. The temporal relation of adherence and alliance to symptom change in cognitive therapy for depression. *J Consult Clin Psychol.* 1999; 67: 578–582.

31. Hollon SD, DeRubeis RJ, Evans MD. Causal mediation of change in treatment for depression: discriminating between nonspecificity and noncausality. *Psychol Bull.* 1987; 102: 139–149.

32. DeRubeis RJ, Evans MD, Hollon SD, et al. How does cognitive therapy work? Cognitive change and symptom change in cognitive therapy and pharmacotherapy for depression. *J Consult Clin Psychol,* 1990; 58: 862–869.

33. Strunk DR, DeRubeis RJ, Chiu AW, Alvarez J. Patients' competence in and performance of cognitive therapy skills: relation to the reduction of relapse risk following treatment for depression. *J Consult Clin Psychol.* 2007; 75: 523–530.

34. Tang TZ, DeRubeis RJ, Hollon SD, et al. Sudden gains in cognitive therapy of depression and relapse/recurrence. *J Consult Clin Psychol.* 2007; 75: 404–408.

35. Hollon SD, DeRubeis RJ. Mediating the effects of cognitive therapy for depression. *Cognit Behav Ther.* 2009; 38(suppl. 1): 43–47.

36. Beck AT, Freeman A, Davis DD. *Cognitive Therapy of Personality Disorders,* 2nd ed. New York: Guilford Press; 2003.

37. Greenberger D, Padesky CA. *Mind over Mood: Change How You Feel by Changing the Way You Think,* (2nd ed.). New York: Guilford Press; 2015.

38. Miller WR. Psychological deficit in depression. *Psychol Bull.* 1975; 82: 238–260.

39. Linehan MM. *Cognitive-Behavior Treatment of Borderline Personality Disorder.* New York: Guilford Press; 1993.

40. Beck JS. *Cognitive Behavior Therapy: Basics and Beyond,* 2nd ed.). New York: Guilford Press; 2011.

/// 17 /// BEHAVIORAL ACTIVATION FOR DEPRESSION

History, Treatment Description,
and Empirical Review

BRETT DAVIS, STEVEN C. DUFOUR,
JESSICA A. JANOS, AND LOUISA G. SYLVIA

17.1. HISTORY OF BEHAVIORAL ACTIVATION

Behavioral activation (BA) has been used to treat depression since the 1970s. This psychotherapeutic approach focuses on increasing patient behaviors that will produce environmental reinforcements to improve thoughts, mood, and overall quality of life.[1] BA can be traced back to B.F. Skinner's work on positive reinforcement and his concept of depression as a consequence of interruptions to healthy behavior and reinforcing stimuli.[2]

In 1974, Peter Lewinsohn described depression as a function of two features: low rates of response-contingent positive reinforcement and inadequate social skills.[3] This conceptualization served as the theoretical underpinning for BA as well as the first published BA-based treatment manual.[4] Specifically, the manual included activity scheduling, social skills training, contingency management strategies, and thought-stopping skills. This BA-based manual influenced the development of other interventions throughout the 1970s and 1980s, including interventions that targeted diverse or minority groups.[5,6]

In 1977, a multi-method assessment study was published that suggested the superiority of cognitive over behavioral techniques.[7] This led Lewinsohn and his students to incorporate cognitive techniques into their research. In 1979, they published a study that demonstrated no differential effectiveness between activity scheduling, skills training, and cognitive techniques,[8] and as such, adopted a cognitive–behavioral rather than a purely behavioral approach.[9] Aaron Beck, the pioneer and developer of cognitive therapy, also included behavioral skills in his updated manual given the growing promise and effectiveness of these techniques.[10] In 1996, Jacobson and colleagues conducted an influential component analysis of Beck's manual that suggested treatment based on his behavioral techniques alone was as effective for improving depressive symptoms as was treatment based on his combined cognitive and behavioral program.[11] Two new behavioral treatment manuals were developed in response to this component analysis: "Behavioral Activation"[12] and the "Brief Behavioral Activation Treatment for Depression,"[13] In this chapter, we will review these treatments, key BA components, and evidence of BA-based therapies for treating depression as well as evidence for delivering these therapies in different formats (e.g., individual vs. group).

17.2. DESCRIPTION OF TREATMENT

17.2.1. A Behaviorist Definition of Depression

In behaviorism, all aspects of human activity, including physical, cognitive, and emotional processes, are regarded as behavior, and the frequency of a behavior is understood to depend on the reinforcement it receives.[2] Depression, or a state of a reduced interest, positive affect, and activity for a period of at least two weeks, is therefore understood to be caused by a reduction in reinforcement of those behaviors.[14] In BA-based treatments, therapists help their clients to increase contact with positive reinforcement through strategic activity scheduling. Performance of non-depressive behaviors and exposure to positive reinforcement drives improvement in depressive emotions and cognitions.

Reviews of existing BA treatment manuals have identified common treatment features.[15,16] The "core" features of BA are present in all of the BA manuals and are considered foundational or essential to the BA approach. There are also supplemental components that may be included to address individual and environmental barriers to activation.

17.2.2. Core Features of BA

17.2.2.1. Activation Activities
All BA manuals encourage clients to complete activities intended to increase contact with sources of positive reinforcement.[16] Some treatment manuals are careful to frame weekly activation goals such that the focus remains on increasing the number of activities opposed to reducing affective symptoms.[12,13] Typically, activities are scheduled in advance, are scheduled during session, are recorded in a calendar or activity log, and are completed outside of session as homework. Some

manuals (e.g., reference 12) recommend practicing activation activities within session to help clients experience the connection between the behavior and a positive reinforcement.

Client and clinician work together to select appropriate assignments, although selection criteria may vary by manual. For example, earlier treatment manuals (e.g., reference 12) often adopt *enjoyment* as the main or sole criterion for selecting activation assignments, even including master lists of common "pleasurable activities" as supplemental materials.[17] Other BA-based manuals encourage activities that provide participants with opportunities to exercise skills and experience mastery (e.g., Chapter 7 of reference 10). More recent BA-based interventions select activities based on a client's goals, values, or specific avoidance behaviors, emphasizing the productive function of the behavior opposed to how pleasurable it is.[12,13]

To assist with appropriate activity selection, some BA-based manuals include defining clients' values, or what is important to them. Some clients may find it helpful to reference a list of generally important life areas (e.g., family relationships, education, work, spirituality) when identifying their values.[18] It is important that the clinician assists with a productive framing of the goals associated with their values, as they should be attainable and within the client's control (i.e., aspects about the client or his or her life that the client can change). The client's goals and values will help to personalize and guide the activation assignments.

17.2.2.2. Self-Monitoring

Behavior monitoring is the skill of tracking one's behaviors and activities between treatment sessions. Typically, an activity log is used to track completion, frequency, and duration of activation behaviors and, sometimes, all activities or avoidance behaviors. Depending on the treatment manual and the specific client needs, activity logs may also track internal experiences that happen during behaviors, such as emotions, thoughts, physical symptoms, or psychological states (e.g., depressed, anxious). Behavior monitoring can serve several functions, including to establish a baseline of activity and common behaviors prior to starting activation assignments, to identify obstacles or barriers to activating behaviors, and to track the connection between behaviors and emotions as well as completion of activation assignments.[19]

17.2.3. Addressing Barriers to Activation

17.2.3.1. Overcoming Environmental Barriers to Activation

Some clients may discover that the reinforcement available in their environment is not adequately supportive of their target behaviors, which can reduce treatment adherence. When this occurs, a BA clinician can provide strategies for modifying environmental reinforcement. One strategy to do this is to make a rewards list, where clients designate appropriate rewards for completing activities or weekly treatment goals. These rewards increase the positive reinforcement of target behaviors.

Another strategy is to form social contracts with friends to modify social rewards for depressive and non-depressive behaviors.[13] Contracts between the client and the client's family and friends can define ways in which they can help to reward healthy behaviors and avoid rewarding unhealthy behaviors. By reducing the relative value of rewards for non-depressive behavior compared to depressive behavior, the frequency of non-depressive behavior is expected to increase.[20]

17.2.3.2. Overcoming Individual Barriers to Activation

Other barriers to BA may relate to an individual's negative emotions or cognitions about changing behaviors or the degree to which an individual possesses certain abilities, such as self-awareness, self-efficacy, or motivation.[21] These individual factors may impact a client's ability to complete activation assignments. For these reasons, certain BA manuals include skills that overcome these individualized barriers, such as (1) social skills training to prepare clients to engage in social activation assignments;[8,22] (2) problem-solving training to prepare clients for issues that arise during activation activities;[22] and (3) relaxation training techniques to address agitation and anxiety clients experience during activation activities.[18,22] Martell and colleagues[12] include mindfulness training in their BA manual, *Depression in Context: Strategies for Guided Action*, to teach clients to bring calm awareness and acceptance of negative feelings and cognitions arising during activation activities.

17.2.4. Current BA Approaches

Today, there are two most commonly used and researched treatment BA manuals: (1) the iteration developed by Martell, Addis, and Jacobson,[12] often referred to simply as "behavioral activation" and (2) the treatment developed by Lejuez, Hopko, and Hopko,[13] called "behavioral activation treatment for depression" (BATD) (Table 17.1).

17.2.4.1. Behavioral Activation (Martell, Addis, and Jacobson)

This BA manual aims to reduce avoidance behaviors in 20 to 24 weekly, 60-minute individual sessions.[23] Avoidance behaviors in the BA approach are depressive symptoms driven by negative reinforcement, such as staying in bed to avoid workplace stress.[24] These behaviors are often problematic in depressed individuals because they may prioritize short- over long-term goals. In BA, avoidance behaviors are explored in a functional analysis that defines their triggers, function, and goal-relevant consequences. During the functional analysis, the clinician presents avoidance behaviors as understandable coping mechanisms responding to environmental triggers, and helps the client identify alternative coping behaviors. The clinician then prompts the client to define specific, attainable goals and values that are within the client's control. Based on a client's goals, values, and avoidance behaviors, a clinician will assign weekly activation activities to promote goal pursuit, regular routines, and alternative coping behaviors. Assignments are reviewed the following

TABLE 17.1. Comparing Core Features and Problem-solving Strategies of Two Current BA Treatment Manuals

	"Behavioral Activation" (Lejuez et al., 2001)[13]	"Breif Behavioral Activation Treatment for Depression" (Martell et al., 2001)[12]
Length	20 to 24 weekly, 60-min individual sessions	10 to 12 weekly, 60-min individual sessions
Activation assignments	Activities assigned by therapist during each sessions; activities selected based on functional assessment and values assesment	Activity hierarchy constructed at beginning of treatment that sets activities for remainder of treatment and is based on structured values assessment
Self-monitoring	Activity logs	Activity logs
Overcoming environmental barriers	Social contracts, reward lists	Social contracts, reward lits
Overcoming individual barriers	Relaxation techniques, mindfulness training, social skills training	Not included

week. This manual recommends adding support strategies to enhance activation assignments, such as mindfulness techniques, relaxation training, and strategies to deal with rumination.[15]

17.2.4.2. BATD (Lejeuz, Hopko, and Hopko)

BATD is delivered in 10 to 12 weekly individual sessions. Sessions initially last for 60 minutes and may shorten over the course of treatment as clients become more comfortable with self-monitoring. This manual is based on the theory of matching law,[20] or the concept that the ratio of performance frequency between two behaviors is equal to the ratio of their reinforcement value. BATD, applying this theory to depression, seeks to reduce the reinforcement value of depressive behavior relative to that of non-depressive behavior. The course of treatment is divided into six units with a unique objective. Unit 1 provides treatment overview, Unit 2 explains depression within the behaviorist paradigm, and Unit 3 explains treatment rationale. In Unit 4, clients prepare for activation assignments by monitoring baseline behaviors and performing a goals and values assessment. Additionally, environmental incentives may be modified in Unit 4 by planning for social contracts and appropriate self-administered rewards, both of which can increase reinforcement of healthy behaviors. In Unit 5, the client constructs a hierarchy of 15 activities, ranging from easy to difficult, that align with the life values and goals identified in Unit 4. As the client executes the activity hierarchy, progress is monitored and adjustments are made in Unit 6.

EMPIRICAL SUPPORT FOR BA

The efficacy and effectiveness of the BA-based manuals have been studied by examining the treatment independently as well as compared to other psychosocial and pharmacotherapy interventions. Efficacy of both traditional and contemporary BA interventions has been strongly supported.[25-27] Meta-analyses also support the effectiveness of BA as an intervention for the treatment of depression in adults. For example, a meta-analysis by Mazzucchelli and colleagues[28] analyzed 34 randomized controlled trials of BA with a total of 2,055 adult participants with depression and found that the overall effect size of BA compared to control conditions was large (0.78).

BA has been compared to cognitive therapy (CT), a structured intervention focused on changing the cognitions in patients that has been used to treat a variety of psychiatric disorders.[10,29] One seminal randomized placebo-controlled trial randomized adults with major depressive disorder to CT, BA, or an antidepressant medication.[30] Among the more severely depressed participants in the study, the researchers found BA to be more efficacious than CT.[30] Additionally, several meta-analyses have supported that BA is as effective as CT for treating depression.[28,31] A recent meta-analysis examining one of the components of BA, activity scheduling, compared to CT found that both treatments were equally effective as well.[32]

BA has also been compared to the impact of cognitive–behavioral therapy (CBT), an intervention that focuses on changing maladaptive thoughts and problematic behavioral patterns,[33,34] in treating depressive symptoms. For example, one landmark study found BA to be as effective as CBT in changing the participants' negative thoughts, even if the participant did not directly discuss the negative thoughts with his or her clinician during the intervention.[11] Several meta-analyses examining studies comparing BA to CBT further support that BA is as effective as CBT up to two years following completion of the intervention.[28,31]

Additional studies have compared BA to other psychosocial interventions. For example, a recent meta-analysis found that BA was as effective for treating symptoms of depression as (1) brief psychotherapy, defined as treatment focusing on insight and development of character through interpersonal relationships, and (2) supportive counseling, defined as interventions in which the clinician works on the development of patient self-awareness through the use of core relationship conditions.[31] Another study, which compared BATD to standard supportive care in an inpatient unit within a hospital setting, found that participants who received BATD had a greater change in depressive symptoms as measured with the Beck Depression Inventory[35] compared to those in the standard care condition, with an effect size of 0.73.[19]

One study also examined the efficacy of BA compared to pharmacotherapy for depression. In this study, BA was compared to CT and antidepressant medication.[30] Researchers found that BA was as efficacious as antidepressant medication for more severely depressed patients, and both the antidepressant medication and

BA conditions were found to be more efficacious than CT alone.[30] These results remained consistent at a two-year follow-up.[36] Additional research is needed to further examine the short- and long-term effects of BA compared to pharmacotherapy.

BA has been appealing as a treatment for depressive symptoms because it is a relatively simple, accessible, and time-efficient treatment intervention for patients to participate in and for therapists to deliver. To emphasize this point, a recent meta-analysis found that better treatment outcomes with BA were not associated with a higher level of qualifications,[31] thus making the treatment a good option for clinicians with limited time to receive training and resources.

Despite these promising data, it remains unclear how many sessions of BA are necessary to improve depression. Most BA manuals suggest at least 10 sessions,[12,13] but participants have demonstrated reductions in depressive symptoms within the first 4 sessions of BA.[37,38] Further research is needed to establish the minimal effective duration of BA.

17.4. ADAPTATIONS OF BA FOR SPECIAL POPULATIONS OR SETTINGS

Preliminary evidence suggests that BA can effectively treat depression in varied populations and settings,[15] including via remote delivery, in group formats, and specific to certain subpopulations.

17.4.1. Telehealth

BA has been adapted to be administered via the phone or web apps. For example, Ly and colleagues[39] adapted BA as an eight-week smartphone app that follows the BA manual developed by Martell and colleagues[12] and Lejuez and colleagues.[13] This BA-based smartphone app was compared to an eight-week mindfulness-based smartphone app treatment. Both groups showed significant improvement in depressive symptoms.[39] O'Mahen and colleagues[40] developed an 11-session web-based BA-based treatment for women with postpartum depression that was developed from Addis and Martel's[41] BA-based manual. This treatment, Postnatal iBA, emphasizes several of the core constructs of BA (e.g., self-monitoring and promotion of alternative behaviors) in the context of behaviors and activities common to new motherhood.[40] There was a significant reduction in depressive symptoms among individuals in the Postnatal iBA group compared to those in the treatment-as-usual group, as measured by the Edinburgh Postnatal Depression Scale (EPDS).[42]

There are promising preliminary data that suggest telehealth adaptations of BA for depression may be beneficial, but future studies are needed. For example, a meta-analysis of 117 commercially available smartphone apps to monitor or treat depression found that only 12 of them contained material specific to CBT or BA, and none of these exceeded the 25% adherence to core BA principles.[43]

17.4.2. Group Therapy

BA manuals have also been developed for delivery in group formats. For example, the Behavioral Activation Group Therapy program was developed for community mental healthcare settings.[44] This group intervention was based on the BA approach examined by Jacobson and colleagues[11] and consisted of 10 95-minute sessions focusing on (1) identifying circumstances surrounding the depression, (2) determining exacerbating behaviors of the depression, and (3) creating a behavior-based treatment plan to improve coping skills and encouraging positive reinforcement.[11] This group-based BA treatment significantly reduced symptoms of depression in a pragmatic setting.[44]

Current research suggests that group-based BA may be helpful for the treatment of depression. For example, a meta-analysis of seven studies examining the efficacy of group-based BA for depression found that it consistently improved outcomes, although protocol heterogeneity across these studies was noted as a key limitation.[45]

17.4.3. Adaptations for Subpopulations

As with many psychotherapies, adaptations of treatment manuals are necessary to be sensitive to the needs of specific subpopulations. Collado and colleagues[46] found success in translating the BATD manual[13] into Spanish and conducted a pilot with 10 Latinos who had limited English proficiency and depressive symptoms. Activity increased and depressive symptoms decreased over the course of the 10 BA-based sessions.[46] In a randomized trial of 43 Spanish-speaking Americans, an adaptation of Martell's manual[12] reduced depressive symptoms only for participants in the treatment group who frequently attended treatment sessions.[47] BA has also been adapted for geriatric populations, with one review finding these adaptations to be effective for treating late-life depression.[48] These studies underscore the potential for BA to be adapted for subpopulations, but more adaptions are needed, as is evidence for their efficacy and effectiveness.

17.5. CONCLUSION AND FUTURE DIRECTIONS

BA, an approach that increases a client's contact with positive reinforcement, is an empirically validated treatment approach for depression. Evidence suggests that BA is as effective as CBT and pharmacotherapy for the treatment of depression. Further research is needed to develop or validate BA adaptations to new formats (e.g., web-based, mobile apps) as well as new populations (e.g., geriatric, adolescent, and specific cultural groups). Further standardization of BA manuals, especially for groups, is also warranted. Finally, there is a need to better understand the dosing of BA, as the minimal duration of BA needed for effective and stable symptom reduction is unknown.

REFERENCES

1. Hopko DR, Lejuez CW, Ruggiero KJ, Eifert GH. Contemporary behavioral activation treatments for depression: Procedures, principles, and progress. *Clin Psychol Rev.* 2003;23(5):699–717. doi:10.1016/S0272-7358(03)00070-9
2. Skinner BF. *About Behaviorism.* New York: Vintage Books; 1974.
3. Lewinsohn PM. A behavioral approach to depression. In: *Essential Papers on Depression.* New York: New York University, 1974:150–172.
4. Lewinsonh PM, Biglan A, Zeiss AM. Behavioral treatment for depression. In: Davidson PO, ed. *Behavioral Management of Anxiety, Depression, and Pain.* New York: Brunner/Mazel; 1976:91–146.
5. Comas-Díaz L. Effects of cognitive and behavioral group treatment on the depressive symptomatology of Puerto Rican women. *J Consult Clin Psychol.* 1981;49(5):627–632. doi:10.1037/0022-006X.49.5.627
6. Padfield M. The comparative effects of two counseling approaches on the intensity of depression among rural women of low socioeconomic status. *J Couns Psychol.* 1976;23(3):209–214. doi:10.1037/0022-0167.23.3.209
7. Shaw BF. Comparison of cognitive therapy and behavior therapy in the treatment of depression. *J Consult Clin Psychol.* 1977;45(4):543–551. doi:10.1037/0022-006X.45.4.543
8. Zeiss AM, Lewinsohn PM, Muñoz RF. Nonspecific improvement effects in depression using interpersonal skills training, pleasant activity schedules, or cognitive training. *J Consult Clin Psychol.* 1979;47(3):427–439.
9. Lewinsohn P, Munoz RF, Youngren M, Zeiss AM, eds. *Control Your Depression.* New York: Fireside; 1986.
10. Beck AT, Rush AJ, eds. *Cognitive Therapy of Depression.* 13th printing. New York: Guilford Press; 1979.
11. Jacobson NS, Dobson KS, Truax PA, et al. A component analysis of cognitive-behavioral treatment for depression. *J Consult Clin Psychol.* 1996;64(2):295–304.
12. Martell CR, Addis ME, Jacobson NS. *Depression in Context: Strategies for Guided Action.* New York: WW Norton; 2001.
13. Lejuez CW, Hopko DR, Hopko SD. A brief behavioral activation treatment for depression: treatment manual. *Behav Modif.* 2001;25(2):255–286. doi:10.1177/0145445501252005
14. American Psychiatric Association. *Diagnostic and Statistical Manual of Mental Disorders (DSM-5).* Washington, DC: American Psychiatric Publishing; 2013.
15. Hopko DR, Ryba MM, McIndoo CC, File A. Behavioral activation. In: Nezu AM, Nezu CM, eds. *The Oxford Handbook of Cognitive and Behavioral Therapies.* New York: Oxford University Press; 2015:229–263.
16. Kanter JW, Manos RC, Bowe WM, Baruch DE, Busch AM, Rusch LC. What is behavioral activation? A review of the empirical literature. *Clin Psychol Rev.* 2010;30(6):608–620. doi:10.1016/j.cpr.2010.04.001
17. Macphillamy DJ, Lewinsohn PM. The pleasant events schedule: studies on reliability, validity, and scale intercorrelation. *J Consult Clin Psychol.* 1982;50(3):363–380.
18. Wilson PH. Combined pharmacological and behavioural treatment of depression. *Behav Res Ther.* 1982;20(2):173–184.
19. Hopko DR, Lejuez CW, Lepage JP, Hopko SD, Mcneil DW. A brief behavioral activation treatment for depression. *Behav Modif.* 2003;27(4):458–469. doi:10.1177/0145445503255489
20. Herrnstein RJ. On the law of effect. *J Exp Anal Behav.* 1970;13(2):243–266. doi:10.1901/jeab.1970.13-243
21. Kanter J, Busch AM, Rusch LC. *Behavioral Activation: Distinctive Features.* London and New York: Routledge; 2009.

22. McLean PD. Decision-making in the behavioral management of depression. In: Davidson PO, ed. *Behavioral Management of Anxiety, Depression, and Pain.* New York: Brunner/Mazel; 1976:91–146.

23. Jacobson NS, Martell CR, Dimidjian S. Behavioral activation treatment for depression: returning to contextual roots. *Clin Psychol Sci Pract.* 2001;8(3):255–270. doi:10.1093/clipsy.8.3.255

24. Ferster CB. A functional analysis of depression. *Am Psychol.* 1973;28(10):857–870.

25. Barrera M. An evaluation of a brief group therapy for depression. *J Consult Clin Psychol.* 1979;47(2):413–415. doi:10.1037/0022-006X.47.2.413

26. Biglan A, Craker D. Effects of pleasant-activities manipulation on depression. *J Consult Clin Psychol.* 1982;50(3):436–438. doi:10.1037/0022-006X.50.3.436

27. McNamara K, Horan JJ. Experimental construct validity in the evaluation of cognitive and behavioral treatments for depression. *J Couns Psychol.* 1986;33(1):23–30. doi:10.1037/0022-0167.33.1.23

28. Mazzucchelli T, Kane R, Rees C. Behavioral activation treatments for depression in adults: a meta-analysis and review. *Clin Psychol Sci Pract.* 2009;16(4):383–411. doi:10.1111/j.1468-2850.2009.01178.x

29. Beck AT. *Cognitive Therapy and the Emotional Disorders.* New York: International Universities Press; 1976.

30. Dimidjian S, Hollon SD, Dobson KS, et al. Randomized trial of behavioral activation, cognitive therapy, and antidepressant medication in the acute treatment of adults with major depression. *J Consult Clin Psychol.* 2006;74(4):658–670. doi:10.1037/0022-006X.74.4.658

31. Ekers D, Richards D, Gilbody S. A meta-analysis of randomized trials of behavioural treatment of depression. *Psychol Med.* 2008;38(05):611–623. doi:10.1017/S0033291707001614

32. Cuijpers P, van Straten A, Warmerdam L. Behavioral activation treatments of depression: a meta-analysis. *Clin Psychol Rev.* 2007;27(3):318–326. doi:10.1016/j.cpr.2006.11.001

33. Beck AT. Cognitive therapy: nature and relation to behavior therapy. *Behav Ther.* 1970;1(2):184–200. doi:10.1016/s0005-7894(70)80030-2

34. Ellis A. *Reason and Emotion in Psychotherapy.* Rev. and updated. Secaucus, NJ: Carol Pub. Group; 1962.

35. Beck AT, Steer RA. *Beck Depression Inventory: Manual.* San Antonio, TX: Psychiatric Corporation; 1987.

36. Dobson KS, Hollon SD, Dimidjian S, et al. Randomized trial of behavioral activation, cognitive therapy, and antidepressant medication in the prevention of relapse and recurrence in major depression. *J Consult Clin Psychol.* 2008;76(3):468–477. doi:10.1037/0022-006X.76.3.468

37. Hopko DR, Armento MEA, Robertson SMC, et al. Brief behavioral activation and problem-solving therapy for depressed breast cancer patients: randomized trial. *J Consult Clin Psychol.* 2011;79(6):834–849. doi:10.1037/a0025450

38. Hopko DR, Robertson SMC, Carvalho JP. Sudden gains in depressed cancer patients treated with behavioral activation therapy. *Behav Ther.* 2009;40(4):346–356. doi:10.1016/j.beth.2008.09.001

39. Ly KH, Trüschel A, Jarl L, et al. Behavioural activation versus mindfulness-based guided self-help treatment administered through a smartphone application: a randomised controlled trial. *BMJ Open.* 2014;4(1):e003440. doi:10.1136/bmjopen-2013-003440

40. O'Mahen HA, Woodford J, McGinley J, et al. Internet-based behavioral activation—treatment for postnatal depression (Netmums): a randomized controlled trial. *J Affect Disord.* 2013;150(3):814–822. doi:10.1016/j.jad.2013.03.005

41. Addis ME, Martell CR. *Overcoming Depression One Step at a Time: The New Behavioral Activation Approach to Getting Your Life Back.* Oakland, CA: New Harbinger Publishing; 2004.

42. Cox JL, Holden JM, Sagovsky R. Detection of postnatal depression: development of the 10-item Edinburgh Postnatal Depression Scale. *Br J Psychiatry J Ment Sci.* 1987;150:782–786.

43. Huguet A, Rao S, McGrath PJ, et al. A systematic review of cognitive behavioral therapy and behavioral activation apps for depression. *PLoS ONE*. 2016;11(5):e0154248. doi:10.1371/journal.pone.0154248

44. Porter JF, Spates CR, Smitham S. Behavioral activation group therapy in public mental health settings: a pilot investigation. *Prof Psychol Res Pract*. 2004;35(3):297–301. doi:10.1037/0735-7028.35.3.297

45. Chan ATY, Sun GYY, Tam WWS, Tsoi KKF, Wong SYS. The effectiveness of group-based behavioral activation in the treatment of depression: an updated meta-analysis of randomized controlled trial. *J Affect Disord*. 2017;208:345–354. doi:10.1016/j.jad.2016.08.026

46. Collado A, Castillo SD, Maero F, Lejuez CW, MacPherson L. Pilot of the brief behavioral activation treatment for depression in Latinos with limited English proficiency: preliminary evaluation of efficacy and acceptability. *Behav Ther*. 2014;45(1):102–115. doi:10.1016/j.beth.2013.10.001

47. Kanter JW, Santiago-Rivera AL, Santos MM, et al. A randomized hybrid efficacy and effectiveness trial of behavioral activation for Latinos with depression. *Behav Ther*. 2015;46(2):177–192. doi:10.1016/j.beth.2014.09.011

48. Polenick CA, Flora SR. Behavioral activation for depression in older adults: theoretical and practical considerations. *Behav Anal*. 2013;36(1):35–55.

PSYCHODYNAMIC AND SUPPORTIVE PSYCHOTHERAPY

DAVID J. HELLERSTEIN
AND ALEXANDER KANE

18.1. PSYCHODYNAMIC PSYCHOTHERAPY

The psychodynamic approach to psychotherapy is perhaps best conceptualized as a broad term that encompasses a number of specific therapeutic strategies bound together by their adherence to a "psychodynamic" understanding of the mind. These therapies rely on the idea that patterns of navigating the world that are established in early life can inform the thoughts, feelings, and behaviors of adults later in life. Historically, psychodynamic psychotherapy (PDT) was born out of Freud's psychoanalytic theory, which posited that very early experiences and memories can become codified in the adult mind just out of reach of consciousness—that is, as unconscious desires, thoughts, defenses, feelings, and conflicts. Indeed, Freud coined the term "psychodynamic" (derived from the Greek words *psyche*, meaning soul or mind, and *dynamis*, meaning force in motion), based on the observation that there seemed to be a constant interplay between these forces that made up the mind—with unconscious elements locked in struggle with the conscious mind, and vice versa, creating internal conflicts that may manifest in psychiatric symptoms or difficulties in adaptation. One of the primary goals and mechanisms of change in PDT is to make these unconscious elements increasingly conscious through the clinician's identification and interpretation of unconscious processes such as transference, defense mechanisms, and resistance.[1] Notably, while there is an enormous range of psychodynamic practices and attendant models of the mind, in this chapter we will focus chiefly on the commonalities of these approaches and the psychodynamic techniques used in the literature that have been demonstrated to be effective, evidence-based interventions for the treatment of depression.

While the roots of PDT remain indebted to the theories of Freud, a growing body of evidence indicates that for many patients, PDT is an effective monotherapy for mild or moderate depression, as well as a potentially useful adjunct to pharmacotherapy in cases of more severe depression.

18.1.1. What Is PDT?

While PDT may take on diverse forms in clinical practice, in the depression literature, PDT is often manualized, and conceptualized as a talking therapy that employs both supportive and interpretive interventions. Supportive interventions seek to bolster adaptive ego functions that are unavailable to the patient due to acute stress or insufficient development of these abilities. When the patient's ego function is relatively stable, interpretive interventions are deployed to draw attention to conscious or unconscious processes or conflicts, with the goal of improving insight into how these elements may sustain and perpetuate difficulties in function or psychopathology. Manualized treatments as used in randomized controlled trials (RCTs; e.g., Luborsky, *Principles of Psychoanalytic Psychotherapy: A Manual for Supportive-Expressive [SE] Treatment*, 2000[2]) incorporate both shorter-term PDT (7–24 sessions) and longer-term PDT (25–49 sessions, with treatment duration as long as 3 years). Notably, in clinical practice PDT is often open-ended in terms of duration and may last several years. As the methodology of RCTs does not lend itself well to the study of PDT as it is often practiced, naturalistic studies have sought to quantify the effectiveness of PDT as it is practiced in the community.[3]

While the specific features of a given PDT treatment may vary, the conceptual focus of PDT is relatively uniform. In both manualized form and in clinical practice, PDT concerns itself with the development of a therapeutic relationship; discussion of past experiences; identifying patterns of avoidance, resistance patterns, and patterns of interpersonal conflict; exploration of fantasies and dreams; and consideration of the processes of transference and countertransference.[4,5]

18.1.2. Theoretical Framework and Key Concepts

Underlying PDT is a particular "dynamic" understanding of how the mind works and an extensive theoretical framework, the most critical concepts of which are reviewed here.

18.1.2.1. Unconscious

In PDT, the unconscious refers to the sum of mental activity that occurs outside of the awareness of the conscious mind. The unconscious comprises memories, feelings, desires, thoughts, and perceptions of self and others that are theorized to be generated by a confluence of genetics, temperament, and early childhood experiences and exposures. Over time, these elements are codified into the way we experience the world—they are hidden from consciousness, in part, to allow for more efficient processing of experiences, but at other times can be kept out of awareness as they may generate feelings of fear, shame, guilt, or anger that are difficult for the conscious mind to tolerate.

18.1.2.2. Defense Mechanisms

Defense mechanisms are a set of strategies that people use, often unconsciously and automatically, to manage distress, anxiety, and conflict and to preserve self-esteem. These coping mechanisms limit a person's awareness or experience of painful affect or conflicts, which are necessary (for all people!) to navigate the world without being continually overwhelmed by negative feelings. Defense mechanisms are often divided into classes of relatively less adaptive and more adaptive defenses. Less adaptive defenses are labeled as such because they preserve good feelings at a high cost—for example, a patient who uses denial to disavow negative emotions may experience frequent chest pain but not present for medical care until he has had a massive heart attack. More adaptive defenses typically rely on repression—that is, painful or unacceptable thoughts or feelings are unconsciously pushed out of awareness to preserve good feelings. Of note, patients' defenses are often heterogeneous—even the high-functioning patient may use less adaptive strategies when under stress, and lower-functioning patients may have domains of function wherein they use more adaptive defenses.[6]

18.1.2.3. Free Association and Resistance

Free association, the patient's attempt to say whatever comes to mind without editing,[6] is used in PDT to elicit unconscious material. In PDT, the patient's free association ideally produces a flow of associations between thoughts, feelings, and memories that may reveal unconscious connections and ultimately lead to material previously outside of awareness. Resistance, on the other hand, consists of those actions the patient takes, consciously or unconsciously, in order to oppose the processes of free association, and more broadly, the processes of therapy that may produce insight and change. It is critical to recognize that patients are often ambivalent about change and about engaging with the uncomfortable thoughts, feelings, and conflicts that may arise in the course of therapy. Resistance in PDT is perhaps best understood as an activation of the patient's defense mechanisms within the therapy to protect against these uncomfortable thoughts, feelings, or conflicts. While resistance may appear, prima facie, to detract from the therapeutic process, it in fact arms the psychodynamic therapist with data regarding the set defense mechanisms the patient uses to defuse painful material.

18.1.2.4. Transference

Transference is the collection of thoughts and feelings, both conscious and unconscious, that a patient has toward the therapist. Transference can be related to the patient's experience of the therapist in the here-and-now, but in PDT, transference perhaps more commonly refers to the displacement of thoughts and feelings that are connected to a prominent figure from the patient's past onto the therapist. Notably, transference is not static nor monolithic, and the therapist may evoke multiple transferences (e.g., maternal, paternal, or sibling transferences), which may evolve and fluctuate over time. By recognizing transference and, when appropriate, making these reactions to the therapist conscious, the psychodynamic therapist and patient may gain insight into how the patient interfaces with others.

18.1.2.5. Countertransference

Conversely, countertransference is a term meant to describe the sum of thoughts and feelings, both conscious and unconscious, that the therapist has toward the patient. Historically, countertransference was thought to be something that interfered with treatment and ought to be minimized, but it is now recognized to be a helpful concept in guiding treatment. It is important to note that countertransference is in fact a broader term that encapsulates two categories of feelings toward the patient: (1) feelings that originate in the therapist and that the therapist may feel toward many patients (e.g., the therapist always feels maternal toward young male patients, who remind her of her son) and (2) feelings that are induced by a specific patient (e.g., a patient who says very little in sessions may induce feelings of frustration in the therapist). The therapist seeks to identify and understand these types of countertransference, which can ultimately decrease the chances that he or she might unconsciously act on these thoughts or feelings, allow the therapist to experience what others in the patient's life might experience, and better understand how the patient functions and relates to others.

18.1.2.6. Interpretation

Interpretations are statements made by the therapist designed to bring unconscious material into consciousness, or identify linkages that were previously outside the patient's awareness, with the goal of enhancing the patient's insight into how his or her mind works. For example, a psychodynamic therapist might make the following interpretation: "I wonder if you might have difficulties opening up to your wife because you're afraid if she learns more about you, she might leave you." Here, the interpretation seeks to explain something that is conscious (i.e., the patient's recognition that he is having difficulty expressing himself to his wife) as being caused by unconscious material (i.e., his fear that his wife will leave him).

18.1.3. Principles of Treatment and Mechanisms of Change in PDT

While stereotypes of PDT in popular culture bring to mind the image of a silent, stoic, and aloof therapist, the contemporary psychodynamic therapist, much like the supportive psychotherapy (SPT) therapist, may be warm, conversational, and spontaneous. Indeed, the therapeutic techniques in PDT fall along the continuum of supportive–interpretive interventions, and the elements of SPT and PDT may overlap considerably (Tables 18.1 and 18.2): Both rely heavily on the fostering of a therapeutic alliance, empathic validation, open-ended questions, maintenance of the treatment

TABLE 18.1. Comparison of SPT and PDT

	PDT	SPT
Conceptual Basis and Goals	1. Ameliorate symptoms and maintain, restore, or improve self-esteem, adaptive skills, and psychological functioning 2. Emphasis on affect and emotional response 3. Identify and confront defense mechanisms 4. Examine the past and its relationship to the present 5. Explore repetitive patterns in behavior, feelings, interpersonal experiences 6. Build insight into internal conflicts, development of more adaptive and more flexible ways of being	1. Ameliorate symptoms and maintain, restore, or improve self-esteem, adaptive skills, and psychological functioning 2. Examine relationships and patients' emotional response and or behavior 3. Respect adaptive defenses 4. Emphasize real relationship
Therapeutic Relationship	1. Therapist generally neutral and expectant, though may take conversational or supportive stance when appropriate 2. Therapist is nondirective, allows patient to free associate 3. Therapist may actively interpret transference relationship or patient's defenses 4. Therapist demonstrates respect and commitment to stick with patient and not reject because he or she does not get well	1. Therapist is conversationally responsive 2. Therapist collaborates in goal setting 3. Agenda can be set by patient or therapist 4. Therapist frames termination similar to an end of an academic course 5. Therapist demonstrates respect and commitment to stick with patient and not reject because he or she does not get well
Interventions	1. Listening 2. Empathic reflection 3. Validation 4. Encouragement to elaborate 5. Clarification 6. Confrontation 7. Observation 8. Interpretation	1. Clarification 2. Confrontation 3. Rationalization 4. Reframing 5. Encouragement 6. Advice 7. Modeling 8. Rehearsal and anticipation 9. Listening

TABLE 18.1. Continued

	PDT	SPT
Application to MDD/PDD	1. Focus on conflicts or ego functions associated with symptoms 2. Ongoing fostering of therapeutic alliance (alliance as predictor of outcome) 3. Addressing situations (interpersonal, behavioral, intrapsychic) that predispose to or maintain depression 4. Accurate interpretations of conflicts or transferences related to symptoms	1. Clear discussion of expectation and clarification of goals with SPT 2. Early (and ongoing) efforts to develop therapeutic alliance 3. Efforts to provide psychoeducation about depression and likely outcomes of treatment, starting from initiation of treatment and continuing throughout course of treatment 4. Ongoing efforts to limit self-destructive behavior; assessment of suicidality risks 5. Support of patient's efforts to deal with symptoms of depression, to re-regulate circadian rhythms, and to maximize daily functioning 6. Addressing situations (interpersonal, behavioral, intrapsychic) that predispose to or maintain depression 7. Treatment should progress from an early focus on acute depressive state (including risk of self-injury); to attaining and maintaining remission from depression; to working toward recovery from depression, including enhancing interpersonal and social skills and problem-solving abilities 8. Work to prevent recurrence of depression and development of chronicity

TABLE 18.2. Characteristics of PDT vs. SPT

Item	PDT	SPT
Empathy	++	++
Reassurance	+	++
Clarification	++	++
Anticipatory guidance	+	++
Normalization	+	++
Reframing	+	++
Limit setting	+	+
Discussion of symptoms and side effects	+	+
Psychoeducation about depressive disorders	+	++
Psychoeducation about interpersonal and psychological issues	++	+++
Extensive assessment of psychiatric disorder and related medical conditions	+	+
Extensive assessment of psychological issues	+++	++
Ongoing detailed discussion of psychological issues	+++	++
Patient and clinician believe they are engaged in ongoing psychotherapy	+++	++
Clinician is aware of transference/therapeutic alliance on ongoing basis	+++	++
Confrontation of defenses	+++	+
Interpretation of transference	+++	+
Focus on past conflicts and childhood experiences	+++	+
Rehearsal and anticipation	+	++
Cognitive restructuring	+	++
Appropriate rationalization	+	++
Examination of relationships and patients' emotional responses and/or behaviors	+++	++
Efforts to limit self-destructive behavior, assessment of suicide risk	++	++
Support patient's efforts to deal with symptoms of disorder	+	++
Systematic attempts to enhance self-esteem, psychological functions, adaptive skills	+	++

frame, therapeutic neutrality, and the use of supportive interventions in order to shore up weakened function. Distinguishing PDT from SPT is the focus on the above dynamic concepts—such as free association, resistance, transference and countertransference, as well as the preferential use of interpretative techniques—in order to draw attention to unconscious thoughts, feelings, patterns of behavior, or linkages between ideas that may be outside of the patient's awareness. PDT presupposes that, in the context of a strong therapeutic alliance, by bringing unconscious material into consciousness, identifying characteristic defense mechanisms, and exploring repetitive patterns that occur both in the transference and outside relationships, the patient builds insight and self-awareness that ultimately contribute to the development of more adaptive and more flexible ways of negotiating the world.

18.1.4. Psychodynamic Explanations of Depression

Most contemporary psychodynamic therapists more comprehensively conceptualize depressive disorders as heterogeneous phenomena that emerge from a complex and unique interplay of biological, psychological, and social factors.[1] With an appropriate patient, however, the psychodynamic therapist will privilege a dynamic understanding of depression. Each of the many psychodynamic theories of mind will have different explanations for distress and depressive states, with each theory's favored elements taking a more central role in the etiology of depression (see reference 7 for further detail). In general, however, PDT takes a more person-focused approach, as opposed to the symptom-guided understanding of depression that one might encounter in the psychopharmacological treatment of depression, and therefore conceptualizes depression as a basic emotional state in all individuals that exists on a continuum ranging from euthymia to mild dysthymia to clinical depression. Broadly speaking, PDT supposes that depression is an affective state that signals a discrepancy between the patient's actual state-of-self and his or her "wished-for state." In this understanding, depression is a set of symptoms that emerge when the patient confronts the gap between his or her actual self and ideal self.[8] Often this gap is generated by persistent interpersonal difficulties, developmental stagnation, distorted self-perceptions, and maladaptive ways of dealing with stress. More contemporary psychodynamic formulations have noted the contributions of specific biopsychosocial elements such as personality traits, self-esteem regulation, characteristic adaptations to stress, attachment style, interpersonal relationships, trauma and stress, among others, to depression;[1] however, the formulation of depression as a problem that emerges when a patient's thoughts, feelings, behaviors or relationships do not align with his or her ideals is one that remains clinically relevant.

18.1.5. Whom to Treat—Selection Criteria for PDT

In PDT, much more so than SPT or cognitive–behavioral therapy (CBT), which seem to be more broadly applicable,[9] effective treatment relies on the particular qualities and abilities of the patient. As such, the selection of appropriate patients is critical for optimization of treatment outcomes. Psychological characteristics that suggest a patient may be a suitable candidate for PDT include being reasonably psychologically minded, intelligent, and able to relate to others in a meaningful and consistent way and to form intimate relationships, with symptoms or distress that seem to arise from intrapsychic conflict driven by competing wishes or desires. Patients should be relatively psychiatrically stable, highly motivated to engage in treatment, and able to tolerate the discomfort and intense affect that may emerge during therapy.[9]

18.1.6. Limitations of PDT

PDT is generally not recommended for patients with major substance abuse, psychosis, severe affective disorders, or active, acute suicidality, as the exploration of painful or uncomfortable experiences and affects in a less supportive setting may precipitate a worsening of symptoms or decrement in function. Patients who are unable to form a trusting therapeutic alliance, such as those with antisocial personality disorder, severe narcissistic personality disorder, or marked paranoia, are unlikely to benefit from PDT. Patients who are less introspective or interested in more explicitly targeting problematic thought and behavioral patterns related to their depression may prefer more structured therapy modalities, such as CBT.

18.1.7. Evidence Basis

18.1.7.1. PDT Monotherapy

When taken from a traditional psychodynamic perspective, the efficacy and outcome of a given course of PDT is determined in part by the psychodynamic characteristics of the patient (e.g., personality structure, array of defenses, degree of insight).[1,3,9] Furthermore, the RCTs included in many meta-analyses of PDT are of variable quality, and the therapy itself, while consistent with the broader conceptual considerations, may vary across trials in both quality and the specific features of the therapy. These caveats notwithstanding, there is a growing body of literature, including manualized RCTs as well as naturalistic studies, demonstrating that PDT's efficacy in the treatment of patients meeting criteria for mild or moderate depression is equivalent to both CBT and SPT.[10] Indeed, one meta-analysis of five trials (with total $n = 435$ patients with depressive disorders) that compared short-term psychodynamic psychotherapy (10–24 weekly sessions) with a control condition (treatment as usual, waiting list, or minimal treatment) found PDT to be an effective treatment for mild or moderate depression as compared to control groups, with a moderate clinical benefit.[11] Likewise, a more robust meta-analysis of 23 RCTs (2,751 patients) showed no significant difference in outcomes between CBT and short-term PDT.[4] More broadly, one study performed seven meta-analyses of 53 randomized trials (2,757 patients with mild to moderate depression) comparing PDT of any duration to six other common psychotherapies and found no clinically significant difference in outcomes between PDT and all other therapies.[12]

18.1.7.2. Combined Treatment

Few studies have tested the efficacy of combining PDT with an antidepressant, either for treating acute unipolar depression or as maintenance treatment for preventing recurrence of depression; however, the limited studies that have been done suggest that the combination of PDT and antidepressants may be superior to medication alone.

In acute depression, very limited data suggest that PDT plus pharmacotherapy may provide superior outcomes compared with pharmacotherapy alone. One randomized trial compared combination treatment (PDT plus clomipramine) with clomipramine alone in 74 patients with unipolar major depression. This study found that significantly fewer patients who received combination treatment, in comparison to clomipramine alone, met criteria for major depression at 10 weeks (9% vs. 28%). In addition, psychosocial functioning was significantly better in patients who received combination treatment.[13]

As maintenance treatment, there is again some evidence to suggest that combination treatment of PDT plus antidepressants may support maintenance of improvements made during early stages of treatment compared to pharmacotherapy alone. In one such study, patients with major depression who had been successfully treated with six months of combination treatment ($n = 41$) or with pharmacotherapy alone ($n = 51$) were then subsequently treated for an additional six months with pharmacotherapy alone. At the end of this six-month period, all treatment was stopped and patients were prospectively followed for up to four years: Recurrence of major depression occurred in significantly fewer patients who had received combined treatment compared with patients who had received pharmacotherapy alone (27% vs. 47%).[14]

18.2. SUPPORTIVE PSYCHOTHERAPY

18.2.1. Why SPT for Treatment of Depression?

SPT is a commonly practiced form of psychotherapy[15] and is adaptable to a wide range of patients. Therapists from various backgrounds, including psychodynamic, cognitive-behavioral, interpersonal, and others, commonly provide SPT to some of their patients. In psychotherapy outcome studies, meta-analyses have shown that SPT has significant efficacy, generally comparable to other treatment approaches such as CBT, interpersonal therapy (IPT), etc.[12] Since mood and anxiety disorders are prevalent among populations of patients seeking psychotherapy, it makes sense to use SPT as a treatment framework for various forms of depression, including major depressive disorder (MDD) and persistent depressive disorder (PDD). SPT can be easily combined with other treatment approaches, such as psychopharmacology, which can add to its utility in treating depression. Since SPT is used for a wide range of conditions, when provided as an antidepressant psychotherapy, it may be beneficial to adapt it specifically for treatment of mood disorders.

18.2.2. What Is Supportive Psychotherapy?

SPT has been defined in various ways by different authors.[2,16-19] Some have described SPT as a treatment with minimal goals that is only suitable for very impaired patients. Karasu,[20] for instance, defines SPT as "the creation of a therapeutic relationship as a temporary buttress or bridge for the deficient patient."

In such models, SPT may not be a stand-alone therapy but instead one pole of a supportive–expressive continuum.[2] SPT may also be defined in a minimal way, as a treatment providing only support and empathy; however, we would call this a "supportive relationship"; it resembles what has been called "nondirective supportive psychotherapy" (NDST), which is often used as an attentional control in psychotherapy studies.[21] While earlier authors such as Rockland[17] and Kernberg[16] defined SPT within a psychoanalytic framework, recent authors[18,19] often define SPT in a way that may be characterized as atheoretical.

In recent models,[18,19] SPT is an active verbal treatment, with a conversational style, which has the goals of maintaining or improving self-esteem, adaptive skills, and psychological functioning (see Tables 18.1 and 18.2). It uses techniques such as clarification, suggestions, praise, reassurance, cognitive restructuring, normalization, and rehearsal and anticipation. Aims include promoting a supportive patient–therapist relationship; enhancing the patient's strengths, coping skills, and abilities to use environmental supports; reducing distress and behavioral dysfunction; achieving independence from psychiatric illness; and maximizing autonomy in treatment decisions.[18] SPT examines relationships and patients' emotional responses and/or behavior with the goal of improving psychosocial functioning. These new models of SPT as a broadly applicable change- and improvement-oriented treatment are in marked contrast to those writers[20] who have viewed SPT as best suited to low-functioning patients and with limited goals of stabilization or preventing decompensation. As an active treatment approach, modern SPT has goals comparable to other modalities such as CBT or IPT.

18.2.2.1. Therapeutic Relationship

The SPT therapist maintains a conversational style, rather than allowing prolonged silences, and demonstrates involvement, empathy, nonjudgmental acceptance, and an appropriate level of interest in the patient's life. SPT therapists respect adaptive defenses or coping mechanisms.[22] In contrast to PDT, in SPT the "real relationship" rather than the transference is emphasized, though the therapist monitors the status of the therapeutic alliance, and may address the therapeutic relationship if the treatment is threatened. There is no effort to enhance the development of what a psychodynamic therapist might call a transference; in fact, this is avoided by trying to decrease the patient's in-session anxiety and to minimize regression. The SPT therapist is not as concerned about anonymity as a psychodynamic therapist might be. He or she might respond briefly to direct questions by the patient and may otherwise use judicious self-disclosure.

18.2.2.2. Goal Setting

The goals of SPT are commonly set in a process of discussion between therapist and patient and may vary over the course of treatment. Goal setting in SPT is a collaborative process based on both the patient's and the clinician's assessment of significant life issues. SPT is primarily present- and future-focused, though it does not ignore past issues. Past experiences are explored in the context of present life issues rather than using the present as a means of entry to exploring past issues.

18.2.2.3. Dealing with Defenses and Transference

Principles of SPT suggest that transference and countertransference issues must be addressed when the frame of the treatment is threatened—for instance, if the patient's attendance of sessions is affected by feelings toward the therapist. Whereas psychodynamic therapists address both positive and negative transference, SPT therapists usually address only the negative transference.

18.2.2.4. Mechanism of Change

The so-called common factors (which include the therapeutic alliance between therapist and client, belief in the treatment, and a clear rationale explaining why the client has developed the problems)[23] contribute to the efficacy of all therapies, including SPT. SPT approaches may have additional benefits—for instance, enabling patients to use existing capabilities that have been obscured by depression. SPT employs ongoing psychoeducation about depression, which may help decrease anxiety and isolation and activate positive coping responses. Many such changes, such as increasing adaptive behaviors and thought patterns, may also occur with other treatments such as CBT, although SPT does not require specific homework assignments or in-session exercises. Though there is a paucity of neuroimaging studies, it is possible that SPT activates brain networks related to executive functioning, increasing top-down regulation of affective states (including fear, anxiety, and sadness), increasing activity of reward networks, and perhaps decreasing hyperactivity of brain networks related to negative ruminations such as the default mode network.[24]

18.2.3 Description of SPT for Depression

SPT does not require major adaptation for use as a specific treatment of depression. It can facilitate recovery from a single episode of MDD or can address the longstanding symptoms of PDD. The main change is a focus on depression as a neuropsychobiological syndrome with common symptoms and significant effects on a patient's perceptions, psychosocial functioning, social relationships, and outlook toward the future. Given that the course of depression is often relapsing and may become chronic, supportive psychotherapy for depression (SPT-D) should focus not only on recovery from an individual episode but on improving long-term outcomes. As a disorder increasing risk of self-injury and suicide, SPT-D should specifically address these issues.

SPT techniques in the context of depression (see Table 18.2) include the following:

- *Reframing*: "You're not a 'bad person'—you have a disorder that changes how people think about themselves and their futures."

- *Normalizing*: "These symptoms [hopelessness, pessimism, self-deprecation, ruminations] are commonly seen in this disorder; they are not your 'fault' "; "It's common for symptoms to last for weeks and gradually improve."
- *Anticipatory guidance*: "If the suicidal ideas come back, how can you plan to cope with them?" "If you have trouble staying asleep, how can you plan to respond?"
- *Confrontation:* "You have a very strong feeling that your life will never get better and you'll never get out of this depression—and yet, you mention that you felt *good* for several hours yesterday, so it's a struggle for you to see that things are actually beginning to improve."
- *Enhancing self-esteem:* "Depression can be seen as a biological illness, so it's not a matter of weakness, it's something that can be coped with successfully."
- *Enhancing psychological functions:* The therapist can help the patient to use more adaptive psychological responses, such as suppression, catharsis, rationalization, humor, and intellectualization.
- *Using adaptive skills:* The therapist can clarify the patient's capacities and what has been helpful in overcoming prior adversities, and can identify the patient's strengths within the context of current symptoms so there is a high likelihood of success, not over-challenging or under-challenging the patient.[25]

SPT may be adapted to address core symptoms of MDD and PDD, including vegetative, cognitive, interpersonal, and affective. Empathy, understanding, and catharsis can increase self-esteem by normalizing the patient's experiences. Vegetative symptoms may be improved by decreasing anxiety and enhancing adaptive behaviors such as diet, decreasing use of stimulants and alcohol, and regularizing sleep. Cognitive symptoms can be addressed by focusing on distortions and by problem solving for concentration and attention problems. Interpersonal symptoms can be addressed by discussing the role of avoidance and isolation as a response to depression that can paradoxically worsen the depression. Modulation of behavior and thoughts may be enhanced by allowing the patient to assume the sickness role, and setting appropriate expectations via reframing of goals at specific phases of treatment. Suicidal risk can be approached by clarification of risk factors and social supports. Anticipatory guidance can help the patient to choose adaptive options when risk increases. SPT can also be combined with case management, family involvement, and clinical outreach services as needed. A course of SPT for a major depressive episode might last approximately 12 to 16 weeks, followed by monthly booster sessions.

Major goals of early treatment include:

- Assessment, diagnosis, formulation
- Crisis management
- Preventing self-injury, suicide

- Tolerating and alleviating symptoms
- Managing side effects
- Setting goals for further treatment

In mid-treatment, psychological and behavioral changes could include:

- Healthy behaviors: exercise, diet, medication compliance, decreasing substance abuse
- Interpersonal skills: increased appropriate risk taking, increased assertiveness, practicing new behavioral interactions, working on modulating interactions with others ("getting what you want and need")
- Addressing residual cognitive and intrapsychic issues, such as low self-esteem, risk averseness, all-or-nothing thinking, catastrophizing.

After several months of treatment, major goals often include:

- Enhancing response: moving from remission toward recovery
- Preventing relapse, recurrence, and chronicity
- Skill development, addressing life goals
- In cases where extended remission of a disorder has been achieved, helping the patient to "extend himself or herself"
- In severe cases, helping patients to tolerate chronic symptoms; realistically optimize adaptation.

SPT's flexible approach can enable clinicians to incorporate techniques and interventions from other psychotherapies. Depression-focused SPT can incorporate techniques from CBT, IPT, and PDT, as well as complementary modalities such as mindfulness meditation or relaxation training.

18.2.4. Combining SPT and Pharmacotherapy

SPT can be easily combined with pharmacotherapy.[26] Psychotherapy can be added to pharmacotherapy with additional benefit as shown by studies of depressed inpatients[27] and outpatients.[28,29] Options include:

- Concurrent treatment (SPT and medication) whether provided by a single clinician or separate clinicians
- Augmentation or sequencing (e.g., add medication to ongoing SPT, or add SPT to ongoing medication)
- Switching (from SPT to psychopharmacological treatment)
- Intermittent use: ongoing pharmacotherapy with intermittent SPT when needed, or ongoing SPT with intermittent use of pharmacotherapy.

Pharmacotherapy may enhance SPT in various ways.[26] Symptom control through medication treatment may enable a patient to work productively in psychotherapy. Improving sleep, normalizing mood, and decreasing anxiety may allow the patient to feel calm and more stable. Selective serotonin reuptake inhibitors (SSRIs) and various mood stabilizers may allow for decreased rejection sensitivity and increased resiliency. On a biological level, medications may decrease hyperarousal of hypothalamic–pituitary–adrenal stress response systems, may lower amygdala activation and enhance adaptive brain plasticity, and may even prompt hippocampal neurogenesis, which has been hypothesized to allow for less black-and-white thinking and more modulated behavioral responses.[24] All of these factors may allow patients to work more productively in psychotherapy.

SPT may also enhance pharmacotherapy, particularly in dealing with individuals with comorbid Axis II diagnoses. Behaviors such as avoidance and social isolation, impulsivity, affective instability, dependency in relationships, black-and-white thinking, and unpracticed social skills may make it difficult for them to keep appointments, take medication regularly, and otherwise become engaged in the patient role. The conversational dialogs of SPT may engage such patients in a therapeutic process to enable them to benefit from pharmacotherapy.

18.2.5. Empirical Studies Supporting the Use of SPT in MDD/PDD

Individual studies of SPT shows benefit in various disorders, including depression and borderline personality disorder, often comparable in efficacy to other treatment approaches.[30,31] The largest body of studies of SPT, however, is for the relatively inactive NDST, which is unlikely to meet standards defined by major writers on SPT.[18,19] In NDST, therapists are instructed only to empathically reflect what the patient tells them[21] rather than participating actively in a psychotherapy as they would in clinical practice. They are prohibited from giving advice or setting treatment goals. Conclusions about the efficacy of SPT from studies of NDST are at best problematic. Nevertheless, there appears to be a common belief that other therapies have been shown to be superior to SPT.

Researcher allegiance to the "active" comparator may play a role both in the conduct of studies and the interpretation of results. For example, in a meta-analysis[32] of 31 studies of NDST, Cuijpers et al. found that NDST "is effective in the treatment of depression in adults. While it was less effective than other psychological treatments (differential effect size $g = -0.20$; 95% CI: -0.32 to -0.08, $p < 0.01$), . . . *these differences were no longer present after controlling for researcher allegiance*" [emphasis added]. Cuijpers et al. concluded that NDST "has a considerable effect on symptoms of depression," mostly from nonspecific factors.

Budge et al.[33] stated:

> Supportive therapy is an established and bona-fide therapy but its implementation
> as a control group for non-specific elements is a treatment that does not resemble

supportive therapy as would be used therapeutically. Allegiance effects . . . are caused by the design of supportive therapy controls, the therapists who deliver supportive therapy, and the patients who are enrolled in the trials.

One might add that individual study reports may be biased toward small differences favoring the researchers' preferred treatment. Indeed, Baardseth et al.[34] found a similar phenomenon in a meta-analysis of anxiety disorders research. Though CBT is commonly believed to be the most effective psychotherapy for anxiety disorders, their meta-analysis found that

> there were no differences between CBT treatments and bona fide non-CBT treatments across disorder-specific and non-disorder specific symptom measures. These analyses, in combination with previous meta-analytic findings, fail to provide corroborative evidence for the conjecture that CBT is superior to bona fide non-CBT treatments.

We are unaware of studies directly comparing NDST to more full-fledged, indeed "bona-fide" SPT, an additional reason that claims a particular psychotherapy is superior to SPT should be viewed with caution.

18.2.5.1. Comparability to Pharmacotherapy

In a meta-analysis of 67 studies of depression ($N = 40$) and anxiety disorders ($N = 27$), pharmacotherapy and psychotherapy had a similar overall effect size. Pharmacotherapy was more efficacious than psychotherapy for dysthymia. Also, pharmacotherapy was more effective than "nondirective counseling,"[35] though in another meta-analysis Cuijpers found that lower effect may be the result of researcher allegiance.[21]

18.2.5.2. Comparison of Different Psychotherapies

In a study comparing the efficacy of various psychotherapies for depression in adults, Cuijpers et al. conducted seven meta-analyses for psychological treatments for mild to moderate adult depression, including CBT, NDST, behavioral activation treatment, psychodynamic treatment, problem-solving therapy, IPT, and social skills training. Each psychotherapy had been studied in at least five RCTs. Overall there was no indication that any of the treatments was more or less successful, except that IPT was somewhat more efficacious ($d = 0.20$) and NDST was somewhat less efficacious ($d = -0.13$). Overall, Cuijpers et al. found no large differences between the major psychotherapies for mild to moderate depression.[12]

18.2.5.3. Outcome of Chronic Depression

In a review of psychotherapy of chronic MDD and dysthymia (what would now be included under the fifth edition of the American Psychiatric Association's *Diagnostic and Statistical Manual of Mental Disorders* [DSM-5] diagnosis of

PDD), Cuijpers et al. conducted a meta-analysis of RCTs, including CBT, IPT, problem-solving therapy, behavioral activation therapy, social skills training, and NDST. They found that "psychotherapy had a small but significant effect ($d = 0.23$) on depression when compared to control groups. Psychotherapy was significantly less effective than pharmacotherapy in direct comparisons ($d = -0.31$), especially SSRIs." Notably, combined psychotherapy and pharmacotherapy was more effective than pharmacotherapy alone ($d = 0.23$) or psychotherapy alone ($d = 0.45$). In dysthymia, SSRIs appeared superior to psychotherapy. No significant differences were found in dropout rates between psychotherapy and the other conditions. Cuijpers et al. concluded that psychotherapy is effective in the treatment of chronic depression and dysthymia, but probably not as effective as pharmacotherapy (particularly the SSRIs). Also of note, Cuijpers et al. found indications that at least 18 treatment sessions were needed to achieve optimal effects of psychotherapy in chronic depression.

18.2.6. Limitations of SPT in MDD/PDD

SPT may be ineffective for some depressed patients. For such patients (e.g., with agitated depression) requiring a higher level of care, such as inpatient hospitalization, weekly psychotherapy may delay use of a more effective treatment. Patients who are unwilling to meet regularly with a therapist or to engage in verbal therapy may be unsuited for SPT. It is worth noting, however, that SPT can be a model for psychotherapy treatments provided in many settings, including day treatment programs and acute inpatient psychiatric settings, and among patients with high levels of symptom severity, if combined with other treatment approaches. Other patients may benefit more from more specific treatment approaches, such as CBT, dialectical behavior therapy, or problem-solving therapy.

Some patients may experience SPT as "superficial" or inadequately intense to meet their expectations and may prefer to explore fantasies, dreams, and in-session affective states; these patients may prefer PDT. Other patients may prefer to work intensively on changing thought and behavior patterns related to their depression and may be more suitable for CBT. However, there is little empirical evidence to determine who such patients may be or whether they receive additional benefit.

Patients who have previously failed to improve with competently performed SPT should be candidates for other treatment approaches.

18.2.7. Who Is Best Suited for SPT?

Most individuals who are willing to enter psychotherapy would be suitable for SPT, since SPT does not require a particular level of motivation (e.g., to do homework, as with CBT) or an ability to be introspective (as for PDT). SPT is worth considering for patients who are reluctant to take medications, as an initial treatment for some (e.g., allowing time to address concerns about medications). SPT approaches are generally useful and may be necessary for depressed patients at suicidal risk.[18] A trial of SPT for MDD may be conducted for a period of weeks or months (but not years) prior to considering other approaches. For some patients SPT may be effective as a solo treatment, with comparable efficacy to other antidepressant psychotherapies.

18.3. SUMMARY AND CONCLUSIONS

In an era favoring somatic therapies, including medications and various methods of brain stimulation, it is important to consider psychotherapy options for depression treatment, including IPT and CBT, but also broadly practiced psychotherapies such as PDT and SPT. A significant body of evidence suggests that both PDT and SPT are helpful for many patients with MDD and other mood disorders.

There is a need for more research on SPT since it is often the default treatment in clinical practice. It is also often a treatment of choice, given the large population of patients with mood disorders, and given the general high level of acceptability of SPT to both practitioners and patients. PDT, though suitable for a narrower range of patients, deserves more study, as it provides an alternative approach that many patients and clinicians prefer, and may be efficacious for patients who do not respond to other approaches.

Psychotherapy researchers should use a robust, active model of SPT (like Novalis,[18] Pinsker,[19] or Rockland's[17] models) when studying putatively more active or specific treatments such as dialectical behavior therapy or CBT, rather than using attentional controls such as NDST. Similarly, they should study robust PDT models that are manualized and that incorporate common PDT approaches.

In clinical settings, practitioners should use robust well-defined psychotherapy models (e.g., bona-fide SPT or PDT) to treat depression and should have clear understandings of treatment goals and defined interventions. They should, in collaboration with patients, define a finite timeframe of treatment, at the end of which other options should be pursued.

Key points are as follows:

- PDT refers to a group of specific therapeutic strategies positing that unconscious content, often related to earlier life experiences, may generate conflicts within a patient, which may manifest as distress or psychiatric symptoms.
- While less broadly applicable than SPT, PDT is an effective monotherapy in patients with mild to moderate depression.
- A subset of patients, including those who are particularly psychologically minded or whose difficulties seem to be driven by intrapsychic conflict, may prefer the exploratory focus of PDT as opposed to more structured therapies, such as CBT.
- SPT is the most commonly practiced form of psychotherapy and is often combined with pharmacotherapy.

- SPT is a broad-spectrum treatment with well-defined techniques and is applicable to a wide range of patients in various treatment settings.
- SPT may be the psychotherapy of choice for many patients with mood disorders.
- There are numerous ways to combine SPT and pharmacotherapy, including concurrent, sequential, and augmenting treatment strategies, and treatment can also include components of other treatments such as CBT.
- There is a need for more research on rigorously performed SPT and PDT, both with and without pharmacotherapy.

REFERENCES

1. Gabbard GO. Techniques of psychodynamic psychotherapy. In: Gabbard GO, ed. *Textbook of Psychotherapeutic Treatments.* Washington, DC: American Psychiatric Press; 2009:43–68.
2. Luborsky L. *Principles of Psychoanalytic Psychotherapy: A Manual for Supportive-Expressive Treatment.* New York: Basic Books, 1984.
3. Leichsenring F. Applications of psychodynamic psychotherapy to specific disorders. In: Gabbard GO, ed. *Textbook of Psychotherapeutic Treatments.* Washington, DC: American Psychiatric Press; 2009:97–132.
4. Steinert C, Munder T, Rabung S, Hoyer J, Leichsenring F. Psychodynamic therapy: as efficacious as other empirically supported treatments? A meta-analysis testing equivalence of outcomes. *Am J Psychiatry.* 2017;174(10):943–953.
5. Shedler J. The efficacy of psychodynamic psychotherapy. *Am Psychol.* 2010;65(2):98.
6. Cabaniss DL. *Psychodynamic Psychotherapy: A Clinical Manual.* New York: John Wiley & Sons; 2016.
7. Gabbard GO. *Psychodynamic Psychiatry in Clinical Practice.* Washington, DC: American Psychiatric Publishing; 2014.
8. Luyten P, Blatt SJ. Psychodynamic treatment of depression. *Psychiatr Clin North Am.* 2012;35(1):111–129.
9. Valbak K. Suitability for psychoanalytic psychotherapy: a review. *Acta Psychiatr Scand.* 2004;109(3):164–178.
10. Leichsenring F, Luyten P, Hilsenroth MJ, et al. Psychodynamic therapy meets evidence-based medicine: a systematic review using updated criteria. *Lancet Psychiatry.* 2015;2(7):648–660.
11. Abbass AA, Kisely SR, Town JM, et al. Short-term psychodynamic psychotherapies for common mental disorders. *Cochrane Database Syst Rev.* 2006;4:CD004687.
12. Cuijpers P, van Straten A, Andersson G, van Oppen P. Psychotherapy for depression in adults: a meta-analysis of comparative outcome studies. *J Consult Clin Psychol.* 2008;76(6):909.
13. Burnand Y, Andreoli A, Kolatte E, et al. Psychodynamic psychotherapy and clomipramine in the treatment of major depression. *Psychiatr Serv.* 2002;53(5):585–590.
14. Maina G, Rosso G, Bogetto F. Brief dynamic therapy combined with pharmacotherapy in the treatment of major depressive disorder: long-term results. *J Affect Disord.* 2009;114(1):200–207.
15. Tanielian TL, Marcus SC, Suarez AP, Pincus HA. Datapoints: trends in psychiatric practice, 1988–1998: II. Caseload and treatment characteristics. *Psychiatr Serv.* 2001;52(7):880.
16. Kernberg O. Supportive psychotherapy: a reevaluation. *Psychiatry.* 1982:480–485.
17. Rockland L. *Supportive Therapy for Borderline Patients: A Psychodynamic Approach.* New York: Guilford; 1992.
18. Novalis PN, Rojcewicz SJ, Peele R. *Clinical Manual of Supportive Psychotherapy.* Washington, DC: American Psychiatric Publishing; 1993.
19. Pinsker H. *A Primer of Supportive Psychotherapy.* Hillsdale, NJ: Analytic Press; 1997.

20. Karasu T. Psychoanalysis and psychoanalytic psychotherapy. In Sadock BJ, Sadock VA, eds. *Kaplan & Sadock's Comprehensive Textbook of Psychiatry.* 8th ed. Philadelphia: Lippincott Williams & Wilkins; 2005:2472–2498.

21. Cuijpers P, Driessen E, Hollon SD, et al. The efficacy of non-directive supportive therapy for adult depression: a meta-analysis. *Clin Psychol Rev.* 2012;32(4):280.

22. Winston A, Rosenthal RN, Pinsker H. *Introduction to Supportive Psychotherapy.* Washington, DC: American Psychiatric Publishing, Inc.; 2004.

23. Spielmans GI, Pasek LF, McFall JP. What are the active ingredients in cognitive and behavioral psychotherapy for anxious and depressed children? A meta-analytic review. *Clin Psychol Rev.* 2007;27(5):642–654.

24. Viamontes GI, Beitman BD. Neural substrates of psychotherapeutic change, part I: The default brain. *Psychiatr Ann.* 2006;36(4):225–236.

25. Rosenthal R. Techniques of individual supportive psychotherapy. In: Gabbard GO, ed. *Textbook of Psychotherapeutic Treatments.* Washington, DC: American Psychiatric Press; 2009:417–446.

26. Hellerstein DJ. Combining supportive psychotherapy with medication. In: Gabbard GO, ed. *Textbook of Psychotherapeutic Treatments.* Washington, DC: American Psychiatric Press; 2009:595–629.

27. Cuijpers P, Clignet F, van Meijel B, et al. Psychological treatment of depression in inpatients: a systematic review and meta-analysis. *Clin Psychol Rev.* 2011;31(3):353–360.

28. Pampallona S, Bollini P, Tibaldi G, et al. Combined pharmacotherapy and psychological treatment for depression: a systematic review. *Arch Gen Psychiatry.* 2004;61(7):714–719.

29. De Jonghe F, Hendricksen M, Van Aalst G, et al. Psychotherapy alone and combined with pharmacotherapy in the treatment of depression. *Br J Psychiatry.* 2004;185(1):37–45.

30. Clarkin J, Levy K, Lenzenweger M, Kernberg O. Evaluating three treatments for borderline personality disorder: a multiwave study. *Am J Psychiatry.* 2007;164(6):922–928.

31. Hellerstein DJ, Rosenthal RN, Pinsker H, et al. A randomized prospective study comparing supportive and dynamic therapies. Outcome and alliance. *J Psychother Pract Res.* 1998;7(4):261–271.

32. Cuijpers P, Driessen E, Hollon SD, et al. The efficacy of non-directive supportive therapy for adult depression: a meta-analysis. *Clin Psychol Rev.* 2012;32(4):280–291.

33. Budge S, Baardseth TP, Wampold BE, Flückiger C. Researcher allegiance and supportive therapy: pernicious effects on results of randomized clinical trials. *Eur J Psychother Couns.* 2010;12(1):23–39.

34. Baardseth TP, Goldberg SB, Pace BT, et al. Cognitive-behavioral therapy versus other therapies: redux. *Clin Psychol Rev.* 2013;33(3):395–405.

35. Cuijpers P, Sijbrandij M, Koole SL, et al. The efficacy of psychotherapy and pharmacotherapy in treating depressive and anxiety disorders: a meta-analysis of direct comparisons. *World Psychiatry.* 2013;12(2):137–148.

/// 19 /// NEUROMODULATION FOR DEPRESSION

State of the Field and Future Directions

JOHN P. COETZEE AND NOLAN WILLIAMS

19.1. INTRODUCTION

Although treatments currently available for depression are diverse, one growing category that holds significant promise for depression, and especially for treatment-resistant depression (TRD), in the near future is neuromodulation. Neuromodulation encompasses a set of interventions, either electrical, chemical, or mechanical in nature, that directly modify the function of the nervous system.[1] The oldest form of neuromodulation, electroconvulsive therapy (ECT), is still one of the most effective treatments available for depression[2,3] and is now supplemented by a variety of newer techniques. The possibility of directly modifying activity in discrete brain areas or systems has a number of advantages over traditional first-line treatments for depression. Not least among these are the focal nature of neuromodulatory treatments, their speed of action, and their potentially lower cost (especially when compared to the cost of untreated or undertreated depression in individuals with TRD).

Neuromodulatory treatments for depression can be divided into two broad categories: invasive and noninvasive. Invasive treatments include procedures such as deep brain stimulation (DBS), vagal nerve stimulation (VNS), and epidural prefrontal cortical stimulation (EpCS) and are typically reserved for the most severe cases, given the risks involved with surgery. The noninvasive techniques, including ECT, transcranial magnetic stimulation (TMS), theta burst stimulation (TBS) (a high-frequency form of patterned TMS), magnetic seizure therapy (MST), and transcranial direct-current stimulation (tDCS), have a potentially broader clinical application than the invasive techniques, given the significantly lower risks and costs associated with them. In this chapter, each of the most common neuromodulatory techniques available at present will be considered, as well as some more novel techniques currently being developed.

19.2. INVASIVE NEUROMODULATION

19.2.1. Deep Brain Stimulation

Surgical treatments for psychiatric disorders suffer from stigma, stemming from the field's troubled history.[4,5] Frontal lobotomy, perhaps most famously, is emblematic of the risks inherent in this kind of treatment.[4] Ablative lesioning therapies for depression have also had significant risks and limited efficacy, and studies employing these methods often suffered from methodological shortcomings.[5] DBS differs in important ways from its predecessors. Unlike ablative or disconnective surgeries, DBS is reversible and adjustable, meaning that sham studies can be easily conducted and that preimplanted devices can be reprogrammed to change the intensity or pattern of stimulation, or even the specific location on the implant of the stimulation.[5] This flexibility has made DBS safer and more scientifically sound than its precursors.

Although the chronic introduction of electrodes into subcortical brain structures for clinical purposes has been practiced in one form or another since at least the 1950s,[6,7] DBS in its modern form was developed in the 1980s to treat intractable motor disorders (e.g., Parkinson's disease, tremor, and dystonia), for which it has proven to be a life-changing treatment.[8,9] This dramatic success led neurosurgeons to explore the possibility of replacing destructive interventions for other disorders with DBS as well, applying DBS successfully for TRD, Tourette's syndrome, obsessive-compulsive disorder, epilepsy, obesity, and cluster headache, among others.[8] It is currently approved by the Food and Drug Administration (FDA) in the United States for the treatment of Parkinson's, essential tremor, and dystonia, and in 2009 the FDA approved DBS for treatment-resistant OCD under a humanitarian device exemption.[10]

With regard to TRD, a variety of potential targets have been tested, and to date there is at least preliminary evidence of both the efficacy and safety of DBS in subgenual anterior cingulate cortex (sgACC), the ventral capsule/ventral striatum, the nucleus accumbens, the lateral habenula, the inferior thalamic peduncle, the medial forebrain bundle, the bed nucleus of the stria terminalis, and the ventral anterior limb of the internal capsule.[11,12] While the ideal target in DBS for TRD is unknown, the evidence for sgACC (Brodmann area 25) is among the strongest, with at least 16 studies demonstrating high rates of response and remission for patients receiving DBS to this structure.[12] By contrast, current published studies supporting the efficacy of other DBS targets for TRD are somewhat smaller in number.[12] Stimulation of the sgACC can result in immediate antidysphoric effects.[13–15] The reduction in depressive symptoms also appears durable, with relief in one study persisting at one year[15] and in another lasting several years.[16] It is possible that the efficacy of sgACC stimulation may be enhanced by individualized target identification using connectomic analysis, although at present this has only been explored in a small pilot study.[17]

DBS has not yet obtained FDA approval as a treatment for depression, and all implementation to date has been off-label.[10] A large multicenter controlled trial, conducted with the aim of gaining FDA approval of DBS for TRD,[18] failed to find a statistically significant difference between groups, although future DBS trials may benefit from allowing time for treatment optimization, which is an influential factor in the effectiveness of DBS.[19] Because DBS requires brain surgery, it comes with significant medical risks, and because of the complexity of the surgery, it requires a multidisciplinary medical team, with years of ongoing monitoring and additional surgeries to replace batteries or move the lead if it has migrated. Given the attendant costs and risks, DBS at this time is primarily an option for the most severe and intractable of cases.

19.2.2. Epidural Prefrontal Cortical Stimulation

Invasive cortical stimulation in humans began as a method for mapping brain functions prior to surgery for epilepsy (or tumor removal).[20] Implantation locations vary, but we can broadly divide implanted electrodes into epidural (on the surface of the brain) or subdural (under the surface), with EpCS falling into the former.[20] As is the case with all forms of electrical neuromodulation, the effects of EpCS largely depend on the characteristics of the pulse being delivered (e.g., frequency, intensity, pulse width, and duty cycle) and on the placement of the electrodes (e.g., location, distance between electrodes, polarity of electrodes).[21] At the stimulation site, fibers tend to be more electrically stimulated than cell bodies,[22,23] which leads to transmission of pulses to the cell bodies from which efferent fibers arrive, and, in the other axonal direction, to the cortical and subcortical targets on which the axons synapse.[20]

EpCS has been used to treat a variety of conditions, such as aphasia,[24,25] tinnitus,[26] and post-stroke recovery,[27] and has recently shown promise for TRD.[28–30] Kopell et al.[28] in 2011 conducted a randomized multisite study on EpCS for major depression that included 12 individuals, with a single electrode placed on left dorsolateral prefrontal cortex (DLPFC), and found a trend but no statistical difference in the blinded phase. In a small study by Nahas et al.[29] in 2010, five patients with TRD underwent EpCS. Seven months later, three were in remission, and one patient had to have the leads removed due to an infection. When these patients were examined again five years later,[30] three of the five were still in remission, with five adverse events, consisting of either suicidal ideation and/or hospitalization (which were determined not to be related to the intervention). One of the two nonresponders was noted to have high-normal impedance values and became a remitter after being reprogrammed.[31]

At this stage, although EpCS shows promise, the number of patients treated with it remains small and more study is needed. It may one day prove an attractive alternative to DBS, given the substantially lower risk involved in implanting an EpCS electrode on the surface of the dura overlying the cortical surface versus implanting a DBS electrode deep inside the brain.[29]

19.2.3. Vagus Nerve Stimulation

Although VNS requires surgery, it is less invasive and safer than either DBS or EpCS.[32] The sgACC, which has shown promise as a target for DBS, connects to the heart via the vagus nerve,[33,34] which has proven to be another useful target for the manipulation of sgACC function in TRD. While the efferent fibers of the vagus primarily originate in the medulla oblongata, and descend to modulate the heart and other internal viscera, the antiseizure and antidepressant benefits of VNS are associated with stimulation to the ascending afferent vagal fibers, which primarily originate in two parasympathetic ganglia found near the base of the skull.[35] These ascending vagal fibers innervate a variety of structures, including the cingulate gyrus and frontal areas.[35,36] Vagal afferents carry somatic and afferent information to the brain, including somatic information from the earlobe (important because the earlobe can also be used as a means of VNS delivery[37]), and make up around 80% of the fibers in the cervical vagus nerve,[35] which is where the stimulating leads are normally placed.[35]

VNS can alter regional cerebral blood in a variety of regions,[36] including amygdala and sgACC.[38] Stimulation of the vagus nerve also reduces inflammatory responses,[39] which are thought to play an important role in the pathogenesis of depression.[40] With regards to efficacy, a large controlled trial found no detectable effect of VNS for TRD,[41] but a subsequent open-label trial found an improvement of 0.45 points per month in the Hamilton Rating Scale for Depression,[42] and it was on the basis of this that the FDA approved VNS for TRD.[43] A recent long-term observational study provided evidence that the effects of VNS are durable as well, with a significantly higher response and remission rate versus treatment as usual at the end of five years.[44]

VNS complications come in two categories: those related to surgery and those related to stimulation.[43] The most common surgical problems are infection (3%–6%), vocal cord paresis (1%), and lower facial weakness (1%).[45] The most common complications related to stimulation include, among others, voice alteration, cough, paresthesia, dyspnea, headache, and pain.[46] These are more common than the surgical complications, with as many as 62% of patients experiencing voice changes, but stimulation issues tend to decline over time, with the proportion of patients experiencing voice problems dropping to 18.7% after five years.[46] VNS is a relatively low-risk alternative to other invasive methods, although judging its efficacy for TRD will require more study.

19.3. NONINVASIVE NEUROMODULATION

19.3.1 Electroconvulsive Therapy

ECT is the oldest and most thoroughly evaluated treatment for TRD, having been in use now for 80 years.[47] It consists, at its most basic level, of the application of electric current to the scalp in order to induce a seizure.[48] Parameters of the current vary widely (duration 0.5–8 s, frequency 20–120 Hz, and pulse width 0.3–1 ms) and are often based on individual seizure threshold.[48] ECT has a well-established and high rate of efficacy for TRD, with a 64% rate of response[49] and a 48% rate of remission.[50] It is especially valuable for the most severe cases of depression, such as those involving catatonia or psychosis.[47] Typically, a series of 9 to 12 seizures are induced over a period of several weeks, with 2 or 3 occurring each week. Treatments are given while the patient is under anesthesia, and may be given either unilaterally or bilaterally, over either the temporal or the frontal cortex.[48] In the United States, a course of 10 treatments can be expected to cost from $10,000 to 15,000.[49]

Although serious complications in ECT are rare,[50] a number of transient adverse events are common, including nausea, headaches, muscle aches, and arrhythmias.[51] The side effects that have played the largest role in limiting the application of ECT, however, are cognitive in nature. These include acute cognitive impairment typically lasting minutes to hours[54] and either retrograde or anterograde amnesia.[55] These are longer lasting when the patient is older and when bitemporal electrode placement is used.[56] Right unilateral ultrabrief pulsed ECT, which was developed in the mid-2000s, demonstrated a marked reduction in cognitive side effects at six months.[57] ECT is also subject to persistent stigma, a consequence of representations of the procedure in popular culture and of how it was administered in the past.[58]

Given that ECT has consistently been found to have superior efficacy for both MDD and TRD compared to other treatments,[59] it is worth asking why this is true. Attempts to clarify the causal pathway of ECT's powerful antidepressant effects have revealed that ECT affects the brain in a large number of ways, many of which interact with each other, which has made pinning down the decisive pathway difficult.[60] As a result of classic studies by Ottosson[61,62] using lidocaine-modified ECT seizures, we know that the seizures appear to be necessary, and studies using low-voltage right unilateral ECT[57] demonstrated that both intensity and anatomical location are critical. Until recently, the dominant explanations of ECT's mechanism of action have focused on the neurobiological level, pointing to the technique's effect on levels of monoamine neurotransmitters,[63] the neuroendocrine system,[64] levels of GABA and seizure thresholds,[65] and levels of brain derived neurotrophic factor.[66] Unfortunately the complexity of the interactions among these mechanisms has made it difficult to say which, if any, may be decisive.

Patients who have benefited from ECT continue to be at high risk for relapse[53] and as such should continue to be treated, with either antidepressants or continuation

ECT.[67] Continuation ECT appears to be more effective at preventing relapse than antidepressants alone.[67] The optimal approach to maintaining remission with ECT and/or antidepressants remains uncertain and in need of further study.[68]

More than any other factor, it is the cognitive deficits that come after ECT that have prevented its wider use.[69] Patients lose memory not only for the time around the treatment itself, but for the period preceding it in a graded fashion.[56] Other impairments of cognition accompany the treatment. These deficits are longer lasting in patients of more advanced age and have much to do with the appeal of more focal methods of neuromodulation for depression.

19.3.2. Transcranial Magnetic Stimulation

In TMS, an electric charge stored in a capacitor is discharged through a wire that is wound around a coil.[70] The electrical current is discharged in an intermittent manner, causing a pulsed magnetic field in the area around the coil. Because this magnetic field is time varying, it will induce an electrical field with a magnitude proportional to the rate of change of the magnetic field (in accordance with Faraday's law).[70] When this coil is placed near the scalp, the electromagnetic field it generates passes through the intervening skin and bone, inducing an electrical current in the brain. The variables of most importance in determining how TMS affects the brain are the shape of the coil, placement of the coil, frequency of the pulsation, and intensity of the magnetic field.[70]

TMS was first developed in the mid-1980s,[71] when it was seen as an appealing alternative to more painful methods of neurostimulation such as transcranial electrical stimulation.[72] Much of the early work involved studies of the motor system.[73] In a crucial milestone, Chen et al.[74] were able to use repetitive TMS (rTMS) to induce long-term changes in excitability. This gave rise to a large number of studies investigating rTMS as a means of inducing either long-term potentiation or long-term depression in the human nervous system, and similar protocols were used for clinical applications as well.[75]

One of the first reports of TMS being used to treat depression was a study by George et al.[76] in which daily rTMS was applied to the left prefrontal cortex of six patients with TRD, resulting in significant reductions in depressive symptoms. Large-scale controlled studies[77,78] later led to FDA approval of high-frequency rTMS for TRD.

Compared to ECT, TMS comes with several advantages. It does not require general anesthesia, which is the most dangerous component of administering ECT.[79] It also does not require the induction of a seizure, which is aversive for many patients. Also, because of the more focal nature of TMS, it is free of the cognitive side effects that tend to come with ECT, and that in older patients may persist for significant periods of time.[56] Finally, TMS does not come with the cultural stigma that still attaches to ECT.[58]

rTMS has repeatedly been found to be more effective for depression than sham[80] but not as effective as ECT.[49] However, given that rTMS is significantly more tolerable than ECT,[49] this is an acceptable tradeoff. A number of large controlled studies have investigated the efficacy of TMS for depression. The first multicenter randomized sham-controlled trial found clinically meaningful improvement on the Montgomery–Asberg Depression Rating Scale (MADRS, $p = 0.06$, standardized effect size = 0.39) as measured at the four-week time point.[78] Another large and comprehensive controlled study by the US National Institutes for Mental Health (NIMH) found that active treatment, relative to sham, had a significant effect on the proportion of remitters.[77] The Brainsway trial, which compared deep TMS to sham, similarly found significant reductions in scores on the Hamilton-21 rating scale compared to sham.[79,80,81] With regard to durability of effects, evidence has also been positive.[82] A consensus report from the Clinical TMS Society[83] that reviewed major controlled trials to date recommended high-frequency left prefrontal TMS given for between four and six weeks as a safe and effective therapy for patients with TRD. There is also evidence that increasing the number of pulses per session may enhance treatment effects, especially in cases of late-life depression.[84]

Some have argued that response and remission rates from rTMS can be increased through the use of personalized targets.[85] A recent study used resting state connectivity to demonstrate the existence of four "biotypes" of depression,[86] which are predictive of rTMS responsiveness. Incorporating information about depression and individual brain connectivity may serve to enhance response to rTMS.

19.3.3. Theta Burst Stimulation

TBS is a patterned form of rTMS first developed by Huang et al.[87] It makes use of theta rhythms (4–7 Hz in human cortex[88]), which are similar to the intrinsic patterns used by the hippocampus in the promotion of long-term depression and long-term potentiation.[89] In TBS, the coil produces triple-pulse bursts at either 50 Hz[87] or 30 Hz,[90] with these bursts being delivered every 200 ms, at 5 Hz. There are two common patterns of TBS: continuous TBS (cTBS), in which this pattern is produced in a continuous manner, and intermittent TBS (iTBS), in which a 2-second burst of TBS is produced every 10 seconds.[87] The behavioral effects of cTBS are primarily inhibitory, while those of iTBS are primarily stimulatory/facilitatory.[70,87] The effects of both types of TBS occur more quickly and last longer than those generated by conventional rTMS.[70]

Both iTBS and cTBS have been tested as a treatment for depression, either unilaterally or bilaterally. Meta-analysis found that TBS was generally superior to sham, and that bilateral (left iTBS and right cTBS) and unilateral left iTBS were the most effective protocols.[91] Importantly, iTBS has been demonstrated to be non-inferior to high-frequency rTMS for depression,[92] even though it can be delivered in substantially less time.

Adverse responses to TBS have been mild and infrequent.[93] There has only been one recorded incident of seizure in a non-epileptic patient, and overall the crude risk for seizure resulting from cTBS is considered to be 0.1%, while the crude risk for any mild adverse event is 5%.[94]

TBS is still a relatively new treatment for depression, but evidence is already accumulating for its effectiveness.[91] New forms of the treatment are also being actively developed.[95,96] TBS is one of the most promising forms of noninvasive depression treatments for the near future.

19.3.4 Transcranial Direct-Current Stimulation

After some interest in transcranial electrical stimulation in the mid-20th century,[97] the technique fell out of favor until a burst of renewed interest in the early 2000s[98] resulting from better understanding of the importance of electrode placement and current strength.[99] tDCS has a number of potential benefits compared to other treatments: It is inexpensive, noninvasive, and painless.[98] The primary obstacle, however, has been the demonstration of efficacy.

tDCS works by applying a weak electric current (0.5–2 mA) to electrodes placed on the scalp above the cortical target.[100] It does not trigger action potentials but rather changes levels of excitability.[100] Specifically, regions of cortex under the cathode become hyperpolarized (and therefore hypoexcitable) while regions under the anode become hypopolarized (and therefore hyperexcitable).[100] Effects can last as long as 60 minutes[101] and are thought to be associated with longer-lasting synaptic changes.[102]

Recent meta-analyses of extant tDCS research examining its safety, efficacy, and tolerability have produced conflicting findings.[100] A review by Kalu et al.[103] of 10 tDCS studies found it to be more effective than sham at reducing depressive symptoms, but also found effects to be highly variable. Berlim et al.,[104] limiting their review to studies including at least 10 sessions of tDCS, found no detectable difference in response or remission between sham and active treatment. Shiozawa et al.,[105] by contrast, found tDCS to be significantly superior to sham in both response and remission rates. Meron et al.[100] concluded that tDCS was an effective treatment for major depressive episodes, but not for TRD. There were significant methodological differences between these reviews. Also, a recent study that compared tDCS to escitalopram failed to establish noninferiority of tDCS,[106] although tDCS did outperform placebo in this study.[107]

While tDCS is safe and may hold promise for depression, the evidence so far regarding its efficacy is mixed. Many of the existing studies have been carried out with very small sample sizes, and our knowledge about tDCS would benefit from larger controlled studies.

19.3.5. Advances in ECT

MST and focally electrically administered seizure therapy (FEAST) are similar to ECT in that all three treatments involve the induction of seizures. MST, which was developed in the early 2000s,[108,109] is carried out using a modified TMS device and generally involves delivering pulses that range in frequency from 40 to 100 Hz.[13] Because it produces tonic-clonic seizures, the patient must be under general anesthesia during the procedure.[111] FEAST, on the other hand, is a modified form of ECT that makes use of polarity control, unidirectional stimulation, and an asymmetrical electrode configuration.[112] Both MST and FEAST are designed to maximize seizure efficacy while minimizing cognitive side effects.

There are important differences between MST and ECT with regard to the mechanism of seizure induction and the type of seizure induced.[111] In ECT much of the electric current is shunted away from the target region by the scalp, and a substantial portion passes through subcortical structures as well, but in MST, the electromagnetic field passes unimpeded through the scalp, and stimulation is more focal, leading to a seizure that tends to be confined to cortex without reaching subcortical layers.[108] As a result, MST produces fewer cognitive side effects than ECT, but it is also less effective for depression.[113] A review of MST studies by Cretaz et al.[111] found that MST produced significant antidepressant effects, with response rates ranging from 40% to 60% and remission rates ranging from 15% to 30%. ECT, by contrast, produces response rates of 50% to 70% when applied to the same conditions.[111] Seizures produced by FEAST are also more focal than those produced by ECT and are produced at a lower threshold.[112,113] As with MST, seizures produced by FEAST tend to affect cortical and frontal areas while sparing subcortical and temporal areas, which reduces cognitive side effects.[115]

A recent review of the extant literature on MST and FEAST concluded that FEAST probably has efficacy similar to ECT, while for MST, efficacy is demonstrated, but not as robustly so as with FEAST.[116] FEAST also demonstrated favorable efficacy in other studies.[115,117] In comparison to FEAST, there are also problems in controlling the dosage with MST because it does not always reliably produce seizures when applied.[116] The two treatments have similar side-effect profiles, both producing fewer cognitive side effects than ECT.[114]

19.4. COMMON MECHANISMS

While neuromodulatory treatments for depression appear diverse, they may produce their antidepressant effects through similar underlying mechanisms. In recent years there has been a growing body of research showing that depression may be best conceptualized as being maintained by pathological patterns of brain connectivity,[86,118,119] either between large brain networks[120–122] or among more specific neural circuits, such as the one containing sgACC and DLPFC.[15,123,124] While this picture of depression as a network pathology does not deny the importance of the underlying neurobiology, a network- or circuit-level approach has important advantages, because it is then possible to selectively intervene by changing discrete functional patterns, either downregulating or upregulating them through the localized injection of electrical, electromagnetic, or mechanical energy, allowing a more precise manipulation of neural function than is possible with pharmaceuticals, which all have systemic effects that extend throughout the brain and body.

With regard to ECT, which is still considered the most efficacious treatment for depression, many brain structures have been implicated in its effects, but two that are of special interest are left DLPFC and sgACC. In an important study by Perrin et al.,[125] researchers used functional connectivity MRI (fcMRI) to identify a set of voxels in and around left DLPFC (specifically, Brodmann areas 44, 45, and 46) that exhibited decreased functional connectivity following successful ECT, a result that is consistent with the so-called hyperconnectivity hypothesis. Under this hypothesis, depressive symptoms are in large part maintained by a pattern of excessive hyperconnectivity between intracortical and corticolimbic circuits.[122]

Some research suggests that depressive symptomatology is closely tied to excessive functional connectivity among three large-scale brain networks:[122] (1) the cognitive control network (also known as the central executive network), which is associated with attention-demanding cognitive tasks,[126] (2) the default mode network, a set of regions with higher activity when the individual is at rest,[127] and (3) the affective network, which is involved in emotional processing.[128,129(p2003),130,131] All of these are thought to be tied together through a hyperconnected or "hotwired" pathway dubbed the dorsal nexus.[122] Convergent evidence from different research strategies appears to support the existence of the dorsal nexus.[122,132,133] Dorsal nexus connectivity also is positively correlated with severity of depression,[134] and selective serotonin reuptake inhibitors (SSRIs)[135] and ECT[125] both reduce connectivity between the dorsal nexus and other brain regions.

At a more granular level, one circuit with special relevance for the treatment of depression (Figure 19.1) involves left DLPFC, sgACC, and the vagus nerve. As mentioned earlier, the sgACC has elevated activity during depression,[136] and activity in sgACC is also a biomarker of effective treatment.[137] A number of studies have found that depression is associated with increased connectivity between sgACC and default mode network sites,[138,139(p201),140,141] as well as cortical[142,143] and limbic sites.[143,144] The sgACC may also serve as the link between inflammatory processes and network connectivity changes in the pathogenesis of depression.[145] The sgACC has also proven to be an important target for DBS, as described earlier.[129]

Unlike sgACC, in depressed individuals the DLPFC has been found to be hypoactive.[15,146] Lower levels of DLPFC activity have also been associated with relapse in a tryptophan depletion-induced relapse paradigm.[147] DLPFC is thought

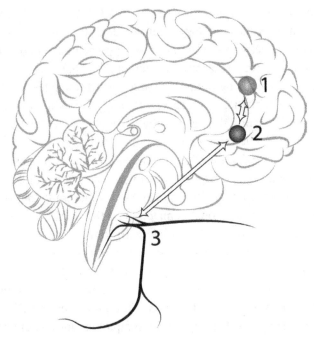

© Image Credited to Austin Guerra

FIGURE 19.1. Tripartate functional circuit proposed to underlie the efficacy of multiple modes of neurostimulation for depression. 1, left DLPFC; 2, sgACC; 3, vagus nerve.

to play an important role in cognitive control, and decreased activity in this region may be related to the uncontrolled rumination that is so often a feature of depression.[130] Left and right DLPFC also play different roles in depression, with hypoactivity in left DLPFC being associated with negative emotional judgment, while hyperactivity in right DLPFC is associated with severity of depression.[148] The opposite associations of depression with the level of activity in DLPFC and in sgACC have turned out to be exploitable for neuromodulation, especially by TMS.[149–151] Some parts of left DLPFC and sgACC are functionally anticorrelated such that a stimulating pattern of TMS pulses administered to areas of left DLPFC results in inhibitory effects on sgACC,[149,152,153] a structure that would normally be out of reach of TMS, for which the proximal effects only reach the outer 2 cm of cortex.[70]

The sgACC is also functionally connected to the heart via the vagus nerve,[33,34] which has proven to be another useful target for the manipulation of sgACC function in depression. As mentioned earlier, VNS can reduce depressive symptoms through stimulation that downregulates activity in sgACC.[154] Efferent fibers of the vagus nerve are also integrated into the DLPFC–sgACC–vagus circuit in such a way that, when TMS is applied to targets in DLPFC that are most effective for the relief of depression (namely, those targets that are also anticorrelated with sgACC function), temporary heart rate deceleration is often observed,[33] consistent with the parasympathetic innervation of the heart by efferent fibers of the vagus nerve.[155]

19.5. FUTURE DIRECTIONS

19.5.1. Accelerated Forms of rTMS

As we discussed, iTBS/rTMS to left DLPFC is one of the most reliably effective treatments for TRD, short of ECT. It may be possible to significantly enhance the effectiveness of these approaches, however, through careful engineering of the treatment components, especially with regard to targeting and dosage. First, left DLPFC is large and has diverse connections to other brain regions, but for the purpose of treating depression, the most important regions of left DLPFC are those that are most functionally anticorrelated with sgACC.[156] Second, because of concerns about avoiding seizure induction, TMS and TBS treatment studies have tended to be conservative regarding the number and intensity of pulses administered.[157] However, just as with pharmaceuticals, there likely exists a dose–response curve for the administration of TMS/TBS, and at present little is known about its exact parameters for depression treatment with this technology.[158,159]

One of the first studies to test a form of accelerated iTBS (aiTBS) was conducted by Duprat et al.[95] The primary innovation of this study was to administer iTBS to left DLPFC five times per day over four days (in contrast to previous studies of iTBS for depression, in which iTBS was administered only once per day[160]). This study also used an intensity that was above 100% of motor threshold and gave patients 1,620 pulses per session, with a gap between sessions of approximately 15 minutes[95] (it is worth noting that the amount of time allowed between sessions for this study was probably not enough to cause additive effects in humans[161]). Although this study showed no statistical difference between sham and active treatments following two weeks of sham and active treatment, patients exhibited a clinical response rate of 26%, and two weeks after the end of the study the response rate had risen to 38%.[95] The study was a crossover design, significantly limiting the interpretation of the study. Patients in this study were also examined for suicidality,[162] for which significant reductions were found, but once again there were no significant differences between active and sham conditions as the study was difficult to interpret due to its design.

A report from Williams et al.[96] described an open-label study of aiTBS that involved some novel elements.

The technique used included a significantly higher dose of aiTBS for depression than most prior studies (1,800 pulses per session, 10 sessions per day for five days for a total of 90,000 pulses/course of iTBS).

It used a targeting technique in which, prior to the administration of iTBS, fcMRI and a specialized algorithm[86,163] were used to locate the subarea of left DLPFC that was most anticorrelated with left sgACC (and to make a subsequent depth adjustment[164]),

A 50-minute delay between aiTBS sessions was used because a delay of this length has been shown to enhance the effects of aiTBS in a nonlinear fashion in animal studies.[165,166]

At the time of the report,[93] the open-label study had completed treatment for six patients with TRD. Among these, there was an average 76% reduction in depressive symptoms from baseline after the final session, with five participants qualifying as responders and four qualifying as being in remission. Reductions in depressive symptoms were accompanied by increased anticorrelation between left DLPFC and sgACC, as revealed by fcMRI.

Another small aiTBS trial was conducted by Bröcker et al.[167] Nine patients (five with MDD and two with bipolar disorder) received 20 sessions of aiTBS targeting their left DLPFC over the course of eight days. Five patients experienced reductions of at least 50% in depressive symptoms, with the only reported adverse effect being mild headaches.

Although still a new technique, aiTBS has promising potential. Given the delayed responses seen in prior randomized studies,[95] future large-scale tests of aiTBS should be conducted as between-groups tests rather than as crossover designs.

19.5.2. Low-Intensity Focused Ultrasound Pulsation

Ultrasound has been used for a variety of industrial and medical applications since World War II, with medical imaging being the most widely known application.[168] High-intensity focused ultrasound (HIFU) has been used for tissue ablation for many years, including in the brain, where ultrasonic waves are able to pass through the skull and be focused on specific intracranial targets, a procedure that is sometimes guided by MRI.[169,170]. Unlike HIFU, which is designed to produce cell death through thermal heating, low-intensity focused ultrasound pulsation (LIFUP) modulates tissue properties through the release of mechanical energy but does not produce tissue damage.[171,172] In the nervous system LIFUP can produce both inhibition and facilitation in targets that cannot be easily reached in other ways.[172] Although LIFUP's mechanism of action is still poorly understood, the effects appear to take place at the axons, and not at the cell bodies, being related to the opening and closing of ion channels via the stretching of lipid bilayers, and not to the thermal properties of the ultrasound pulsation.[172]

LIFUP is still a young technology, and at the present time most existing studies have been conducted in nonhuman animals. These include applications to produce antidepressant effects[173] and to transiently open the blood–brain barrier[174] in rats, as well as to stimulate increased production of new cells in the dentate gyrus.[175] Research using LIFUP in humans is still comparatively rare, but a few early studies have been completed. These include applications to modulate activity in motor cortex,[176] as well as in thalamus,[177] and clinical applications such as the use of LIFUP to "wake up" vegetative patients.[178] Hameroff et al.[179] conducted a study in humans in which they successfully used transcranial ultrasound to improve mood and global affect ratings at the 10- and 40-minute time points, as well as to reduce pain ratings.

There is substantial evidence that LIFUP is safe. The intensities at which LIFUP is administered are far lower than those for HIFU, and throughout multiple studies using LIFUP in both human and nonhuman animals, no tissue damage has been detectable.[172] In addition, in studies that use HIFU, no damage has been found to tissue outside the focal area, even though ultrasound intensities experienced by those areas are much higher than what is used in LIFUP.[172]

An important advantage that focused ultrasound has over TMS is that its area of stimulation can extend significantly deeper into the brain, meaning that it is possible to do noninvasive stimulation of subcortical structures such as sgACC directly, instead of indirectly, as is done with TMS. Taking all this into account, LIFUP and other forms of focused ultrasound have great promise for the treatment of depression.

19.6. CONCLUSIONS

There are a variety of invasive and noninvasive forms of neuromodulation available for the treatment of depression, and these are especially relevant for TRD. When choosing a treatment for a particular patient, the clinician should consider the likely efficacy of the technique, as well as its side-effect profile, risk, and cost. In general, noninvasive approaches should be tried prior to invasive ones, given the lower levels of associated risk. At present, ECT is still the most efficacious treatment available for depression, although the possibility of cognitive side effects must be taken into consideration.

Many neuromodulatory treatments produce antidepressant effects through action on one or more components of a functionally connected circuit that includes, among others, left DLPFC, sgACC, and vagus nerve.[33,145,154,180] Newer techniques being developed are targeting this circuit more explicitly.[95,96,162]

The field of neurostimulation is growing[1] and offers a set of treatments that can complement traditional first-line therapies as well as being reasonable alternatives to them. In the near future we can expect the effectiveness, tolerability, and precision of these techniques to grow, which will be a benefit to both clinicians and patients.

REFERENCES

1. Krames ES, Hunter Peckham P, Rezai A, Aboelsaad F. Chapter 1: What is neuromodulation? In: Krames ES, Peckham PH, Rezai AR, eds. *Neuromodulation*. San Diego: Academic Press; 2009:3–8. doi:10.1016/B978-0-12-374248-3.00002-1

2. Kellner CH, Knapp RG, Petrides G, et al. Continuation electroconvulsive therapy vs pharmacotherapy for relapse prevention in major depression: a multisite study from the Consortium for Research in Electroconvulsive Therapy (CORE). *Arch Gen Psychiatry*. 2006;63(12):1337–1344. doi:10.1001/archpsyc.63.12.1337

3. Milev RV, Giacobbe P, Kennedy SH, et al. Canadian Network for Mood and Anxiety Treatments (CANMAT) 2016 clinical guidelines for the management of adults with major depressive disorder: section 4. Neurostimulation treatments. *Can J Psychiatry*. 2016;61(9):561–575. doi:10.1177/0706743716660033

4. Mashour GA, Walker EE, Martuza RL. Psychosurgery: past, present, and future. *Brain Res Rev*. 2005;48(3):409–419. doi:10.1016/j.brainresrev.2004.09.002

5. Morishita T, Fayad SM, Higuchi M, et al. Deep brain stimulation for treatment-resistant depression: systematic review of clinical outcomes. *Neurotherapeutics*. 2014;11(3):475–484. doi:10.1007/s13311-014-0282-1

6. Delgado JR. Evaluation of permanent implantation of electrodes within the brain. *Electroencephalogr Clin Neurophysiol*. 1955;7(4):637–644.

7. Lüscher C. Dark past of deep-brain stimulation. *Nature*. 2018;555(7696):306–307.

8. Coffey RJ. Deep brain stimulation devices: a brief technical history and review. *Artif Organs*. 2009;33(3):208–220. doi:10.1111/j.1525-1594.2008.00620.x

9. Williams NR, Okun MS. Deep brain stimulation (DBS) at the interface of neurology and psychiatry. *J Clin Invest*. 2013;123(11):4546–4556. doi:10.1172/JCI68341

10. Dougherty DD. Deep brain stimulation: clinical applications. *Psychiatr Clin North Am*. 2018;41(3):385–394. doi:10.1016/j.psc.2018.04.004

11. Bergfeld IO, Mantione M, Hoogendoorn MLC, et al. Deep brain stimulation of the ventral anterior limb of the internal capsule for treatment-resistant depression: a randomized clinical trial. *JAMA Psychiatry*. 2016;73(5):456–464. doi:10.1001/jamapsychiatry. 2016.0152

12. Drobisz D, Damborská A. Deep brain stimulation targets for treating depression. *Behav Brain Res*. 2019;359:266–273. doi:10.1016/j.bbr.2018.11.004

13. Lozano AM, Giacobbe P, Hamani C, et al. A multicenter pilot study of subcallosal cingulate area deep brain stimulation for treatment-resistant depression. *J Neurosurg*. 2012;116(2):315–322. doi:10.3171/2011.10.JNS102122

14. Lozano AM, Mayberg HS, Giacobbe P, et al. Subcallosal cingulate gyrus deep brain stimulation for treatment-resistant depression. *Biol Psychiatry*. 2008;64(6):461–467. doi:10.1016/j.biopsych.2008.05.034

15. Mayberg HS, Lozano AM, Voon V, et al. Deep brain stimulation for treatment-resistant depression. *Neuron*. 2005;45(5):651–660. doi:10.1016/j.neuron.2005.02.014

16. Kennedy SH, Giacobbe P, Rizvi SJ, et al. Deep brain stimulation for treatment-resistant depression: follow-up after 3 to 6 years. *Am J Psychiatry*. 2011;168(5):502–510. doi:10.1176/appi.ajp.2010.10081187

17. Riva-Posse P, Choi KS, Holtzheimer PE, et al. A connectomic approach for subcallosal cingulate deep brain stimulation surgery: prospective targeting in treatment-resistant depression. *Mol Psychiatry*. 2018;23(4):843–849. doi:10.1038/mp.2017.59

18. Holtzheimer PE, Husain MM, Lisanby SH, et al. Subcallosal cingulate deep brain stimulation for treatment-resistant depression: a multisite, randomised, sham-controlled trial. *Lancet Psychiatry*. 2017;4(11):839–849. doi:10.1016/S2215-0366(17)30371-1

19. Zhang C, Denys D, Voon V, Sun B. Reshaping the deep brain stimulation trial for treatment-resistant depression. *Brain Stimulat*. 2018;11(3):628–630. doi:10.1016/j.brs.2018.01.005

20. Lefaucheur J-P. Principles of therapeutic use of transcranial and epidural cortical stimulation. *Clin Neurophysiol*. 2008;119(10):2179–2184. doi:10.1016/j.clinph.2008.07.007

21. Ranck JB. Which elements are excited in electrical stimulation of mammalian central nervous system: a review. *Brain Res*. 1975;98(3):417–440.

22. McIntyre CC, Grill WM. Extracellular stimulation of central neurons: influence of stimulus waveform and frequency on neuronal output. *J Neurophysiol*. 2002;88(4):1592–1604. doi:10.1152/jn.2002.88.4.1592

23. Nowak LG, Bullier J. Axons, but not cell bodies, are activated by electrical stimulation in cortical gray matter. II. Evidence from selective inactivation of cell bodies and axon initial segments. *Exp Brain Res*. 1998;118(4):489–500.

24. Balossier A, Etard O, Descat C, et al. Epidural cortical stimulation as a treatment for poststroke aphasia: a systematic review of the literature and underlying neurophysiological mechanisms. *Neurorehabil Neural Repair*. 2016;30(2):120–130. doi:10.1177/1545968315606989

25. Cherney LR, Harvey RL, Babbitt EM, et al. Epidural cortical stimulation and aphasia therapy. *Aphasiology*. 2012;26(9):1192–1217. doi:10.1080/02687038.2011.603719

26. Balossier A, Carron R, Régis J. Epidural cortical stimulation for the treatment of chronic resistant tinnitus. *Brain Stimul Basic Transl Clin Res Neuromodulation*. 2017;10(2):484.

27. Brown JA, Lutsep H, Cramer SC, Weinand M. Motor cortex stimulation for enhancement of recovery after stroke: case report. *Neurol Res*. 2003;25(8):815–818.

28. Kopell BH, Halverson J, Butson CR, et al. Epidural cortical stimulation of the left dorsolateral prefrontal cortex for refractory major depressive disorder. *Neurosurgery*. 2011;69(5):1015–29– discussion 1029. doi:10.1227/NEU.0b013e318229cfcd

29. Nahas Z, Anderson BS, Borckardt J, et al. Bilateral epidural prefrontal cortical stimulation for treatment-resistant depression. *Biol Psychiatry*. 2010;67(2):101–109. doi:10.1016/j.biopsych.2009.08.021

30. Williams NR, Short EB, Hopkins T, et al. Five-year follow-up of bilateral epidural prefrontal cortical stimulation for treatment-resistant depression. *Brain Stimulat*. 2016;9(6):897–904. doi:10.1016/j.brs.2016.06.054

31. Williams NR, Bentzley BS, Hopkins T, et al. Optimization of epidural cortical stimulation for treatment-resistant depression. *Brain Stimulat*. 2018;11(1):239–240. doi:10.1016/j.brs.2017.09.001

32. Schachter SC. Vagus nerve stimulation therapy summary five years after FDA approval. *Neurology*. 2002;59(6 suppl 4):S15–S29.

33. Iseger TA, Padberg F, Kenemans JL, et al. Neuro-cardiac-guided TMS (NCG-TMS): probing DLPFC-sgACC-vagus nerve connectivity using heart rate—first results. *Brain Stimulat*. 2017;10(5):1006–1008.

34. Lane RD, Weidenbacher H, Smith R, et al. Subgenual anterior cingulate cortex activity covariation with cardiac vagal control is altered in depression. *J Affect Disord*. 2013;150(2):565–570.

35. Henry TR. Therapeutic mechanisms of vagus nerve stimulation. *Neurology*. 2002;59(6 suppl 4):S3–S14.

36. Conway CR, Sheline YI, Chibnall JT, et al. Cerebral blood flow changes during vagus nerve stimulation for depression. *Psychiatry Res Neuroimaging*. 2006;146(2):179–184.

37. Ellrich J, others. Transcutaneous vagus nerve stimulation. *Eur Neurol Rev*. 2011;6(4):262–264.

38. Zobel A, Joe A, Freymann N, et al. Changes in regional cerebral blood flow by therapeutic vagus nerve stimulation in depression: an exploratory approach. *Psychiatry Res Neuroimaging*. 2005;139(3):165–179.

39. Borovikova LV, Ivanova S, Zhang M, et al. Vagus nerve stimulation attenuates the systemic inflammatory response to endotoxin. *Nature*. 2000;405(6785):458.

40. Leonard BE. Inflammation, depression and dementia: are they connected? *Neurochem Res*. 2007;32(10):1749–1756.

41. Rush AJ, Marangell LB, Sackeim HA, et al. Vagus nerve stimulation for treatment-resistant depression: a randomized, controlled acute phase trial. *Biol Psychiatry*. 2005;58(5):347–354.

42. Rush AJ, Sackeim HA, Marangell LB, et al. Effects of 12 months of vagus nerve stimulation in treatment-resistant depression: a naturalistic study. *Biol Psychiatry*. 2005;58(5):355–363.

43. Ben-Menachem E, Revesz D, Simon B, Silberstein S. Surgically implanted and non-invasive vagus nerve stimulation: a review of efficacy, safety and tolerability. *Eur J Neurol*. 2015;22(9):1260–1268.

44. Aaronson ST, Sears P, Ruvuna F, et al. A 5-year observational study of patients with treatment-resistant depression treated with vagus nerve stimulation or treatment as usual: comparison of response, remission, and suicidality. *Am J Psychiatry*. 2017;174(7):640–648. doi:10.1176/appi.ajp.2017.16010034

45. Ben-Menachem E. Vagus-nerve stimulation for the treatment of epilepsy. *Lancet Neurol*. 2002;1(8):477–482.

46. Ben-Menachem E. Vagus nerve stimulation, side effects, and long-term safety. *J Clin Neurophysiol.* 2001;18(5):415–418.

47. Moksnes K. Electroconvulsive therapy without consent. *Tidsskr Den Nor Laegeforening Tidsskr Prakt Med Ny Raekke.* 2013;133(19):2047–2050.

48. Swartz CM, Nelson A. Rational electroconvulsive therapy electrode placement. *Psychiatry (Edgmont).* 2005; 2(7):37.

49. Cusin C, Dougherty DD. Somatic therapies for treatment-resistant depression: ECT, TMS, VNS, DBS. *Biol Mood Anxiety Disord.* 2012;2(1):14.

50. Cristancho MA, Alici Y, Augoustides JG, O'Reardon JP. Uncommon but serious complications associated with electroconvulsive therapy: Recognition and management for the clinician. *Current Psychiatry Reports.* 2008 Dec 1;10(6):474–480.

51. Datto CJ. Side effects of electroconvulsive therapy. *Depression and Anxiety.* 2000;12(3):130–134.

52. Ren J, Li H, Palaniyappan L, et al. Repetitive transcranial magnetic stimulation versus electroconvulsive therapy for major depression: a systematic review and meta-analysis. *Prog Neuropsychopharmacol Biol Psychiatry.* 2014;51:181–189. doi:10.1016/j.pnpbp.2014.02.004

53. Jelovac A, Kolshus E, McLoughlin DM. Relapse following successful electroconvulsive therapy for major depression: a meta-analysis. *Neuropsychopharmacology.* 2013;38(12):2467–2474. doi:10.1038/npp.2013.149

54. Yen T, Khafaja M, Lam N, et al. Post-electroconvulsive therapy recovery and reorientation time with methohexital and ketamine: a randomized, longitudinal cross-over design trial. *J ECT.* 2015;31(1):20–25. doi:10.1097/YCT.0000000000000132

55. Semkovska M, McLoughlin DM. Objective cognitive performance associated with electroconvulsive therapy for depression: a systematic review and meta-analysis. *Biol Psychiatry.* 2010;68(6):568–577. doi:10.1016/j.biopsych.2010.06.009

56. Sackeim HA, Prudic J, Fuller R, et al. The cognitive effects of electroconvulsive therapy in community settings. *Neuropsychopharmacology.* 2007;32(1):244–254. doi:10.1038/sj.npp.1301180

57. Sackeim HA, Prudic J, Nobler MS, et al. Effects of pulse width and electrode placement on the efficacy and cognitive effects of electroconvulsive therapy. *Brain Stimulat.* 2008;1(2):71–83. doi:10.1016/j.brs.2008.03.001

58. Payne NA, Prudic J. Electroconvulsive therapy part II: a biopsychosocial perspective. *J Psychiatr Pract.* 2009;15(5):369.

59. Pagnin D, de Queiroz V, Pini S, Cassano GB. Efficacy of ECT in depression: a meta-analytic review. *J ECT.* 2004;20(1):13–20.

60. McCall WV, Andrade C, Sienaert P. Searching for the mechanism(s) of ECT's therapeutic effect. *J ECT.* 2014;30(2):87–89. doi:10.1097/YCT.0000000000000121

61. Cronholm B, Ottosson J-O. Experimental studies of the therapeutic action of electroconvulsive therapy in endogenous depression: the role of the electrical stimulation and of the seizure studied by variation of stimulus intensity and modification by lidocaine of seizure discharge. *Acta Psychiatr Scand.* 1960;35(S145):69–101.

62. Ottosson J-O. Seizure characteristics and therapeutic efficiency in electroconvulsive therapy: an analysis of the antidepressive efficiency of grand mal and lidocaine-modified seizures. *J Nerv Ment Dis.* 1962;135(3):239–251.

63. Heninger G, Delgado P, Charney D. The revised monoamine theory of depression: a modulatory role for monoamines, based on new findings from monoamine depletion experiments in humans. *Pharmacopsychiatry.* 1996;29(01):2–11.

64. Kamil R, Joffe RT. Neuroendocrine testing in electroconvulsive therapy. *Psychiatr Clin North Am.* 1991;14(4):961–970.

65. Sackeim HA. The anticonvulsant hypothesis of the mechanisms of action of ECT: current status. *J ECT.* 1999;15(1):5–26.

66. Chen F, Madsen TM, Wegener G, Nyengaard JR. Repeated electroconvulsive seizures increase the total number of synapses in adult male rat hippocampus. *Eur Neuropsychopharmacol.* 2009;19(5):329–338.

67. Gagné Jr GG, Furman MJ, Carpenter LL, Price LH. Efficacy of continuation ECT and antidepressant drugs compared to long-term antidepressants alone in depressed patients. *Am J Psychiatry.* 2000;157(12):1960–1965.

68. Lisanby SH. Electroconvulsive therapy for depression. *N Engl J Med.* 2007;357(19):1939–1945. doi:10.1056/NEJMct075234

69. Sackeim HA. Modern electroconvulsive therapy: vastly improved yet greatly underused. *JAMA Psychiatry.* 2017;74(8):779–780. doi:10.1001/jamapsychiatry.2017.1670

70. Rossi S, Hallett M, Rossini PM, Pascual-Leone A. Safety, ethical considerations, and application guidelines for the use of transcranial magnetic stimulation in clinical practice and research. *Clin Neurophysiol.* 2009;120(12):2008–2039. doi:10.1016/j.clinph.2009.08.016

71. Barker AT, Jalinous R, Freeston IL. Non-invasive magnetic stimulation of human motor cortex. *Lancet.* 1985;325(8437):1106–1107.

72. Merton P, Morton H, Hill D, Marsden C. Scope of a technique for electrical stimulation of human brain, spinal cord, and muscle. *Lancet.* 1982;320(8298):597–600.

73. Kujirai T, Caramia MD, Rothwell JC, et al. Corticocortical inhibition in human motor cortex. *J Physiol.* 1993;471:501–519.

74. Chen R, Classen J, Gerloff C, et al. Depression of motor cortex excitability by low-frequency transcranial magnetic stimulation. *Neurology.* 1997;48(5):1398–1403. doi:10.1212/WNL.48.5.1398

75. Ziemann U. Thirty years of transcranial magnetic stimulation: where do we stand? *Exp Brain Res.* 2017;235(4):973–984.

76. George MS, Wassermann EM, Williams WA, et al. Daily repetitive transcranial magnetic stimulation (rTMS) improves mood in depression. *Neuroreport Int J Rapid Commun Res Neurosci.* 1995;6(14):1853–1856.

77. George MS, Lisanby SH, Avery D, et al. Daily left prefrontal transcranial magnetic stimulation therapy for major depressive disorder: a sham-controlled randomized trial. *Arch Gen Psychiatry.* 2010;67(5):507–516. doi:10.1001/archgenpsychiatry.2010.46

78. O'Reardon JP, Solvason HB, Janicak PG, et al. Efficacy and safety of transcranial magnetic stimulation in the acute treatment of major depression: a multisite randomized controlled trial. *Biol Psychiatry.* 2007;62(11):1208–1216.

79. Lagasse RS. Anesthesia safety: model or myth? A review of the published literature and analysis of current original data. *Anesthesiology.* 2002;97(6):1609–1617.

80. Loo CK, Mitchell PB. A review of the efficacy of transcranial magnetic stimulation (TMS) treatment for depression, and current and future strategies to optimize efficacy. *J Affect Disord.* 2005;88(3):255–267.

81. Levkovitz Y, Isserles M, Padberg F, et al. Efficacy and safety of deep transcranial magnetic stimulation for major depression: a prospective multicenter randomized controlled trial. *World Psychiatry.* 2015;14(1):64–73.

82. Janicak PG, Nahas Z, Lisanby SH, et al. Durability of clinical benefit with transcranial magnetic stimulation (TMS) in the treatment of pharmacoresistant major depression: assessment of relapse during a 6-month, multisite, open-label study. *Brain Stimulat.* 2010;3(4):187–199.

83. Perera T, George MS, Grammer G, et al. The Clinical TMS Society consensus review and treatment recommendations for TMS therapy for major depressive disorder. *Brain Stimulat.* 2016;9(3):336–346.

84. Kaster TS, Daskalakis ZJ, Noda Y, et al. Efficacy, tolerability, and cognitive effects of deep transcranial magnetic stimulation for late-life depression: a prospective randomized controlled trial. *Neuropsychopharmacology.* 2018;43(11):2231–2238. doi:10.1038/s41386-018-0121-x

85. Downar J, Daskalakis ZJ. New targets for rTMS in depression: a review of convergent evidence. *Brain Stimulat.* 2013;6(3):231–240. doi:10.1016/j.brs.2012.08.006

86. Drysdale AT, Grosenick L, Downar J, et al. Resting-state connectivity biomarkers define neurophysiological subtypes of depression. *Nat Med.* 2017;23(1):28–38. doi:10.1038/nm.4246

87. Huang Y-Z, Edwards MJ, Rounis E, et al. Theta burst stimulation of the human motor cortex. *Neuron.* 2005;45(2):201–206. doi:10.1016/j.neuron.2004.12.033

88. Klimesch W. EEG alpha and theta oscillations reflect cognitive and memory performance: a review and analysis. *Brain Res Rev.* 1999;29(2–3):169–195.

89. Hölscher C, Anwyl R, Rowan MJ. Stimulation on the positive phase of hippocampal theta rhythm induces long-term potentiation that can be depotentiated by stimulation on the negative phase in area CA1 in vivo. *J Neurosci.* 1997;17(16):6470–6477.

90. Wu SW, Shahana N, Huddleston DA, Gilbert DL. Effects of 30 Hz theta burst transcranial magnetic stimulation on the primary motor cortex. *J Neurosci Methods.* 2012;208(2): 161–164.

91. Berlim MT, McGirr A, dos Santos NR, et al. Efficacy of theta burst stimulation (TBS) for major depression: an exploratory meta-analysis of randomized and sham-controlled trials. *J Psychiatr Res.* 2017;90:102–109.

92. Blumberger DM, Vila-Rodriguez F, Thorpe KE, et al. Effectiveness of theta burst versus high-frequency repetitive transcranial magnetic stimulation in patients with depression (THREE-D): a randomised non-inferiority trial. *Lancet.* 2018;391(10131):1683–1692. doi:10.1016/S0140-6736(18)30295-2

93. Oberman L, Edwards D, Eldaief M, Pascual-Leone A. Safety of theta burst transcranial magnetic stimulation: a systematic review of the literature. *J Clin Neurophysiol.* 2011;28(1):67–74. doi:10.1097/WNP.0b013e318205135f

94. Rossi S, Hallett M, Rossini PM, Pascual-Leone A, Safety of TMS Consensus Group. Safety, ethical considerations, and application guidelines for the use of transcranial magnetic stimulation in clinical practice and research. *Clin Neurophysiol.* 2009;120(12):2008–2039. doi:10.1016/j.clinph.2009.08.016

95. Duprat R, Desmyter S, Rudi DR, et al. Accelerated intermittent theta burst stimulation treatment in medication-resistant major depression: a fast road to remission? *J Affect Disord.* 2016;200:6–14. doi:10.1016/j.jad.2016.04.015

96. Williams NR, Sudheimer KD, Bentzley BS, et al. High-dose spaced theta-burst TMS as a rapid-acting antidepressant in highly refractory depression. *Brain J Neurol.* 2018;141(3):e18. doi:10.1093/brain/awx379

97. Lolas F. Brain polarization: behavioral and therapeutic effects. *Biol Psychiatry.* 1977;12(1):37–47.

98. Fregni F, Boggio PS, Nitsche MA, et al. Treatment of major depression with transcranial direct current stimulation. *Bipolar Disord.* 2006;8(2):203–204.

99. Nitsche MA, Liebetanz D, Antal A, et al. Modulation of cortical excitability by weak direct current stimulation—technical, safety and functional aspects. *Clin Neurophysiol.* 2003;56:255–276.

100. Meron D, Hedger N, Garner M, Baldwin DS. Transcranial direct current stimulation (tDCS) in the treatment of depression: systematic review and meta-analysis of efficacy and tolerability. *Neurosci Biobehav Rev.* 2015;57:46–62. doi:10.1016/j.neubiorev.2015.07.012

101. Brunoni AR, Nitsche MA, Bolognini N, et al. Clinical research with transcranial direct current stimulation (tDCS): challenges and future directions. *Brain Stimulat.* 2012;5(3):175–195.

102. Brunoni AR, Ferrucci R, Fregni F, et al. Transcranial direct current stimulation for the treatment of major depressive disorder: a summary of preclinical, clinical and translational findings. *Prog Neuropsychopharmacol Biol Psychiatry.* 2012;39(1):9–16.

103. Kalu UG, Sexton CE, Loo CK, Ebmeier KP. Transcranial direct current stimulation in the treatment of major depression: a meta-analysis. *Psychol Med.* 2012;42(9):1791–1800. doi:10.1017/S0033291711003059

104. Berlim MT, Van den Eynde F, Daskalakis ZJ. Clinical utility of transcranial direct current stimulation (tDCS) for treating major depression: a systematic review and meta-analysis of randomized, double-blind and sham-controlled trials. *J Psychiatr Res*. 2013;47(1):1–7. doi:10.1016/j.jpsychires.2012.09.025

105. Shiozawa P, Fregni F, Benseñor IM, et al. Transcranial direct current stimulation for major depression: an updated systematic review and meta-analysis. *Int J Neuropsychopharmacol*. 2014;17(9):1443–1452. doi:10.1017/S1461145714000418

106. Brunoni AR, Moffa AH, Sampaio-Junior B, et al. Trial of electrical direct-current therapy versus escitalopram for depression. *N Engl J Med*. 2017;376(26):2523–2533. doi:10.1056/NEJMoa1612999

107. Lisanby SH. Noninvasive brain stimulation for depression: the devil is in the dosing. *N Engl J Med*. 2017;376(26):2593–2594. doi:10.1056/NEJMe1702492

108. Lisanby SH, Luber B, Schlaepfer TE, Sackeim HA. Safety and feasibility of magnetic seizure therapy (MST) in major depression: randomized within-subject comparison with electroconvulsive therapy. *Neuropsychopharmacology*. 2003;28(10):1852–1865. doi:10.1038/sj.npp.1300229

109. Lisanby SH, Schlaepfer TE, Fisch H-U, Sackeim HA. Magnetic seizure therapy of major depression. *Arch Gen Psychiatry*. 2001;58(3):303–305.

110. Engel A, Kayser S. An overview on clinical aspects in magnetic seizure therapy. *J Neural Transm*. 2016;123(10):1139–1146.

111. Cretaz E, Brunoni AR, Lafer B. Magnetic seizure therapy for unipolar and bipolar depression: a systematic review. *Neural Plast*. 2015;2015.

112. Spellman T, Peterchev AV, Lisanby SH. Focal electrically administered seizure therapy: a novel form of ECT illustrates the roles of current directionality, polarity, and electrode configuration in seizure induction. *Neuropsychopharmacology*. 2009;34(8):2002–2010. doi:10.1038/npp.2009.12

113. Lisanby SH. Update on magnetic seizure therapy: a novel form of convulsive therapy. *J ECT*. 2002;18(4):182–188.

114. Chahine G, Short B, Spicer K, et al. Regional cerebral blood flow changes associated with focal electrically administered seizure therapy (FEAST). *Brain Stimulat*. 2014;7(3):483–485. doi:10.1016/j.brs.2014.02.011

115. Sahlem GL, Short EB, Kerns S, et al. Expanded safety and efficacy data for a new method of performing electroconvulsive therapy. *J ECT*. 2016;32(3):197–203. doi:10.1097/YCT.0000000000000328

116. Sackeim HA, Short EB, Salem GL, et al. Focal and spatially-targeted ECT: comparison of MST and FEAST. *Brain Stimul Basic Transl Clin Res Neuromodulation*. 2017;10(2):358–359. doi:10.1016/j.brs.2017.01.056

117. Nahas Z, Short B, Burns C, et al. A feasibility study of a new method for electrically producing seizures in man: focal electrically administered seizure therapy (FEAST). *Brain Stimulat*. 2013;6(3):403–408. doi:10.1016/j.brs.2013.03.004

118. Fox MD, Snyder AZ, Vincent JL, et al. The human brain is intrinsically organized into dynamic, anticorrelated functional networks. *Proc Natl Acad Sci USA*. 2005;102(27):9673–9678. doi:10.1073/pnas.0504136102

119. Zeng L-L, Shen H, Liu L, et al. Identifying major depression using whole-brain functional connectivity: a multivariate pattern analysis. *Brain J Neurol*. 2012;135(Pt 5):1498–1507. doi:10.1093/brain/aws059

120. Menon V. Large-scale brain networks and psychopathology: a unifying triple network model. *Trends Cogn Sci*. 2011;15(10):483–506. doi:10.1016/j.tics.2011.08.003

121. Sheline YI, Barch DM, Price JL, et al. The default mode network and self-referential processes in depression. *Proc Natl Acad Sci USA*. 2009;106(6):1942–1947. doi:10.1073/pnas.0812686106

122. Sheline YI, Price JL, Yan Z, Mintun MA. Resting-state functional MRI in depression unmasks increased connectivity between networks via the dorsal nexus. *Proc Natl Acad Sci USA*. 2010;107(24):11020–11025. doi:10.1073/pnas.1000446107

123. Cooney RE, Joormann J, Eugène F, et al. Neural correlates of rumination in depression. *Cogn Affect Behav Neurosci*. 2010;10(4):470–478. doi:10.3758/CABN.10.4.470

124. Rogers MA, Kasai K, Koji M, et al. Executive and prefrontal dysfunction in unipolar depression: a review of neuropsychological and imaging evidence. *Neurosci Res*. 2004;50(1):1–11. doi:10.1016/j.neures.2004.05.003

125. Perrin JS, Merz S, Bennett DM, et al. Electroconvulsive therapy reduces frontal cortical connectivity in severe depressive disorder. *Proc Natl Acad Sci USA*. 2012;109(14):5464–5468. doi:10.1073/pnas.1117206109

126. Corbetta M, Shulman GL. Control of goal-directed and stimulus-driven attention in the brain. *Nat Rev Neurosci*. 2002;3(3):201–215. doi:10.1038/nrn755

127. Shulman GL, Fiez JA, Corbetta M, et al. Common blood flow changes across visual tasks: II. Decreases in cerebral cortex. *J Cogn Neurosci*. 1997;9(5):648–663. doi:10.1162/jocn.1997.9.5.648

128. Bush G, Luu P, Posner MI. Cognitive and emotional influences in anterior cingulate cortex. *Trends Cogn Sci*. 2000;4(6):215–222.

129. Johansen-Berg H, Gutman DA, Behrens TEJ, et al. Anatomical connectivity of the subgenual cingulate region targeted with deep brain stimulation for treatment-resistant depression. *Cereb Cortex*. 2008;18(6):1374–1383. doi:10.1093/cercor/bhm167

130. Mayberg HS, Liotti M, Brannan SK, et al. Reciprocal limbic-cortical function and negative mood: converging PET findings in depression and normal sadness. *Am J Psychiatry*. 1999;156(5):675–682. doi:10.1176/ajp.156.5.675

131. Ongür D, Ferry AT, Price JL. Architectonic subdivision of the human orbital and medial prefrontal cortex. *J Comp Neurol*. 2003;460(3):425–449. doi:10.1002/cne.10609

132. Nixon NL, Liddle PF, Nixon E, et al. Biological vulnerability to depression: linked structural and functional brain network findings. *Br J Psychiatry J Ment Sci*. 2014;204:283–289. doi:10.1192/bjp.bp.113.129965

133. Norbury R, Mannie Z, Cowen PJ. Imaging vulnerability for depression. *Mol Psychiatry*. 2011;16(11):1067–1068. doi:10.1038/mp.2011.44

134. Peng D, Liddle EB, Iwabuchi SJ, et al. Dissociated large-scale functional connectivity networks of the precuneus in medication-naïve first-episode depression. *Psychiatry Res*. 2015;232(3):250–256. doi:10.1016/j.pscychresns.2015.03.003

135. McCabe C, Mishor Z, Filippini N, et al. SSRI administration reduces resting state functional connectivity in dorso-medial prefrontal cortex. *Mol Psychiatry*. 2011;16(6):592–594. doi:10.1038/mp.2010.138

136. Hamani C, Mayberg H, Stone S, et al. The subcallosal cingulate gyrus in the context of major depression. *Biol Psychiatry*. 2011;69(4):301–308. doi:10.1016/j.biopsych.2010.09.034

137. Pizzagalli DA. Frontocingulate dysfunction in depression: toward biomarkers of treatment response. *Neuropsychopharmacology*. 2011;36(1):183–206. doi:10.1038/npp.2010.166

138. Alexopoulos GS, Hoptman MJ, Kanellopoulos D, et al. Functional connectivity in the cognitive control network and the default mode network in late-life depression. *J Affect Disord*. 2012;139(1):56–65. doi:10.1016/j.jad.2011.12.002

139. Berman MG, Peltier S, Nee DE, et al. Depression, rumination and the default network. *Soc Cogn Affect Neurosci*. 2011;6(5):548–555. doi:10.1093/scan/nsq080

140. Greicius MD, Flores BH, Menon V, et al. Resting-state functional connectivity in major depression: abnormally increased contributions from subgenual cingulate cortex and thalamus. *Biol Psychiatry*. 2007;62(5):429–437. doi:10.1016/j.biopsych.2006.09.020

141. Zhou Y, Yu C, Zheng H, et al. Increased neural resources recruitment in the intrinsic organization in major depression. *J Affect Disord*. 2010;121(3):220–230. doi:10.1016/j.jad.2009.05.029

142. Davey CG, Yücel M, Allen NB, Harrison BJ. Task-related deactivation and functional connectivity of the subgenual cingulate cortex in major depressive disorder. *Front Psychiatry.* 2012;3:14. doi:10.3389/fpsyt.2012.00014

143. de Kwaasteniet B, Ruhe E, Caan M, et al. Relation between structural and functional connectivity in major depressive disorder. *Biol Psychiatry.* 2013;74(1):40–47. doi:10.1016/j.biopsych.2012.12.024

144. Connolly CG, Wu J, Ho TC, et al. Resting-state functional connectivity of subgenual anterior cingulate cortex in depressed adolescents. *Biol Psychiatry.* 2013;74(12):898–907. doi:10.1016/j.biopsych.2013.05.036

145. Harrison NA, Brydon L, Walker C, et al. Inflammation causes mood changes through alterations in subgenual cingulate activity and mesolimbic connectivity. *Biol Psychiatry.* 2009;66(5):407–414. doi:10.1016/j.biopsych.2009.03.015

146. Gotlib IH, Hamilton JP. Neuroimaging and depression: current status and unresolved issues. *Curr Dir Psychol Sci.* 2008;17(2):159–163. doi:10.1111/j.1467-8721.2008.00567.x

147. Bremner JD, Innis RB, Salomon RM, et al. Positron emission tomography measurement of cerebral metabolic correlates of tryptophan depletion-induced depressive relapse. *Arch Gen Psychiatry.* 1997;54(4):364–374.

148. Grimm S, Beck J, Schuepbach D, et al. Imbalance between left and right dorsolateral prefrontal cortex in major depression is linked to negative emotional judgment: an fMRI study in severe major depressive disorder. *Biol Psychiatry.* 2008;63(4):369–376. doi:10.1016/j.biopsych.2007.05.033

149. Fox MD, Liu H, Pascual-Leone A. Identification of reproducible individualized targets for treatment of depression with TMS based on intrinsic connectivity. *NeuroImage.* 2013;66:151–160. doi:10.1016/j.neuroimage.2012.10.082

150. Philip NS, Barredo J, Aiken E, Carpenter LL. Neuroimaging mechanisms of therapeutic transcranial magnetic stimulation for major depressive disorder. *Biol Psychiatry Cogn Neurosci Neuroimaging.* 2018;3(3):211–222. doi:10.1016/j.bpsc.2017.10.007

151. Tik M, Hoffmann A, Sladky R, et al. Towards understanding rTMS mechanism of action: stimulation of the DLPFC causes network-specific increase in functional connectivity. *NeuroImage.* 2017;162:289–296. doi:10.1016/j.neuroimage.2017.09.022

152. Cash RFH, Zalesky A, Thomson RH, et al. Subgenual functional connectivity predicts antidepressant treatment response to transcranial magnetic stimulation: independent validation and evaluation of personalization. *Biol Psychiatry.* 2019 [Epub before print]. doi:10.1016/j.biopsych.2018.12.002

153. Weigand A, Horn A, Caballero R, et al. Prospective validation that subgenual connectivity predicts antidepressant efficacy of transcranial magnetic stimulation sites. *Biol Psychiatry.* 2018;84(1):28–37. doi:10.1016/j.biopsych.2017.10.028

154. Pardo JV, Sheikh SA, Schwindt GC, et al. Chronic vagus nerve stimulation for treatment-resistant depression decreases resting ventromedial prefrontal glucose metabolism. *NeuroImage.* 2008;42(2):879–889. doi:10.1016/j.neuroimage.2008.04.267

155. Warner HR, Cox A. A mathematical model of heart rate control by sympathetic and vagus efferent information. *J Appl Physiol.* 1962;17:349–355. doi:10.1152/jappl.1962.17.2.349

156. Petrides M, Pandya DN. Dorsolateral prefrontal cortex: comparative cytoarchitectonic analysis in the human and the macaque brain and corticocortical connection patterns. *Eur J Neurosci.* 1999;11(3):1011–1036.

157. Schrader LM, Stern JM, Koski L, et al. Seizure incidence during single- and paired-pulse transcranial magnetic stimulation (TMS) in individuals with epilepsy. *Clin Neurophysiol.* 2004;115(12):2728–2737. doi:10.1016/j.clinph.2004.06.018

158. Modirrousta M, Meek BP, Wikstrom SL. Efficacy of twice-daily vs once-daily sessions of repetitive transcranial magnetic stimulation in the treatment of major depressive disorder: a retrospective study. *Neuropsychiatr Dis Treat.* 2018;14:309–316. doi:10.2147/NDT.S151841

159. Sonmez AI, Camsari DD, Nandakumar AL, et al. Accelerated TMS for depression: a systematic review and meta-analysis. *Psychiatry Res.* 2019;273:770–781. doi:10.1016/j.psychres.2018.12.041

160. Li C-T, Chen M-H, Juan C-H, et al. Efficacy of prefrontal theta-burst stimulation in refractory depression: a randomized sham-controlled study. *Brain J Neurol.* 2014;137(Pt 7):2088–2098. doi:10.1093/brain/awu109

161. Nettekoven C, Volz LJ, Kutscha M, et al. Dose-dependent effects of theta burst rTMS on cortical excitability and resting-state connectivity of the human motor system. *J Neurosci.* 2014;34(20):6849–6859. doi:10.1523/JNEUROSCI.4993-13.2014

162. Desmyter S, Duprat R, Baeken C, et al. Accelerated intermittent theta burst stimulation for suicide risk in therapy-resistant depressed patients: a randomized, sham-controlled trial. *Front Hum Neurosci.* 2016;10:480. doi:10.3389/fnhum.2016.00480

163. Fox MD, Buckner RL, White MP, et al. Efficacy of TMS targets for depression is related to intrinsic functional connectivity with the subgenual cingulate. *Biol Psychiatry.* 2012;72(7):595–603. doi:10.1016/j.biopsych.2012.04.028

164. Stokes MG, Chambers CD, Gould IC, et al. Simple metric for scaling motor threshold based on scalp-cortex distance: application to studies using transcranial magnetic stimulation. *J Neurophysiol.* 2005;94(6):4520–4527. doi:10.1152/jn.00067.2005

165. Kramár EA, Babayan AH, Gavin CF, et al. Synaptic evidence for the efficacy of spaced learning. *Proc Natl Acad Sci USA.* 2012;109(13):5121–5126. doi:10.1073/pnas.1120700109

166. Lynch G, Kramár EA, Babayan AH, et al. Differences between synaptic plasticity thresholds result in new timing rules for maximizing long-term potentiation. *Neuropharmacology.* 2013;64:27–36. doi:10.1016/j.neuropharm.2012.07.006

167. Bröcker E, van den Heuvel L, Seedat S. Accelerated theta-burst repetitive transcranial magnetic stimulation for depression in South Africa: a series of nine cases. *South Afr J Psychiatry.* 2018;24(0). doi:10.4102/sajpsychiatry.v24i0.1272

168. Rezayat E, Toostani IG. A review on brain stimulation using low-intensity focused ultrasound. *Basic Clin Neurosci.* 2016;7(3):187–194. doi:10.15412/J.BCN.03070303

169. Jolesz FA. MRI-guided focused ultrasound surgery. *Annu Rev Med.* 2009;60:417–430. doi:10.1146/annurev.med.60.041707.170303

170. Villamar MF, Santos Portilla A, Fregni F, Zafonte R. Noninvasive brain stimulation to modulate neuroplasticity in traumatic brain injury. *Neuromodulation.* 2012;15(4):326–337. doi:10.1111/j.1525-1403.2012.00474.x

171. Baek H, Pahk KJ, Kim H. A review of low-intensity focused ultrasound for neuromodulation. *Biomed Eng Lett.* 2017;7(2):135–142. doi:10.1007/s13534-016-0007-y

172. Bystritsky A, Korb AS, Douglas PK, et al. A review of low-intensity focused ultrasound pulsation. *Brain Stimulat.* 2011;4(3):125–136. doi:10.1016/j.brs.2011.03.007

173. Zhang D, Li H, Sun J, et al. Antidepressant-like effect of low-intensity transcranial ultrasound stimulation. *IEEE Trans Biomed Eng.* 2019;66(2):411–420. doi:10.1109/TBME.2018.2845689

174. Mooney ME, Herin DV, Specker S, et al. Pilot study of the effects of lisdexamfetamine on cocaine use: a randomized, double-blind, placebo-controlled trial. *Drug Alcohol Depend.* 2015;153:94–103. doi:10.1016/j.drugalcdep.2015.05.042

175. Scarcelli T, Jordão JF, O'Reilly MA, et al. Stimulation of hippocampal neurogenesis by transcranial focused ultrasound and microbubbles in adult mice. *Brain Stimulat.* 2014;7(2):304–307. doi:10.1016/j.brs.2013.12.012

176. Gibson BC, Sanguinetti JL, Badran BW, et al. Increased excitability induced in the primary motor cortex by transcranial ultrasound stimulation. *Front Neurol.* 2018;9:1007. doi:10.3389/fneur.2018.01007

177. Legon W, Ai L, Bansal P, Mueller JK. Neuromodulation with single-element transcranial focused ultrasound in human thalamus. *Hum Brain Mapp.* 2018;39(5):1995–2006. doi:10.1002/hbm.23981

178. Monti MM, Schnakers C, Korb AS, et al. Non-invasive ultrasonic thalamic stimulation in disorders of consciousness after severe brain injury: a first-in-man report. *Brain Stimulat.* 2016;9(6):940–941. doi:10.1016/j.brs.2016.07.008

179. Hameroff S, Trakas M, Duffield C, et al. Transcranial ultrasound (TUS) effects on mental states: a pilot study. *Brain Stimulat.* 2013;6(3):409–415. doi:10.1016/j.brs.2012.05.002

180. Avissar M, Powell F, Ilieva I, et al. Functional connectivity of the left DLPFC to striatum predicts treatment response of depression to TMS. *Brain Stimulat.* 2017;10(5):919–925. doi:10.1016/j.brs.2017.07.002

Novel, Nontraditional Treatment Strategies for Depression

/// 20 /// EXERCISE AS A TREATMENT FOR DEPRESSION

CHAD D. RETHORST

20.1. INTRODUCTION

Initial evidence of the association between physical activity and depression came from epidemiological studies. Analyzing data from the National Health and Nutrition Examination Survey, Farmer et al. (1988) reported a cross-sectional association between low levels of self-reported physical activity and elevated depressive symptoms. Furthermore, engaging in little or no physical activity doubled the risk of incident depression eight years later. These findings have generalized across populations, most recently demonstrated in a population-based study of 36 low- and middle-income countries (Stubbs, Koyanagi, et al., 2016).

These findings have also been replicated in studies using objective measures of physical activity. Vallance et al. (2011) found that those with depression engaged in 50% less moderate to vigorous physical activity compared to those without depression. Individuals in the bottom quartile of moderate to vigorous physical activity were more than twice as likely to have depression. In an analysis from the Hispanic Community Health Study/Study of Latinos, Rethorst et al. (2017) found that objectively measured vigorous physical activity was associated with lower depressive symptoms.

Depressive symptoms have also been associated with lower cardiorespiratory fitness. In the Aerobics Center Longitudinal Study (ACLS), Galper et al. (2006) reported an inverse association between cardiorespiratory fitness and depressive symptoms. In another analysis of the ACLS cohort, Dishman et al. (2012) found evidence of the importance in maintaining cardiorespiratory fitness to reduce depression risk. In this analysis, age-related decreases in cardiorespiratory fitness were associated with increased risk of incident depression. Similarly, a recent meta-analysis evaluated the prospective association between physical activity and incident depression. This analysis combined the results of 49 studies that included over 266,000 individuals and concluded that higher levels of physical activity reduced the odds of incident depression by 17% (Schuch et al., 2018).

A study by Harvey et al. (2018) used data from the HUNT Cohort Study to evaluate the dose and intensity of physical activity necessary for protective effects against depression. They found that engaging in any physical activity reduced the risk of depression; engaging in at least one hour of weekly physical activity resulted in significant reductions in risk of depression, regardless of the intensity of the activity.

20.2. EXERCISE AS A TREATMENT FOR DEPRESSION

20.2.1. Aerobic Exercise

The epidemiological evidence described in Section 20.1 clearly demonstrates an association of physical activity with lower levels of depressive symptoms and a lower prevalence and incidence of depressive disorders. However, this does not provide evidence for the utility of exercise as a treatment for depressive disorders. Trials examining the potential antidepressant effects of exercise began in the 1980s. These smaller trials, many only published as dissertations, provided preliminary evidence of the treatment effects of aerobic exercise (Burrus, 1984; Epstein, 1987; Kanner, 1991; Levin, 1984; Martinsen, Medhus, & Sandvik, 1985; McCann & Holmes, 1984; McNeil, LeBlanc, & Joyner, 1991; Veale et al., 1992).

One of the first larger trials was conducted in 156 older adults, who were randomized to receive exercise, sertraline, or exercise plus sertraline. All three treatment arms demonstrated significant reductions in depressive symptoms. Participants in the sertraline condition experienced a more rapid reduction in depressive symptoms (1–2 weeks), but the three treatment conditions were not significantly different at the end of the 16-week trial (Blumenthal et al., 1999). In a second trial, Blumenthal et al. (2007) randomized older adults to one of four treatment groups: home-based exercise, supervised exercise, sertraline, or placebo pill. At the end of the 16-week study, all three active treatment groups demonstrated significantly lower depressive symptoms compared to the placebo pill group.

A trial conducted by Dunn et al. (2005) evaluated the dose–response relationship of exercise with depression. Participants in the study were randomized to two doses of exercise, equivalent to 150 or 75 minutes per week of moderate to vigorous activity, completed in either three or five sessions per week, or an attentional control group. The results supported the hypothesized dose–response relationship, with participants in the high-dose exercise group experiencing greater reductions in depressive symptoms; however, exercise frequency did not differentially affect depressive symptoms. The low-dose group and the control group did not differ at the end of the 12-week trial.

Further support for a dose–response relationship comes from the Regassa study. In this randomized controlled trial, 946 patients scoring more than 9 on the Patient Health Questionnaire (PHQ)-9 were recruited from primary care clinics and randomized to one of three treatment conditions: exercise, internet-based cognitive–behavioral therapy, or treatment as usual. After three months, patients in the internet-based cognitive–behavioral therapy and exercise groups experienced greater reductions in depressive symptoms compared to treatment as usual (Hallgren et al., 2015). Within the exercise group, patients were further randomized to receive one of three exercise programs: (1) "light exercise" (yoga or stretching classes), (2) "moderate exercise" (moderate-intensity aerobics classes), or (3) "vigorous exercise" (high-intensity aerobics/strength training classes). All three exercise conditions reduced depressive symptoms significantly compared to treatment as usual, and there was no significant difference in treatment effect between the three exercise groups (Helgadottir, Hallgren, Ekblom, & Forsell, 2016).

The studies just described primarily focused on exercise as a standalone treatment for depression, but another set of studies have evaluated exercise as an augmentation treatment strategy. Mather et al. (2002) enrolled 83 older adults who still had significant depressive symptoms (>10 on the Geriatric Depression Scale) despite at least six weeks of antidepressant medication treatment. Participants were randomized to either twice-weekly group exercise classes or twice-weekly health education classes. At the end of the 10-week intervention, 55% of participants in the exercise group demonstrated a treatment response (depressive symptoms reduced by 30%) compared to 33% in the health education group. In a similar study, Trivedi et al. (2011) examined exercise as an augmentation treatment in adults who had significant residual depressive symptoms ($\geq$14 on the Hamilton Rating Scale for Depression) despite at least two months of antidepressant medication treatment. Participants were randomized to one of two exercise doses, equivalent to approximately 150 or 45 minutes per week. The covariate-adjusted remission rate for the high-dose group was 28.3% compared to 15.5% in the low-dose group. Though the difference was not statistically significant, the remission rate observed in the high-dose group is comparable to remission rates observed for augmentation strategies in the STAR*D trial (A. Rush, 2006; A. J. Rush et al., 2006).

20.2.2. Resistance Training

The studies described in Section 20.2.1 by Mather (2002) and Hallgren (2015) incorporated some resistance training in their exercise programs. However, these studies do not provide clear evidence for the potential of resistance training in the treatment of depression. Though not as extensively studied as aerobic exercise, there is at least preliminary evidence on resistance training. Epidemiological studies have demonstrated an association of grip strength, which provides a valid proxy measure of overall muscle strength, with reduced prevalence and incidence of depression (Fukumori et al., 2015; Hamer, Batty, & Kivimaki, 2015; McDowell, Gordon,

& Herring, 2018; Taekema, Gussekloo, Maier, Westendorp, & de Craen, 2010; Veronese et al., 2017). However, the most compelling evidence comes from two randomized controlled trials conducted in older adults by Singh et al. In the first study, 32 participants were randomized to either progressive resistance training or an attentional control group. At the end of the 10-week trial, participants in the exercise group experienced a greater reduction in depressive symptoms (Singh, Clements, & Fiatarone, 1997). In a follow-up phase, participants in the exercise group were asked to continue their resistance training in unsupervised sessions for an additional 10 weeks. At the end of that unsupervised period, participants in the exercise condition continued to have lower levels of depressive symptoms compared to the control group. This significant difference in depressive symptoms remained at a 26-month follow-up assessment (Singh, Clements, & Singh, 2001). In the second study, Singh et al. examined the dose–response relationship of resistance training by randomizing participants to either high-intensity resistance training (80% of maximum load), low-intensity resistance training (20% of maximum load), or treatment as usual. As hypothesized, the high-intensity resistance training resulted in greater reductions in depressive symptoms compared to both the low-intensity resistance training and treatment-as-usual groups, while the low-intensity resistance training resulted in greater reductions in depressive symptoms compared to the treatment-as-usual group (Singh et al., 2005).

20.2.3. Meta-analyses

The results of the studies described in Sections 20.2.1 and 20.2.2, along with other trials examining exercise as a treatment for depression, have been summarized in numerous meta-analyses (Cooney et al., 2013; Lawlor & Hopker, 2001; C. D. Rethorst, Wipfli, & Landers, 2009; Schuch, Vancampfort, et al., 2016; Stathopoulou, Powers, Berry, Smits, & Otto, 2006). Overall, these meta-analyses have reported moderate to large effect sizes supporting the use of exercise in the treatment of depression.

20.3. MAINTENANCE OF TREATMENT EFFECTS

Follow-up analyses of the two Blumenthal et al. (1999; 2007) studies suggest improved long-term outcomes with exercise treatment. In a follow-up of the SMILE I that randomized participants to exercise, sertraline, or a combination of the two, the exercise group demonstrated lower rates of depression relapse compared to the sertraline group ($p < .01$). Furthermore, participants who self-reported engaging in at least 50 minutes of weekly physical activity during the six-month follow-up period were 50% less likely to be depressed at the end of the follow-up (Babyak et al., 2000). A follow-up to SMILE II reported similar findings. Initial treatment group (home-based exercise, supervised exercise, sertraline, placebo pill) was not related to depression status at a one-year follow-up. This result is difficult to interpret as there was significant treatment crossover: During the follow-up period one-third of patients randomized to non-medication groups reported taking an antidepressant medication and 40% of participants in the non-exercise groups reported engaging in exercise during the follow-up period. Antidepressant medication use during the follow-up period was not associated with depression status. On the other hand, a dose–response relationship between exercise and depression status was observed, such that engaging in more exercise increased the likelihood of depression remission. The benefit of exercise peaked at approximately 180 minutes/week, as those who reported at least 180 minutes of exercise per week were three times more likely to be in remission compared to those who engaged in no exercise during the follow-up period (Hoffman et al., 2011).

Helgadottir et al. (2017) examined 12-month follow-up data from the Regassa study. Compared to treatment as usual, only the light exercise group demonstrated significantly lower depressive symptoms compared to treatment as usual. Additionally, compared to the moderate exercise group, both light exercise and vigorous exercise resulted in lower depressive symptoms at the 12-month follow-up.

20.4. PHYSICAL HEALTH BENEFITS

Beyond alleviating depressive symptoms, exercise has positive physical health benefits that may be particularly important for persons with depression. Physical conditions such as type 2 diabetes and coronary heart disease are common medical comorbidities in persons with depression, resulting in poorer disease outcomes and premature mortality. In a study by Rethorst et al. (2017), persons with depression had an increased mortality risk that was exacerbated by metabolic syndrome. However, the effects of both depression and metabolic syndrome on mortality were attenuated by improved cardiorespiratory fitness. Levels of cardiorespiratory fitness are lower in persons with depression but can be improved with exercise training (Stubbs, Rosenbaum, Vancampfort, Ward, & Schuch, 2016).

20.5. EXERCISE IN CLINICAL CARE SETTINGS

The evidence supporting exercise as an effective treatment for depression has resulted in its inclusion in many treatment guidelines. The American Psychiatric Association's *Practice Guideline for the Treatment of Patients with Major Depressive Disorder* supports exercise as a first-line treatment (Gelenberg et al., 2010). Similarly, the Canadian Network for Mood and Anxiety Treatments supports exercise as a "a first- or second-line treatment" (Ravindran et al., 2016), the National Institute for Health and Clinic Excellence (NICE) recommends exercise as an initial treatment for mild to moderate depression (NICE, 2009), and the Royal Australian & New Zealand College of Psychiatrists suggests lifestyle interventions, including exercise, be used as a "Step 0," prior to psychotherapy or pharmacotherapy (Malhi et al., 2015).

Yet, exercise remains underused as a treatment in clinical settings. In a survey of practitioners in the United Kingdom, only 5% include exercise as one of their top three treatment options for patients (NICE, 2009), and in a survey of patients receiving care in an outpatient mental health clinic, only 37% reported their providers discussed the benefits of exercise (Janney et al., 2017). The lack of exercise advice from providers is not only in contradiction of practice guidelines, but also contradicts the desires of patients with depression. Approximately 84% patients completing this survey reported noticing a link between their activity and their mental health, and 85% indicated an interest in becoming more active. In another survey of patients seeking treatment for depression, 96% expressed an interest in exercise as part of their treatment (Busch et al., 2016).

One barrier to implementation of exercise as a treatment for depression in the clinical setting is the lack of training providers receive in exercise prescription (Hebert, Caughy, & Shuval, 2012). Analyses of medical training programs in several countries have highlighted the virtual nonexistence of training in exercise prescription (Stoutenberg et al., 2015; Strong et al., 2017). A paper by Rethorst and Trivedi (2013) provides practical guidance for clinicians interested in prescribing exercise as a treatment for their patients with depression. The F.I.T.T. model for exercise prescription requires providing an exercise prescription that includes Frequency, Intensity, Time, and Type. Based on the existing evidence, Rethorst and Trivedi recommend prescription of an exercise program for patients with depression with a frequency of three to five sessions per week, at a moderate to vigorous intensity (50% to 85% maximum heart rate), each session lasting 45 to 60 minutes. As for the type of exercise, both aerobic exercise and resistance training have proven efficacious in the treatment of depression. Therefore, the type of exercise prescribed should be based on patient preference.

Clinical decision making about which patients are appropriate presents another challenge in providing exercise treatment in clinical settings. In a qualitative study, general practitioners note that a patient's motivation, resources, and life circumstances all contribute to his or her ability to act on exercise advice (Searle et al., 2012). As a result, clinicians often indicate a preference to refer patient to exercise professionals for exercise advice (Ampt et al., 2009; Laws et al., 2009; Persson, Brorsson, Ekvall Hansson, Troein, & Strandberg, 2013). While this is feasible in many countries, such as the United Kingdom and Australia, there are no reimbursable referral options available in the United States.

Another challenge in choosing the appropriate patients for exercise treatment involves identifying those who are most likely to benefit. Depression is a heterogeneous disorder, and that heterogeneity is reflected in treatment response. It is well established that only a subset of patients with depression will respond to an initial treatment with a selective serotonin reuptake inhibitor (Rush, 2006; Rush et al., 2006). Similarly, it appears that only a subset of patients will experience a reduction in depressive symptoms following exercise treatment, with remission rates equivalent to those of antidepressant medications. Therefore, an important step in optimizing the use of exercise treatment in clinical settings is predicting which patients will experience a treatment benefit.

Secondary analysis of completed randomized controlled trials provides preliminary evidence of treatment outcome predictors. Herman et al. (2002) identified clinical factors that predicted treatment response in the SMILE trial. Secondary analysis of the TREAD study has identified demographic (Trivedi et al., 2011), clinical (Greer et al., 2016; Rethorst, Sunderajan, et al., 2013; Rethorst, Tu, Carmody, Greer, & Trivedi, 2016), and biological predictors (Rethorst, Toups, et al., 2013; Toups et al., 2011) of treatment outcomes. Results of these analyses and others are summarized in a meta-analysis by Schuch et al. (2016) suggesting the potential for both clinical and biological factors as predictors of treatment response to exercise.

What is clear from these studies is that while several factors have been identified as statistically significant predictors of treatment response to exercise, no one factor predicts treatment outcomes with enough certainty to be of clinical utility. Instead, clinical utility will be derived from combining the predictive capability of multiple factors. As a proof-of-concept, an analysis of the TREAD study found a set of four predictors could predict treatment outcomes at a level sufficient to inform clinical decision making (Rethorst, South, Rush, Greer, & Trivedi, 2017).

20.6. FUTURE DIRECTIONS

As we have discussed, substantial evidence supports the use of exercise in the treatment of depression. Therefore, future research should focus on how exercise can be used in clinical settings. Specifically, strategies need to be developed to enhance the effectiveness of exercise prescription to ensure that patients are able to complete their prescribed exercise dose. Optimal use of exercise in clinical settings will also require a personalized medicine approach (Collins & Varmus, 2015) in which only those patients most likely to benefit would be prescribed exercise. Finally, more research is needed on exercise as a complement to other depression treatments. The SMILE trials have examined the effects of exercise combined with antidepressant medications but were likely not sufficiently powered to detect differences between active treatments. Less research has examined the combined effects of exercise and psychotherapy. Results from a recent trial indicate a possible benefit of exercise with cognitive–behavioral therapy in smoking cessation (Smits et al., 2016). Exercise might also serve as an intervention to maintain benefits from novel acute treatments like brain stimulation and ketamine.

REFERENCES

Ampt, A. J., Amoroso, C., Harris, M. F., McKenzie, S. H., Rose, V. K., & Taggart, J. R. (2009). Attitudes, norms and controls influencing lifestyle risk factor management in general practice. *BMC Family Practice, 10*, 59. doi:10.1186/1471-2296-10-59

Babyak, M., Blumenthal, J. A., Herman, S., Khatri, P., Doraiswamy, M., Moore, K., . . . Krishnan, K. R. (2000). Exercise treatment for major depression: Maintenance of therapeutic benefit at 10 months. *Psychosomatic Medicine, 62*(5), 633–638.

Blumenthal, J. A., Babyak, M. A., Doraiswamy, P. M., Watkins, L., Hoffman, B. M., Barbour, K. A., . . . Sherwood, A. (2007). Exercise and pharmacotherapy in the treatment of major depressive disorder. *Psychosomatic Medicine, 69*(7), 587–596. doi:10.1097/PSY.0b013e318148c19a

Blumenthal, J. A., Babyak, M. A., Moore, K. A., Craighead, W. E., Herman, S., Khatri, P., . . . Krishnan, K. R. (1999). Effects of exercise training on older patients with major depression. *Archives of Internal Medicine, 159*(19), 2349–2356.

Burrus, M. J. (1984). *The effects of a running treatment program on depressed adolescents.* University of Miami.

Busch, A. M., Ciccolo, J. T., Puspitasari, A. J., Nosrat, S., Whitworth, J. W., & Stults-Kolehmainen, M. (2016). Preferences for exercise as a treatment for depression. *Mental Health & Physical Activity, 10*, 68–72. doi:10.1016/j.mhpa.2015.12.004

Collins, F. S., & Varmus, H. (2015). A new initiative on precision medicine. *New England Journal of Medicine, 372*(9), 793–795.

Cooney, G. M., Dwan, K., Greig, C. A., Lawlor, D. A., Rimer, J., Waugh, F. R., . . . Mead, G. E. (2013). Exercise for depression. *Cochrane Database Syst Rev, 9*(9), CD004366. doi:10.1002/14651858.CD004366.pub6

Dishman, R. K., Sui, X., Church, T. S., Hand, G. A., Trivedi, M. H., & Blair, S. N. (2012). Decline in cardiorespiratory fitness and odds of incident depression. *American Journal of Preventive Medicine, 43*(4), 361–368. doi:10.1016/j.amepre.2012.06.011

Dunn, A. L., Trivedi, M. H., Kampert, J. B., Clark, C. G., & Chambliss, H. O. (2005). Exercise treatment for depression: Dfficacy and dose response. *American Journal of Preventive Medicine, 28*(1), 1–8. doi:10.1016/j.amepre.2004.09.003

Epstein, D. (1987). Aerobic activity versus group cognitive therapy: An evaluative study of contrasting interventions for the alleviation of clinical depression. University of Nevada, Reno.

Farmer, M. E., Locke, B. Z., Moscicki, E. K., Dannenberg, A. L., Larson, D. B., & Radloff, L. S. (1988). Physical activity and depressive symptoms: The NHANES I Epidemiologic Follow-up Study. *American Journal of Epidemiology, 128*(6), 1340–1351.

Fukumori, N., Yamamoto, Y., Takegami, M., Yamazaki, S., Onishi, Y., Sekiguchi, M., . . . Fukuhara, S. (2015). Association between hand-grip strength and depressive symptoms: Locomotive Syndrome and Health Outcomes in Aizu Cohort Study (LOHAS). *Age and Ageing, 44*(4), 592–598. doi:10.1093/ageing/afv013

Galper, D. I., Trivedi, M. H., Barlow, C. E., Dunn, A. L., & Kampert, J. B. (2006). Inverse association between physical inactivity and mental health in men and women. *Medicine and Science in Sports and Exercise, 38*(1), 173–178. doi:10.1249/01.mss.0000180883.32116.28

Gelenberg, A. J., Freeman, M. P., Markowitz, J. C., Rosenbaum, J. F., Thase, M. E., Trivedi, M. H., . . . Fawcett, J. A. (2010). *Practice guidelines for the treatment of patients with major depressive disorder* (3rd ed.). Arlington, VA: American Psychiatric Association.

Greer, T. L., Trombello, J. M., Rethorst, C. D., Carmody, T. J., Jha, M. K., Liao, A., . . . Trivedi, M. H. (2016). Improvements in psychosocial functioning and health-related quality of life following exercise augmentation in patients with treatment response but nonremitted major depressive disorder: results from the TREAD Study. *Depression and Anxiety, 33*(9), 870–881. doi:10.1002/da.22521

Hallgren, M., Kraepelien, M., Ojehagen, A., Lindefors, N., Zeebari, Z., Kaldo, V., & Forsell, Y. (2015). Physical exercise and internet-based cognitive-behavioural therapy in the treatment of depression: Randomised controlled trial. *British Journal of Psychiatry, 207*(3), 227–234. doi:10.1192/bjp.bp.114.160101

Hamer, M., Batty, G. D., & Kivimaki, M. (2015). Sarcopenic obesity and risk of new onset depressive symptoms in older adults: English Longitudinal Study of Ageing. *International Journal of Obesity, 39*(12), 1717–1720. doi:10.1038/ijo.2015.124

Harvey, S. B., Overland, S., Hatch, S. L., Wessely, S., Mykletun, A., & Hotopf, M. (2018). Exercise and the prevention of depression: Results of the HUNT Cohort Study. *American Journal of Psychiatry*, *175*(1), 28–36. doi:10.1176/appi.ajp.2017.16111223

Hebert, E. T., Caughy, M. O., & Shuval, K. (2012). Primary care providers' perceptions of physical activity counselling in a clinical setting: A systematic review. *British Journal of Sports Medicine*, *46*(9), 625–631. doi:10.1136/bjsports-2011-090734

Helgadottir, B., Forsell, Y., Hallgren, M., Moller, J., & Ekblom, O. (2017). Long-term effects of exercise at different intensity levels on depression: A randomized controlled trial. *Preventive Medicine*, *105*, 37–46. doi:10.1016/j.ypmed.2017.08.008

Helgadottir, B., Hallgren, M., Ekblom, O., & Forsell, Y. (2016). Training fast or slow? Exercise for depression: A randomized controlled trial. *Preventive Medicine*, *91*, 123–131. doi:10.1016/j.ypmed.2016.08.011

Herman, S., Blumenthal, J. A., Babyak, M., Khatri, P., Craighead, W. E., Krishnan, K. R., & Doraiswamy, P. M. (2002). Exercise therapy for depression in middle-aged and older adults: Predictors of early dropout and treatment failure. *Health Psychology*, *21*(6), 553–563.

Hoffman, B. M., Babyak, M. A., Craighead, W. E., Sherwood, A., Doraiswamy, P. M., Coons, M. J., & Blumenthal, J. A. (2011). Exercise and pharmacotherapy in patients with major depression: One-year follow-up of the SMILE study. *Psychosomatic Medicine*, *73*(2), 127–133. doi:10.1097/PSY.0b013e31820433a5

Janney, C. A., Brzoznowski, K. F., Richardson, C. R., Dopp, R. R., Segar, M. L., Ganoczy, D., . . . Valenstein, M. (2017). Moving towards wellness: Physical activity practices, perspectives, and preferences of users of outpatient mental health service. *General Hospital Psychiatry*, *49*, 63–66. doi:10.1016/j.genhosppsych.2017.07.004

Kanner, K. D. (1991). High versus low-intensity exercise as part of an inpatient treatment program for childhood and adolescent depression. Ph.D. thesis, California School of Professional Psychology, San Diego.

Lawlor, D. A., & Hopker, S. W. (2001). The effectiveness of exercise as an intervention in the management of depression: Systematic review and meta-regression analysis of randomised controlled trials. *BMJ*, *322*(7289), 763–767.

Laws, R. A., Kemp, L. A., Harris, M. F., Davies, G. P., Williams, A. M., & Eames-Brown, R. (2009). An exploration of how clinician attitudes and beliefs influence the implementation of lifestyle risk factor management in primary healthcare: A grounded theory study. *Implementation Science*, *4*, 66. doi:10.1186/1748-5908-4-66

Levin, S. J. (1984). The effects of a ten-week jogging program as an adjunctive treatment for patients in a social rehabilitation clinic. Dissertation, Adelphi University.

Malhi, G. S., Bassett, D., Boyce, P., Bryant, R., Fitzgerald, P. B., Fritz, K., . . . Singh, A. B. (2015). Royal Australian and New Zealand College of Psychiatrists clinical practice guidelines for mood disorders. *Australian and New Zealand Journal of Psychiatry*, *49*(12), 1087–1206. doi:10.1177/0004867415617657

Martinsen, E. W., Medhus, A., & Sandvik, L. (1985). Effects of aerobic exercise on depression: a controlled study. *British Medical Journal (Clinical Research Ed.)*, *291*(6488), 109.

Mather, A. S., Rodriguez, C., Guthrie, M. F., McHarg, A. M., Reid, I. C., & McMurdo, M. E. (2002). Effects of exercise on depressive symptoms in older adults with poorly responsive depressive disorder: Randomised controlled trial. *British Journal of Psychiatry*, *180*, 411–415.

McCann, I. L., & Holmes, D. S. (1984). Influence of aerobic exercise on depression. *Journal of Personality and Social Psychology*, *46*(5), 1142–1147.

McDowell, C. P., Gordon, B. R., & Herring, M. P. (2018). Sex-related differences in the association between grip strength and depression: Results from the Irish Longitudinal Study on Ageing. *Experimental Gerontology*, *104*, 147–152. doi:10.1016/j.exger.2018.02.010

McNeil, J. K., LeBlanc, E. M., & Joyner, M. (1991). The effect of exercise on depressive symptoms in the moderately depressed elderly. *Psychology and Aging, 6*(3), 487–488.

National Institute for Health and Care Excellence (NICE). (2009). Depression: Treatment and management of depression in adults. Clinical Guideline 90. Retrieved from http://www.nice.org.uk.

Persson, G., Brorsson, A., Ekvall Hansson, E., Troein, M., & Strandberg, E. L. (2013). Physical activity on prescription (PAP) from the general practitioner's perspective—a qualitative study. *BMC Family Practice, 14*, 128. doi:10.1186/1471-2296-14-128

Ravindran, A. V., Balneaves, L. G., Faulkner, G., Ortiz, A., McIntosh, D., Morehouse, R. L., . . . CANMAT Depression Work Group. (2016). Canadian Network for Mood and Anxiety Treatments (CANMAT) 2016 clinical guidelines for the management of adults with major depressive disorder: Section 5. Complementary and alternative medicine treatments. *Canadian Journal of Psychiatry. Revue Canadienne de Psychiatrie, 61*(9), 576–587. doi:10.1177/0706743716660290

Rethorst, C. D., Leonard, D., Barlow, C. E., Willis, B. L., Trivedi, M. H., & DeFina, L. F. (2017). Effects of depression, metabolic syndrome, and cardiorespiratory fitness on mortality: Results from the Cooper Center Longitudinal Study. *Psychological Medicine, 47*(14), 2414–2420. doi:10.1017/S0033291717000897

Rethorst, C. D., Moncrieft, A. E., Gellman, M. D., Arredondo, E. M., Buelna, C., Castaneda, S. F., . . . Stoutenberg, M. (2017). Isotemporal analysis of the association of objectively measured physical activity with depressive symptoms: Results from Hispanic Community Health Study/Study of Latinos (HCHS/SOL). *Journal of Physical Activity and Health, 14*(9), 733–739. doi:10.1123/jpah.2016-0648

Rethorst, C. D., South, C. C., Rush, A. J., Greer, T. L., & Trivedi, M. H. (2017). Prediction of treatment outcomes to exercise in patients with nonremitted major depressive disorder. *Depression and Anxiety, 34*(12), 1116–1122. doi:10.1002/da.22670

Rethorst, C. D., Sunderajan, P., Greer, T. L., Grannemann, B. D., Nakonezny, P. A., Carmody, T. J., & Trivedi, M. H. (2013). Does exercise improve self-reported sleep quality in nonremitted major depressive disorder? *Psychological Medicine, 43*(4), 699–709. doi:10.1017/S0033291712001675

Rethorst, C. D., Toups, M. S., Greer, T. L., Nakonezny, P. A., Carmody, T. J., Grannemann, B. D., . . . Trivedi, M. H. (2013). Pro-inflammatory cytokines as predictors of antidepressant effects of exercise in major depressive disorder. *Molecular Psychiatry, 18*(10), 1119–1124. doi:10.1038/mp.2012.125

Rethorst, C. D., & Trivedi, M. H. (2013). Evidence-based recommendations for the prescription of exercise for major depressive disorder. *Journal of Psychiatric Practice, 19*(3), 204–212. doi:10.1097/01.pra.0000430504.16952.3e

Rethorst, C. D., Tu, J., Carmody, T. J., Greer, T. L., & Trivedi, M. H. (2016). Atypical depressive symptoms as a predictor of treatment response to exercise in major depressive disorder. *Journal of Affective Disorders, 200*, 156–158. doi:10.1016/j.jad.2016.01.052

Rethorst, C. D., Wipfli, B. M., & Landers, D. M. (2009). The antidepressive effects of exercise: A meta-analysis of randomized trials. *Sports Medicine, 39*(6), 491–511. doi:10.2165/00007256-200939060-00004

Rush, A. (2006). Acute and longer-term outcomes in depressed outpatients requiring one or several treatment steps: A STAR*D report. *American Journal of Psychiatry, 163*(11), 1905. doi:10.1176/ajp.2006.163.11.1905

Rush, A. J., Trivedi, M. H., Wisniewski, S. R., Stewart, J. W., Nierenberg, A. A., Thase, M. E., . . . Team, S. D. S. (2006). Bupropion-SR, sertraline, or venlafaxine-XR after failure of SSRIs for depression. *New England Journal of Medicine, 354*(12), 1231–1242. doi:10.1056/NEJMoa052963

Schuch, F. B., Dunn, A. L., Kanitz, A. C., Delevatti, R. S., & Fleck, M. P. (2016). Moderators of response in exercise treatment for depression: A systematic review. *Journal of Affective Disorders*, *195*, 40–49. doi:10.1016/j.jad.2016.01.014

Schuch, F. B., Vancampfort, D., Firth, J., Rosenbaum, S., Ward, P. B., Silva, E. S., . . . Stubbs, B. (2018). Physical activity and incident depression: A meta-analysis of prospective cohort studies. *American Journal of Psychiatry*, *175*(7), 631–648. doi:10.1176/appi. ajp.2018.17111194

Schuch, F. B., Vancampfort, D., Richards, J., Rosenbaum, S., Ward, P. B., & Stubbs, B. (2016). Exercise as a treatment for depression: A meta-analysis adjusting for publication bias. *Journal of Psychiatric Research*, *77*, 42–51. doi:10.1016/j.jpsychires.2016.02.023

Searle, A., Calnan, M., Turner, K. M., Lawlor, D. A., Campbell, J., Chalder, M., & Lewis, G. (2012). General practitioners' beliefs about physical activity for managing depression in primary care. *Mental Health and Physical Activity*, *5*(1), 13–19. doi:10.1016/j.mhpa.2011.11.001

Singh, N. A., Clements, K. M., & Fiatarone, M. A. (1997). A randomized controlled trial of progressive resistance training in depressed elders. *Journals of Gerontology. Series A: Biological Sciences and Medical Sciences*, *52*(1), M27–35.

Singh, N. A., Clements, K. M., & Singh, M. A. (2001). The efficacy of exercise as a long-term antidepressant in elderly subjects: A randomized, controlled trial. *Journals of Gerontology. Series A: Biological Sciences and Medical Sciences*, *56*(8), M497–M504.

Singh, N. A., Stavrinos, T. M., Scarbek, Y., Galambos, G., Liber, C., & Fiatarone Singh, M. A. (2005). A randomized controlled trial of high versus low intensity weight training versus general practitioner care for clinical depression in older adults. *Journals of Gerontology. Series A: Biological Sciences and Medical Sciences*, *60*(6), 768–776.

Smits, J. A., Zvolensky, M. J., Davis, M. L., Rosenfield, D., Marcus, B. H., Church, T. S., . . . Baird, S. O. (2016). The efficacy of vigorous-intensity exercise as an aid to smoking cessation in adults with high anxiety sensitivity: A randomized controlled trial. *Psychosomatic Medicine*, *78*(3), 354–364. doi:10.1097/psy.0000000000000264

Stathopoulou, G., Powers, M. B., Berry, A. C., Smits, J. A. J., & Otto, M. W. (2006). Exercise interventions for mental health: A quantitative and qualitative review. *Clinical Psychology: Science and Practice*, *13*(2), 179–193. doi:10.1111/j.1468-2850.2006.00021.x

Stoutenberg, M., Stasi, S., Stamatakis, E., Danek, D., Dufour, T., Trilk, J. L., & Blair, S. N. (2015). Physical activity training in US medical schools: Preparing future physicians to engage in primary prevention. *The Physician and Sportsmedicine*, *43*(4), 388–394. doi:10.1080/00913847.2015.1084868

Strong, A., Stoutenberg, M., Hobson-Powell, A., Hargreaves, M., Beeler, H., & Stamatakis, E. (2017). An evaluation of physical activity training in Australian medical school curricula. *Journal of Science and Medicine in Sport*, *20*(6), 534–538. doi:10.1016/j.jsams.2016.10.011

Stubbs, B., Koyanagi, A., Schuch, F. B., Firth, J., Rosenbaum, S., Veronese, N., . . . Vancampfort, D. (2016). Physical activity and depression: A large cross-sectional, population-based study across 36 low- and middle-income countries. *Acta Psychiatrica Scandinavica*, *134*(6), 546–556. doi:10.1111/acps.12654

Stubbs, B., Rosenbaum, S., Vancampfort, D., Ward, P. B., & Schuch, F. B. (2016). Exercise improves cardiorespiratory fitness in people with depression: A meta-analysis of randomized control trials. *Journal of Affective Disorders*, *190*, 249–253. doi:10.1016/j.jad.2015.10.010

Taekema, D. G., Gussekloo, J., Maier, A. B., Westendorp, R. G., & de Craen, A. J. (2010). Handgrip strength as a predictor of functional, psychological and social health. A prospective population-based study among the oldest old. *Age and Ageing*, *39*(3), 331–337. doi:10.1093/ageing/afq022

Toups, M. S., Greer, T. L., Kurian, B. T., Grannemann, B. D., Carmody, T. J., Huebinger, R., . . . Trivedi, M. H. (2011). Effects of serum brain derived neurotrophic factor on exercise augmentation treatment of depression. *Journal of Psychiatric Research, 45*(10), 1301–1306. doi:10.1016/j.jpsychires.2011.05.002

Trivedi, M. H., Greer, T. L., Church, T. S., Carmody, T. J., Grannemann, B. D., Galper, D. I., . . . Blair, S. N. (2011). Exercise as an augmentation treatment for nonremitted major depressive disorder: A randomized, parallel dose comparison. *Journal of Clinical Psychiatry, 72*(5), 677–684. doi:10.4088/JCP.10m06743

Vallance, J. K., Winkler, E. A., Gardiner, P. A., Healy, G. N., Lynch, B. M., & Owen, N. (2011). Associations of objectively-assessed physical activity and sedentary time with depression: NHANES (2005-2006). *Preventive Medicine, 53*(4-5), 284–288. doi:10.1016/j.ypmed.2011.07.013

Veale, D., Le Fevre, K., Pantelis, C., de Souza, V., Mann, A., & Sargeant, A. (1992). Aerobic exercise in the adjunctive treatment of depression: a randomized controlled trial. *Journal of the Royal Society of Medicine, 85*(9), 541–544.

Veronese, N., Stubbs, B., Trevisan, C., Bolzetta, F., De Rui, M., Solmi, M., . . . Sergi, G. (2017). Poor physical performance predicts future onset of depression in elderly people: Progetto Veneto Anziani Longitudinal Study. *Physical Therapy, 97*(6), 659–668. doi:10.1093/ptj/pzx017

/// 21 /// THERAPEUTIC MINDFULNESS AND DEPRESSION

EVAN COLLINS AND ZINDEL SEGAL

21.1. INTRODUCTION

Currently, there is considerable scientific and popular interest in therapeutic mindfulness-based interventions (MBI) for a variety of clinical conditions. Some of the most robust findings are for depression in its various forms, and this chapter will review the knowledge base to date. Starting with the history and development of the clinical use of mindfulness, we will explore the various MBIs used in depression, review the supporting evidence and putative mechanisms, and discuss future directions.

Mindfulness is one translation of the ancient Pali word *sati*, describing an awareness arising from certain forms of meditation practice. Although present in many Buddhist traditions, it was introduced as a secular therapeutic modality in 1979 by Jon Kabat-Zinn[1,2] when he developed mindfulness-based stress reduction (MBSR) as a group-based treatment for chronically ill patients not responding to traditional medical therapies. MBSR was envisioned as a trans-diagnostic intervention targeting those with chronic pain and other chronic physical conditions not well addressed by a medical model focused on cure. Despite being focused on chronic physical conditions MBSR inevitably dealt with mental health distress like depression and anxiety associated with these conditions.[3]

Although Kabat-Zinn had begun to formally evaluate MBSR for both mental health symptoms secondary to chronic pain[1] and to primary anxiety disorder,[4] its utility in depression began with the work of John Teasdale, Mark Williams, and Zindel Segal in the 1990s. Funded to develop an adaptation of cognitive therapy to target depressive relapse, they studied MBSR with Kabat-Zinn and went on to develop mindfulness-based cognitive therapy (MBCT) as the first focused MBI for depression. In doing so they also emphasized the need to standardize the modality and rigorously assess it through randomized controlled trials (RCTs).[5]

One operational definition of mindfulness is "the awareness that emerges through paying attention on purpose, in the present moment, non-judgementally, to things as they are."[6] This denotes an awareness practice that arises from intentional training of attention and supported by attitudes of nonjudgment, curiosity, and acceptance. This speaks to a model of mindfulness comprising three components (intention, attention, and attitude[7]), which lead to increased awareness and a re-perceiving of experience. This training of attentional focus and investigation of experience through mindfulness practice is thought to result in increases in cognitive, emotional, and behavioral flexibility and regulation; distress tolerance; and the capacity for decentering from negative mental states. These metacognitive skills that regulate distressing thoughts and emotions in depression are thought to develop through observing thoughts in mindfulness meditation similar to the strategy of cognitive appraisal in traditional cognitive therapy.[8]

21.2. MINDFULNESS AND DEPRESSION SYMPTOMS, SYNDROMES, AND DISORDERS

Whereas MBSR groups are trans-diagnostic and only more recently targeted toward specific patient groups like cancer, pain, and addiction,[9] MBCT was originally designed and researched for prevention of relapse in remitted patients with recurrent depression. More recently MBCT has been offered to other groups, including other mood disorders or physical conditions with secondary depressive symptoms[10] as well as more trans-diagnostic groups including mixed mood and anxiety disorders.[11] By and large, despite the heterogeneity in group composition and application, the focus of MBSR remains stress, whereas in MBCT the lens is mood.

Even within a homogeneous MBCT group of remitted patients with recurrent depression, there will always be a range of symptomatic heterogeneity, from complete remission to more severe residual depressive symptoms.[12] From a diagnostic perspective, the mood disorders that MBIs (chiefly MBCT) have been studied in include (1) recurrent major depressive disorder (MDD) in full or partial remission,[8] (2) residual depressive symptoms,[13] treatment-resistant depression,[14] and suicide ideation,[15] (3) depression, whether MDD or syndromal, in specific populations like adolescents[16] or geriatric populations,[17] (4) other depressive disorders as outlined in the fifth edition of the American Psychiatric Association's *Diagnostic and Statistical Manual of Mental Disorders* (DSM-5), including bipolar depression,[18] dysthymia,[19] and depression secondary to or comorbid with substance use,[20] and (4) depressive symptoms in medically ill populations like cancer[21] or chronic pain.[22]

Other group-based MBIs that address these mood disorders aside from MBCT, and to the degree participants with depression are enrolled, include mindfulness-based relapse prevention (MBRP) targeting substance use relapse;[23] mindful self-compassion, a group therapy focused on self-compassion;[24] and MBSR.[25] Individual therapies that have explicit components of mindfulness, although not necessarily training in meditation practices, include acceptance and commitment therapy, which is commonly used to treat depression;[26] dialectical behavioral therapy, which uses aspects of mindfulness to treat borderline personality and associated mood manifestations like depressive episodes, emotional dysregulation, and suicidality;[27] and other mindfulness-informed individual psychotherapies either totally focused on mindfulness or integrating mindfulness practices and constructs into relational or psychodynamic modalities.[28]

21.3. THE EVIDENCE BASE

There has been an exponential increase in published research of mindfulness and in particular RCTs in a rapidly increasing breadth of clinical populations. With increasing RCTs there are now a number of systematic reviews and meta-analyses from which to draw conclusions. In this chapter we focus on the MBIs that have training in mindfulness meditation as a core feature, specifically MBSR, MBCT, and their variations. Most of the research, and the strongest evidence in mood disorders, is with MBCT; this is not surprising given it was originally designed to target depression. Each review offers a different lens for understanding the impact of MBI on depression, whether symptom, syndrome, or clinical disorder. In what follows we focus on the results on depression, even though most studies assessed multiple outcomes. Taken together they demonstrate a growing evidence base for therapeutic mindfulness.

Goyal et al.[29] conducted a systematic review and meta-analysis on stress-related outcomes, including depression, in diverse clinical populations. Assessing 47 studies of 3,320 patients, they found low-moderate effect sizes in mindfulness meditation reducing depression at eight weeks ($d = 0.30$) and lower effects ($d = 0.23$) at three to six months. In separating out those studies using active controls they found low evidence of no effect, or insufficient evidence for differences between MBIs and control conditions, but noted most studies were not sufficiently powered to detect differences or non-inferiority.

A more recent meta-analysis by Goldberg et al.[30] examined the efficacy of MBI on clinical symptoms for heterogeneous psychiatric disorders and included 171 RCTs comprising 12,005 participants from 2000 to 2016. Given past criticism around mindfulness research trial design, the authors differentiated between five different control conditions: (1) no treatment (e.g., waitlist control), (2) minimal treatment, denoting brief or low-intensity interventions, (3) nonspecific active controls, in which no mechanism or rationale was identified, (4) specific active controls with rationale but minimal evidence, and (5) evidence-based treatments based on American Psychological Association's recommendations for the specific disorder. The strongest findings were for MBI effects on depression, with some supporting evidence for pain, smoking, and other addiction disorders. At post-treatment, MBI was superior in treating depression to no treatment ($d = 0.59$) and specific active controls ($d = 0.37$); however, it showed no difference with evidence-based treatments ($d = -0.01$). At follow-up the results were similar, with MBI superiority to no treatment and specific controls ($d = 0.55$ and 0.35 respectively) but equivalency with evidence-based treatments ($d = 0.04$).

In studying the effects of standardized MBIs in healthcare, Gotnick et al.[31] provided an overview of systematic reviews and meta-analyses and broke down their results into specific clinical populations. In summarizing MBI effects in cancer populations they reported 16 RCTs comprising 1,668 cancer patients and found significant improvements in mental health but not physical symptoms, with effect sizes for reducing depression ranging from 0.37 to 0.44 (standardized mean difference [SMD]). In nine studies of 577 patients with cardiovascular disease, improvements in depressive symptoms showed SMD = 0.35. In 13 RCTs studying 722 patients with chronic pain, depression change showed SMD = 0.26, and in 16 studies of 1,331 patients with various chronic somatic conditions, depression change was SMD = 0.45 for MBSR and SMD = 0.64 for MBCT.

The above studies were a mix of MBIs, including MBCT. Assessing MBSR specifically and its effects on depression, a Campbell Collaboration systematic review[32] pooled 96 studies encompassing 7,647 patients. Of these studies 22 trials targeted mild to moderate mental health problems, 47 somatic conditions, and 32 from the general population. MBSR showed moderate effect sizes in various mental health outcomes, and in the 11 studies using established measures of depression the effect size was moderate in studies with inactive controls ($g = 0.53$) and low ($g = 0.22$) in studies using active controls.

Looking specifically at MBIs in those meeting diagnostic criteria for depression with current symptoms, Strauss et al.[33] conducted a meta-analysis of 12 studies among 575 patients. There were significant between-group differences in favor of MBI ($g = -0.073$) in treating depression irrespective of primary diagnosis, whereas no significant findings were found in treating anxiety symptoms. However, when studies using inactive and active controls were separated, large significant effect sizes were evidenced with inactive controlled studies ($g = -1.03$) but not with active controls ($g = 0.03$). Six of the studies were MBCT, and these showed significant differences in treating depression ($g = 0.39$) versus the five studies using MBSR.

Another systematic review of MBIs and other meditation therapies for depressive disorders, including yoga, was conducted by Jain et al.[34] Assessing 18 RCTs (of which 8 were MBCT) among 1,173 participants, they found moderate to large effect sizes in studies with waitlist or treatment-as-usual controls, as well as nonspecific active controls like psychoeducation, but no significant differences when the meditation modality was controlled with an evidence-based treatment. As Goyal et al. cautioned in their meta-analysis, Jain et al. also recommend that studies that compared MBIs with other evidence-based treatments for depression need to be adequately powered and pre-hoc criteria identified as to how differences or noninferiority will be determined.

Again, some of the strongest evidence is with MBCT in preventing depressive relapse in those with histories of recurrent major depression. In studying this, Kuyken et al.[35] pooled 1,258 remitted patients from nine studies. In comparing MBCT with any non-MBCT treatment, the hazard ratio (HR) for depressive relapse was 0.69; in comparing MBCT with active treatments in five studies the HR was 0.79; and in comparing MBCT with antidepressant maintenance the HR was 0.77, but it did not reach statistical significance. From this body of findings, there seems to be a significantly reduced rate of relapse/recurrence over 60 weeks but equivalence compared with usual care including antidepressants. In exploring moderators for effect they found no evidence that MBCT had differential effects based on demographics; however, data suggest that treatment effects were larger in those with higher depressive scores at baseline, adding support to previous work that suggests MBCT is most beneficial in those with a greater number of past depressive relapse episodes[36] and those who report a history of childhood adversity.[37]

In a systematic review of MBCT to treat major depression,[38] the authors synthesized 17 studies and distinguished between MBCT monotherapy and adjunctive therapy, as well between prevention of depressive relapse and treatment of active symptoms in MDD. Their review supported the use of adjunctive MBCT for both relapse prevention and active treatment but found insufficient evidence for monotherapy, although a large trial since then[37] showed MBCT with discontinuation of antidepressants to be equivalent to maintenance antidepressant treatment. Their critique of current research is that there is a need for larger sample sizes to allow for stratification of disease severity and better monitoring of adverse effects, and to account for dropout rates by using intention-to-treat analyses.

In studying the effect of different nonpharmacologic therapies to prevent depressive relapse,[39] a meta-analysis of 22 studies and 4,216 subjects identified seven studies as MBCT and the others being cognitive therapy, interpersonal therapy, and various service-level interventions. Cognitive therapy showed a risk reduction for depressive relapse of 25%, interpersonal therapy 22%, and MBCT 21%, although differences between the modalities were not significant. Since then a recent head-to-head RCT between MBCT and cognitive therapy also showed equivalence between rates or time to relapse of major depression over 24 months of follow-up.[6]

There have been a number of reviews studying the impact of MBI in specific populations, including youth,[16] the elderly,[17] and family caregivers of those with dementia,[40] among others, all of which have assessed depression as one of the outcome measures. Additionally, there are reviews specific to depressive symptoms in mental health and physical conditions like MBRP for substance use disorders[41] and MBSR or MBCT in chronic pain patients[22] or patients with cancer.[21] By and large, all these studies report the same results as those we have already reviewed: MBIs tend to show moderate effect sizes in treating depression but effect size lessens when MBIs are compared with active controls and lessens further or disappears when compared to evidence-based treatments for depression. An exception is the review of MBRP,[41] where there are no significant findings supporting mindfulness reducing depression in this population.

Specific to depression in bipolar disorder, a recent meta-analysis[18] assessed 12 MBCT studies, of which only 3 were controlled. Although overall, in pre–post assessments of 142 patients, MBCT improved depression and anxiety but not mania or cognition, in the three RCTs with treatment-as-usual controls among 132 patients, there were no significant between-group differences. The authors conclude that there is tentative evidence for MBCT in bipolar disorder but more larger-scale research needs to be done. At the very least MBCT appears to be feasible and acceptable in this population.

As the evidence base matures, there is the need for research to expand from efficacy to effectiveness in terms of economic evaluations, generalizability to community settings, and implementation science.[42] To this end, Kuyken et al.[37] conducted a large trial of MBCT for prevention of depressive relapse in general practices in the community. As part of this study, in which 424 patients were followed for 60 weeks and received either MBCT with tapering or discontinuation of antidepressants compared to those receiving antidepressants alone, an economic assessment was added. Although MBCT added additional costs due to its group format, the overall increase was minimal. Other health care and societal costs were similar in the two arms, and any cost differences were not statistically significant.

In general, MBIs have been shown to be feasible and safe for many clinical populations, including those with symptomatic MDD, although only a minimum of studies have systematically assessed the adverse effects of mindfulness.[38] The relative feasibility and safety of MBIs in depressed populations is important as there were concerns early on that those with active depression might not be suitable for participation in mindfulness groups as their cognitive, physical, or mood symptoms might limit participation. Related to safety is the body of work applying MBCT to reducing suicidal ideation in depressive disorders.[15] The research investigating this suggests that MBCT might decouple the association between suicidal cognitions and other depressive symptoms. The few RCTs testing this hypothesis show some benefit, with small to moderate effect sizes independent of other depressive symptoms.[43]

As most MBIs are group modalities there is a potential for cost-efficiency, although challenges to access (e.g., expense, waitlists, and geographic distance) remain. As with other time-limited psychotherapies, online formats are being developed as one route to increase access. A 2016 meta-analysis of online MBI synthesized 15 RCTs, of which 8 had active controls.[44] Depression effect sizes were small but significant ($g = 0.29$), although seven of the studies were in nonclinical populations, and of the three studies in anxiety or depression, the effect size for depression change was $g = 0.41$. Clearly more research is needed to evaluate whether the potential increased reach of digital therapies can be justified even if they provide a lower level of overall efficacy.

In summarizing the evidence base, the research shows moderate effect sizes in addressing depressive relapse and treatment of active depression (be it MDD or comorbid, syndromal depression) with reduced effect sizes or no difference in comparing MBIs with alternative evidence-based treatments. Further research is needed with active controls that match the MBI in time and intensity; larger samples powered to detect differences or non-inferiority; longer follow-ups; reports of treatment fidelity and adverse effects; procedures that support data sharing between studies; and attention to generalizability, including community-based studies. It would also help for studies to explore mediating and moderating variables supporting a better understanding of mechanisms and potential differences in treatment effect. At minimum, studies should report on key background variables, including demographics and clinical history of depression.

21.4. DEPRESSION TREATMENT GUIDELINE RECOMMENDATIONS

As a consequence of its growing evidence base, MBCT is being increasingly recommended in national and other depression treatment guidelines. These include the 2009 National Institute for Health and Care Excellence (NICE) guidelines for depression in the United Kingdom (last updated in 2018),[45] which recommend MBCT "for people who are currently well but have experienced three or more previous episodes of depression." In the Canadian Mood and Anxiety Treatment (CANMAT) guidelines in Canada,[46] "MBCT is recommended as sequential first-line treatment (Level 1 Evidence) after a course of antidepressants, and MBCT is recommended as a second-line alternative to long-term maintenance antidepressant treatment (Level 2 Evidence)." The US Veterans Affairs and Department of Defense Clinical Management Guideline for Management of Major Depression[47] recommends that MBCT

> should be used during the continuation phase of treatment with patients at high risk for relapse (i.e., two or more prior episodes, double depression, unstable remission status) to reduce the risk of subsequent relapse/recurrence. This can occur after pharmacotherapy has ended or as a combined intervention for patients continuing pharmacotherapy. This is rated [A] as a strong recommendation."

Finally, the Royal Australian and New Zealand College of Psychiatrists' clinical practice guidelines for mood disorders[48] cite MBCT as a maintenance treatment for depression and prevention of depressive relapse.

21.5. POTENTIAL MECHANISMS OF ACTION

In understanding the mechanisms underlying the therapeutic effect of mindfulness in depression, it is helpful to explore the theoretical underpinnings of MBCT. Whereas cognitive therapy is premised on the impact of negative thinking on mood perpetuated by dysfunctional schemas, MBCT arose from work of Teasdale et al., who studied the impact of negative mood on thinking versus thinking on mood.[49]

Together with Segal and Williams, Teasdale posited a model of cognitive vulnerability that viewed individuals with recurrent depression as having unique patterns of negative thinking.[50] According to this model, in those with a history of depression, minor mood fluctuations that others might experience as normal everyday sadness would precipitate a reinstatement of thinking patterns experienced when depressed so that small changes in mood trigger large changes in negative thinking. This model was expanded to include two other mechanisms observed in individuals prone to depressive relapse: (1) a neurobiological activation threshold posited by Post[51] that decreases the more episodes of depression an individual experiences· and (2) employment of a ruminative thinking style as a response to depression. This rumination response style, first proposed by Nolen-Hoeksema,[52] is an attempt to cope with depression by problem solving and "thinking oneself out of depression" and has repeatedly been shown to be a dysfunctional response style that perpetuates more rumination and depressive feelings.

These three concurrent mechanisms of increased vulnerability through both cognitive reactivity and a lower neurobiological threshold, as well as the maladaptive coping style of depressive rumination, formed the basis for understanding how mindfulness might address depression relapse risk. Whereas the cognitive therapy model focuses on the *content* of thought though an identification and reinterpretation of cognitions, the mindfulness model explores one's *relationship* to thoughts in seeing them as mere mental events and components of experience that pass through the mind and over which one can exercise a choice in taking them up or not. While both emphasize a decentered stance, the mindfulness model focuses less on changing the content of thoughts and more about decentering as an end in itself from which to observe experience in mindful awareness and decrease reactivity. As part of this process, the participant explores how other components of experience, like somatic sensation and emotion, interplay with thinking and impact behavior.

The mindfulness model is predicated on contrasting two modes of mind for the depressed individual: (1) the *doing* mode, which is used to accomplish tasks that are necessary for achieving goals in the impersonal, external world but are less useful in our personal and internal worlds, especially in dealing with mental states like sadness and (2) the *being* mode, in which one practices direct experience of whatever is present, be it pleasant, unpleasant, or neutral, knowing that like all aspects of experience it will pass and in most cases need not be avoided or held onto. The being mode situates one in the present moment as opposed to the future, which can seed anxious preoccupation, or the past, which fuels depressive rumination. This is not to say there is anything wrong with the doing mode and its necessity for daily functioning, or that the being mode is some transcendental state devoid of activity. Both are modes of mind that can accompany any activity or lack of activity; however, the being mode is a direct experiential form of cognitive self-focus distinct from the analytical and conceptual processing of experience of the doing mode, which promotes reactivity and is maladaptive with depression.[53]

Research that supports this model includes neuroimaging studies such as those done by Farb et al.,[54] in which mindfulness training was associated with greater processing of experience through present moment attention evidenced by decreases in medial prefrontal cortex (mPFC) activity, a region associated with self-evaluation and task-oriented processing, while waitlist controls were more likely to employ a narrative self-reference with increased mPFC activity. This suggested that interoceptive awareness could prevent hijacking of thought into rumination. Other support for this model came from Brewer et al.,[55] who showed that mindfulness training was associated with decreased activation in mPFC and posterior cingulate cortex, regions making up the default mode network known to be associated with depression.[56]

In a supporting vein, a neuroimaging study of individuals at risk for depression[57] had subjects view sad and neutral film clips to assess cognitive reactivity. Following exposure to the mood challenge there was increased activity in the mPFC along with decreased activity in the visual cortex. Those individuals with the largest discrepancy between prefrontal and visual reactivity showed the greatest risk of relapse over 18 months of follow-up, suggesting that attention to somatosensory foci when exposed to negative mood might lessen cognitive reactivity and rumination.

Taken together, neuroimaging supports a model in which mindfulness training enhances present moment awareness through recruitment of sensory pathways over more cognitive evaluation through the prefrontal cortices. Favoring nonconceptual sensory pathways over habitual cognitive reappraisal responses to negative stimuli seems to lead to an emotional regulation characterized by lessened negative self-evaluation, increased distress tolerance, and greater self-compassion and empathy.[58]

To further explore potential mechanisms, a systematic review of MBCT studies was conducted by van der Velden et al.[59] Twenty-three studies were included, of which 12 showed some support for mindfulness as a construct, negative cognitions like worry and rumination, cognitive reactivity, self-compassion and meta-awareness or decentering in predicting response to MBCT. Regarding depressogenic thinking, worry showed a clearer signal than rumination. More preliminary evidence was found for attention regulation, memory specificity, self-discrepancy, emotional reactivity, and momentary positive and negative affect. The authors also suggested that other neural or genetic factors are important targets in need of further study.

In a systematic review and meta-analysis of meditation studies by Gu et al.[60], 9 MBCT and 11 MBSR studies were examined. In applying structural equation modeling to pooled meta-analytic results they found strong and consistent evidence for cognitive and emotional reactivity as mediators, while mindfulness and repetitive negative thinking yielded moderate but consistent support. In addition, there was preliminary but insufficient evidence for psychological flexibility and self-compassion as mechanisms. In their modeling with mental health outcomes, especially depression, there was stronger evidence for mindfulness and repetitive negative thinking as significant mediators.

Another review of MBSR and MBCT mechanisms examined 4 studies of co-morbid physical and psychological conditions and 14 studies of psychological conditions alone.[61] They identified a number of potential mechanisms, including mindfulness, worry, and rumination in the physical health studies, and mindfulness skills, rumination, worry, affect and self-compassion, cognitive and emotional reactivity, and attentional processing in the studies focused on psychological conditions. Of these, the strongest evidence was for mindfulness, although in general few of the studies met established criteria for mechanism studies. Similar to the two reviews cited above, there was a call for more rigorous methodologies to better understand mechanisms of mindfulness.

Table 21.1 summarizes this work and lists potential moderators that may strengthen or weaken the relationship between MBIs and depression. Regarding mediators, there is some evidence for mindfulness and negative cognitions and preliminary evidence for the others. On the moderator side, there is evidence for three or more past depressive episodes,[36] history of childhood adversities,[37] depressive symptoms at baseline,[62] and concurrent antidepressant use[38] predicting better response to MBCT in preventing depressive relapse. The other moderators have not been tested.

Specific to MBCT, a large trial comparing cognitive therapy to MBCT with 24 months of follow-up and a primary outcome of relapse/recurrence of major depression showed equivalency between the two modalities.[6] A secondary analysis of this trial[63] highlighted the importance of three regulatory skills at work in both CT and MBCT: the cognitive skill of decentering, the attitudinal skill of distress tolerance, and degree of residual symptoms. Improvements over time were seen with in both decentering and distress tolerance but not residual symptoms, while decentering was the one factor that significantly predicted relapse/recurrence while controlling for past episodes of depression and other variables. Specific to the role of home

TABLE 21.1. Potential Mediators and Moderators to Relationship Between MBI and Response

Potential Mediators	Potential Moderators
Cognitive reactivity	>3 depressive episodes
Emotional regulation/reactivity	Childhood adversities
Mindfulness skills	Baseline depressive symptoms
Repetitive negative thinking—worry	Type of depression
Repetitive negative thinking—rumination	Concurrent treatment (e.g., antidepressants)
Meta-awareness/decentering	Demographics
Psychological flexibility	Adherence (e.g., class attendance)
Self-compassion	Meditation "dose"
Attention regulation	Therapist training
Momentary positive and negative affect	Fidelity to model
Memory specificity	Sequencing of MBI
Neural mechanisms and genetics could be both.	

practice to support these regulatory skills, degree of practice during active treatment did not predict eventual relapse/recurrence, although it did predict degree of practice after intervention. Practice during follow-up was indirectly related to relapse/recurrence through the degree it predicted growth in decentering.

21.6. FUTURE DIRECTIONS

Two recent reviews of the research make concrete recommendations regarding what is needed to strengthen the evidence base and mature the field. A mapping review of MBIs[42] (using the National Institutes of Health Stage Model for behavioral interventions[64]) argues that most research continues to be either basic research exploring mindfulness as a construct or mechanisms of change (25% of studies) or early stage pilot and feasibility studies with nonrandomized designs and minimal follow-up (45%). Twenty percent of studies mapped were RCTs with passive controls, and only 9% were RCTs using active controls in research settings. Less than 1% of studies were RCTs in community settings, with equally small numbers researching effectiveness (1%) or implementation and dissemination (<1%). The authors make a number of recommendations for maturing of clinical mindfulness research, including the need to have more rigorous RCTs using active control conditions and to move beyond efficacy to effectiveness measures and implementation science.

A second review of methodological rigor in mindfulness research[65] assessed 142 published studies for six measures of key methodological standards: active control conditions, larger sample sizes, adequate follow-up assessment, assessment of treatment fidelity, reporting of therapist training, and intent-to-treat analyses. They found only modest improvements in research quality over the 16 years of publication, although their assessment of improving standards was skewed by one high-quality RCT[66] conducted early in their timeframe of analysis. Taken together, one can conclude from the above two reviews that with the explosion of scientific interest and research into MBI, there is now a need for quality over quantity.

Along with the call for increased rigor in evaluative research, there is a similar need to better understand the mechanisms underlying the therapeutic benefit in depression through large-scale evaluative trials that also measure meditators of effect, or mechanistic studies alone. In addition to more studies exploring psychological mediators of effect along with neural, genetic, and other biological factors, researchers need to better understand potential moderators listed in Table 21.1. The issue of meditation "dosage" and understanding how much mindfulness practice in class or through home practice is required to maximize benefit is an especially important area of study and was partially addressed by the recent trial of MBCT and cognitive therapy.[63] Where MBCT fits in relation to other therapies is also important to study. With the work on sequential integration models by Guidi et al.,[67] we need to know what combination of biological and psychological therapies, and in what order, works for different types of depression. Conflicting evidence exists for whether MBCT needs be offered concurrently to antidepressants or whether MBI monotherapy is sufficient.

Although more work is needed, the growing evidence base suggests that MBIs, chiefly MBCT, can be an effective therapy for depression. The strongest evidence is for prevention of relapse in recurrent depression, with more preliminary evidence for symptomatic or treatment-resistant depression. Effect sizes tend to be moderate and at least equivalent to treatments like antidepressants and cognitive therapy. MBSR shows some evidence for reducing depressive distress in a number of physical conditions and in nonclinical populations with low to moderate effect sizes. Although there is much work to be done to fully understand the place of mindfulness in mental health care, MBIs and especially MBCT are well on their way to becoming established modalities for treating and understanding depression in its various forms.

REFERENCES

1. Kabat-Zinn J, Lipworth L, Burney R. The clinical use of mindfulness meditation for the self-regulation of chronic pain. *J Behav Med.* 1985; 8(2): 163–190.
2. Kabat-Zinn J. *Full catastrophe living: using the wisdom of your body and mind to face stress, pain, and illness.* New York: Bantam Books; 2013.
3. Kabat-Zinn J. Mindfulness-based interventions in context: past, present, and future. *Clin Psych Sci Prac.* 2003; 10(2): 144–156.
4. Miller JJ, Fletcher K, Kabat-Zinn J. Three-year follow-up and clinical implications of a mindfulness meditation-based stress reduction intervention in the treatment of anxiety disorders. *Gen Hosp Psychiatry.* 1995; 17(3): 192–200.
5. Segal ZV, Teasdale JD, Williams JMG. *Mindfulness-based cognitive therapy for depression: a new approach to preventing relapse.* New York: Guilford; 2002, 2013.
6. Williams JMG, Teasdale J, Segal ZV, Kabat-Zinn J. *The mindful way through depression.* New York: Guilford; 2007.
7. Shapiro SL, Carlson LE, Astin JA, Freedman B. Mechanisms of mindfulness. *J Clin Psychol.* 2006; 62(3): 373–386.
8. Farb N, Anderson A, Ravindran A, et al. Prevention of relapse/recurrence in major depressive disorder with either mindfulness-based cognitive therapy or cognitive therapy. *J Consult Clin Psychol.* 2018; 86(2): 200–204. doi.org/10.1037/ccp0000266.
9. Crowe M, Jordan J, Burrell B, et al. Mindfulness-based stress reduction for long-term physical conditions: a systematic review. *Aust N Z J Psychiatry.* 2015; 50(1): 21–32.
10. Metcalfe CA, Dimidjian S. Extensions and mechanisms of mindfulness-based cognitive therapy: a review of the evidence. *Aust Psychol.* 2014; 49: 271–279.
11. Newby JM, Mckinnon A, Kuyken W, Gilbody S, Dalgleish T. Systematic review and meta-analysis of transdiagnostic psychological treatments for anxiety and depressive disorders in adulthood. *Clin Psychol Rev.* 2015; 40: 91–110.
12. Segal ZV, Walsh KM. Mindfulness-based cognitive therapy for residual depressive symptoms and relapse prophylaxis. *Curr Opin Psychiatry.* 2016; 29(1): 7–12.
13. Chiesa A, Mandelli L, Serretti A. Mindfulness-based cognitive therapy versus psychoeducation for patients with major depression who did not achieve remission following antidepressant treatment: a preliminary analysis. *J Alt Compl Med.* 2012; 18(8): 756–760.
14. Eisendrath SJ, Gillung E, Delucchi KL, et al. A randomized controlled trial of mindfulness-based cognitive therapy for treatment-resistant depression. *Psychother Psychosom.* 2016; 85(2): 99–110.

15. Williams JM, Fennell MJ, Barnhofer T, et al. *Mindfulness-based cognitive therapy with people at risk of suicide*. New York: Guilford; 2017.

16. Zoogman S, Goldberg SB, Hoyt WT, Miller L. Mindfulness interventions with youth: a meta-analysis. *Mindfulness*. 2015; 6(2): 290–302.

17. Kishita N, Takei Y, Stewart I. A meta-analysis of third wave mindfulness-based cognitive behavioral therapies for older people. *Int J Geriatr Psychiatry*. 2017; 32(12): 1352–1361.

18. Chu C-S, Stubbs B, Chen T-Y, et al. The effectiveness of adjunct mindfulness-based intervention in treatment of bipolar disorder: a systematic review and meta-analysis. *J Affect Disord*. 2018; 225: 234–245.

19. Hamadian S, Omidi A, Mousavinsab SM, Naziri G. The effect of combining mindfulness-based cognitive therapy with pharmacotherapy on depression and emotion regulation of patients with dysthymia: a clinical study. *Iran J Psychiatry*. 2016; 11(3): 166–172.

20. Zemestani M, Ottaviani C. Effectiveness of mindfulness-based relapse prevention for co-occurring substance use and depression disorders. *Mindfulness*. 2016; 7(6): 1347–1355.

21. Haller H, Winkler MM, Klose P, et al. Mindfulness-based interventions for women with breast cancer: an updated systematic review and meta-analysis. *Acta Oncol*. 2017; 56(12): 1665–1676.

22. Hilton L, Hempel S, Ewing BA, et al. Mindfulness meditation for chronic pain: systematic review and meta-analysis. *Ann Behav Med*. 2017; 51(2): 199–213.

23. Li W, Howard MO, Garland EL, et al. Mindfulness treatment for substance misuse: a systematic review and meta-analysis. *J Subst Abuse Treat*. 2017; 75: 62–96.

24. Neff KD, Germer CK. A pilot study and randomized controlled trial of the mindful self-compassion program. *J Clin Psychol*. 2013; 69(1): 28–44.

25. Serpa JG, Taylor SL, Tillisch K. Mindfulness-based stress reduction (MBSR) reduces anxiety, depression, and suicidal ideation in veterans. *Med Care*. 2014; 52(12 Suppl 5): S19–S24.

26. Ost LG. The efficacy of acceptance and commitment therapy: an updated systematic review and meta-analysis. *Behav Res Ther*. 2014; 61: 105–121.

27. Elices M, Soler J, Feliu-Soler A, et al. Combining emotion regulation and mindfulness skills for preventing depression relapse: a randomized-controlled study. *Borderline Personal Disord Emot Dysreg*. 2017; 4: 13.

28. Pollak SM, Pedulla T, Siegel RD, *Sitting together: essential skills for mindfulness-based psychotherapy* New York: Guilford; 2014.

29. Goyal M, Singh S, Sibinga E, et al. Meditation programs for psychological stress and well-being: a systematic review and meta-analysis. *JAMA Intern Med*. 2014; 174(3): 357–368.

30. Goldberg SB, Tucker RP, Greene PA, et al. Mindfulness-based interventions for psychiatric disorders: a systematic review and meta-analysis. *Clin Psychol Rev*. 2018; 59: 52–60.

31. Gotink RA, Chu P, Busschbach JJV, et al. Standardised mindfulness-based interventions in healthcare: an overview of systematic reviews and meta-analyses of RCTs. *PLoS One*. 2015; 10(4): e0124344.

32. de Vibe M, Bjørndal A, Fattah S, et al. Mindfulness-based stress reduction (MBSR) for improving health, quality of life and social functioning in adults: a systematic review and meta-analysis. *Campbell Systematic Reviews*, 2017. https://campbellcollaboration.org/library/mindfulness-stress-reduction-for-adults.html.

33. Strauss C, Cavanagh K, Oliver A, et al. Mindfulness-based interventions for people diagnosed with a current episode of an anxiety or depressive disorder: a meta-analysis of randomised controlled trials. *PLoS One*. 2014; 9: e96110.

34. Jain FA, Walsh RN, Eisendrath SJ, et al. Critical analysis of the efficacy of meditation therapies for acute and subacute phase treatment of depressive disorders: a systematic review. *Psychosomatics*. 2015; 56(2): 140–152.

35. Kuyken W, Warren FC, Taylor RS, et al. Efficacy of mindfulness-based cognitive therapy in prevention of depressive relapse. *JAMA Psychiatry*. 2016; 73(6): 565.

36. Segal ZV, Bieling P, Young T, et al. Antidepressant monotherapy vs. sequential pharmaco-therapy and mindfulness-based cognitive therapy, or placebo, for relapse prophylaxis in recurrent depression. *Arch Gen Psychiatry.* 2010; 67(12): 1256–1264.

37. Kuyken W, Hayes R, Barrett B, et al. Effectiveness and cost-effectiveness of mindfulness-based cognitive therapy compared with maintenance antidepressant treatment in the prevention of depressive relapse or recurrence (PREVENT): a randomised controlled trial. *Lancet.* 2015; 386(9988): 63–73.

38. Sorbero M E, Ahluwalia S, Reynolds K, et al. *A systematic review of mindfulness-based cognitive therapy for major depressive disorder.* RAND Corporation, 2015. www.jstor.org. myaccess.library.utoronto.ca/stable/10.7249/j.ctt19w7254.

39. Clarke K, Mayo-Wilson E, Kenny J, Pilling S. Can non-pharmacological interventions prevent relapse in adults who have recovered from depression? A systematic review and meta-analysis of randomised controlled trials. *Clin Psychol Rev.* 2015; 39: 58–70.

40. Liu Z, Chen QL, Sun YY. Mindfulness training for psychological stress in family caregivers of persons with dementia: a systematic review and meta-analysis of randomized controlled trials. *Clin Interv Aging.* 2017; 12: 1521–1529.

41. Grant S, Colaiaco B, Motala A, et al. Mindfulness-based relapse prevention for substance use disorders: a systematic review and meta-analysis. *J Addict Med.* 2017; 11(5): 386–396.

42. Dimidjian S, Segal ZV. Prospects for a clinical science of mindfulness-based intervention. *Am Psychol.* 2015; 70(7): 593–620. doi:10.1037/a0039589.

43. Forkmann T, Brakemeier EL, Teismann T, et al. The effects of mindfulness-based cognitive therapy and cognitive behavioral analysis system of psychotherapy added to treatment as usual on suicidal ideation in chronic depression: results of a randomized-clinical trial. *J Affect Disord.* 2016; 200: 51–57.

44. Spijkerman MPJ, Pots WTM, Bohlmijer ET. Effectiveness of online mindfulness-based interventions in improving mental health: a review and meta-analysis of randomised controlled trials *Clin Psychol Rev.* 2016; 45: 102–114.

45. National Collaborating Centre for Mental Health. Depression in adults: the treatment and management of depression in adults. Ch. 1.9. http:// www.nice.org.uk/guidance/cg90/chapter/1- recommendations#continuation-and-relapse-prevention.

46. Parikh SV, Quilty LC, Ravitz P, et al. Canadian Network for Mood and Anxiety Treatments (CANMAT) 2016 clinical guidelines for the management of adults with major depressive disorder. Section 2. Psychological treatments. *Can J Psychiatry.* 2016; 61(9): 524–539.

47. VA/DoD clinical practice guideline for management of major depressive disorder. Washington, DC: Department of Veterans Affairs; 2009. http://www.healthquality.va.gov/guidelines/MH/mdd/MDDFULL053013.pdf.

48. Mahli GS, Bassett D, Boyce P, et al. Royal Australian and New Zealand College of Psychiatrists clinical guidelines for mood disorders. https://www.ranzcp.org/files/resources/college_statements/clinician/cpg/mood-disorders-cpg.aspx.

49. Teasdale JD. Change in cognition during depression—psychopathological implications: discussion paper. *J R Soc Med.* 1983; 76(12): 1038–1044.

50. Teasdale JD, Segal Z, Williams JM. How does cognitive therapy prevent depressive relapse and why should attentional control (mindfulness) training help? *Behav Res Ther.* 1995; 33(1): 25–39.

51. Post RM. Transduction of psychological stress into the neurobiology of recurrent affective disorder. *Am J Psychiatry.* 1992; 149: 999–1010.

52. Nolen-Hoeksema, S. Responses to depression and their effects on the duration of depressive episodes. *J Abnorm Psychol.* 1991; 100: 569–582.

53. Watkins E, Teasdale J. Adaptive and maladaptive self-focus in depression. *J Affect Disord.* 2004; 8(2): 1–8.

54. Farb NAS, Segal ZV, Mayberg H, et al. Attending to the present: mindfulness meditation reveals distinct neural modes of self-reference. *Soc Cogn Affect Neurosci.* 2007; 2: 313–322. doi:10.1093/ scan/nsm030.

55. Brewer JA, Worhunsky PD, Gray JR, et al. Meditation experience is associated with differences in default mode network activity and connectivity. *Proc Nat Acad Sci USA.* 2011; 108: 20254–20259. doi:10.1073/pnas.1112029108.

56. Coutinho JF, Fernandesl SV, Soares JM, et al. Default mode network dissociation in depressive and anxiety states. *Brain Imaging Behav.* 2016; 10(1): 147–157.

57. Farb NA, Anderson AK, Bloch RT, Segal ZV. Mood-linked responses in medial prefrontal cortex predict relapse in patients with recurrent unipolar depression. Biol Psychiatry. 2011; 70(4): 366–372.

58. Farb NAS, Anderson AK, Segal ZV. The mindful brain and emotion regulation. *Can J Psychiatry.* 2012; 57(2): 70–77.

59. Van der velden AM, Kuyken W, Wattar U, et al. A systematic review of mechanisms of change in mindfulness-based cognitive therapy in the treatment of recurrent major depressive disorder. *Clin Psychol Rev.* 2015; 37: 26–39.

60. Gu J, Strauss C, Bond R, Cavanagh K. How do mindfulness-based cognitive therapy and mindfulness-based stress reduction improve mental health and wellbeing? A systematic review and meta-analysis of mediation studies. *Clin Psychol Rev.* 2015; 37: 1–12.

61. Alsubaie M, Abbott R, Dunn B, et al. Mechanisms of action in mindfulness-based cognitive therapy (MBCT) and mindfulness-based stress reduction (MBSR) in people with physical and/or psychological conditions: a systematic review. *Clin Psychol Rev.* 2017; 55: 74–91.

62. Manicavasgar V, Parker G, Perich T. Mindfulness-based cognitive therapy vs. cognitive behaviour therapy as a treatment for non-melancholic depression. *J Affect Disord.* 2011; 130(1-2): 138–144.

63. Segal ZV, Anderson AK, Gulamani T, et al. Practice of therapy acquired regulatory skills and depressive relapse/recurrence prophylaxis following cognitive therapy or mindfulness based cognitive therapy. *J Consult Clin Psychol,* 2019; 87(2): 161–170. doi: 10.1037/ccp000035.

64. Onken LS, Carroll KM, Shoham V, et al. Reenvisioning clinical science: unifying the discipline to improve the public health. *Clin Psychol Sci.* 2014; 2(1): 22–34.

65. Goldberg SB, Tucker RP, Greene PA, et al. Is mindfulness research methodology improving over time? A systematic review. *PLoS One.* 2017; 12(10): e0187298. doi:10.1371/journal. pone.0187298

66. Teasdale JD, Segal ZV, Williams JM, et al. Prevention of relapse/recurrence in major depression by mindfulness-based cognitive therapy. *J Consult Clin Psychol.* 2000; 68: 615–623.

67. Guidi J, Tomba E, Fava GA. The sequential integration of pharmacotherapy and psychotherapy in the treatment of major depressive disorder: a meta-analysis of the sequential model and a critical review of the literature. *Am J Psychiatry.* 2016; 173(2): 128–137.

/// 22 /// PROBIOTICS AND NUTRACEUTICALS

BRITTANY L. MASON AND ANDREW H. CZYSZ

22.1. INTRODUCTION

Growing evidence that nutritional intake and mood are intrinsically linked has given rise to the field of nutritional psychiatry. This field seeks to expand understanding of how diet and nutrition influences the risk for psychiatric disorders, including depression, as well as provide new insights to guide the prevention and treatment of psychiatric illness (Marx, Moseley et al. 2017). Diet is an exceedingly difficult environmental factor to study. A number of different methodologies are used to try to quantify how diet, nutrition, and dietary elements may impact mood and the risk for developing depression. Many of these approaches will be discussed here. While dietary elements and nutrients can directly affect the brain, diet can also influence mood through more indirect means, such as through modulation of gut microbiota distribution. In addition to a more comprehensive understanding of how diet can impact mood, continued examination of the role of the gut microbiota provides new avenues for treatment development and a deeper understanding of the physiology that underlies depression. This chapter will provide a broad perspective on the knowledge of how nutrition influences depression and some emerging probiotic and nutraceutical treatment strategies.

22.2. NUTRITION AND DEPRESSION

Diet is a key factor affecting health and is a possible environmental variable that can be modulated to improve health. However, understanding *how* diet affects health is a particularly complicated endeavor. Diets across the world vary greatly in their content. Leaving aside the serious issue of malnutrition, the actual composition of various diets can have greatly different impacts on human physiology. Given the desire to find optimal nutrition for humans, different regional diets have been examined for their contribution to good health and longevity. When examined for their role in helping provide good mental health, particular dietary patterns have been associated with a decreased risk for depression. Consistently, these diets consist of a high intake of vegetables, fruit, fish, whole grains, nuts, and seeds with a limited intake of processed foods and red meat, and unhealthy diets mainly consist of a high intake of processed, high-fat, high-sugar food (Psaltopoulou, Sergentanis et al. 2013; Lai, Hiles et al. 2014; Opie, O'Neil et al. 2015). A significant challenge to dietary research is the complexity in determining dietary intake, including both caloric load and nutritional content. The SMILES trial was specifically designed to see if general improvements in diet could improve depression symptoms, using intensive dietary intervention compared to a social support control group (Jacka, O'Neil et al. 2017). Though the sample sizes were small ($n = 33$ in dietary intervention and $n = 34$ in control), the dietary intervention group had significantly greater improvement after 12 weeks as measured by the Montgomery–Asberg Depression Rating Scale compared to the control group, and the number needed to treat based on remission scores was 4.1 (Jacka, O'Neil et al. 2017). The results appeared to be independent of changes in body mass index, self-efficacy, smoking, or physical activity. Thus, these data support the hypothesis that there is some component of diet, independent of those metabolic impacts directly related to dietary improvement.

Broad examination of a regional diet also provides some insight into which types of foods may support good mental health. The Invecchiare in Chianti study made progress in determining the specific foods that may impact depression. This longitudinal study of over 1,000 Italians used clear quantification of dietary intake, a food frequency questionnaire, and an established scale to measure depressive symptoms, the Center for Epidemiologic Studies Depression scale (CES-D). They determined that fish intake was negatively associated with CES-D scores and that sweet food intake was positively associated with those scores. Higher CES-D scores were associated with decreases in intake of vegetables and red and processed meat and increases in intake of dairy products and savory snacks over a three-year period (Elstgeest, Visser et al. 2019). This study gives a good rationale for continuing to examine how these specific dietary elements can affect the development of depression. However, given the challenge in finding and prescribing an ideal diet for all humans, not all dietary studies are able to find clear evidence to support their role in good mental health.

The Mediterranean diet has been studied for its role in risk for developing depression; however, support for its role in improving mental health is not entirely clear. This diet is characterized by high consumption of olive oil, whole grains, and plants; low intake of saturated fat and sugar; and moderate consumption of fish, dairy, and red wine, and is generally perceived to be one of the more healthful and longevity-associated diets. A Mediterranean-style dietary intervention (MedDiet) for adults self-reporting depression (HELFIMED study) was compared to social group activity. At three months, those in the MedDiet group were consuming more vegetables, fruit, nuts, legumes, and whole grains and fewer unhealthy snacks, red meat, and chicken. The MedDiet group also had great reductions in depression and improved quality-of-life scores, with these improvements being sustained at six months, and reduced depression being correlated with increased MedDiet score (Parletta, Zarnowiecki et al. 2019). Importantly, those in the MedDiet group also were supplemented with fish oil, a supplement containing high levels of omega-3 fatty acids, which are discussed in more detail below. Higher adherence to the Mediterranean diet at midlife has been associated with a lower risk for depressive symptoms in French men, but not women (Adjibade, Assmann et al. 2018), suggesting that the Mediterranean diet is not sufficient to prevent depression in all cases. A meta-analysis on the impact of diet on depression symptoms of 24 independent cohorts was able to support the findings that adherence to a high-quality diet was associated with lower risk for depression and that consumption of fish and vegetables played a role (Molendijk, Molero et al. 2018). However, the other specific food groups could not be identified by this analysis, and adherence to low-quality diets was not associated with a higher incidence of depression. In addition, those studies that controlled for depressive severity or used formal diagnoses did not show statistically significant findings. With the suggestion that a healthy diet may be beneficial for mental health, it leaves the question if an unhealthy diet is a risk factor for developing depression. Examination of the high-sugar, high-saturated-fat "Western" diet was examined in a cohort of British men and women. No association was found with this dietary pattern and the onset or recurrence of depressive symptoms (Vermeulen, Knuppel et al. 2018). Therefore, it is likely that specific dietary elements drive these relationships, and future research will need to determine which particular nutritional aspects are most beneficial, and for what groups of people with depression.

A first attempt has been made at this, using a systematic review to identify nutrients with demonstrated support for having antidepressant effects. Thirty-four essential nutrients for humans were compiled based on the Institute of Medicine's Dietary Reference Intake and then refined to create an evidence-based list of antidepressant nutrients, which were then ranked by the level of evidence available for their efficacy. These were then incorporated into the top antidepressant foods, based on the availability of the antidepressant nutrients available in the evaluated foods, creating an antidepressant food score. The top-scoring foods were seafood, leafy greens, cruciferous vegetables, and nuts (LaChance and Ramsey 2018). The authors noted that no other health or dietary information was considered in these rankings, such as cholesterol, saturated fat, or sodium. Therefore, it is very likely that particular aspects of diet may reduce the risk of developing depression and others may increase that risk; however, it remains unclear which aspects of diet may be the best to implement for prevention. In general, the old adage of "an apple a day keeps the doctor away" might be updated to say "a bunch of kale and a tin of sardines a day keeps the psychiatrist at bay."

22.3. NUTRACEUTICALS FOR DEPRESSION AND ANXIETY

Given that it may be exceedingly difficult to get people to shift the entire composition of their diet, researchers have worked to determine if particular dietary elements or nutrients may be efficacious for depression treatment or prevention. In addition, it is easier to try to understand how specific dietary elements may affect mood, and therefore research using these components can provide some clarity. These dietary elements that are commonly taken used as supplements but suggested to function in some ways like medication are referred to as nutraceuticals. Those with the most support as nutraceuticals for depression are detailed here. Though this is not an exhaustive list, attention has been paid to those which to date have the most support for their use as antidepressant agents. A brief section details other candidates that have some evidence for support, but that researchers cannot fully suggest are effective at this stage.

An important caveat around the use of nutraceuticals as treatment agents is dosing. Due to their status normally as supplements that are not regulated by the US Food and Drug Administration and thus not as regulated pharmaceuticals, there are fewer controls and regulations placed on the conformity of the final product. Many of the substances discussed here will be chemical compounds or products made up of various components, the efficacy of which may not be equivalent. Thus the product that may be available on the shelf could contain vastly different units or different mixes of related products. For example, the product marketed under the generic term "fish oil" may contain less of the seemingly efficacious omega-3 fatty acid than thought to provide antidepressant action and may be more enriched in those that are less supported as antidepressant agents. Although some of the listed products are now associated with dosing that supports treatment effects, that actual dose may be harder to obtain simply based on the heterogeneity of various products on the market.

22.3.1. Omega-3 Fatty Acids

Omega-3 fatty acids, also known as long-chain polyunsaturated fatty acids (PUFAs), are essential dietary acids that must be obtained from dietary sources. Although there are a number of omega-3 fatty acids, eicosapentaenoic acid (EPA) and docosahexaenoic acid (DHA) are the most studied forms that seem to provide some benefit for depression. The parent version from which EPA and DHA are synthesized is α-linoleic acid, contained in walnuts, flaxseed, and canola oil. Because endogenous conversion of dietary α-linoleic acid to EPA and DHA is believed to be rather inefficient and only reaches about 10% to 15%, it is supplementation of EPA and DHA specifically that shows the most promise for being beneficial for mood. Naturally occurring sources of EPA and DHA are primarily seafood, with supplementation likely occurring in a distilled version often referred to as "fish oil." A wide demographic shift in diet across recent generations has led epidemiologists to look to the associations between fish consumption and the prevalence of depression. They found some evidence that higher consumption of fish seems to reduce the incidence of depression and lower consumption of fish is associated with increased incidence of depression in a variety of global populations (Parker, Gibson et al. 2006). This dietary shift from foods containing omega-3 fatty acids to foods containing omega-6 fatty acids affects the ratio of these, going from a 1:1 representation to overrepresentation of omega-6 fatty acids, with now more than a 10:1 ratio. This shift has consequences for the downstream production of bioactive compounds, such as arachidonic acid and inflammatory eicosanoids (Parker, Gibson et al. 2006). A higher ratio of arachidonic acid (synthesized from omega-6 fatty acids) to EPA was significantly correlated with depression symptoms, supporting the hypothesis that this shift may be implicated in the development of depression, although this difference was not entirely explained by dietary intake (Adams, Lawson et al. 1996).

The PREDIMED-Plus trial, designed specifically to ascertain the relationship among fish consumption, omega-3 fatty acid intake, and prevalence of depression, found that moderate consumption of fish and omega-3 fatty acid was associated with a lower incidence of depression, but not high intake (Sanchez-Villegas, Alvarez-Perez et al. 2018). Further studies in multiple cohorts of participants with depression support that omega-3 does seem to reduce depressive symptom; however, the effects are not always consistent across types of omega-3 fatty acids nor populations studied (Parker, Gibson et al. 2006). The HELFIMED dietary intervention trial used fish oil supplementation in addition to the MedDiet. In the MedDiet group, which had improved depression symptoms as well as quality of life, there were also some correlations with increased omega-3s, decreased omega-6s, and improved mental health (Parletta, Zarnowiecki et al. 2019). The mechanisms by which omega-3 seem to prevent or help depression are still unclear, but it is hypothesized to be via anti-inflammatory action or through some currently unknown direct role of omega-3s (Parker, Gibson et al. 2006). Systematic review of the clinical trials using omega-3s as adjunctive treatment with antidepressants found positive results and generally supported their use (Sarris, Murphy et al. 2016). The Canadian Network for Mood and Anxiety Treatments (CANMAT) revised guidelines for 2016 also included omega-3 fatty acids in their recommended treatments, as either first- or second-line treatments, for mild to moderate depression (Ravindran, Balneaves et al. 2016). Administration of omega-3 fatty acids is not without risks, with reported association with prostate cancer risk, albeit weak, and higher doses suspected to increase bleeding; impair immune functioning and lipid and glucose metabolism; and increase lipid peroxidation (EFSA Panel on Dietetic Products, Nutrition and Allergies 2012; Fu, Zheng et al. 2015).

22.3.2. *S*-adenosylmethionine (SAMe)

SAMe is a naturally occurring molecule that is able to participate in a number of important metabolic pathways, primarily methylation, transulfuration, and transaminopropylation (De Berardis, Orsolini et al. 2016). The majority of these interactions involve its reactive methyl group and acting as a methyl donor but also as part of folate-mediated one-carbon metabolism. Distinct aspects of this complex biological pathway are contained within mitochondria, the cytoplasm, and the nucleus, but it is believed that the same pool of folate cofactors are used in each pathway; therefore, a shift in this common pool could affect any part of this important biological cycle (Fox and Stover 2008). SAMe specifically is implicated in gene regulation, protein localization, and catabolism of small molecules, but one-carbon metabolism can also be impaired by deficiencies in folate and various forms of vitamin B (Fox and Stover 2008). Impaired folate metabolism has been implicated in a wide variety of diseases, including neural tube defects, cardiovascular disease, and cancer, and also mood disorders (Fox and Stover 2008).

SAMe has been evaluated as both adjunctive treatment and monotherapy for depression. Multiple trials, including open-label, placebo-controlled, and antidepressant-comparison, have shown SAMe to be efficacious for reducing depressive symptoms and having similar or improved efficacy over established antidepressants (De Berardis, Orsolini et al. 2016). Systematic review of clinical trials that evaluated the efficacy of a number of nutraceuticals involved in one-carbon metabolism, including SAMe, folic acid (or related folinic acid or methylfolate), B6, and B12, found their antidepressant treatment effects supported by the majority of studies (Sarris, Murphy et al. 2016). A meta-analysis of those studies that used folic acid did not support the use of this nutraceutical for depression, but the data for methylfolate did seem somewhat more positive. However, not all data support this and use of SAMe as monotherapy. Thus, it is suggested for those with mild depression but should be avoided as monotherapy in cases of severe depression. Most side effects reported were fairly mild, including mild gastrointestinal (GI) symptoms, sweating, irritability, and tachycardia; however, there are risks for serotonin syndrome when combined with some common medications. In addition, the chance for increased restlessness and anxiety may make them unusable in some psychiatric patients (De Berardis, Orsolini et al. 2016). There is also some evidence that SAMe can induce hypomanic or manic switching in some depressed patients, primarily those already diagnosed with bipolar disorder, with elevated risk after intravenous or intramuscular administration (Sarris, Murphy et al. 2016). Given these data, SAMe was included in the CANMAT 2016 guidelines as a second-line adjunctive treatment for those with mild or moderate depression (Ravindran, Balneaves et al. 2016).

22.3.3 Acetyl-L-Carnitine

Acetyl-L-carnitine is an endogenously produced molecule shown to be critical for hippocampal function. It modulates synaptic plasticity, likely via histone acetylation of key genes that regulate the expression of important factors such as the pro-neurogenic brain-derived neurotrophic factor (BDNF), and through regulation of synaptic glutamate release through the metabotropic glutamate receptor of class-2, mGlu2 (Nasca, Xenos et al. 2013; Wang, Lu et al. 2015;, Lau, Bigio et al. 2016). Levels of acetyl-L-carnitine, and not those of free carnitine, were seen to be decreased in depressed patients compared with age- and sex-matched healthy controls (Nasca, Bigio et al. 2018). The effects of acetyl-L-carnitine were comparable to fluoxetine in an elderly dysthymic population, and the positive mood changes occurred more quickly with acetyl-L-carnitine (Bersani, Meco et al. 2013). Additional randomized control trials also showed comparable or a more efficacious effect compared to traditional antidepressants for dysthymia or in other medically comorbid depressed populations (Wang, Han et al. 2014). Acetyl-L-carnitine has been suggested to be most useful in these populations more risk for side effects or adverse events associated with traditional antidepressant use. The CANMAT 2016 guidelines included acetyl-L-carnitine as a recommended third-line treatment monotherapy (Ravindran, Balneaves et al. 2016).

22.3.4. St. John's Wort

St. John's wort (*Hypericum perforatum*) is an herbaceous perennial plant commonly found in Europe and Asia. St. John's wort has been used as treatment for depression by practitioners of Traditional Chinese Medicine for many years and has been widely prescribed for depression in a number of European countries. A recent meta-analysis examined 27 clinical trials using St. John's wort for the treatment of depression across China, Germany, Denmark, Brazil, and the United States (Ng, Venkatanarayanan et al. 2017). They found that the use of St. John's wort as an antidepressant agent could be supported with comparable response and remission rates and significantly lower discontinuation or dropout rate to selective serotonin reuptake inhibitors. The evidence suggested that St. John's wort could be most useful in those with mild to moderate depression, and it seems to produce fewer side effects leading to discontinuation. However, St. John's wort has some notable and very problematic drug–drug interactions that make its use more difficult in those who are more medically or psychiatrically ill. In addition, the variations between preparations and the lack of regulation around its distribution make it a difficult product to use, given noted differences in potency and ingredients across manufacturers.

22.3.5. Additional Products Under Study

Other nutraceuticals have received some attention but cannot currently be supported by data. One of these is vitamin D, an essential vitamin that can be obtained from dietary sources, although the majority comes from bioconversion in the skin from sunlight exposure (Parker, Brotchie et al. 2017). Although there are reasonable data suggesting that deficiency in vitamin D is associated with increased risk for developing depression and perhaps with depression severity, the data are much less supportive of the role of supplementation with vitamin D being efficacious as an antidepressant (Parker, Brotchie et al. 2017). The previously mentioned systematic review did find two studies testing vitamin D as an adjunctive treatment to support the efficacy of vitamin D (Sarris, Murphy et al. 2016); however, a more comprehensive meta-analysis was unable to support vitamin D as a successful antidepressant agent (Gowda, Mutowo et al. 2015). Vitamin D may provide more reliable antidepressant effects in those with established deficiencies in vitamin D and in those with more clinically established or moderate to severe depression. It may also play a role in the overall system of regulation as noted above for one of the probiotic studies; however, at this stage, the data are insufficient to support its role as an antidepressant agent.

One of the major neurotransmitters implicated in depression is serotonin, so compounds involved in the synthesis of serotonin have been evaluated for antidepressant effects. 5-hydroxytryptophan (5-HTP) is an intermediate of serotonin (5-HT) that is derived from the essential amino acid L-tryptophan. Although the earliest preclinical studies seemed to support supplementation of these compounds having antidepressant effects, more recent work does not provide clear support for either L-tryptophan or 5-HTP as beneficial for depression. Some work supports that monotherapy may be superior to placebo, but not greater than existing antidepressants, nor as adjunctive treatment. Further study is needed to determine if there may be a population that would most benefit from these supplements and whether they could provide an adequate increase in antidepressant response (Sarris, Murphy et al. 2016). 5-HTP is still being investigated as a component of a multi-nutrient supplement for adjunctive treatment for treatment-resistant depression (Ravindran, Balneaves et al. 2016; Dome, Tombor et al. 2019).

Another compound that has received some attention is saffron, the world's most expensive spice, which is derived from the *Crocus sativus* plant. Though a systematic review was able to find positive support for saffron and its bioactive compounds as an antidepressant agent, all studies evaluated came from the same research group (Lopresti and Drummond 2014). Therefore, replication of these findings is needed before saffron could be recommended as a treatment for depression. A recent study using a novel saffron extract from a different research group did find some improvement in mood and related symptoms in healthy controls after one month, with larger changes in their high-dose group (Kell, Rao et al. 2017). This suggests that further examination of saffron as a mood-lifting agent is warranted.

Other dietary elements that have received some attention include a number of minerals, including zinc and magnesium, as well as amino acids and creatine, which are unlikely to be singular antidepressant agents but may play a role in determining the overall value of a particular diet or supplement.

22.4. THE BRAIN–GUT AXIS

As our understanding of how dietary elements can impact the human body, and specifically how they can regulate mood, it has required a more comprehensive understanding of how the GI system integrates with the brain. To regulate this dynamic system, the GI tract and the brain must maintain constant communication and direct feedback must be provided to the central nervous system (CNS) regarding the status of the peripheral body. The presence of the blood–brain barrier limits a majority of circulating hormones from reaching brain parenchyma, but the more permeable vessels of the circumventricular organs allow for these peripheral signals to reach the brain (Benarroch 2011). Therefore, direct neuronal innervation, in addition to extensive hormonal signaling, assists with rapid bidirectional communication. This direct relationship has become known as the gut–brain axis. Autonomic neural pathways originating in the CNS innervate the GI system, including the esophagus, stomach, small and large intestine, liver, and pancreas (Udit and Gautron 2013). Peripheral information is received by the brain in the dorsal vagal complex, integrating information from the sensory afferent signals carried by the vagus nerve informing of gastric stretch, levels of glucose and lipids in the liver, and circulating signals, and this information is then transmitted into deep brain structures (Saper, Chou et al. 2002; Mason, Wang et al. 2014). This allows for the status of the gut to be relayed directly to the brain and for the necessary CNS control to be modulated accordingly. Given that the status of the gut, energy balance, and metabolism are monitored and regulated almost constantly by the body, it is becoming more apparent that we must integrate these processes into our understanding of how the nutritional status can affect mood. An increasingly important component that determines the status of the gut is the gut microbiota, which may also provide a new avenue for our understanding of how depression may develop.

22.5. THE GUT MICROBIOTA

Humans have coexisted with microbial species, including bacteria, viruses, eukaryotes, and archaea, for our entire evolution (Human Microbiome Project Consortium 2012a). Although considerably smaller in mass, the number of bacterial cells is roughly equivalent to human cells in the body (Sender, Fuchs et al. 2016) and distinct microbial communities thrive both on and inside the human body at major bodily sites, including the gut (Human Microbiome Project Consortium 2012b). The gut microbiota consist of 10^{13} to 10^{14} total microorganisms, including four major phyla of bacterial life: Firmicutes, Bacteriodetes, Actinobacteria, and Proteobacteria (Grenham, Clarke et al. 2011; Tlaskalova-Hogenova, Stepankova et al. 2011), which interact with the host in a variety of ways. A single person's microbiota distribution is specific and unique, yet the microbiota distributions of those from a shared environment are highly similar (Human Microbiome Project Consortium 2012b). The development of one's microbial community begins at birth, with the human infant being generally sterile and accumulating its personal bacterial distribution through interactions with its environment, caregivers, and diet in the first months and years of life. This developmental period largely determines the final adult microbiome, which is relatively stable and remains close to the population that was established in early life, though the specific biomass of the various microbial populations may shift due to factors such as antibiotics and diet (Forsythe, Sudo et al. 2010; Grenham, Clarke et al. 2011; Faith, Guruge et al. 2013). Importantly, the gut microbiota is responsive to diet, taking what we eat and turning it into other products. Ultimately, the gut microbiota works to use the remaining undigested alimentary compounds from indigestible dietary fiber and function as a potent bioreactor, producing simple sugars, short-chain fatty acids, nutrients, and antioxidants, and contribute to the synthesis of vitamins (Bengmark 2013; Davila, Blachier et al. 2013). It is hypothesized these reactions can have a significant influence on human mood regulation. Also, those bacteria that rely on particular factors to survive will be unable to thrive in the gut that does not regularly supply these life-sustaining compounds.

22.6. GUT MICROBIOTA CHANGES IN DEPRESSION

Recently, an expanding field of research has begun to explore changes in the gut microbiota and their association with mood. Antibiotic administration is associated with higher risk for depression, with increasing odds for repeated courses, and a similar association is observed for anxiety (Lurie, Yang et al. 2015). Examination of the gut microbiota in adults with depression has found decreased microbial diversity (Kelly, Borre et al. 2016) and different abundance of bacterial groups compared to healthy controls (Chen, Zheng et al. 2018). Once the specific bacterial groups are quantified, it becomes less clear which may be beneficial for mood and which may be detrimental. Bifidobacteria and Lactobacillus counts have been shown to be lower in those with depression compared to healthy controls (Aizawa, Tsuji et al. 2016). Reduced Bacteroidetes have been seen in patients with depression compared to healthy controls, with no other significant differences in taxonomic associations (Naseribafrouei, Hestad et al. 2014). Metaproteomics in a small sample of depressed Chinese participants showed found less abundance of Bacteroidetes and Proteobacteria and greater abundance of Firmicutes and Actinobacteria compared to healthy controls (Chen, Li et al. 2018). However, a previous study also in Chinese participants showed that Bacteroidetes, Proteobacteria, and Actinobacteria are increased in patients with depression, whereas Firmicutes were decreased (Jiang, Ling et al. 2015). Lachnospiraceae in depressed participants were decreased in the first study and increased in the second study.

Given the association of particular bacterial groups and the diet of their human host, the specific groups of people who are examined may explain some of the inconsistencies in the findings. However, a recent study has tried to explain more of the function of particular bacterial groups, which could clarify the role that gut bacteria could play in mood regulation. Examination of the gut microbiota of those with depression indicated that relative abundance of fecal Bacteroides was negatively correlated with brain signatures associated with depression and was a contributor to GABA-producing pathways (Strandwitz, Kim et al. 2019). As GABA is a primary neurotransmitter associated with mood, this could be a first indication of how the gut microbiota could directly impact the brain and change mood. Although these findings are not entirely consistent, they do suggest that changes in

Bacteroides, phylum: Bacteroidetes, are associated with depression. Future research will confirm these findings and determine if encouraged growth of Bacteroides is beneficial for depression. Although diet is a major factor in gut microbiota composition, none of the above studies specifically examined or integrated dietary status into their analyses. A cohort of depressed Taiwanese patients were compared to healthy controls using 16S rRNA sequencing and specific quantification of dietary nutrient content. Actinobacteria and Firmicutes were overrepresented in depressed patients; there was a high abundance of Bifidobacterium and Blautia in those with depression and a high abundance of Prevotella in controls. Blautia, Sutterella, and Eggerthella were moderately correlated with depression scores; interestingly, Holdemania showed a moderate correlation with anxiety and perceived stress more in those with depression but not in controls (Ella Chung, Chen et al. 2019). These data continue to present a complex picture of the gut microbiota that may be present in those with depression. Like many other explorations for biomarkers of depression, differences in gut microbiota may indicate specific subgroups within the diagnosis. Confirmation of more homogenous changes in those with depression may help to target treatments or presentation strategies.

22.7. PROBIOTICS FOR DEPRESSION AND ANXIETY

Although the gut microbiota distribution that is most associated with depression is still under study, attempts to supplement with probiotics have been evaluated to see if they may be efficacious for depression. This comes from the hypothesis that some beneficial bacteria may be missing from the gut of those with depression, and therefore supplementation could replenish this important group. The two most studied probiotics for depression to date are Bifidobacteria and Lactobacillus. These may have been the first candidates given their wide availability in existing probiotic preparations and some evidence that they were beneficial in other disease states, such as inflammatory bowel disease (Coqueiro, Raizel et al. 2018). Various formulations of species have been evaluated and are briefly detailed here.

The first evaluation of a probiotic as an antidepressant involved *Bifidobacterium infantis*, which is one of the earliest bacteria to colonize the infant gut and is believed to be a beneficial species for a host of disease states. Although it was not seen to affect depression-like behavior in rats, it did significantly affect a number of systems associated with depression, including a reduction in pro-inflammatory cytokine response and changes in the serotonin biosythesis pathway seen in both plasma and brain (Desbonnet, Garrett et al. 2008). Further testing of *B. infantis* supported and expanded these findings using maternal separation as a model of depression (Desbonnet, Garrett et al. 2010).

Work in humans started first with Lactobacillus species, which is widely available for human consumption and has shown some effects on mood. Healthy adults who reported more depressed mood at baseline showed a significant improvement in mood scores after consuming a fermented yogurt drink containing *Lactobacillus casei* for three weeks (Benton, Williams et al. 2007). Thirty-nine patients with chronic fatigue syndrome but not diagnosed depression who consumed *L. casei* for eight weeks showed reduced scores on the Beck Anxiety Inventory, though depression scores remained unchanged compared to those who consumed the placebo (Rao, Bested et al. 2009). It is now understood that various bacteria in the gut share some cross-function and that products from one species can be used by another. It is interesting, then, that combinations of these two bacterial groups have also shown some effects on mood and in some different ways. *Lactobacillus helveticus R0052* and *Bifidobacterium longum R0175* were shown to reduce psychological distress in humans, indicated by reductions in day-to-day depression, anxiety, anger scores, and cortisol levels (Messaoudi, Lalonde et al. 2011). Use of a multispecies probiotic in healthy, nondepressed individuals consisting of *Bifidobacterium bifidum W23*, *Bifidobacterium lactis W52, Lactobacillus acidophilus W37, Lactobacillus brevis W63, Lactobacillus casei W56, Lactobacillus salivarius W24,* and *Lactococcus lactis (W19* and *W58)* showed a significant reduction in overall cognitive reactivity to sad mood, largely accounted for by reduced rumination and aggressive thoughts (Steenbergen, Sellaro et al. 2015).

There are fewer positive trials in those with diagnosed depression or low mood. Administration of *L. acidophilus, L. casei,* and *B. bifidum* to depressed participants was shown have significantly greater reductions on the Beck Depression Inventory compared to placebo, as well as decreased serum insulin, a measurement of insulin resistance (HOMA-IR), and the inflammatory marker high-sensitivity C-reactive protein (CRP), and increased antioxidant glutathione (Akkasheh, Kashani-Poor et al. 2016). *L. helveticus* and *B. longum* were able to produce a significant reduction in the Beck Depression Inventory score for those with depression compared to placebo (Kazemi, Noorbala et al. 2019). Though a number of these studies provide some evidence that these probiotics can improve mood, it is still unclear how effective probiotics could be as an antidepressant treatment, or for which person. Other studies have not found these probiotics to be beneficial. Participants with at least moderate scores on self-report mood measures and not currently taking psychotropic medications were randomly allocated to *L. helveticus* and *B. longum* or a matched placebo for eight weeks. No differences were found for any of the psychological assessments; however, baseline vitamin D levels did show a moderate treatment effect for a number of the outcome measures (Romijn, Rucklidge et al. 2017). *Lactobacillus plantarum* 299v was given to depressed patients as an adjunct to selective serotonin uptake inhibitors, and even though no significant differences were found for depression scores or pro-inflammatory cytokines, the probiotic did improve cognitive performance and reduce the concentration of a marker of inflammatory activity, kynurenine, compared to placebo (Rudzki, Ostrowska et al. 2019). Thus, it may suggest that probiotics could be useful as adjunctive treatments for depression in concert with traditional antidepressants or to manage specific symptom domains that may be present in some but not all patients with depression.

Extensive work from the Alimentary Pharmabotic Center (APC) Microbiome Institute in Cork, Ireland, has examined the ability of some probiotics to improve mood and attempted to test the physiological systems they could target. These researchers have termed these compounds "psychobiotics." The first to show some efficacy was *Bifidobacterium longum* 1714. This probiotic was given to healthy volunteers and reduced cortisol output and subjective anxiety after a stressful task, as well as improving hippocampal-dependent visuospatial memory performance (Allen, Hutch et al. 2016). However, another probiotic, *L. rhamnosus* (JB-1), which had shown promise in preclinical models of an anxious mouse strain, failed to improve mood, anxiety, stress, or sleep quality or attenuate any stress response (Kelly, Allen et al. 2017). These researcher take a number of their preclinical findings and work to implement them in human studies, and this particular failure highlights the difficulty in translating these findings to humans. Given that humans are a different host than the rodents on which many preclinical findings are based, this provides a clear need to truly understand how these systems operate in humans. Nevertheless, probiotics and manipulation of the gut microbiota for the management of depression are worthy for further research and development.

22.8. A COMPREHENSIVE PICTURE

Given the complexity of nutritional intake and metabolism, it is highly unlikely that any single compound or organism mentioned here is a panacea for all cases of depression. The integration of consumed food into the body and the complex pathways involved in converting that to energy, storing that energy, and mobilizing its use means that a holistic view of the system will provide a greater opportunity toward finding solutions for depression. Current understanding supports the idea that gut bacteria live not in isolation, but instead in dynamic communities that interact and regulate one another. These interactions affect the host and the system in which the bacteria live, and these bacteria can affect the metabolism of diet and the inflammatory tone of the host and actively affect pharmacokinetics of drug disposition. Therefore, a comprehensive understanding of the status of the person, mind, and body will help guide us toward personalized medicine that will likely include dietary adjustments and probiotic supplementation in an effort to treat and prevent depression.

REFERENCES

Adams, P. B., S. Lawson, A. Sanigorski and A. J. Sinclair (1996). "Arachidonic acid to eicosapentaenoic acid ratio in blood correlates positively with clinical symptoms of depression." *Lipids 31* (Suppl): S157–161.

Adjibade, M., K. E. Assmann, V. A. Andreeva, C. Lemogne, S. Hercberg, P. Galan and E. Kesse-Guyot (2018). "Prospective association between adherence to the Mediterranean diet and risk of depressive symptoms in the French SU.VI.MAX cohort." *Eur J Nutr 57*(3): 1225–1235.

Aizawa, E., H. Tsuji, T. Asahara, T. Takahashi, T. Teraishi, S. Yoshida, M. Ota, N. Koga, K. Hattori and H. Kunugi (2016). "Possible association of Bifidobacterium and Lactobacillus in the gut microbiota of patients with major depressive disorder." *J Affect Disord 202*: 254–257.

Akkasheh, G., Z. Kashani-Poor, M. Tajabadi-Ebrahimi, P. Jafari, H. Akbari, M. Taghizadeh, M. R. Memarzadeh, Z. Asemi and A. Esmaillzadeh (2016). "Clinical and metabolic response to probiotic administration in patients with major depressive disorder: a randomized, double-blind, placebo-controlled trial." *Nutrition 32*(3): 315–320.

Allen, A. P., W. Hutch, Y. E. Borre, P. J. Kennedy, A. Temko, G. Boylan, E. Murphy, J. F. Cryan, T. G. Dinan and G. Clarke (2016). "Bifidobacterium longum 1714 as a translational psychobiotic: modulation of stress, electrophysiology and neurocognition in healthy volunteers." *Transl Psychiatry 6*: e939.

Benarroch, E. E. (2011). "Circumventricular organs: receptive and homeostatic functions and clinical implications." *Neurology 77*(12): 1198–1204.

Bengmark, S. (2013). "Gut microbiota, immune development and function." *Pharmacol Res 69*(1): 87–113.

Benton, D., C. Williams and A. Brown (2007). "Impact of consuming a milk drink containing a probiotic on mood and cognition." *Eur J Clin Nutr 61*(3): 355–361.

Bersani, G., G. Meco, A. Denaro, D. Liberati, C. Colletti, R. Nicolai, F. S. Bersani and A. Koverech (2013). "L-Acetylcarnitine in dysthymic disorder in elderly patients: a double-blind, multicenter, controlled randomized study vs. fluoxetine." *Eur Neuropsychopharmacol 23*(10): 1219–1225.

Chen, J. J., P. Zheng, Y. Y. Liu, X. G. Zhong, H. Y. Wang, Y. J. Guo and P. Xie (2018). "Sex differences in gut microbiota in patients with major depressive disorder." *Neuropsychiatr Dis Treat 14*: 647–655.

Chen, Z., J. Li, S. Gui, C. Zhou, J. Chen, C. Yang, Z. Hu, H. Wang, X. Zhong, L. Zeng, K. Chen, P. Li and P. Xie (2018). "Comparative metaproteomics analysis shows altered fecal microbiota signatures in patients with major depressive disorder." *Neuroreport 29*(5): 417–425.

Coqueiro, A. Y., R. Raizel, A. Bonvini, J. Tirapegui and M. M. Rogero (2018). "Probiotics for inflammatory bowel diseases: a promising adjuvant treatment." *Int J Food Sci Nutr* [Epub ahead of print]. doi:10.1080/09637486.2018.1477123.

Davila, A. M., F. Blachier, M. Gotteland, M. Andriamihaja, P. H. Benetti, Y. Sanz and D. Tome (2013). "Intestinal luminal nitrogen metabolism: role of the gut microbiota and consequences for the host." *Pharmacol Res 68*(1): 95–107.

De Berardis, D., L. Orsolini, N. Serroni, G. Girinelli, F. Iasevoli, C. Tomasetti, A. de Bartolomeis, M. Mazza, A. Valchera, M. Fornaro, G. Perna, M. Piersanti, M. Di Nicola, M. Cavuto, G. Martinotti and M. Di Giannantonio (2016). "A comprehensive review on the efficacy of S-adenosyl-L-methionine in major depressive disorder." *CNS Neurol Disord Drug Targets 15*(1): 35–44.

Desbonnet, L., L. Garrett, G. Clarke, J. Bienenstock and T. G. Dinan (2008). "The probiotic *Bifidobacteria infantis*: an assessment of potential antidepressant properties in the rat." *J Psychiatr Res 43*(2): 164–174.

Desbonnet, L., L. Garrett, G. Clarke, B. Kiely, J. F. Cryan and T. G. Dinan (2010). "Effects of the probiotic *Bifidobacterium infantis* in the maternal separation model of depression." *Neuroscience 170*(4): 1179–1188.

Dome, P., L. Tombor, J. Lazary, X. Gonda and Z. Rihmer (2019). "Natural health products, dietary minerals and over-the-counter medications as add-on therapies to antidepressants in the treatment of major depressive disorder: a review." *Brain Res Bull 146*: 51–78.

EFSA Panel on Dietetic Products, Nutrition and Allergies (2012). "Scientific opinion on the tolerable upper intake level of eicosapentaenoic acid (EPA), docosahexaenoic acid (DHA) and docosapentaenoic acid (DPA)." *EFSA J 10*(7): 2815.

Ella Chung, Y.-C., H.-C. Chen, H.-C. Lori Chou, I. M. Chen, M.-S. Lee, L.-C. Chuang, Y.-W. Liu, M.-L. Lu, C.-H. Chen, C.-H. Wu, M.-C. Huang, S.-C. Liao, Y.-H. Ni, M.-S. Lai, W.-L. Shih and P.-H. Kuo (2019). "Exploration of microbiota targets for major depressive disorder and mood related traits." *J Psychiatr Res 111*: 74–82.

Elstgeest, L. E. M., M. Visser, B. Penninx, M. Colpo, S. Bandinelli and I. A. Brouwer (2019). "Bidirectional associations between food groups and depressive symptoms: longitudinal findings from the Invecchiare in Chianti (InCHIANTI) study." *Br J Nutr 121*(4): 439–450.

Faith, J. J., J. L. Guruge, M. Charbonneau, S. Subramanian, H. Seedorf, A. L. Goodman, J. C. Clemente, R. Knight, A. C. Heath, R. L. Leibel, M. Rosenbaum and J. I. Gordon (2013). "The long-term stability of the human gut microbiota." *Science 341*(6141): 1237439.

Forsythe, P., N. Sudo, T. Dinan, V. H. Taylor and J. Bienenstock (2010). "Mood and gut feelings." *Brain Behav Immun 24*(1): 9–16.

Fox, J. T. and P. J. Stover (2008). "Folate-mediated one-carbon metabolism." *Vitam Horm 79*: 1–44.

Fu, Y. Q., J. S. Zheng, B. Yang and D. Li (2015). "Effect of individual omega-3 fatty acids on the risk of prostate cancer: a systematic review and dose-response meta-analysis of prospective cohort studies." *J Epidemiol 25*(4): 261–274.

Gowda, U., M. P. Mutowo, B. J. Smith, A. E. Wluka and A. M. Renzaho (2015). "Vitamin D supplementation to reduce depression in adults: meta-analysis of randomized controlled trials." *Nutrition 31*(3): 421–429.

Grenham, S., G. Clarke, J. F. Cryan and T. G. Dinan (2011). "Brain-gut-microbe communication in health and disease." *Front Physiol 2*: 94.

Human Microbiome Project Consortium (2012a). "A framework for human microbiome research." *Nature 486*(7402): 215–221.

Human Microbiome Project Consortium (2012b). "Structure, function and diversity of the healthy human microbiome." *Nature 486*(7402): 207–214.

Jacka, F. N., A. O'Neil, R. Opie, C. Itsiopoulos, S. Cotton, M. Mohebbi, D. Castle, S. Dash, C. Mihalopoulos, M. L. Chatterton, L. Brazionis, O. M. Dean, A. M. Hodge and M. Berk (2017). "A randomised controlled trial of dietary improvement for adults with major depression (the 'SMILES' trial)." *BMC Medicine 15*(1): 23.

Jiang, H., Z. Ling, Y. Zhang, H. Mao, Z. Ma, Y. Yin, W. Wang, W. Tang, Z. Tan, J. Shi, L. Li and B. Ruan (2015). "Altered fecal microbiota composition in patients with major depressive disorder." *Brain Behav Immun 48*: 186–194.

Kazemi, A., A. A. Noorbala, K. Azam, M. H. Eskandari and K. Djafarian (2019). "Effect of probiotic and prebiotic vs placebo on psychological outcomes in patients with major depressive disorder: a randomized clinical trial." *Clin Nutr 38*(2): 522–528.

Kell, G., A. Rao, G. Beccaria, P. Clayton, A. M. Inarejos-García and M. Prodanov (2017). "Affron®, a novel saffron extract (*Crocus sativus* L.), improves mood in healthy adults over 4 weeks in a double-blind, parallel, randomized, placebo-controlled clinical trial." *Compl Ther Med 33*: 58–64.

Kelly, J. R., A. P. Allen, A. Temko, W. Hutch, P. J. Kennedy, N. Farid, E. Murphy, G. Boylan, J. Bienenstock, J. F. Cryan, G. Clarke and T. G. Dinan (2017). "The potential psychobiotic Lactobacillus rhamnosus (JB-1) fails to modulate stress or cognitive performance in healthy male subjects." *Brain Behav Immun 61*: 50–59.

Kelly, J. R., Y. Borre, C. O' Brien, E. Patterson, S. el Aidy, J. Deane, P. J. Kennedy, S. Beers, K. Scott, G. Moloney, A. E. Hoban, L. Scott, P. Fitzgerald, P. Ross, C. Stanton, G. Clarke, J. F. Cryan and T. G. Dinan (2016). "Transferring the blues: depression-associated gut microbiota induces neurobehavioural changes in the rat." *J Psychiatr Res 82*: 109–118.

LaChance, L. R. and D. Ramsey (2018). "Antidepressant foods: an evidence-based nutrient profiling system for depression." *World J Psychiatry 8*(3): 97–104.

Lai, J. S., S. Hiles, A. Bisquera, A. J. Hure, M. McEvoy and J. Attia (2014). "A systematic review and meta-analysis of dietary patterns and depression in community-dwelling adults." *Am J Clin Nutr 99*(1): 181–197.

Lau, T., B. Bigio, D. Zelli, B. S. McEwen and C. Nasca (2016). "Stress-induced structural plasticity of medial amygdala stellate neurons and rapid prevention by a candidate antidepressant." *Mol Psychiatry 22*: 227.

Lopresti, A. L. and P. D. Drummond (2014). "Saffron (*Crocus sativus*) for depression: a systematic review of clinical studies and examination of underlying antidepressant mechanisms of action." *Hum Psychopharmacol Clin Exp 29*(6): 517–527.

Lurie, I., Y. X. Yang, K. Haynes, R. Mamtani and B. Boursi (2015). "Antibiotic exposure and the risk for depression, anxiety, or psychosis: a nested case-control study." *J Clin Psychiatry 76*(11): 1522–1528.

Marx, W., G. Moseley, M. Berk and F. Jacka (2017). "Nutritional psychiatry: the present state of the evidence." *Proc Nutr Soc 76*(4): 427–436.

Mason, B. L., Q. Wang and J. M. Zigman (2014). "The central nervous system sites mediating the orexigenic actions of ghrelin." *Annu Rev Physiol 76*: 519–533.

Messaoudi, M., R. Lalonde, N. Violle, H. Javelot, D. Desor, A. Nejdi, J. F. Bisson, C. Rougeot, M. Pichelin, M. Cazaubiel and J. M. Cazaubiel (2011). "Assessment of psychotropic-like properties of a probiotic formulation (Lactobacillus helveticus R0052 and Bifidobacterium longum R0175) in rats and human subjects." *Br J Nutr 105*(5): 755–764.

Molendijk, M., P. Molero, F. Ortuno Sanchez-Pedreno, W. Van der Does and M. Angel Martinez-Gonzalez (2018). "Diet quality and depression risk: a systematic review and dose-response meta-analysis of prospective studies." *J Affect Disord 226*: 346–354.

Nasca, C., B. Bigio, F. S. Lee, S. P. Young, M. M. Kautz, A. Albright, J. Beasley, D. S. Millington, A. A. Mathe, J. H. Kocsis, J. W. Murrough, B. S. McEwen and N. Rasgon (2018). "Acetyl-L-carnitine deficiency in patients with major depressive disorder." *Proc Natl Acad Sci USA 115*(34): 8627–8632.

Nasca, C., D. Xenos, Y. Barone, A. Caruso, S. Scaccianoce, F. Matrisciano, G. Battaglia, A. A. Mathé, A. Pittaluga, L. Lionetto, M. Simmaco and F. Nicoletti (2013). "L-acetylcarnitine causes rapid antidepressant effects through the epigenetic induction of mGlu2 receptors." *Proc Natl Acad Sci USA 110*(12): 4804–4809.

Naseribafrouei, A., K. Hestad, E. Avershina, M. Sekelja, A. Linlokken, R. Wilson and K. Rudi (2014). "Correlation between the human fecal microbiota and depression." *Neurogastroenterol Motil.*

Ng, Q. X., N. Venkatanarayanan and C. Y. X. Ho (2017). "Clinical use of *Hypericum perforatum* (St John's wort) in depression: a meta-analysis." *J Affect Disord 210*: 211–221.

Opie, R. S., A. O'Neil, C. Itsiopoulos and F. N. Jacka (2015). "The impact of whole-of-diet interventions on depression and anxiety: a systematic review of randomised controlled trials." *Public Health Nutr 18*(11): 2074–2093.

Parker, G., H. Brotchie and R. K. Graham (2017). "Vitamin D and depression." *J Affect Disord 208*: 56–61.

Parker, G., N. A. G. Gibson, H. Brotchie, G. Heruc, A.-M. Rees and D. Hadzi-Pavlovic (2006). "Omega-3 fatty acids and mood disorders." *Am J Psychiatry 163*(6): 969–978.

Parletta, N., D. Zarnowiecki, J. Cho, A. Wilson, S. Bogomolova, A. Villani, C. Itsiopoulos, T. Niyonsenga, S. Blunden, B. Meyer, L. Segal, B. T. Baune and K. O'Dea (2019). "A Mediterranean-style dietary intervention supplemented with fish oil improves diet quality and mental health in people with depression: a randomized controlled trial (HELFIMED)." *Nutr Neurosci 22*(7): 474–487.

Psaltopoulou, T., T. N. Sergentanis, D. B. Panagiotakos, I. N. Sergentanis, R. Kosti and N. Scarmeas (2013). "Mediterranean diet, stroke, cognitive impairment, and depression: a meta-analysis." *Ann Neurol 74*(4): 580–591.

Rao, A. V., A. C. Bested, T. M. Beaulne, M. A. Katzman, C. Iorio, J. M. Berardi and A. C. Logan (2009). "A randomized, double-blind, placebo-controlled pilot study of a probiotic in emotional symptoms of chronic fatigue syndrome." *Gut Pathog 1*(1): 6.

Ravindran, A. V., L. G. Balneaves, G. Faulkner, A. Ortiz, D. McIntosh, R. L. Morehouse, L. Ravindran, L. N. Yatham, S. H. Kennedy, R. W. Lam, G. M. MacQueen, R. V. Milev and S. V. Parikh (2016). "Canadian Network for Mood and Anxiety Treatments (CANMAT) 2016 clinical guidelines for the management of adults with major depressive disorder. Section 5. Complementary and alternative medicine treatments." *Can J Psychiatry 61*(9): 576–587.

Romijn, A. R., J. J. Rucklidge, R. G. Kuijer and C. Frampton (2017). "A double-blind, randomized, placebo-controlled trial of Lactobacillus helveticus and Bifidobacterium longum for the symptoms of depression." *Aust N Z J Psychiatry 51*(8): 810–821.

Rudzki, L., L. Ostrowska, D. Pawlak, A. Malus, K. Pawlak, N. Waszkiewicz and A. Szulc (2019). "Probiotic Lactobacillus Plantarum 299v decreases kynurenine concentration and improves cognitive functions in patients with major depression: a double-blind, randomized, placebo controlled study." *Psychoneuroendocrinology 100*: 213–222.

Sanchez-Villegas, A., J. Alvarez-Perez, E. Toledo, J. Salas-Salvado, C. Ortega-Azorin, M. D. Zomeno, J. Vioque, J. A. Martinez, D. Romaguera, J. Perez-Lopez, J. Lopez-Miranda, R. Estruch, A. Bueno-Cavanillas, F. Aros, J. A. Tur, F. J. Tinahones, O. Lecea, V. Martin, M. Ortega-Calvo, C. Vazquez, X. Pinto, J. Vidal, L. Daimiel, M. Delgado-Rodriguez, P. Matia, D. Corella, A. Diaz-Lopez, N. Babio, M. A. Munoz, M. Fito, M. Garcia de la Hera, I. Abete, A. Garcia-Rios, E. Ros, M. Ruiz-Canela, M. A. Martinez-Gonzalez, M. Izquierdo and L. Serra-Majem (2018). "Seafood consumption, omega-3 fatty acids intake, and lifetime prevalence of depression in the PREDIMED-Plus trial." *Nutrients 10*(12). doi:10.3390/nu10122000.

Saper, C. B., T. C. Chou and J. K. Elmquist (2002). "The need to feed: homeostatic and hedonic control of eating." *Neuron 36*(2): 199–211.

Sarris, J., J. Murphy, D. Mischoulon, G. I. Papakostas, M. Fava, M. Berk and C. H. Ng (2016). "Adjunctive nutraceuticals for depression: a systematic review and meta-analyses." *Am J Psychiatry 173*(6): 575–587.

Sender, R., S. Fuchs and R. Milo (2016). "Revisiting the ratio of bacterial to host cells in humans." *Cell 164*(3): 337–340.

Steenbergen, L., R. Sellaro, S. van Hemert, J. A. Bosch and L. S. Colzato (2015). "A randomized controlled trial to test the effect of multispecies probiotics on cognitive reactivity to sad mood." *Brain Behav Immun 48*: 258–264.

Strandwitz, P., K. H. Kim, D. Terekhova, J. K. Liu, A. Sharma, J. Levering, D. McDonald, D. Dietrich, T. R. Ramadhar, A. Lekbua, N. Mroue, C. Liston, E. J. Stewart, M. J. Dubin, K. Zengler, R. Knight, J. A. Gilbert, J. Clardy and K. Lewis (2019). "GABA-modulating bacteria of the human gut microbiota." *Nature Microbiol 4*(3): 396–403.

Tlaskalova-Hogenova, H., R. Stepankova, H. Kozakova, T. Hudcovic, L. Vannucci, L. Tuckova, P. Rossmann, T. Hrncir, M. Kverka, Z. Zakostelska, K. Klimesova, J. Pribylova, J. Bartova, D. Sanchez, P. Fundova, D. Borovska, D. Srutkova, Z. Zidek, M. Schwarzer, P. Drastich and D. P. Funda (2011). "The role of gut microbiota (commensal bacteria) and the mucosal barrier in the pathogenesis of inflammatory and autoimmune diseases and cancer: contribution of germ-free and gnotobiotic animal models of human diseases." *Cell Mol Immunol 8*(2): 110–120.

Udit, S. and L. Gautron (2013). "Molecular anatomy of the gut-brain axis revealed with transgenic technologies: implications in metabolic research." *Front Neurosci 7*: 134.

Vermeulen, E., A. Knuppel, M. J. Shipley, I. A. Brouwer, M. Visser, T. Akbaraly, E. J. Brunner and M. Nicolaou (2018). "High-sugar, high-saturated-fat dietary patterns are not associated with depressive symptoms in middle-aged adults in a prospective study." *J Nutr 148*(10): 1598–1604.

Wang, S. M., C. Han, S. J. Lee, A. A. Patkar, P. S. Masand and C. U. Pae (2014). "A review of current evidence for acetyl-L-carnitine in the treatment of depression." *J Psychiatr Res* *53*: 30–37.

Wang, W., Y. Lu, Z. Xue, C. Li, C. Wang, X. Zhao, J. Zhang, X. Wei, X. Chen, W. Cui, Q. Wang and W. Zhou (2015). "Rapid-acting antidepressant-like effects of acetyl-L-carnitine mediated by PI3K/AKT/BDNF/VGF signaling pathway in mice." *Neuroscience* *285*: 281–291.

/// 23 /// CHRONOBIOLOGICAL TREATMENTS

Sleep and Light Therapies

RAYMOND W. LAM

23.1. INTRODUCTION

Chronobiology refers to the study of biological and circadian rhythms, oscillating events that recur about every 24 hours and that are observable at molecular, cellular, organ, hormonal, and behavioral levels. In humans, a central biological clock or pacemaker controls many circadian rhythms, including cortisol, growth hormone, and thyroid stimulating hormone. The biological clock is also involved in regulating the daily sleep–wake cycle. Given that sleep symptoms are intimately associated with depressive disorders, it may not be surprising that circadian rhythm disturbances have been implicated in the neurobiology of major depressive disorder (MDD) and that chronotherapeutics, or interventions targeting the circadian system, are effective treatments. In this chapter, we briefly review the circadian system and its dysfunction in MDD and present the evidence for chronotherapeutic interventions, specifically manipulation of the sleep–wake cycle and bright light therapy.

23.2. CIRCADIAN RHYTHMS AND DEPRESSION

In humans, the central biological pacemaker is located in the brain, within the suprachiasmatic nucleus (SCN) of the hypothalamus (1). A complex neural pathway leads from the SCN to the pineal gland, which secretes melatonin, a neurohormone that is implicated in sleep and reproductive function. Melatonin is only secreted at night; the onset of melatonin secretion occurs near 8 p.m., with levels rising steadily through the night. Melatonin offset occurs in the morning hours, and there are very low circulating melatonin levels during the day. The biological clock is externally regulated by zeitgebers (a German word meaning synchronizers), including the light/dark cycle, external bright light, dietary habits, and social or activity cues. Light is the strongest zeitgeber. The circadian effects of light are transmitted through the eyes, but not via visual rod or cone photoreceptors. Instead, the circadian light signal is transduced by melanopsin, a photopigment contained in retinal ganglia cells. A retinohypothalamic tract directly connects the retina to the SCN. The molecular clock mechanism, which is remarkably conserved from one-celled organisms through to humans, has been well studied and many clock genes have been identified.

Circadian rhythms can be generally characterized by amplitude (the difference between peak and trough of the rhythm), phase (the time of an event; e.g., the peak time, relative to external time or to another rhythm), and period (time between each event; e.g., peak to peak). For example, core body temperature is under control of the biological clock and has a distinct circadian rhythm, with peak temperatures occurring in the afternoon and trough temperatures (minima) occurring in the early morning, about two to four hours before awakening. Well-established clinical markers of circadian rhythms include the time of core body temperature minima and the time of melatonin onset (measured under dim light conditions, since melatonin secretion is suppressed by bright light).

Many circadian rhythms are disrupted in depression, with evidence for both circadian phase shifts and decreased amplitude of rhythms (1,2). Circadian phase shifts can be likened to jet lag after crossing time zones, in which internal biological rhythms are misaligned with the new external clock time. These circadian disturbances may be caused by primary dysfunction of the biological clock (e.g., dysfunctional clock genes) or by secondary disruption of zeitgebers such as stress-induced changes in sleep, photic (light) exposure, or social behavior (Figure 23.1). Circadian theories are also intimately associated with seasonal affective disorder (SAD), a pattern of recurrent depressive episodes that start and stop during particular seasons. The

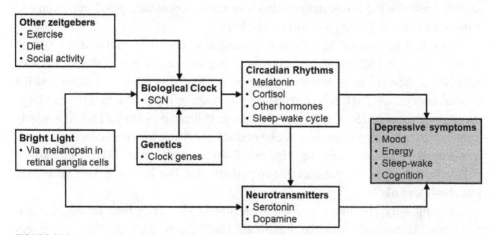

FIGURE 23.1. Potential circadian influences on depressive symptoms.

usual SAD pattern consists of winter depressions with spring/summer remission of symptoms. A winter phase-delay hypothesis seeks to explain the "atypical" depressive symptoms experienced by patients with SAD, including hypersomnia, difficulty arising in the morning, fatigue, and overeating.

The sleep–wake cycle can also be considered a circadian rhythm because we regularly go to sleep and wake up at about the same time every 24 hours. The prevailing theory of sleep–wake cycle regulation involves a two-process model with both homeostatic and circadian factors (3). The homeostatic process is an internal need for sleep, which increases the longer that we are awake. For example, the longer that we have been awake past midnight, the sleepier we get, the more easily we fall asleep, and the longer we sleep (homeostatic process). The circadian process is an oscillating propensity for sleepiness and wakefulness that varies with different times in the circadian cycle: Maximal sleepiness occurs near the body temperature minima at about 4 a.m., while maximal wakefulness occurs at about 8 a.m. In the previous example, if we stay up all night (as in post night-call) past 8 a.m., we find that we become less sleepy, have a harder time falling asleep, and sleep fewer hours because we are now in a wakeful time in the circadian cycle. It is this interaction between the homeostatic and circadian processes that dictates how easily we fall asleep and how long we sleep. Disruptions in the sleep–wake cycle can lead to circadian sleep disorders such as delayed sleep phase syndrome (DSPS), in which the time of sleep onset and waking occur later than usual.

23.3. SLEEP DEPRIVATION (WAKE THERAPY)

Since disturbances in sleep and wake are cardinal symptoms of depression, it is not surprising that manipulation of the sleep–wake cycle has been investigated as a treatment in MDD (3,4). Depressed patients often will say, "If only I had more sleep, I would feel better." Surprisingly, keeping them awake all night is more likely to improve their mood. Total sleep deprivation (TSD, now known as wake therapy to better describe the active intervention) can result in dramatic mood improvement, with some patients feeling a return to baseline.

Since first recognized as a clinical treatment in the early 1940s, many studies have shown that TSD improves depression in a substantial proportion of patients with MDD. Several meta-analyses based on unblinded studies have supported the clinical benefits of TSD, with a response rate ranging from 37% to 53% and large pre–post effect sizes (5). However, the evidence is limited by the fact that it is nearly impossible to design a sham or placebo control condition for sleep deprivation, and so a placebo response cannot be ruled out. Conversely, because TSD as a treatment is so counterintuitive to patients, the hypothesis that the TSD response is entirely placebo is less likely.

Unfortunately, the mood improvement after TSD is not long lasting. Several reviews of sleep deprivation studies found that 80% to 85% of TSD responders relapsed the next day after a recovery sleep (6). Relapse can occur even after brief naps. However, it is interesting that up to 15% of patients appear to have sustained TSD responses, up to two weeks or longer, even after a recovery sleep. Other studies have sought to prolong the transient response to wake therapy, with some evidence suggesting that combining TSD with medications such as lithium or antidepressants, or with bright light therapy, can sustain the response to wake therapy (7).

The main problem with wake therapy is adherence, since many patients do not have the motivation to stay awake all night. A regimen in which an all-night sleep deprivation is alternated with nights of regular sleep may make it easier to implement as an outpatient. Alternatively, partial sleep deprivation, in which patients are restricted to sleep only from 10 p.m. to 2 a.m., may also be effective and may make it easier for patients to comply with wake therapy.

23.4. BRIGHT LIGHT THERAPY

The use of bright light as a chronotherapeutic intervention for depression was first investigated over 35 years ago by Daniel Kripke and colleagues (8) but it was the seminal study of phototherapy for SAD (9) that sparked clinical interest in the antidepressant effects of light. Since then, many studies and meta-analyses (e.g., reference 10) have concluded that light therapy, consisting of daily exposure to bright, artificial light, is an effective treatment for SAD (recurrent major depressive episodes with a seasonal pattern, in the terminology of the fifth edition of the American Psychiatric Association's *Diagnostic and Statistical Manual of Mental Disorders*), with effects comparable to selective serotonin reuptake inhibitor (SSRI) antidepressants. More recent studies have shown that light therapy is also effective in non-seasonal depression (11), both alone (12) and in combination with antidepressant medications (13). The combination of light and an SSRI antidepressant appears to be more efficacious than either monotherapy.

Based on this evidence, clinical guidelines now recommend light therapy as a first-line treatment for SAD and as a second-line adjunctive treatment for non-seasonal MDD (14). Light therapy has also been investigated for other conditions such as bipolar disorder, peripartum depression, premenstrual depressive disorder, attention-deficit/hyperactivity disorder, bulimia nervosa, and behavioral disturbances in dementia. Light therapy is also used for sleep–wake disorders such as DSPS. Other studies have combined light therapy with sleep deprivation approaches in unipolar and bipolar depression (6,15).

Major hypotheses for the therapeutic effect of light therapy in SAD involve circadian rhythm regulation, since light is the strongest synchronizer of the circadian pacemaker in the brain. (16). However, bright light has also been shown to have direct effects on neurotransmitter receptors, including serotonin and dopamine (17,18), which may explain its effectiveness in non-seasonal MDD.

The clinical parameters for light therapy include dose (intensity, wavelength, and duration of daily exposure) and timing (time of day for exposure) (19). The standard recommended procedure is 10,000 lux white light for 30 minutes in the

TABLE 23.1. Standard Protocol for Light Therapy

Parameter	Protocol
Intensity	10,000 lux
Wavelength	White light, no ultraviolet wavelengths
Duration	30 minutes
Timing	Early morning
Onset of effect	In SAD, usually within 1–2 weeks; in non-seasonal MDD, usually within 2–4 weeks

early morning (Table 23.1). Lux is a photometric measure of illumination intensity. The antidepressant effect of light is mediated through the eyes, but patients do not need to be staring at the light—they can read, eat, or work on their mobile device or computer during light therapy. Fluorescent light is usually used because incandescent light is too hot, but devices with light-emitting diode (LED) lights are now available. Most commercial light devices have ultraviolet filters because the ultraviolet wavelengths are not necessary for the antidepressant effects and long-term ultraviolet exposure has potential harmful effects. Newer research is investigating the chronobiological effects of low-intensity blue light. Melanopsin, the retinal photopigment that transduces the circadian light signal, is more sensitive to blue light, and low-intensity blue light shifts circadian rhythms similarly to higher-intensity white light. However, there is still limited research comparing the antidepressant effects of low-intensity blue light to bright white light.

Light boxes remain the gold standard device (Figure 23.2), but smaller light "books" and light glasses or visors are also available. Light therapy devices usually cost $100 to $300 and can be purchased at many pharmacies or medical supply stores, or on the internet. Several academic organizations have internet sites with useful information about light therapy (e.g., www.UBCsad.ca, www.CET.org). Users should ensure that a light device has been properly tested and that the dose of light is specified. Because the lux intensity falls dramatically with distance, the light device should specify the correct distance to achieve a specified lux rating. The smaller devices, although more compact and portable, require more careful positioning to ensure that the proper dose of light reaches the eyes.

Adverse effects reported for light therapy are generally mild and self-limited, but may include headache, nausea, eyestrain, agitation, and insomnia. There are also case reports of manic induction with bright light; hence, patients with bipolar disorder should use the same cautions with light therapy as with other antidepressants. Patients with bipolar disorder type I (with manic episodes) should be taking mood stabilizers if light is used. There are no harmful ocular effects with long-term use of bright white light. However, relative contraindications to using bright light include preexisting retinal disease, macular degeneration, and use of retinal photosensitizing

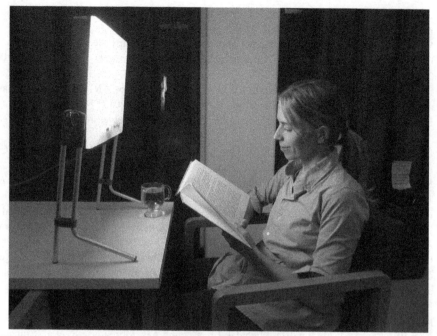

FIGURE 23.2. Example of a fluorescent light box used for light therapy.

drugs (e.g., thioridazine). An ophthalmological consultation prior to light therapy is not routinely required unless retinal risk factors are present.

23.5. SUMMARY

Chronobiological treatments offer noninvasive, well-tolerated alternatives to pharmacotherapy and psychotherapy in patients with MDD. Although wake therapy lacks placebo-controlled evidence, TSD can be considered as adjunctive treatment for patients with MDD, especially those who require rapid response and can be monitored (e.g., hospitalized patients, acutely suicidal patients). In contrast, light therapy is regarded as an evidence-based, first-line treatment for SAD. Although its evidence base for efficacy in non-seasonal MDD is more limited, light therapy can be considered as a first-line treatment for patients with mild to moderate depression severity when standard treatments are not tolerated, or as adjunctive treatment with antidepressants.

REFERENCES

1. McClung CA. How might circadian rhythms control mood? Let me count the ways. *Biol Psychiatry* 2013; 74:242–249.
2. Harvey AG. Sleep and circadian functioning: critical mechanisms in the mood disorders? *Annu Rev Clin Psychol.* 2011; 7:297–319.

3. Borbely AA, Daan S, Wirz-Justice A, Deboer T. The two-process model of sleep regulation: a reappraisal. *J Sleep Res.* 2016; 25:131–143.

4. Wirz-Justice A, Benedetti F, Berger M, Lam RW, Martiny K, Terman M, et al. Chronotherapeutics (light and wake therapy) in affective disorders. *Psychol Med.* 2005; 35:939–944.

5. Boland EM, Rao H, Dinges DF, Smith RV, Goel N, Detre JA, et al. Meta-analysis of the antidepressant effects of acute sleep deprivation. *J Clin Psychiatry* 2017; 78:e1020–e1034.

6. Dallaspezia S, Benedetti F. Sleep deprivation therapy for depression. *Curr Top Behav Neurosci.* 2015; 25:483–502.

7. Dallaspezia S, Suzuki M, Benedetti F. Chronobiological therapy for mood disorders. *Curr Psychiatry Rep.* 2015; 17:95–106.

8. Kripke DF, Risch SC, Janowsky D. Bright white light alleviates depression. *Psychiatry Res.* 1983; 10:105–112.

9. Rosenthal NE, Sack DA, Gillin JC, Lewy AJ, Goodwin FK, Davenport Y, et al. Seasonal affective disorder. A description of the syndrome and preliminary findings with light therapy. *Arch Gen Psychiatry* 1984; 41:72–80.

10. Golden RN, Gaynes BN, Ekstrom RD, Hamer RM, Jacobsen FM, Suppes T, et al. The efficacy of light therapy in the treatment of mood disorders: a review and meta-analysis of the evidence. *Am J Psychiatry* 2005; 162:656–662.

11. Perera S, Eisen R, Bhatt M, Bhatnagar N, de Souza R, Thabane L, et al. Light therapy for non-seasonal depression: systematic review and meta-analysis. *BJPsych Open* 2016; 2:116–126.

12. Lam RW, Levitt AJ, Levitan RD, Michalak EE, Cheung AH, Morehouse R, et al. Efficacy of bright light treatment, fluoxetine, and the combination in patients with nonseasonal major depressive disorder: a randomized clinical trial. *JAMA Psychiatry* 2016; 73:56–63.

13. Penders TM, Stanciu CN, Schoemann AM, Ninan PT, Bloch R, Saeed SA. Bright light therapy as augmentation of pharmacotherapy for treatment of depression: a systematic review and meta-analysis. *Prim Care Companion CNS Disord.* 2016; 18(5). doi:10.4088/PCC.15r01906.

14. Ravindran AV, Balneaves L, Faulkner G, Ortiz A, McIntosh D, Morehouse R, et al. CANMAT 2016 clinical guidelines for the management of adults with major depressive disorder. Section 5. Complementary and alternative medicine treatments. *Can J Psychiatry* 2016; 61:576–587.

15. Wu JC, Kelsoe JR, Schachat C, Bunney BG, DeModena A, Golshan S, et al. Rapid and sustained antidepressant response with sleep deprivation and chronotherapy in bipolar disorder. *Biol Psychiatry* 2009; 66:298–301.

16. Levitan RD. The chronobiology and neurobiology of winter seasonal affective disorder. *Dialog Clin Neurosci.* 2007; 9:315–324.

17. Sohn CH, Lam RW. Update on the biology of seasonal affective disorder. *CNS Spectr.* 2005; 10:635–646.

18. Tyrer AE, Levitan RD, Houle S, Wilson AA, Nobrega JN, Rusjan PM, et al. Serotonin transporter binding is reduced in seasonal affective disorder following light therapy. *Acta Psychiatr Scand.* 2016; 134:410–419.

19. Lam RW, Tam EM. *A Clinician's Guide to Using Light Therapy.* Cambridge, UK: Cambridge University Press; 2009.

Special Populations in Depression

/// 24 /// CHILD AND ADOLESCENT DEPRESSION

ANDREW DIEDERICH, JESSICA M. JONES, AND GRAHAM J. EMSLIE

24.1. INTRODUCTION

Depression is prevalent in youth, with estimates ranging from around 2% in childhood to 4% to 8% of adolescents.[1,2] Population surveys estimate between 11% and 18% of youth will experience a depressive disorder by age 18.[3] Depression causes significant impairment in psychosocial functioning, as well as morbidity and mortality among youth. In 2016 suicide was the third leading cause of death among youth between the ages of 10 and 14 and the second leading cause of death among individuals between the ages of 15 and 34.[4]

Evidence-based psychosocial and psychopharmacological treatments are available for depressed youth, but many children and adolescents do not receive sufficient treatment. Stigma continues to impact both identification and management and greatly impacts time to care as well as treatment implementation. When depression is undertreated, the consequences can be serious, increasing risk for substance abuse, eating disorders, adolescent pregnancy, suicidal thoughts, suicide attempts, and death by suicide.

This chapter focuses on features specific to the pediatric population. We will review the diagnosis and symptomatology, epidemiology, and treatment of early onset depression.

24.2. DIAGNOSIS AND SYMPTOMATOLOGY

24.2.1. Assessment

Diagnostic criteria for depression in youth are essentially the same as those employed in adult populations, though the process for assessment differs in fundamental
ways. Youth typically do not self-present for treatment, but rather are more often
brought to care by a parent or caregiver. Clinicians use information from multiple
informants to understand the nature and duration of depressive symptoms in youth.
Youth often have difficulties reporting the frequency and duration of symptoms accurately; thus, the temporal aspects of reporting on symptoms over the course of
illness often necessitates input from adult sources. However, parents and youth often
do not agree in their reporting symptoms of depression, emotional distress, and suicidality.[5-8] Youth tend to report more accurately on the internalizing symptoms of
the disorder, while caregivers report more accurately on externalizing or behavior-
focused symptoms.[9] A combination of validated clinician-rated and parent and self-
report rating scales is often helpful in assessing the severity of a youth's depression
during a diagnostic evaluation, as well as throughout treatment to measure change in
severity of symptoms over time. Table 24.1 lists validated measures commonly used
for assessing depression in youth.

Pediatric and adult depressive disorders involve essentially the same symptoms,
with the exception of irritability, as depressed youth may present with irritable mood
in the absence of explicit sadness. While there is conflicting evidence on the association of age and anhedonia, hypersomnia and concentration difficulties are more
frequently reported in adolescents, while sadness and feelings of worthlessness are
more frequently endorsed in younger children.[18]

In 2016, the US Preventive Services Task Force issued a recommendation that
all adolescents in primary care be screened for depression.[19] A comprehensive

TABLE 24.1. Rating Scales for Assessing Depression in Youth

Rating Scales	Completed by
Beck Depression Inventory (BDI)[10]	Youth
Center for Epidemiologic Studies Depression Scale (CESD) and CESD-R[11]	Youth
Children's Depression Inventory (CDI)[12]	Youth
Children's Depression Rating Scale-Revised (CDRS-R)[13]	Clinician
Mood and Feelings Questionnaire (MFQ)[14]	Youth, parent
Patient Health Questionnaire-9 Adolescent (PHQ-A)[15]	Youth
Quick Inventory of Depressive Symptomatology-Adolescents (QIDS-A)[16]	Youth, parent, clinician
Reynolds Adolescent Depression Scale (RADS) and RADS-2[17]	Youth

assessment also necessitates a detailed biological family history, including first-, second-, and third-degree relatives. In early onset depression there is a familial aggregation effect with depression, alcoholism, anxiety, and other psychiatric diagnoses in first- and second-degree relatives,[20,21] and youth with a family history of affective and anxiety disorders have a threefold increased risk of developing early onset depression.[22] Chronic depression has been shown to be familial, particularly in cases of preadolescent onset.[23] The current mental state of the caregiver is significant as well, as the youth's treatment outcome may be impacted by parental disorders, particularly maternal depression. Parents may not identify the disorder in themselves[24] and may benefit from their own referral for assessment and treatment. Significant clinical acumen is necessary to synthesize the information obtained.

24.2.2. Course of Illness

Early onset depression has a similar course to adult depression. Over 90% of youth recover from an initial episode of depression within one to two years of onset.[25] However, 40% to 70% of youth treated for a depressive episode will experience a relapse or recurrence of depression.[2,26,27] Factors contributing to relapse and recurrence in depressed youth include higher levels of baseline depression severity, comorbidities, and residual symptoms, such as sleep disturbance and irritability at the end of acute treatment.[28]

24.2.3. Comorbidities and Differential Diagnoses

The assessment and management of comorbid medical conditions in depressed youth are critical, both for the accuracy of diagnoses and functional improvement. Medical diagnoses across a number of organ systems are associated with high rates of pediatric depression, including asthma, diabetes mellitus, and multiple neurological conditions.[29] Hypothyroidism and systemic lupus erythematosus can mimic depression, making these important aspects of the differential. Multiple studies have identified strong comorbidity of psychiatric disorders in youth with neurological conditions such as brain injury, epilepsy, migraine headache, and learning disabilities.[29] Additionally, medications can induce depression, though in the specific case of Accutane (isotretinoin), recent meta-analysis refutes prior assertions that this medication does so.[30]

Coexisting psychiatric conditions, including anxiety, behavior disorders, attention-deficit/hyperactivity disorder, and substance use, are common in depressed youth. Avenevoli and colleagues found that 63.7% of adolescents with major depressive disorder (MDD) had a comorbid psychiatric disorder, with anxiety disorders and behavior disorders most strongly associated with MDD.[1] Because several symptoms of these disorders overlap, evaluating each diagnosis is essential.

Substance abuse is often a feature of adolescent depression, with rates from 25% to 48%.[31,32] Positive response to short-term depression treatment has been associated with reduced likelihood of substance use disorders, though not alcohol use disorders.[33]

Depression in adolescents is also highly correlated with a myriad of poor outcomes in adulthood, including later alcohol, nicotine, and substance use disorders;[34] increased medical problems;[35] poorer overall physical well-being;[36] poorer health; higher healthcare utilization; increased health-related work impairment;[37] failure to complete secondary school; unemployment; and unplanned pregnancy/parenthood.[38] Reducing the psychosocial impairments within the episode, shortening the episode, and preventing relapse and recurrence in pediatric depression are essential to reduce subsequent difficulties across the lifespan.

24.3. EPIDEMIOLOGY

Major mood disorders often begin in early life.[39] In the National Comorbidity Survey, the prevalence rate of MDD in adolescents was 11%.[1] Rates of depression are similar in males and females during childhood.[40] At puberty, depression becomes more prevalent in females, with rates of depression two to three times higher than in males.[2,41] This gender difference remains consistent throughout adulthood and is consistent across cultures.[41] Studies of early onset depression throughout the world are limited, though several have found prevalence rates similar to the United States. Canals[42] suggests that psychosocial similarities across cultures and culture-independent risk factors for depression, such as biological factors, could explain the similar depression rates in Europe and the United States. Stewart and colleagues reported similar rates of depression among adolescents in Hong Kong (2.2%) and the United States (2.2%), though US adolescents reported more irritability and Hong Kong adolescents reported more fatigue.[43] Polaino and Domenech[44] found that 1.8% of a sample of nine-year-olds in Spain met criteria for major depression. Bailly[45] reported a 4.4% prevalence of depression in French adolescents, while Spanish adolescent depression rates range from 1.4% in males to 3.3% in females.[42]

24.4. TREATMENT

24.4.1. General Considerations

Factors to consider in treatment planning include the course and severity of depressive illness, relevant psychosocial factors, medical and/or psychiatric comorbidities, family and cultural factors, and caregiver/youth treatment preferences. Youth would likely benefit from psychotherapeutic intervention, which can be provided by psychologists, social workers, or licensed professional counselors. If the depression is moderate to severe, a primary care clinician might begin pharmacological treatment or refer to child psychiatry for specialty care. It is critical to educate youth and their families on effective treatment options, potential side effects, and treatment expectations so that they are informed during the decision-making process. To date, the combination of pharmacotherapy and psychotherapy, specifically treatment with selective serotonin reuptake inhibitors (SSRIs) and cognitive–behavioral therapy (CBT), appears to be the most efficacious treatment for moderate to severe depression in youth,[46] though several effective treatment options are available.[47,48]

Psychoeducation is a critical component of any depression treatment and should include educating the youth and family that depression is an illness, with biological and genetic bases, and that it is treatable. Psychoeducation about the course of illness and risks of untreated depression is important. It is important to provide information about suicide risk, warning signs for suicidality, crisis procedures, and safety precautions, including increased supervision and restricting access to lethal means of self-harm. Youth and parents should understand the treatment options, including their risks and benefits. Providing parents with information about how they can support depressed youth can have a significant augmenting effect on the youth's treatment. This includes reducing high expressed emotion in the home, which is associated with poorer treatment response and increased risk of relapse, as well as addressing other preventable stressors.[49] Parents can also help by supporting youth's treatment adherence. In cases when a parent is also depressed, it is important to educate parents that remission of maternal depression is associated with decrease in youth symptoms and problem behaviors.[50] It is often helpful for clinicians to communicate with the youth's school, with parental permission, to inform the school counselor about the nature of the youth's illness, as well as regarding accommodations to support the youth during treatment.

24.4.2. Pharmacological Treatment

24.4.2.1. Acute Treatment

Current treatment guidelines, based on the Texas Children's Medication Algorithm Project (CMAP), provide clinicians with a structured, evidence-based framework for managing pharmacological treatment of depression in youth.[51] The design provides initial strategies of individual antidepressant medications with favorable efficacy/safety profiles. Treatment progresses to subsequent, stepwise strategies in cases of nonresponse or partial response (defined as <50% improvement in depressive symptoms) or medication intolerance. If a depressed youth responds to a particular medication (defined as ≥50% improvement in depressive symptoms), treatment progresses to continuation treatment. If a depressed youth does not respond or only partially responds to an antidepressant, the algorithm recommends switching to a different antidepressant or adding an augmenting agent. Generally, switching is for minimal or nonresponders or those with side effects, and augmentation is for youth who partially respond to an antidepressant but have not achieved full response or remission. The most common augmenting agents are bupropion and atypical antipsychotics, such as aripiprazole, quetiapine, and risperidone. Mood stabilizers, such as lamotrigine and lithium, are less commonly used.[52] However, none of these have been systematically studied in depressed youth.

The algorithm in Figure 24.1 is intended as a decision-making guide for clinicians rather than a rigid set of rules. It is important to note that the goal of acute treatment is to treat to remission (having minimal or no depressive symptoms) so as to reduce risk of future relapse and/or recurrence. One caveat is that it is often difficult to distinguish side effects from continued or worsening depression. For example, antidepressants may cause apathy, sleep disturbance, or appetite changes, but these symptoms are also present in depression, resulting in difficulty distinguishing ongoing or worsening symptoms (due to insufficient treatment) from medication side effects.

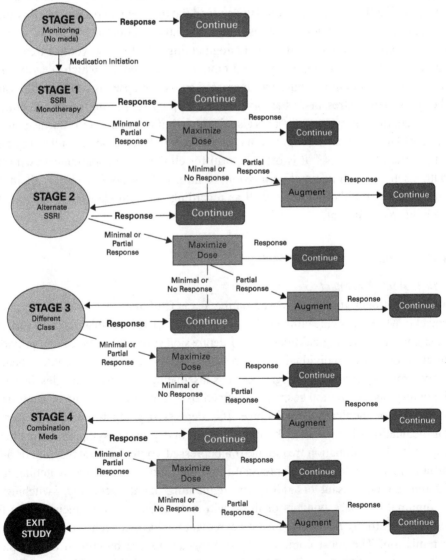

FIGURE 24.1. Treatment of depression in children and adolescents: an algorithm.

SSRIs are considered the first line of medication treatment for depressed youth.[2,51,53] (Table 24.2). These recommendations are based on antidepressant trials conducted in children and adolescents with MDD. Of note, no double-blinded, placebo-controlled studies have been conducted in youth with other depressive disorders (e.g., dysthymia, depression not otherwise specified). A 2007 meta-analysis of 27 randomized controlled trials (RCTs) for MDD in youth showed an average response rate of 61% for SSRIs and 50% for placebo.[54] Fluoxetine showed a larger difference between medication and placebo than other antidepressants in children younger than 12.

To date, fluoxetine is the only antidepressant with a US Food and Drug Administration (FDA) indication for treatment of both children and adolescents (ages eight years and older) with MDD. Escitalopram has an FDA indication for adolescents (ages 12 years and older) with MDD. No other antidepressants have an FDA indication for treatment of depression in youth, although some have indications for other psychiatric conditions. The FDA requires two positive studies of an individual antidepressant to obtain an indication for the treatment of pediatic depression. Other SSRIs have been shown to be effective only in single studies, largely due to high placebo response rates. In comparing placebo rates in RCTs of SSRIs and newer antidepressants, youth have been shown to be more responsive to placebo than adults (36%), resulting in more failed trials of antidepressants.[55] The mean placebo response rate in Bridge's 2009 meta-analysis of antidepressant RCTs was significantly higher than that in Hazell's 1995 meta-analysis (48% vs. 37%, respectively),[56,57] suggesting that placebo response rates in depressed youth have increased over time. Higher placebo response was associated with lower baseline depression severity and younger age.

There are limited data on second-line antidepressants. For youth who fail to respond to an initial trial of an SSRI, the algorithm recommends switching to an alternate SSRI. This recommendation is based on results from the Treatment of Resistant Depression in Adolescents (TORDIA) study, which was the only study of adolescents who have failed to respond to one SSRI. In the TORDIA study, 334 adolescents with SSRI-resistant depression were randomized to either a medication

TABLE 24.2. SSRI Formulations and Dosing

Medication	Formulations	Initial Dose	Target Dose		Max. Dose
			Children	Adolescents	
Fluoxetine	10, 20, 40 mg	10–20	20–40	20–40	40 mg/day
	20 mg/5 mL	mg/day	mg/day	mg/day	
Escitalopram	5, 10, 20 mg	5–10	10–20	10–20	20 mg/day
	5 mg/5 mL	mg/day	mg/day	mg/day	
Citalopram	10, 20, 40 mg	10–20	20–40	20–40	40 mg/day
	10 mg/5 mL	mg/day	mg/day	mg/day	
Sertraline	25, 50, 100 mg	12.5–25	50–200	50–200	200 mg/day
	20 mg/mL	mg/day	mg/day	mg/day	

switch alone (alternate SSRI or venlafaxine) or a medication switch plus CBT. Results after 12 weeks showed similar improvement rates for a second SSRI or a non-SSRI (venlafaxine), although SSRIs had a slightly better adverse event profile. In addition, switching antidepressants and adding CBT was superior to a medication switch alone (55% for medication switch plus CBT vs. 41% for medication switch alone) with respect to clinical response, although not pace of response or attainment of remission.[58] Importantly, combined treatment may also protect against suicidality in patients taking an antidepressant, though this has not been shown in all the studies of combination treatment versus antidepressant medication alone.

Third-line treatment options for youth who have not fully responded to two adequate trials of SSRIs would be to switch to a non-SSRI. To date, there are no studies of youth who have failed to respond to two antidepressants and no positive studies of other antidepressant classes, including serotonin–norepinephrine reuptake inhibitors (SNRIs) (Table 24.3). Due to limited evidence of efficacy and unfavorable side-effect profiles, tricyclic antidepressants (TCAs) are not considered a second- or third-line treatment option, though they might be considered in cases where multiple agents have failed or when other family members have had a positive response. Small trials of newer antidepressants, such as vilazodone, vortioxetine, and levomilnacipran, show promise, and larger studies in youth are ongoing.

Approximately 55% to 65% of youth will respond to treatment with an SSRI, though remission rates are much lower (around 30% to 41%).[59–61] In a review of three large studies examining psychopharmacological and psychosocial treatment, several clinical characteristics were linked to nonresponse to an antidepressant in all three studies, including more severe depression, poorer functioning, higher rates of suicidal ideation and hopelessness, and more comorbid psychiatric conditions.[62]

The goal of acute treatment, either with psychotherapy or pharmacology, is symptom remission, not just symptom improvement. Remission may take up to 12 weeks of acute treatment. Regardless of the treatment, once remission is established, the patient enters the continuation and maintenance phases of treatment.

24.4.2.2. Continuation and Maintenance Treatment

Current guidelines recommend that all youth continue treatment, with psychotherapy and/or antidepressants, for at least six to nine months following acute response. Youth who do not achieve remission or who have continuing residual symptoms following acute treatment experience higher rates of relapse and recurrence.[26,63–65] In a double-blinded, randomized discontinuation study, 102 youth who responded to 12 weeks of acute treatment with fluoxetine were randomized to continue fluoxetine treatment or to placebo. After six months of follow-up, those who received continued fluoxetine treatment were significantly less likely to relapse than those who received placebo (42% vs. 69.2%, respectively). In addition, time to relapse was significantly shorter in the placebo group compared with the fluoxetine group. Youth with residual symptoms after 12 weeks of acute fluoxetine treatment were more likely to relapse

TABLE 24.3. Atypical Antidepressant Formulations and Dosing

Medication	Formulations	Initial Dose	Target Dose		Max. Dose
			Children	Adolescents	
Bupropion	75, 100 mg	100 mg/day	150–300 mg/day	300 mg/day	300 mg/day
Bupropion SR	100,150, 200 mg				
Bupropion XL	150, 300 mg	150 mg/day	150–300 mg/day	450 mg/day	450 mg/day
Desvenlafaxine	50, 100 mg	50 mg/day	50 mg/day	50–100 mg/day	100 mg/day
Duloxetine	20, 30, 60 mg	20 mg/ b.i.d.	40–60 mg/day	40–60 mg/day	60 mg/day
Levomilnacipran	20, 40, 80, 120 mg	20 mg/b.i.d. for 2 days, then 40 mg/day	40–120 mg/day	40–120 mg/day	120 mg/day
Mirtazapine	15, 30, 45 mg[a]	7.5–15 mg/day	15–45 mg/day	15–45 mg/day	45 mg/day
Trazadone	50, 100, 150, 300 mg	25–50 mg/day	100–150 mg/day	100–150 mg/day	150 mg/day
Venlafaxine XR	37.5, 75, 150 mg	37.5 mg/day	150–225 mg/day	150–225 mg/day	300 mg/day
Vilazodone	10, 20, 40 mg	10 mg/day	15–30 mg/day	30–40 mg/day	40 mg/day
Vortioxetine	5, 10, 15, 20 mg	10 mg/day	20 mg/day	20 mg/day	20 mg/day

[a] Both non-dissolving and dissolving tablet available in these doses.

during the six months of follow-up treatment regardless of whether they were receiving fluoxetine or placebo.[26]

There are limited data on antidepressant maintenance treatment in youth, though Cheung and colleagues in 2008 found that youth who received 52 weeks of sertraline maintenance treatment remained well when compared with those treated with placebo.[66] The burden of determining the need for maintenance pharmacotherapy falls to the clinician, who must consider if treatment is indicated as well as the type and duration of treatment. It is generally held that youth with chronic/severe depression or more than two depressive episodes should continue maintenance treatment for at least one year. Many additional factors may support the need for maintenance treatment, including suicidality, family mental illness, and lack of community resources. When discontinuing treatment, providers should consider psychosocial stressors and protective factors, such as family support, school requirements, etc. Following discontinuation of medication, youth should be reassessed within one to two weeks to assess for side effects and return of depressive symptoms.

24.4.2.3. Antidepressants and Suicidality

Youth with depression are much more likely to think about suicide and to attempt it than nondepressed youth. Most adolescents with a lifetime history of suicidal ideation (89.3%) and attempts (96.1%) have at least one psychiatric disorder, with most having a depressive disorder.[67] The controversy around increases in suicidality in adolescents treated with antidepressants warrants special consideration, as initial reports suggested increased activation, agitation, and suicidal behavior. This resulted in the FDA requesting an independent reanalysis of the adverse event data. Despite findings that suicidality occurred in 4% of children on antidepressants compared with 2% on placebo, prospectively collected rating scales from those studies did not demonstrate any difference in suicidality between active treatment and placebo groups.[54,68] No youth completed suicide during the course of these studies. In a meta-analysis examining this issue, Hetrick and colleagues reported an "increased risk of suicidal ideation and behavior in those receiving an SSRI compared with those receiving a placebo," though the rates of suicidality observed were very low compared with those seen in community studies.[69] Others concur that SSRI-induced suicidality in adolescents presents a weak but statistically significant effect, a risk that must be weighed against the risks of untreated depression.[70,71] While there is no clear consensus on the underlying mechanism of the relationship between antidepressants and suicidality, these findings highlight the need for ongoing monitoring for adverse events during treatment. All depressed youth must be assessed for the presence and severity of suicidality and overall suicide risk as part of their evaluation and treatment plan, as well as throughout treatment.

24.4.3. Psychotherapy

Acute treatment studies of psychotherapy alone for the treatment of pediatric depression show mixed results. Weersing and colleagues conducted a meta-analysis of 42 psychotherapy RCTs published between 1998 and 2014.[72] Results suggest that the evidence for interventions in adolescents is significantly stronger than for children. While CBT was classified as "possibly efficacious" for depressed children, both CBT and interpersonal therapy (IPT) were classified as "well-established" for depressed adolescents. Furthermore, there is a great deal of empirical support for the effectiveness of specific psychotherapies, particularly CBT, IPT, attachment-based family therapy, and dialectical behavior therapy (DBT) in the treatment of early onset depression. To learn more about specific psychotherapy components, please refer to the other chapters on various psychotherapies.

CBT is the most commonly used, widely studied specific therapy for pediatric depression. Several studies have demonstrated CBT's effectiveness for depressed youth.[73,74] Some evidence suggests that CBT is most effective when combined with antidepressant medication, particularly for more severely depressed youth or those with treatment-resistant depression. Guidelines indicate that CBT alone may be an appropriate first-line treatment for those with mild depression.[2] Data from the TORDIA study suggest that augmenting pharmacotherapy with CBT may also enhance response during acute treatment.[58] Additionally, group CBT has been extensively studied and appears to be an effective treatment for depressed youth.[75]

Insomnia is frequently comorbid with depression, with approximately 75% of those with depression reporting symptoms of sleep disturbance.[76] Insomnia often persists after treatment, as it is one of the most common residual symptoms in youth treated for depression.[61] Insomnia has been found to be associated with poorer treatment outcomes in depressed adolescents and has been associated with death by suicide in adolescents.[77,78] Depression treatments targeting insomnia have been found to be effective in adults, and CBT for insomnia (CBT-I) has been adapted for depressed adolescents, with promising pilot data.[79–81]

IPT has demonstrated effectiveness in the treatment of depressive symptoms in adolescents.[82,83] IPT has also been shown to be effective in Puerto Rican populations and appears to have consonance with Puerto Rican cultural values.[84] Rosselló and colleagues randomized adolescents to IPT, CBT, or waitlist control. IPT and CBT were found to significantly reduce depressive symptoms when compared with the waitlist condition. Clinical significance tests suggested that 82% of adolescents in IPT and 59% of those in CBT were functional after treatment.[84] A recent meta-analysis suggests that IPT is an effective treatment for depressed adolescents, though limited data exist on the effectiveness of IPT to reduce suicide risk.[85]

Group IPT has been shown to be effective in reducing depression severity and improving social functioning in depressed adolescents in US school-based mental health clinics, and it has also been adapted to Taiwanese and Puerto Rican populations, with positive outcomes.[86–88] Family-based IPT (FB-IPT), which involves parents and specifically targets parent–child conflict, has demonstrated feasibility and acceptability as well as high rates of treatment compliance and reductions in depressive and anxiety symptoms in children. In a recent RCT, depressed children (ages 7–12) who received FB-IPT had higher remission rates, greater depressive symptom reduction, and greater reduction in interpersonal impairment than those who received client-centered therapy.[89]

DBT has been adapted for adolescents, particularly those with suicidal ideation and/or borderline personality disorder (BPD) features.[90] Two RCTs have demonstrated that DBT is effective in reducing self-harm in adolescents with BPD characteristics.[91,92] These results are significant, as they support DBT as the first evidence-based treatment for reducing repeat suicide attempts and non-suicidal self-injury in adolescents.

Family factors appear to play a role in relapse, though clinical trials of family therapy for depressed youth are difficult to evaluate, due to the diversity of interventions studied. Attachment-based family therapy (ABFT), the first manualized family therapy, specifically targets disruptive family processes associated with depression and suicide. ABFT focuses on improving family problem solving and affect regulation, while strengthening family cohesion. Two RCTs have demonstrated significantly superior effects of ABFT compared with controls in reducing depressive symptoms and suicidality, though only those youth without MDD saw significant reductions in suicidality.[93,94]

While much of the literature in pediatric psychiatry has focused on the treatment of illness, growing evidence supports the promotion of wellness and resilience. Early work in this area was been spearheaded by the positive psychology movement.[95] A positive approach includes the enhancement of strengths, positive experiences, mood, and cognitions. The focus of treatment is not only to achieve the absence of illness, but to promote the presence of wellness. Specific strategies include mastery, positive self-regard, goal setting, quality relations/social problem solving, and optimism.[95–97]

More recent work has been done to promote wellness and adaptive coping strategies to enhance well-being in youth successfully treated for depression.[98,99] Based on traditional CBT, relapse prevention CBT (RP-CBT) is a brief manualized, individual intervention with a family component. RP-CBT uses cognitive-behavioral techniques to target residual symptoms and other risk factors for relapse (negative attributional style, family conflict, expressed emotion). RP-CBT incorporates six wellness strategies: self-acceptance (positive self-schemas and helpful explanatory style), social wellness (social skills and social problem solving), success (autonomy and mastery), self-goals (sense of purpose), spirituality (optimism, gratitude, and altruism), and soothing (relaxation). Kennard and colleagues in 2014 conducted an RCT of depressed youth (ages 7–17) who had responded to six weeks of acute fluoxetine treatment. Youth were randomized to RP-CBT plus continued medication management and medication management alone. During the 30-week treatment period, youth receiving RP-CBT had lower relapse rates compared to those receiving medication management (9% vs. 26.5%). Those treated with RP-CBT also had greater percent time well and required lower antidepressant doses.[99]

24.4.4. Other Treatments

Evidence suggests that exercise is associated with lower rates of depressive symptoms in youth. In a prospective, longitudinal community sample, youth with greater levels of exercise had lower levels of depressive symptoms.[100] In clinical samples, exercise has been shown to be a promising alternative treatment strategy for depression.[101,102] Results from a recent meta-analysis suggest that exercise reduces depressive symptoms in adolescents, particularly in clinical samples.[103]

The use of alternative or complementary medications is popular among pediatric patients, though there is little empirical evidence. The most commonly used agents are St. John's wort, omega-3 fatty acids, and S-adenosylmethionine

(SAMe). Transcranial magnetic stimulation (TMS) has also been studied in adolescents with treatment-resistant depression. The majority of TMS studies have been open-label, and one RCT of TMS is ongoing (for review see reference 104). Intravenous ketamine has also been studied in an open-label study in adolescents with treatment resistant depression (TRD).[105] No RCTs of ketamine have been conducted.

24.4.5. Barriers to Treatment

Efficacious evidence-based psychosocial and psychopharmacological treatments are available for depressed youth, but many youth do not receive sufficient treatment. Stigma is one widely recognized barrier to receipt, continuity, and outcomes of mental health care.[106] Youth's perceived barriers to care, including stigma and uncertainty about the family's response, have been associated with decreased use of treatment, particularly antidepressants.[107] Additional barriers include an adolescent's difficulty accepting a depression diagnosis, treatment cost, lack of awareness in families or health care providers, and effectiveness of available treatments.

24.5. CONCLUSION

It is widely recognized that depression is prevalent in youth and is frequently underrecognized and undertreated, resulting in substantial morbidity and mortality. With appropriate assessment, depression can be identified and effective evidence-based treatments are available. Given the paucity of new approaches to treatment, it is important to maximize the potential effectiveness of existing treatments. This can be achieved by improving depression screening, improving access to adequate evidence-based treatments, and treating to remission through ongoing measure-based care. Despite a promising approach to individualized depression treatment, biomarker research has been complicated by the heterogeneity of depression. Continued refinement and optimization of biomarker research has the potential to tailor depression treatment to individual patients, potentially opening the door to faster, more specific, and more efficacious treatments.

REFERENCES

1. Avenevoli S, Swendsen J, He JP, et al. Major depression in the National Comorbidity Survey-Adolescent Supplement: prevalence, correlates, and treatment. *J Am Acad Child Adolesc Psychiatry.* 2015;54(1):37–44.
2. Birmaher B, Brent D, Bernet W, et al. Practice parameter for the assessment and treatment of children and adolescents with depressive disorders. *J Am Acad Child Adolesc Psychiatry.* 2007;46(11):1503–1526.
3. Coyle JT, Pine DS, Charney DS, et al. Depression and Bipolar Support Alliance consensus statement on the unmet needs in diagnosis and treatment of mood disorders in children and adolescents. *J Am Acad Child Adolesc Psychiatry.* 2003;42(12):1494–1503.

4. National Institute of Mental Health. Suicide is a leading cause of death in the United States. 2016; Data courtesy of the CDC. Available at: https://www.nimh.nih.gov/health/statistics/suicide.shtml. Accessed January 23, 2019.

5. Jensen PS, Rubio-Stipec M, Canino G, et al. Parent and child contributions to diagnosis of mental disorder: are both informants always necessary? *J Am Acad Child Adolesc Psychiatry.* 1999;38(12):1569–1579.

6. Makol BA, Polo AJ. Parent–child endorsement discrepancies among youth at chronic risk for depression. *J Abnorm Child Psychol.* 2018;46(5):1077–1088.

7. Kim C, Choi H, Ko H, Park CG. Agreement between parent proxy reports and self-reports of adolescent emotional distress. *J School Nurs.* 2018 [Epub before print]. doi:10.1177/1059840518792073.

8. Klaus NM, Mobilio A, King CA. Parent–adolescent agreement concerning adolescents' suicidal thoughts and behaviors. *J Clin Child Adolesc Psychol.* 2009;38(2):245–255.

9. Herjanic B, Reich W. Development of a structured psychiatric interview for children: agreement between child and parent on individual symptoms. *J Abnorm Child Psychol.* 1997;25(1):21–31.

10. Beck AT, Steer RA, Brown GK. *BDI-II, Beck Depression Inventory: Manual.* San Antonio, TX: Psychological Corporation; 1996.

11. Eaton WW, Smith C, Ybarra M, et al. Center for Epidemiologic Studies Depression Scale: review and revision (CESD and CESD-R). In: *The Use of Psychological Testing for Treatment Planning and Outcomes Assessment: Instruments for Adults.* Vol. 3, 3rd ed. Mahwah, NJ: Lawrence Erlbaum Associates Publishers; 2004:363–377.

12. Kovacs M. The Children's Depression, Inventory (CDI). *Psychopharmacol Bull.* 1985;21(4):995–998.

13. Poznanski EO, Mokros HB. *Children's Depression Rating Scale, Revised (CDRS-R).* Los Angeles: Western Psychological Services; 1996.

14. Daviss WB, Birmaher B, Melhem NA, et al. Criterion validity of the Mood and Feelings Questionnaire for depressive episodes in clinic and non-clinic subjects. *J Child Psychol Psychiatry.* 2006;47(9):927–934.

15. Richardson LP, McCauley E, Grossman DC, et al. Evaluation of the Patient Health Questionnaire-9 Item for detecting major depression among adolescents. *Pediatrics.* 2010;126(6):1117–1123.

16. Moore HK, Hughes CW, Mundt JC, et al. A pilot study of an electronic, adolescent version of the Quick Inventory of Depressive Symptomatology. *J Clin Psychiatry.* 2007;68(9):1436–1440.

17. Osman A, Gutierrez PM, Bagge CL, et al. Reynolds Adolescent Depression Scale, second edition: a reliable and useful instrument. *J Clin Psychol.* 2010;66(12):1324–1345.

18. Sorensen MJ, Nissen JB, Mors O, Thomsen PH. Age and gender differences in depressive symptomatology and comorbidity: an incident sample of psychiatrically admitted children. *J Affect Disord.* 2005;84(1):85–91.

19. Forman-Hoffman V, McClure E, McKeeman J, et al. Screening for major depressive disorder in children and adolescents: a systematic review for the U.S. Preventive Services Task Force. *Ann Intern Med.* 2016;164(5):342–349.

20. Goes FS, McCusker MG, Bienvenu OJ, et al. Co-morbid anxiety disorders in bipolar disorder and major depression: familial aggregation and clinical characteristics of co-morbid panic disorder, social phobia, specific phobia and obsessive-compulsive disorder. *Psychol Med.* 2012;42(7):1449–1459.

21. Klein DN, Lewinsohn PM, Seeley JR, Rohde P. A family study of major depressive disorder in a community sample of adolescents. *Arch Gen Psychiatry.* 2001;58(1):13–20.

22. Williamson DE, Birmaher B, Axelson DA, et al. First episode of depression in children at low and high familial risk for depression. *J Am Acad Child Adolesc Psychiatry.* 2004;43(3):291–297.

23. Mondimore FM, Zandi PP, Mackinnon DF, et al. Familial aggregation of illness chronicity in recurrent, early-onset major depression pedigrees. *Am J Psychiatry.* 2006;163(9):1554–1560.

24. Luby JL, Heffelfinger AK, Mrakotsky C, et al. The clinical picture of depression in preschool children. *J Am Acad Child Adolesc Psychiatry.* 2003;42(3):340–348.

25. Emslie GJ, Rush AJ, Weinberg WA, et al. Recurrence of major depressive disorder in hospitalized children and adolescents. *J Am Acad Child Adolesc Psychiatry.* 1997;36(6):785–792.

26. Emslie GJ, Kennard BD, Mayes TL, et al. Fluoxetine versus placebo in preventing relapse of major depression in children and adolescents. *Am J Psychiatry.* 2008; 165(4):459–467.

27. Kennard BD, Emslie GJ, Mayes TL, Hughes JL. Relapse and recurrence in pediatric depression. *Child Adolesc Psychiatr Clin North Am.* 2006;15(4):1057–1079.

28. Kennard BD, Mayes TL, Chahal Z, et al. Predictors and moderators of relapse in children and adolescents with major depressive disorder. *J Clin Psychiatry.* 2018 [Epub before print]. doi:10.4088/JCP.15m10330.

29. Chapman MR, Hughes JL, Kennard BD, et al. Psychopharmacological treatment for depression in children and adolescents: promoting recovery and resilience. In: M Hodes, S Gau, eds., *Positive Mental Health, Fighting Stigma and Promoting Resiliency for Children and Adolescents.* San Diego: Elsevier Academic Press; 2016:205–235.

30. Huang YC, Cheng YC. Isotretinoin treatment for acne and risk of depression: a systematic review and meta-analysis. *J Am Acad Dermatol.* 2017;76(6):1068–1076.

31. Deykin EY, Buka SL, Zeena TH. Depressive illness among chemically dependent adolescents. *Am J Psychiatry.* 1992;149(10):1341–1347.

32. Rao U, Ryan ND, Dahl RE, et al. Factors associated with the development of substance use disorder in depressed adolescents. *J Am Acad Child Adolesc Psychiatry.* 1999;38(9):1109–1117.

33. Curry J, Silva S, Rohde P, et al. Onset of alcohol or substance use disorders following treatment for adolescent depression. *J Consult Clin Psychol.* 2012;80(2):299–312.

34. Groenman AP, Janssen TWP, Oosterlaan J. Childhood psychiatric disorders as risk factor for subsequent substance abuse: a meta-analysis. *J Am Acad Child Adolesc Psychiatry.* 2017;56(7):556–569.

35. Bardone AM, Moffitt TE, Caspi A, et al. Adult physical health outcomes of adolescent girls with conduct disorder, depression, and anxiety. *J Am Acad Child Adolesc Psychiatry.* 1998;37(6):594–601.

36. Lewinsohn PM, Rohde P, Seeley JR, et al. Psychosocial functioning of young adults who have experienced and recovered from major depressive disorder during adolescence. *J Abnorm Psychol.* 2003;112(3):353–363.

37. Keenan-Miller D, Hammen CL, Brennan PA. Health outcomes related to early adolescent depression. *J Adolesc Health.* 2007;41(3):256–262.

38. Clayborne ZM, Varin M, Colman I. Systematic review and meta-analysis: adolescent depression and long-term psychosocial outcomes. *J Am Acad Child Adolesc Psychiatry.* 2019;58(1):72–79.

39. Kessler RC, Avenevoli S, Ries Merikangas K. Mood disorders in children and adolescents: an epidemiologic perspective. *Biol Psychiatry.* 2001;49(12):1002–1014.

40. Lewinsohn PM, Gotlib IH. Behavioral theory and treatment of depression. In: EE Beckham, WR Leber, eds., *Handbook of Depression*, 2nd ed. New York: Guilford Press; 1995:352–375.

41. Wade TJ, Cairney J, Pevalin DJ. Emergence of gender differences in depression during adolescence: national panel results from three countries. *J Am Acad Child Adolesc Psychiatry.* 2002;41(2):190–198.

42. Canals J, Domenech E, Carbajo G, Blade J. Prevalence of DSM-III-R and ICD-10 psychiatric disorders in a Spanish population of 18-year-olds. *Acta Psychiatr Scand.* 1997;96(4):287–294.

43. Stewart SM, Lewinsohn PM, Lee PWH, et al. Symptom patterns in depression and "subthreshold" depression among adolescents in Hong Kong and the United States. *J Cross Cultural Psychol.* 2002;33(6):559–576.

44. Polaino-Lorente A, Domenech E. Prevalence of childhood depression: results of the first study in Spain. *J Child Psychol Psychiatry.* 1993;34(6):1007–1017.

45. Bailly D, Beuscart R, Collinet C, et al. Sex differences in the manifestations of depression in young people: a study of French high school students: I. Prevalence and clinical data. *Eur Child Adolesc Psychiatry.* 1992;1(3):135–145.

46. March J, Silva S, Petrycki S, et al. Fluoxetine, cognitive-behavioral therapy, and their combination for adolescents with depression: Treatment for Adolescents With Depression Study (TADS) randomized controlled trial. *JAMA.* 2004;292(7):807–820.

47. Sakolsky D, Birmaher B. Developmentally informed pharmacotherapy for child and adolescent depressive disorders. *Child Adolesc Psychiatr Clin North Am.* 2012;21(2):313–325.

48. Tompson MC, Boger KD, Asarnow JR. Enhancing the developmental appropriateness of treatment for depression in youth: integrating the family in treatment. *Child Adolesc Psychiatr Clin North Am.* 2012;21(2):345–384.

49. Peris TS, Miklowitz DJ. Parental expressed emotion and youth psychopathology: new directions for an old construct. *Child Psychiatry Hum Devel.* 2015;46(6):863–873.

50. Wickramaratne P, Gameroff MJ, Pilowsky DJ, et al. Children of depressed mothers 1 year after remission of maternal depression: findings from the STAR*D-Child Study. *Am J Psychiatry.* 2011;168(6):593–602.

51. Hughes CW, Emslie GJ, Crismon ML, et al. Texas Children's Medication Algorithm Project: update from Texas Consensus Conference Panel on Medication Treatment of Childhood Major Depressive Disorder. *J Am Acad Child Adolesc Psychiatry.* 2007;46(6):667–686.

52. Zia Z, Chanhal Z, Mayes T, et al. Treatment of unremitted depression in children and adolescents: does switching treatment or augmenting strategies help in symptom reduction? Poster presented at the Annual Meeting of the American Society of Clinical Psychopharmacology, Miami, FL. June 21–25,2015.

53. Cheung AH, Zuckerbrot RA, Jensen PS, et al. Guidelines for Adolescent Depression in Primary Care (GLAD-PC): II. Treatment and ongoing management. *Pediatrics.* 2007;120(5):e1313.

54. Bridge JA, Iyengar S, Salary CB, et al. Clinical response and risk for reported suicidal ideation and suicide attempts in pediatric antidepressant treatment: a meta-analysis of randomized controlled trials. *JAMA.* 2007;297(15):1683–1696.

55. Meister R, Abbas M, Antel J, et al. Placebo response rates and potential modifiers in double-blind randomized controlled trials of second- and newer-generation antidepressants for major depressive disorder in children and adolescents: a systematic review and meta-regression analysis. *Eur Child Adolesc Psychiatry.* 2018 [Epub before print]. doi: 10.1007/s00787-018-1244-7.

56. Bridge JA, Birmaher B, Iyengar S, et al. Placebo response in randomized controlled trials of antidepressants for pediatric major depressive disorder. *Am J Psychiatry.* 2009;166(1):42–49.

57. Hazell P, O'Connell D, Heathcote D, et al. Efficacy of tricyclic drugs in treating child and adolescent depression: a meta-analysis. *BMJ (Clin Res).* 1995;310(6984):897–901.

58. Brent D, Emslie G, Clarke G, et al. Switching to another SSRI or to venlafaxine with or without cognitive behavioral therapy for adolescents with SSRI-resistant depression: the TORDIA randomized controlled trial. *JAMA.* 2008;299(8):901–913.

59. Emslie GJ, Rush AJ, Weinberg WA, et al. A double-blind, randomized, placebo-controlled trial of fluoxetine in children and adolescents with depression. *Arch Gen Psychiatry.* 1997;54(11):1031–1037.

60. Emslie GJ, Heiligenstein JH, Wagner KD, et al. Fluoxetine for acute treatment of depression in children and adolescents: a placebo-controlled, randomized clinical trial. *J Am Acad Child Adolesc Psychiatry.* 2002;41(10):1205–1215.

61. Kennard B, Silva S, Vitiello B, et al. Remission and residual symptoms after short-term treatment in the Treatment of Adolescents with Depression Study (TADS). *J Am Acad Child Adolesc Psychiatry.* 2006;45(12):1404–1411.

62. Emslie GJ, Kennard BD, Mayes TL. Predictors of treatment response in adolescent depression. *Pediatr Ann.* 2011;40(6):300–306.

63. Curry J, Silva S, Rohde P, et al. Recovery and recurrence following treatment for adolescent major depression. *Arch Gen Psychiatry.* 2011;68(3):263–269.

64. Emslie GJ, Mayes T, Porta G, et al. Treatment of Resistant Depression in Adolescents (TORDIA): week 24 outcomes. *Am J Psychiatry.* 2010;167(7):782–791.

65. Vitiello B, Emslie G, Clarke G, et al. Long-term outcome of adolescent depression initially resistant to selective serotonin reuptake inhibitor treatment: a follow-up study of the TORDIA sample. *J Clin Psychiatry.* 2011;72(3):388–396.

66. Cheung A, Kusumakar V, Kutcher S, et al. Maintenance study for adolescent depression. *J Child Adolesc Psychopharmacol.* 2008;18:389–394.

67. Nock MK, Green JG, Hwang I, et al. Prevalence, correlates, and treatment of lifetime suicidal behavior among adolescents: results from the National Comorbidity Survey Replication Adolescent Supplement. *JAMA Psychiatry.* 2013;70(3):300–310.

68. Hammad TA, Laughren T, Racoosin J. Suicidality in pediatric patients treated with antidepressant drugs. *Arch Gen Psychiatry.* 2006;63(3):332–339.

69. Hetrick SE, McKenzie JE, Merry SN. The use of SSRIs in children and adolescents. *Curr Opin Psychiatry.* 2010;23(1):53–57.

70. Dudley M, Goldney R, Hadzi-Pavlovic D. Are adolescents dying by suicide taking SSRI antidepressants? A review of observational studies. *Australas Psychiatry.* 2010;18(3):242–245.

71. Reeves RR, Ladner ME. Antidepressant-induced suicidality: an update. *CNS Neurosci Ther.* 2010;16(4):227–234.

72. Weersing VR, Jeffreys M, Do MT, et al. Evidence base update of psychosocial treatments for child and adolescent depression. *J Clin Child Adolesc Psychol.* 2017;46(1):11–43.

73. Brent DA, Holder D, Kolko D, et al. A clinical psychotherapy trial for adolescent depression comparing cognitive, family, and supportive therapy. *Arch Gen Psychiatry.* 1997;54(9):877–885.

74. Curry J. Specific psychotherapies for child and adolescent depression. *Biol Psychiatry.* 2001;49:1091–1100.

75. Keles S, Idsoe T. A meta-analysis of group cognitive behavioral therapy (CBT) interventions for adolescents with depression. *J Adolesc.* 2018;67:129–139.

76. Ivanenko A, Crabtree VM, Gozal D. Sleep in children with psychiatric disorders. *Pediatr Clin North Am.* 2004;51(1):51–68.

77. Emslie GJ, Kennard BD, Mayes TL, et al. Insomnia moderates outcome of serotonin-selective reuptake inhibitor treatment in depressed youth. *J Child Adolesc Psychopharmacol.* 2012;22(1):21–28.

78. Goldstein TR, Bridge JA, Brent DA. Sleep disturbance preceding completed suicide in adolescents. *J Consult Clin Psychol.* 2008;76(1):84–91.

79. Manber R, Edinger JD, Gress JL, et al. Cognitive behavioral therapy for insomnia enhances depression outcome in patients with comorbid major depressive disorder and insomnia. *Sleep.* 2008;31(4):489–495.

80. Clarke G, Harvey AG. The complex role of sleep in adolescent depression. *Child Adolesc Psychiatr Clin North Am.* 2012;21(2):385–400.

81. Conroy DA, Czopp AM, Dore-Stites DM, et al. Modified cognitive behavioral therapy for insomnia in depressed adolescents: a pilot study. *Behav Sleep Med.* 2017 [Epub before print]. doi:10.1080/15402002.2017.1299737.

82. Mufson L, Weissman MM, Moreau D, Garfinkel R. Efficacy of interpersonal psychotherapy for depressed adolescents. *Arch Gen Psychiatry.* 1999;56(6):573–579.

83. Santor DA, Kusumakar V. Open trial of interpersonal therapy in adolescents with moderate to severe major depression: effectiveness of novice IPT therapists. *J Am Acad Child Adolesc Psychiatry.* 2001;40(2):236–240.

84. Rosselló J, Bernal G. The efficacy of cognitive-behavioral and interpersonal treatments for depression in Puerto Rican adolescents. *J Consult Clin Psychol.* 1999;67(5):734–745.

85. Pu J, Zhou X, Liu L, et al. Efficacy and acceptability of interpersonal psychotherapy for depression in adolescents: a meta-analysis of randomized controlled trials. *Psychiatry Res.* 2017;253:226–232.

86. Tang TC, Jou SH, Ko CH, et al. Randomized study of school-based intensive interpersonal psychotherapy for depressed adolescents with suicidal risk and parasuicide behaviors. *Psychiatry Clin Neurosci.* 2009;63(4):463–470.

87. Rosselló J, Bernal G, Rivera-Medina C. Individual and group CBT and IPT for Puerto Rican adolescents with depressive symptoms. *Cultur Divers Ethnic Minor Psychol.* 2008;14(3):234–245.

88. Mufson L, Dorta KP, Wickramaratne P, et al. A randomized effectiveness trial of interpersonal psychotherapy for depressed adolescents. *Arch Gen Psychiatry.* 2004;61(6):577–584.

89. Dietz LJ, Weinberg RJ, Brent DA, Mufson L. Family-based interpersonal psychotherapy for depressed preadolescents: examining efficacy and potential treatment mechanisms. *J Am Acad Child Adolesc Psychiatry.* 2015;54(3):191–199.

90. Rathus JH, Miller AL. Dialectical behavior therapy adapted for suicidal adolescents. *Suicide Life Threat Behav.* 2002;32(2):146–157.

91. Mehlum L, Tormoen AJ, Ramberg M, et al. Dialectical behavior therapy for adolescents with repeated suicidal and self-harming behavior: a randomized trial. *J Am Acad Child Adolesc Psychiatry.* 2014;53(10):1082–1091.

92. McCauley E, Berk MS, Asarnow JR, et al. Efficacy of dialectical behavior therapy for adolescents at high risk for suicide: a randomized clinical trial. *JAMA Psychiatry.* 2018;75(8):777–785.

93. Diamond GS, Reis BF, Diamond GM, et al. Attachment-based family therapy for depressed adolescents: a treatment development study. *J Am Acad Child Adolesc Psychiatry.* 2002;41(10):1190–1196.

94. Diamond GS, Wintersteen MB, Brown GK, et al. Attachment-based family therapy for adolescents with suicidal ideation: a randomized controlled trial. *J Am Acad Child Adolesc Psychiatry.* 2010;49(2):122–131.

95. Seligman ME, Csikszentmihalyi M. Positive psychology: an introduction. *Am Psychol.* 2000;55(1):5–14.

96. Segal ZV, Williams JM, Teasdale JD. *Mindfulness-Based Cognitive Therapy for Depression*, 2nd ed. New York: Guilford Press; 2012.

97. Snyder CR, Lopez SJ. *Handbook of Positive Psychology.* New York: Oxford University Press; 2005.

98. Kennard BD, Emslie GJ, Mayes TL, et al. Cognitive-behavioral therapy to prevent relapse in pediatric responders to pharmacotherapy for major depressive disorder. *J Am Acad Child Adolesc Psychiatry.* 2008;47(12):1395–1404.

99. Kennard BD, Emslie GJ, Mayes TL, et al. Sequential treatment with fluoxetine and relapse--prevention CBT to improve outcomes in pediatric depression. *Am J Psychiatry.* 2014;171(10):1083–1090.

100. Rothon C, Edwards P, Bhui K, et al. Physical activity and depressive symptoms in adolescents: a prospective study. *BMC Med.* 2010;8(1):32.

101. Dopp RR, Mooney AJ, Armitage R, King C. Exercise for adolescents with depressive disorders: a feasibility study. *Depress Res Treat.* 2012;2012:257472.

102. Hughes CW, Barnes S, Barnes C, et al. Depressed Adolescents Treated with Exercise (DATE): a pilot randomized controlled trial to test feasibility and establish preliminary effect sizes. *Ment Health Phys Act.* 2013;6(2). doi:10.1016/j.mhpa.2013.06.006.

103. Carter T, Morres ID, Meade O, Callaghan P. The effect of exercise on depressive symptoms in adolescents: a systematic review and meta-analysis. *J Am Acad Child Adolesc Psychiatry.* 2016;55(7):580–590.

104. Croarkin PE, MacMaster FP. Transcranial magnetic stimulation for adolescent depression. *Child Adolesc Psychiatr Clin North Am.* 2019;28(1):33–43.

105. Cullen KR, Amatya P, Roback MG, et al. Intravenous ketamine for adolescents with treatment-resistant depression: an open-label study. *J Child Adolesc Psychopharmacol.* 2018;28(7):437–444.

106. Georgakakou-Koutsonikou N, Williams JM. Children and young people's conceptualizations of depression: a systematic review and narrative meta-synthesis. *Child Care Health Dev.* 2017;43(2):161–181.

107. Meredith LS, Stein BD, Paddock SM, et al. Perceived barriers to treatment for adolescent depression. *Med Care.* 2009;47(6):677–685.

/// 25 /// DEPRESSION IN OLDER ADULTS

HANADI AJAM OUGHLI, JORDAN F. KARP, AND ERIC J. LENZE

25.1. INTRODUCTION

Late-life depression (LLD), defined as major depressive disorder (MDD) in those aged 65 years and older, is quite common, with prevalence ranging from 1% to 5% in older adults living in the community and 6% to 9% in primary care settings.[1] Its occurrence is associated with deleterious health outcomes in older adults, as LLD leads to both an increased risk and worsening of incident cerebrovascular, cardiovascular, and metabolic diseases, as well as an increased risk of cognitive impairment and the development of dementia.[2,3] Additionally, LLD exacerbates frailty and functional decline and contributes to all-cause mortality.[1]

Late-onset major depressive disorder, on the other hand, is a depressive disorder with first onset after the age of 50 years.[4] Late-onset depression may have unique age-related etiologies, including neurodegenerative disease that may involve hippocampal volume loss, decreased total brain volume, microvascular ischemic disease, and disrupted cortical tracts relevant for mood regulation.[4–6] Depressive symptoms associated with age-related vascular changes, also known as vascular depression, often have a chronic and insidious course and patients may have less insight into their mood symptoms.[7] It is often characterized by executive dysfunction, difficulties with decision making, slowed speed of information processing, and impairments in concentration and attention.[7] It is usually cognitive complaints that first trigger a clinical evaluation versus depressive symptoms.[7] Despite this interesting etiologic difference between early and late-onset depression in older adults, no treatment-relevant subtypes of depression have emerged to guide treatment based on age of onset or specific biomarkers such as structural and functional neuroimaging.

25.2. CLINICAL PRESENTATION OF LLD

The diagnosis of depression does not change with age. It is often assumed that depression in older adults is more prevalent than at younger ages due to the unique challenges associated with aging, including loss of independence, reduced financial status, loneliness, grief, and changes in physical and cognitive abilities.[8] However, the literature has been consistent in demonstrating that the incidence and prevalence rates for depression in community-living older adults are significantly lower than in younger adults and in middle age.[8] Depression, though, is very common in medically ill older adults in settings such as hospitals, perioperatively, and nursing homes, where the syndrome often presents as clinically significant depressive symptoms not meeting full criteria for MDD.[9]

LLD tends to have a chronic course, with frequent recurrences and relapses. The median time to recurrence is shortest among older adults,[1,8,10] and this unstable state of remission may be because of high number of previous episodes, elevated medical burden, comorbid anxiety, or neurodegenerative disease. In terms of phenomenology, somatic and emotional symptoms associated with depression present similarly across young, middle, and older adulthood.[8,11] Several studies have shown that older age and chronic somatic diseases are not associated with elevated somatic symptoms in depression.[11] Additionally, the severity of depressive symptoms in older adults tends to be lower when compared to young adults with MDD.[8]

In terms of response to treatment, LLD is equally responsive to treatment as in younger adults.[8] Numerous studies have supported the efficacy of treatment for LLD, including pharmacotherapy, psychotherapy, and neurostimulation (e.g., electroconvulsive therapy [ECT], transcranial magnetic stimulation [TMS]). There is evidence that the acute phase of depression is not more difficult to treat in older adults than in younger adults.[8] However, there remains the challenge of maintaining remission among older adults given the increased likelihood of relapse and recurrence.[8]

25.3. DIFFERENTIAL DIAGNOSIS

The diagnostic criteria for MDD in older adults are the same as they are for younger adults. Older adults, however, suffer from chronic illnesses and are susceptible to a number of neurological conditions that may interfere with making a diagnosis, in part because some neurological conditions (e.g., stroke) can produce mood changes such as apathy that can be confused with depression. In addition, many acute and chronic medical illnesses can cause symptoms such as fatigue or sleep impairment that overlap with diagnostic criteria for MDD. Geriatric mental health specialists often work within a team approach to care, and psychiatric assessments often include a medical workup as well as neurological and neuropsychological assessments. It is also crucial to review depressed patients' medications, as some—such as cholinesterase inhibitors, beta-blockers, and chronic use of opioids—may be associated with depressive symptoms.[12,13] For clinicians focusing on geriatrics, a useful rule of thumb is "always suspect the medications" since older adults are more prone to medication-induced neuropsychiatric problems and this is the one etiology of depression that is easiest to reverse (simply by stopping the offending medication).[14]

To make the diagnosis of depression in older adults, it is essential to ascertain that the patients do not have a medical or metabolic disorder that better explains the symptoms and they are abstaining from (or at least not abusing) drugs and alcohol. Certain medical conditions, such as cardiovascular disease, thyroid and parathyroid disorders, vitamin B12 and vitamin D deficiency, dehydration, Addison's disease, and infectious diseases, can contribute to depressive symptoms. On the other hand, MDD is not usually a diagnosis of exclusion in older adults: The common comorbidity of medical conditions and depression in older adults is mostly explained by fact that both are common in this age group, and that depressive symptoms can increase as part of a psychosocial stress response to illness. In such cases, MDD is still the diagnosis; the diagnosis of "depression due to medical illness" is made only if there is a direct causal and physiological link from the medical illness to the depressive symptoms. For some of these conditions, such as thyroid disease, treatment can alleviate troubling symptoms of depression such as fatigue.

In addition, many neurological conditions share mood symptoms. For instance, Parkinson's disease can manifest with mood (and anxiety) symptoms.[15] Similarly, frontal temporal dementia resembles a mood disorder as it may be characterized by personality changes, impulsivity, agitation, irritability, and compulsive behavior, with memory impairment presenting in the later phases of the illness.[16] Assessment of depression in older adults with moderate to severe dementia is challenging and requires reliance on observation of behavior and reports from caregivers and other collaterals. Two mood scales are useful in quantifying depressive symptoms in older adults with cognitive impairments, the Cornell Scale for Depression[17] and the Dementia Mood Assessment.[18] Both of these scales are completed in an interview format with the patient and caregivers who are familiar with the patient and can accurately describe changes in his or her behavior.

25.4. ASSESSMENT OF TREATMENT-RESISTANT DEPRESSION

A consensus definition of treatment-resistant depression (TRD) is the presence of MDD with continued depressive symptoms despite at least two adequate antidepressant trials (typically one current and one or more past trials). An adequate trial is defined by dose and duration—it should be at least four weeks in duration at a dose that is known to be efficacious; in this way, treatment resistance should be distinguished from "pseudoresistance," which is failure to receive (or tolerate) an adequate trial.[19] Some empirical evidence suggests this definition predicts which older adults are unlikely to response to selective serotonin reuptake inhibitors (SSRIs) or serotonin–norepinephrine reuptake inhibitors (SNRIs) but may be good candidates for augmentation pharmacotherapy with second-generation antipsychotics.[20] It might be argued that depression can be considered "treatment resistant" only when it fails to respond to two trials of different classes of antidepressants (e.g., an SSRI and an SNRI). Little research exists to guide treatment of LLD in such cases, although studies are ongoing to help address this.

With apparent TRD, it is critical to consider several underlying causes. First, a review of the diagnosis is essential as the differential diagnosis of depression includes MDD, dementia, a mood disorder due to a general medical condition (i.e., hypothyroidism, low vitamin B12 levels, sleep apnea), and substance-induced mood disorder, which can occur in alcoholism or opioid dependence. The second step is to assess adherence and compliance with medication treatment. It is important to confirm that the patients are taking their medications every day; many patients do not, due to cognitive impairment, ambivalence, lack of insight, fear of medication side effects, or the misguided concern that antidepressants are addictive. Patients who do not take their medications as prescribed may benefit from adherence counseling,[21] and those who have even a mild degree of cognitive impairment likely will need help in the form of prompts or having a family member administer the medication.

25.5. DIAGNOSTIC AND SCREENING TOOLS

Measurement-based care is highly effective for depression in older adults.[22,23] Several instruments can be used for this purpose, including the Beck Depression Inventory and the Geriatric Depression Scale. The Patient Health Questionnaire (PHQ) depression module PHQ-9[24] is a self-administered nine-item depression measure that queries the frequency of depressive symptoms over the past two weeks. It is a useful screening and severity-rating tool at initial evaluation, and it is also valuable for tracking the severity of symptoms in follow-up assessments to measure response to treatment. It should be noted that measurement-based care of depression (vs. care that is not measurement-based) has an effect size far larger than any single antidepressant's efficacy.[25] This highlights the importance of using measurement tools in routine care to guide treatment, whether in primary care or specialty mental health settings.

Also, these measures track suicidal ideation, and patients who report suicidal thoughts should always be assessed further to determine their risk. Of note, thoughts of death in older adults can occur independently of depression, and many older adults have "normative" thoughts about their death,[26] generally reported in a manner such as "I've had a good long life and if death comes, I'm not afraid—I'm ready." However, patients with specific suicidal intent or plans,[27] those with prior suicide attempts, and patients whose reasons for dying outweigh their reasons for living need to be monitored closely and managed appropriately.[27] Several modifiable and nonmodifiable risk factors have been identified that make suicide more likely.[27] The nonmodifiable risk factors include old age; male gender; being widowed or divorced; previous suicide attempts or attempts at self-harm; and loss of health, status, independence, or significant relations.[27] The potentially modifiable risk factors include social isolation, the presence of chronic pain, alcohol or drug abuse, the presence of hopelessness, the severity of depressive symptoms, and access to means such as firearms or stockpiling medications.[27] Certain behaviors can also be potential clues to suicidal ideation or intent: agitation, giving away personal possessions, reviewing one's will, increase in alcohol consumption, noncompliance with medications, taking unnecessary risks, and preoccupation with death.[27] As well, treatment-emergent suicidal thoughts are not uncommon during antidepressant treatment for LLD—one recent study puts it at 10%[28]—and though this is likely due to the underlying depressive illness (rather than an adverse effect of medication per se), it still highlights the critical need to monitor for suicidal ideation throughout treatment.

Depression at all ages is associated with cognitive complaints, but in older adults it is frequently associated with overt cognitive impairment.[29] The impairments include memory, executive function, and information processing speed—what can be called "fluid intelligence" (as contrasted with crystallized intelligence, aka IQ).[29] The relationship is complex and bidirectional. The co-occurrence of cognitive impairment does not change depression treatment—antidepressants[30] are still used—but it does guide management, including the need for a careful search for potentially reversible/treatable causes of the cognitive impairment (in particular, sedating and otherwise cognitive-toxic medications) as well as management of adherence and other daily living and safety issues.

25.6. TREATMENT

Figure 25.1 provides a suggested treatment algorithm for antidepressant use in older adults as well as general guidelines. This is based on our clinical experience and a review of the literature.

25.6.1. Pharmacotherapy

SSRIs are considered to be the first-line medication treatment for depression in older adults due to their efficacy, safety, tolerability, ease of use, and absence of off-target sedative and cognitive effects.[31] In addition, they ameliorate anxiety symptoms, which often co-occur with depressive symptoms.[32,33] SSRIs have been studied extensively in randomized controlled trials (RCTs) in older adults with variable results.[34–38] Several clinical trials in LLD have shown greater response to fluoxetine,[38] sertraline,[37] and paroxetine[36] than placebo; however, large clinical trials failed to show greater response to escitalopram[34,35] and citalopram than placebo. The reason for this heterogeneity in LLD clinical trials is not apparent; however, meta-analyses have shown that SSRIs as a class were more effective than placebo, with no clear differences in efficacy between specific SSRIs.[39,40] The point here is that, although some specific medications have shown a lack of evidence in LLD clinical trials, SSRIs as a class are considered to be effective.

Several safety concerns have been raised with the use of SSRIs in older adults, including an increased risk of falls, fall-related fractures, and bone loss.[41] This has

Antidepressant Treatment Algorithm

(Note: + = augment for partial responder; Δ =switch for non responder)

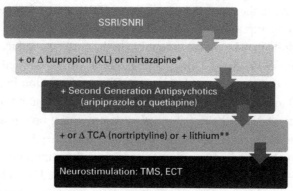

* Other strategies: + buspirone; + or Δ vortioxetine
** Other strategy: T3

FIGURE 25.1. Antidepressant treatment algorithm in older adults. High-quality medication management for LLD must include all of the following: being encouraging and providing a sense of hope, encouraging aerobic activity, eliminating nuisance medications, engaging caregivers, teaching coping skills, involving community resources, teaching and promoting healthy sleep, screening for cognitive impairment, working with primary care physicians to ensure cardiac and metabolic health, and minimizing barriers to medication adherence.

Abbreviations: SSRI, selective serotonin reuptake inhibitors; SNRI, serotonin and norepinephrine reuptake inhibitors; XL, extended release; TMS, transcranial magnetic stimulation; ECT, electroconvulsive therapy.

led to a 2012, 2015, and 2019 update of the Beers criteria that categorize SSRIs (and SNRIs) as potentially inappropriate medications for older adults because of fall risk.[42] However, no large-scale experimental (i.e., RCT) data either support or refute these assertions, and depression itself is associated with falls and accelerated bone loss.[43] Large-scale observational studies often help identify adverse drug effects; however, the caveat is for the adverse effects of the drug to be different from the disease itself.[44] Confounding by indication or indication bias is a possible cause of these medication-associated risks, and it is doubtful that observational studies alone would be sufficient to determine these risks[44] accurately. Therefore the field awaits a better estimate of causal effect; one approach would be to conduct RCTs when feasible that include biomarkers of bone health and remodeling.

Other concerns with SSRIs include hyponatremia due to syndrome of inappropriate antidiuretic hormone (SIADH), which has an incidence ranging from less than 1% to 40%.[45,46] Hyponatremia can lead to deleterious sequelae such as delirium, confusion, seizures, and increased rate of hospitalization.[46] Older adults with chronic kidney disease or congestive heart failure and those receiving diuretics are at a greater risk for hyponatremia.[46] Thus, monitoring serum sodium concentrations at baseline or soon after starting an SSRI is recommended, especially if SIADH has previously occurred or if it is suggested by a patient's presentation.[46]

Additionally, SSRIs increase the risk of bleeding by lowering platelet serotonin levels and altering the efficiency of platelet-driven hemostasis.[47] The upper gastrointestinal tract is the most common site of SSRI-induced bleeding, which may be reduced by concurrent use of acid-suppressing drugs.[47]

Older adults may be more susceptible to the cardiac conduction effects of SSRIs. In 2011, the US Food and Drug Administration (FDA) warned that citalopram was associated with a dose-dependent risk of QTc prolongation in adults older than 60. Doses of 30 mg/day were associated with a QTc prolongation of more than 30 msec from baseline.[48] Nevertheless, it remains controversial how practitioners should act on this warning,[49] and it seems that few practitioners heed it.[50]

SNRIs such as venlafaxine, desvenlafaxine, duloxetine, and milnacipran are a logical second-line treatment when an SSRI trial has failed.[51,52] They reasonably could be used as a first-line treatment for certain patients, such as those with comorbid pain conditions. However, as has been demonstrated with venlafaxine, patients whose depression has failed to respond to multiple antidepressants are unlikely to respond to SNRIs.[20]

Bupropion, a norepinephrine and dopamine reuptake inhibitor, and is commonly used as a monotherapy as well as an adjunct therapy in LLD.[53] Its side-effect profile does not include sedation, cognitive impairment, weight gain, or sexual dysfunction. However, it has a narrow therapeutic index and is associated with emergent anxiety and an increased risk of seizures at doses of more than 450 mg; it also can cause ataxia and falls in the elderly, particularly when combined with a drug that blocks its metabolism via cytochrome P450 2B6 such as paroxetine.[54] This highlights a larger point in LLD treatment—avoid, when possible, medication combinations with drug–drug interactions, as older adults may be more susceptible to adverse drug reactions from these interactions due to their reduced physiological reserve and cognitive reserve, and increased rates of polypharmacy. This is important in depression treatment because older adults, like younger adults, often require augmentation approaches, as discussed later in the chapter.

Mirtazapine is a noradrenergic and a specific serotonin antidepressant; it directly and potently blocks postsynaptic $5HT_2$ and $5HT_3$ receptors,[55] which may account for its anxiolytic and hypnotic effects.[56] It has an early onset of antidepressant action, with relief of symptoms often appearing within two weeks.[57] Overall, mirtazapine is generally tolerable, with its main side effects being sedation and increased appetite, making it a preferable choice in older adults with intolerance to SSRIs, poor sleep, and reduced appetite. One puzzling issue about mirtazapine is that it has a strong antihistaminergic effect and so would be expected to cause cognitive impairment and an increased risk of delirium in older adults, yet these effects appear to be relatively uncommon.[58]

Tricyclic antidepressants (TCAs) have been studied extensively in older adults with LLD,[59,60] and although there appears to be no evidence of superior efficacy of TCAs to SSRIs,[31,61] they are still often used as second-line treatments in depression and frequently for somatic conditions such as chronic pain (at sub-antidepressant doses). Their use in older adults is limited due to a number of safety and tolerability concerns, such as their anticholinergicity, cardiotoxicity, sedating properties, and tendency to cause orthostatic hypotension. TCAs are divided into two categories: (1) tertiary amines, which have two methyl groups at the end of the side chain, such as amitriptyline, clomipramine, doxepin, imipramine, and trimipramine; and (2) secondary amines, which have one methyl group at the end of the side chains, such as desipramine (active metabolite of imipramine), nortriptyline (active metabolite of amitriptyline), and protriptyline. Tertiary amines are more potent in blocking serotonin reuptake and have more anticholinergic and antihistaminergic side effects, whereas secondary amines are more potent in blocking norepinephrine reuptake. Therefore, if a TCA were to be used for treatment of LLD, it should almost always be a secondary amine agent. Among the secondary amine agents, nortriptyline is particularly favored in LLD because extensive clinical trials have defined a therapeutic window—drug levels of 80 to 120 ng/ml, which define its optimal dose.

Monoamine oxidase inhibitors (MAOIs) are rarely used in older adults due to numerous safety and tolerability concerns, including sedation, orthostatic hypotension, problems with dietary and medication co-administration, and narrow therapeutic index. The selegiline patch has fewer safety and tolerability concerns than the rest of the MAOIs; however, there are no current studies looking at its efficacy in LLD.

Other medications have been considered as augmentation agents in the treatment of LLD, including stimulants and donepezil; however, there are few data to guide these suggestions. One large-scale RCT of donepezil augmentation in LLD found that it improved global cognition; however, it also increased recurrence of depressive episodes, making for an overall unacceptable risk/benefit ratio.[13] Another similar RCT found no benefits of donepezil augmentation.[62] Stimulant treatment in combination with an SSRI may have greater antidepressant efficacy than an SSRI alone;[63] however, stimulants can exacerbate anxiety as well as cause elevations in heart rate, and their US Drug Enforcement Administration (DEA) designation as Schedule II limits their use.

The primary goal of treatment of LDD is remission of depressive symptoms. However, there is a substantial placebo response in depression treatment. If a course of treatment is presented credibly by a physician, patients often are relieved that they are receiving the appropriate help and feel better as a result.[64,65] Other explanations include naturalistic changes in mood, or perhaps the initial diagnosis of major depression was inaccurate. Even properly diagnosed major depression can remit spontaneously, especially when it is of short duration.

Optimizing the dose of the antidepressant and treating for an adequate time is vital. Generally, this is defined as "use the full dosing range as necessary and as tolerated and give at least four to six weeks at the maximal dose." Following this guidance prevents a common problem of undertreatment in LLD: when a patient is kept on an inadequate dose despite persistent symptoms. If a patient has symptoms that do not remit during the first trial of antidepressants, there are several options to consider, such as within-class switches, between-class switches, and augmentation.

For example, if one adequate trial of an SSRI has failed, a trial of another SSRI can be considered. However, a preferable option is switching to another class, such as an SNRI, mirtazapine, and bupropion. The choice of a between-class rather than a within-class switch has little solid evidence and is rather based on expertise and solid deduction; if a patient does not respond to an adequate trial of an SSRI, it would be wise to switch to a medication with a different mechanism of action. Alternatively, when choosing between mirtazapine and bupropion, it may be best to consider the side effects of the medication that match to the patient. For a patient complaining of anxiety, insomnia, and weight loss, a trial of mirtazapine, with its sedating, anti-anxiety, and appetite stimulant properties, might be beneficial. However, if a patient is complaining of fatigue, weight gain, and/or sexual dysfunction, a trial of bupropion, with its stimulant-like properties, might be recommended.

Augmentation strategies are frequently used in LLD just as in younger adults.[66] They are intuitively appealing when a patient has a partial response to the initial medication. One common augmentation strategy is to add a low dose of second-generation antipsychotic. The FDA has approved augmentation with aripiprazole, quetiapine, and brexpiprazole for depression. Augmentation with aripiprazole has been investigated in the elderly[67] with doses starting at 2 mg daily and dose increases done every two weeks to a maximum of 10 to 15 mg daily as tolerated. Quetiapine has also been shown to benefit older adults with LLD, with standard doses starting at 25 to 50 mg at night and increasing in 50-mg intervals to a maximum dose of 300 mg daily as tolerated. The same applies to brexipiprazole, which has a more favorable profile in terms of side effects such as akathisia as compared to aripiprazole. The main concern regarding the use of antipsychotics in older adults is their greater propensity to develop akathisia, parkinsonism, and tardive dyskinesia.[67] Greater depression severity may predict treatment-emergent akathisia with aripiprazole augmentation pharmacotherapy, but it is typically of mild severity and responds to dose reduction.[68]

An additional augmentation strategy is adding a second antidepressant from a different class than the index one. Bupropion and mirtazapine may be added in combination with SSRIs and SNRIs. A third strategy is to add a low dose of lithium to the primary antidepressant. Lithium at lower doses, targeting a blood level of 0.3 to 0.6 mEq, is an evidence-based option for treatment of LLD.[69] Long-term monitoring for hypothyroidism and chronic kidney disease is necessary when augmenting with lithium.

One main concern with augmentation is polypharmacy. Older adults taking two antidepressants are vulnerable to the cumulative risks and adverse events of each medication, plus some augmentation strategies have drug–drug interactions that might lead to severe side effects.[54,70] This includes pharmacokinetic drug interactions (where one drug affects the metabolism of another, raising its concentration in the body) and pharmacodynamic interactions (e.g., taking multiple sedatives or multiple anticholinergics and suffering the cumulative or synergistic effects of them). Thus, using augmentation therapy in geriatric patients requires a firm understanding of both the pharmacokinetic and pharmacodynamic interactions among medications.[71] Non-pharmacological treatments—both somatic, such as repetitive TMS, and psychosocial, such as therapy—and promoting increased physical activity[72] should be considered as augmentation strategies to antidepressants as well.

Long-term maintenance antidepressant treatment prevents the relapse and recurrence of depression.[59,73] Older adults placed on two years of maintenance treatment with SSRIs were less likely to have a recurrence of depression compared to those receiving placebo.[73] In addition to symptomatic remission, the benefits of maintenance treatment extend to improved quality of life and social adjustment.[74]

25.6.2. Novel Mechanism Pharmacotherapies

Several novel mechanism agents for depression exist. In 2013 the FDA approved vortioxetine for treatment of depression in older adults.[75] This serotonergic (5-HT) antidepressant has pharmacological effects beyond the traditional 5-HT reuptake blockade; it is a full $5HT_{1A}$ agonist and a $5HT_{1B}$ partial agonist.[75] In addition, it antagonizes $5HT1_D$, $5HT_3$, and $5HT_7$ receptors.[75] In vivo, nonclinical studies have shown an increase in serotonin, noradrenaline, dopamine, acetylcholine, and histamine neurotransmitters in specific brain areas.[76] It has a good safety and tolerability profile, with nausea being the most common adverse effect.[75] Vortioxetine also appears to have pro-cognitive effects for information processing speed, executive functioning, and attention as well as memory and delayed recall. This improvement in cognition may be due to its modulation of serotonin receptor subtypes[77] that are involved in cognitive processes.[76]

Other novel mechanism pharmacotherapies for LLD target inflammation. Depression is associated with increased levels of inflammatory cytokines such as tumor necrosis factor alpha (TNFα), interleukin-6 (IL-6), and IL-1 beta (IL-1β).[78] In addition, aging puts the body in a pro-inflammatory state.[79] Several potential explanations have emerged regarding elevated levels of inflammatory cytokines in depression, including alterations in the hypothalamic–pituitary–adrenal axis activity, as well as differences in the immune system's exposure to microorganisms.[78] Both mechanisms may lead to increased production of inflammatory cytokines, thereby eliciting depressive symptoms.[78] Antidepressant treatment for depression reduces IL-1β and IL-6 levels significantly.[78] Vilazodone was approved by the FDA for treatment of depression in 2011.[80] It increases serotonin levels by inhibiting the serotonin transporter (SERT), and it is a $5HT_{1A}$ partial agonist, which also enhances its anxiolytic effects.[80] Vilazodone has been shown to significantly downregulate pro-inflammatory genes in comparison to other SSRIs.[81] Monocytes and dendritic cells were the primary cellular origins of transcript reductions with vilazodone treatment.[81] Thus, both vilazodone, with its anti-inflammatory effect, and vortioxetine, with its pro-cognitive effects, are intriguing options in older adults with LLD.

Ketamine, an anesthetic drug with N-methyl-D-aspartate (NMDA) glutamate receptor antagonism activity, provides a novel antidepressant mechanism. Several studies have shown that brief low-dose infusions of ketamine in unipolar depression significantly and rapidly (within hours) reduce depressive symptoms; effects last approximately one week. Side effects of ketamine include sympathomimetic effects such as hypertension, dissociation, confusion, and psychosis, which are often mitigated by co-administration of clonidine, an alpha-2 agonist.[82] The clinical significance of ketamine in older adults awaits further study.[83,84]

Modulation of the opiate system may also be a novel treatment approach for treatment of LLD.[85] Buprenorphine is a partial agonist at the μ opiate receptor and an antagonist of κ opiate receptors.[86] It is believed that buprenorphine's kappa antagonism accounts for its antidepressant effects; it has an acceptable safety profile, with a low risk of respiratory depression and euphoria because of only partial mu agonism. A small open-label pilot study found that buprenorphine augmentation significantly improved depressive symptoms in older adults with TRD.[86] Additionally, buprenorphine was safe and well tolerated, with constipation and nausea being the most common side effects.[86] A recent placebo-controlled functional magnetic resonance imaging (fMRI) study in LLD found that low-dose buprenorphine increased emotional activation but not reward activity.[87] Further studies are needed to develop buprenorphine as a novel therapeutic augmentation strategy for depression.

25.6.3. Neurostimulation

ECT is the most effective treatment of depression in younger and older adults and has been shown to be a safe option.[88] ECT has a more rapid response than medications and is considered to be cost-effective, associated with shorter and less costly hospital stays.[89] ECT should be considered as a first-line treatment for patients who are severely ill, acutely suicidal, or so incapacitated that they need hospitalization (e.g., unable to eat)[90] and tends to be more effective earlier during the depressive episode.[91] The main concerns regarding ECT are temporary memory impairments[92] and a high rate of relapse in the six months after the treatment is stopped. However, this risk of relapse may be minimized by ongoing maintenance ECT with or without antidepressant pharmacotherapy.[93]

Repetitive TMS is safe, well tolerated, and efficacious in the treatment of depression in older adults.[94] It has pro-cognitive effects that are independent of mood changes and was found to improve executive functioning in older patients.[94] A primary limitation is availability and feasibility, as it may be difficult to get older patients to attend a TMS center multiple times weekly for four or more consecutive weeks.

25.6.4. Psychosocial Treatment

Nonpharmacological options for treatment of depression in older adults should also be considered as augmentation strategies; these include exercise programs and psychotherapy.[72] These options can be used alone or in combination with antidepressants. Exercise may improve brain health and reduce symptoms of depression in older adults, likely through multiple neurobiological and psychosocial pathways such as producing changes in endorphin and monoamine levels, decreasing cortisol levels, behavioral activation, and, when in groups, social connectedness.[95] More research is needed for this promising treatment, both to maximize its putative benefits and, especially, to increase its reach and sustainability.

The IMPACT (Improving Mood: Providing Access to Collaborative Treatment) study showed that older adults tend to find psychotherapy to be preferable than medications.[96] Cognitive–behavioral therapy, interpersonal therapy, and problem-solving therapy are all effective psychotherapies for older adults that can be adapted to accommodate associated mild cognitive impairments. Maintenance treatment with a combination of psychotherapy and pharmacotherapy is associated with a lower relapse rate than either therapy alone.[59] More recent data suggest that mind–body treatments such as mindfulness training are effective in LLD for both symptoms and co-occurring cognitive dysfunction.[97,98]

25.7. SUMMARY

While research has advanced the clinical care of depression in late life, in truth the evidence on treatment of LLD is limited, and much of our knowledge is based on work with younger adults and simply using the basic principles of geriatrics.[99] While there have been a few innovations in the pharmacotherapy of LLD over the past decade, there is a notable absence of a truly novel antidepressant treatment that is geriatric specific. This runs counter to the fact that numerous studies over the past several decades have found important differences in geriatric depression, including accelerated physiological and biological aging, small-vessel cerebrovascular disease, and high risk for Alzheimer's disease. Thus, much more work is needed to translate these findings into treatments that work for geriatric depression.

REFERENCES

1. Hall CA, Reynolds III CF. Late-life depression in the primary care setting: challenges, collaborative care, and prevention. *Maturitas.* 2014;79(2):147–152.
2. Valkanova V, Ebmeier KP. Vascular risk factors and depression in later life: a systematic review and meta-analysis. *Biol Psychiatry.* 2013;73(5):406–413.
3. Diniz BS, Butters MA, Albert SM, et al. Late-life depression and risk of vascular dementia and Alzheimer's disease: systematic review and meta-analysis of community-based cohort studies. *Br J Psychiatry.* 2013;202(5):329–335.
4. Geerlings MI, Gerritsen L. Late-life depression, hippocampal volumes, and hypothalamic-pituitary-adrenal axis regulation: a systematic review and meta-analysis. *Biol Psychiatry.* 2017;82(5):339–350.
5. Mahgoub N, Alexopoulos GS. Amyloid hypothesis: is there a role for antiamyloid treatment in late-life depression? *Am J Geriatr Psychiatry.* 2016;24(3):239–247.
6. Alves GS, Carvalho AF, Sudo FK, et al. Structural neuroimaging findings in major depressive disorder throughout aging: a critical systematic review of prospective studies. *CNS Neurol Disord Drug Targets.* 2014;13(10):1846–1859.

7. Taylor WD, Schultz SK, Panaite V, Steffens DC. Perspectives on the management of vascular depression. *Am J Psychiatry.* 2018;175(12):1169–1175.

8. Haigh EAP, Bogucki OE, Sigmon ST, Blazer DG. Depression among older adults: a 20-year update on five common myths and misconceptions. *Am J Geriatr Psychiatry.* 2018;26(1):107–122.

9. Lenze EJ, Avidan MS. Pride and prejudice in the treatment of depression and anxiety in acutely ill older adults. *Am J Geriatr Psychiatry.* 2019;27(4):391–394.

10. Mueller TI, Kohn R, Leventhal N, et al. The course of depression in elderly patients. *Am J Geriatr Psychiatry.* 2004;12(1):22–29.

11. Hegeman JM, de Waal MW, Comijs HC, et al. Depression in later life: a more somatic presentation? *J Affect Disord.* 2015;170:196–202.

12. Dhondt T, Derksen P, Hooijer C, et al. Depressogenic medication as an aetiological factor in major depression: an analysis in a clinical population of depressed elderly people. *Int J Geriatr Psychiatry.* 1999;14(10):875–881.

13. Reynolds CF, Butters MA, Lopez O, et al. Maintenance treatment of depression in old age: a randomized, double-blind, placebo-controlled evaluation of the efficacy and safety of donepezil combined with antidepressant pharmacotherapy. *Arch Gen Psychiatry.* 2011;68(1):51–60.

14. Pollock BG. Primum non nocere: prescription of potentially inappropriate psychotropic medications to older adults. *Am J Geriatr Psychiatry.* 2019;27(2):186–187.

15. Dobkin RD, Mann SL, Interian A, et al. Cognitive-behavioral therapy improves diverse profiles of depressive symptoms in Parkinson's disease. *Int J Geriatr Psychiatry.* 2019;34(5):722–729.

16. Swartz JR, Miller BL, Lesser IM, et al. Behavioral phenomenology in Alzheimer's disease, frontotemporal dementia, and late-life depression: a retrospective analysis. *J Geriatr Psychiatry Neurol.* 1997;10(2):67–74.

17. Alexopoulos GS, Abrams RC, Young RC, Shamoian CA. Cornell Scale for Depression in Dementia. *Biol Psychiatry.* 1988;23(3):271–284.

18. Onega LL, Abraham IL. Factor structure of the Dementia Mood Assessment Scale in a cohort of community-dwelling elderly. *Int Psychogeriatr.* 1997;9(4):449–457.

19. Cristancho P, Lenze EJ, Dixon D, et al. Executive function predicts antidepressant treatment noncompletion in late-life depression. *J Clin Psychiatry.* 2018;79(3). doi:10.4088/JCP.16m11371.

20. Hsu JH, Mulsant BH, Lenze EJ, et al. Impact of prior treatment on remission of late-life depression with venlafaxine and subsequent aripiprazole or placebo augmentation. *Am J Geriatr Psychiatry.* 2016;24(10):918–922.

21. Sirey JA, Banerjee S, Marino P, et al. Adherence to depression treatment in primary care: a randomized clinical trial. *JAMA Psychiatry.* 2017;74(11):1129–1135.

22. Bruce ML, Ten Have TR, Reynolds CF, et al. Reducing suicidal ideation and depressive symptoms in depressed older primary care patients: a randomized controlled trial. *JAMA.* 2004;291(9):1081–1091.

23. Unützer J, Katon W, Callahan CM, et al. Collaborative care management of late-life depression in the primary care setting: a randomized controlled trial. *JAMA.* 2002;288(22):2836–2845.

24. Phelan E, Williams B, Meeker K, et al. A study of the diagnostic accuracy of the PHQ-9 in primary care elderly. *BMC Fam Pract.* 2010;11:63.

25. Guo T, Xiang YT, Xiao L, et al. Measurement-based care versus standard care for major depression: a randomized controlled trial with blind raters. *Am J Psychiatry.* 2015;172(10):1004–1013.

26. Szanto K, Lenze EJ, Waern M, et al. Research to reduce the suicide rate among older adults: methodology roadblocks and promising paradigms. *Psychiatr Serv.* 2013;64(6):586–589.

27. Canadian Coalition for Seniors' Mental Health. National guidelines for seniors' mental health: the assessment and treatment of depression. 2006. https://ccsmh.ca/national-guidelines-for-seniors-mental-health-project/.

28. Cristancho P, O'Connor B, Lenze EJ, et al. Treatment-emergent suicidal ideation in depressed older adults. *Int J Geriatr Psychiatry.* 2017;32(6):596–604.

29. Steinberg M, Shao H, Zandi P, et al. Point and 5-year period prevalence of neuropsychiatric symptoms in dementia: the Cache County Study. *Int J Geriatr Psychiatry.* 2008;23(2):170–177.

30. Leong C. Antidepressants for depression in patients with dementia: a review of the literature. *Consult Pharm.* 2014;29(4):254–263.

31. Alexopoulos GS, Katz IR, Reynolds CF, et al. Pharmacotherapy of depressive disorders in older patients. *Postgrad Med.* 2001;Spec No Pharmacotherapy:1–86.

32. Lenze EJ, Mulsant BH, Shear MK, et al. Efficacy and tolerability of citalopram in the treatment of late-life anxiety disorders: results from an 8-week randomized, placebo-controlled trial. *Am J Psychiatry.* 2005;162(1):146–150.

33. Lenze EJ, Wetherell JL. Bringing the bedside to the bench, and then to the community: a prospectus for intervention research in late-life anxiety disorders. *Int J Geriatr Psychiatry.* 2009;24(1):1–14.

34. Bose A, Li D, Gandhi C. Escitalopram in the acute treatment of depressed patients aged 60 years or older. *Am J Geriatr Psychiatry.* 2008;16(1):14–20.

35. Kasper S, de Swart H, Friis Andersen H. Escitalopram in the treatment of depressed elderly patients. *Am J Geriatr Psychiatry.* 2005;13(10):884–891.

36. Rapaport MH, Schneider LS, Dunner DL, et al. Efficacy of controlled-release paroxetine in the treatment of late-life depression. *J Clin Psychiatry.* 2003;64(9):1065–1074.

37. Schneider LS, Nelson JC, Clary CM, et al. An 8-week multicenter, parallel-group, double-blind, placebo-controlled study of sertraline in elderly outpatients with major depression. *Am J Psychiatry.* 2003;160(7):1277–1285.

38. Tollefson GD, Bosomworth JC, Heiligenstein JH, et al. A double-blind, placebo-controlled clinical trial of fluoxetine in geriatric patients with major depression. The Fluoxetine Collaborative Study Group. *Int Psychogeriatr.* 1995;7(1):89–104.

39. Kok RM, Nolen WA, Heeren TJ. Efficacy of treatment in older depressed patients: a systematic review and meta-analysis of double-blind randomized controlled trials with antidepressants. *J Affect Disord.* 2012;141(2-3):103–115.

40. Tedeschini E, Levkovitz Y, Iovieno N, et al. Efficacy of antidepressants for late-life depression: a meta-analysis and meta-regression of placebo-controlled randomized trials. *J Clin Psychiatry.* 2011;72(12):1660–1668.

41. Macri JC, Iaboni A, Kirkham JG, et al. Association between antidepressants and fall-related injuries among long-term care residents. *Am J Geriatr Psychiatry.* 2017;25(12):1326–1336.

42. American Geriatrics Society updated Beers Criteria for potentially inappropriate medication use in older adults. *J Am Geriatr Soc.* 2012;60(4):616–631.

43. Gebara MA, Shea ML, Lipsey KL, et al. Depression, antidepressants, and bone health in older adults: a systematic review. *J Am Geriatr Soc.* 2014;62(8):1434–1441.

44. Gebara MA, Lipsey KL, Karp JF, et al. Cause or effect? Selective serotonin reuptake inhibitors and falls in older adults: a systematic review. *Am J Geriatr Psychiatry.* 2015;23(10):1016–1028.

45. Fabian TJ, Amico JA, Kroboth PD, et al. Paroxetine-induced hyponatremia in the elderly due to the syndrome of inappropriate secretion of antidiuretic hormone (SIADH). *J Geriatr Psychiatry Neurol.* 2003;16(3):160–164.

46. Gandhi S, Shariff SZ, Al-Jaishi A, et al. Second-generation antidepressants and hyponatremia risk: a population-based cohort study of older adults. *Am J Kidney Dis.* 2017;69(1):87–96.

47. Andrade C, Sharma E. Serotonin reuptake inhibitors and risk of abnormal bleeding. *Psychiatr Clin North Am.* 2016;39(3):413–426.

48. Drye LT, Spragg D, Devanand DP, et al. Changes in QTc interval in the citalopram for agitation in Alzheimer's disease (CitAD) randomized trial. *PLoS One.* 2014;9(6):e98426.

49. Gerlach LB, Kim HM, Yosef M, et al. Electrocardiogram monitoring after the Food and Drug Administration sarnings for citalopram: unheeded alerts? *J Am Geriatr Soc.* 2018;66(8):1562–1566.

50. Zivin K, Pfeiffer PN, Bohnert AS, et al. Evaluation of the FDA warning against prescribing citalopram at doses exceeding 40 mg. *Am J Psychiatry.* 2013;170(6):642–650.

51. Raskin J, Wiltse CG, Siegal A, et al. Efficacy of duloxetine on cognition, depression, and pain in elderly patients with major depressive disorder: an 8-week, double-blind, placebo-controlled trial. *Am J Psychiatry.* 2007;164(6):900–909.

52. Schatzberg A, Roose S. A double-blind, placebo-controlled study of venlafaxine and fluoxetine in geriatric outpatients with major depression. *Am J Geriatr Psychiatry.* 2006;14(4):361–370.

53. Dew MA, Whyte EM, Lenze EJ, et al. Recovery from major depression in older adults receiving augmentation of antidepressant pharmacotherapy. *Am J Psychiatry.* 2007;164(6):892–899.

54. Joo JH, Lenze EJ, Mulsant BH, et al. Risk factors for falls during treatment of late-life depression. *J Clin Psychiatry.* 2002;63(10):936–941.

55. de Boer T. The pharmacologic profile of mirtazapine. *J Clin Psychiatry.* 1996;57(Suppl 4):19–25.

56. Holm KJ, Markham A. Mirtazapine: a review of its use in major depression. *Drugs.* 1999;57(4):607–631.

57. Schatzberg AF, Kremer C, Rodrigues HE, et al. Double-blind, randomized comparison of mirtazapine and paroxetine in elderly depressed patients. *Am J Geriatr Psychiatry.* 2002;10(5):541–550.

58. Nelson JC, Hollander SB, Betzel J, et al. Mirtazapine orally disintegrating tablets in depressed nursing home residents 85 years of age and older. *Int J Geriatr Psychiatry.* 2006;21(9):898–901.

59. Reynolds CF, Frank E, Perel JM, et al. Nortriptyline and interpersonal psychotherapy as maintenance therapies for recurrent major depression: a randomized controlled trial in patients older than 59 years. *JAMA.* 1999;281(1):39–45.

60. Reynolds CF, Perel JM, Frank E, et al. Three-year outcomes of maintenance nortriptyline treatment in late-life depression: a study of two fixed plasma levels. *Am J Psychiatry.* 1999;156(8):1177–1181.

61. Mulsant BH, Pollock BG, Nebes R, et al. A twelve-week, double-blind, randomized comparison of nortriptyline and paroxetine in older depressed inpatients and outpatients. *Am J Geriatr Psychiatry.* 2001;9(4):406–414.

62. Devanand DP, Pelton GH, D'Antonio K, et al. Donepezil treatment in patients with depression and cognitive impairment on stable antidepressant treatment: a randomized controlled trial. *Am J Geriatr Psychiatry.* 2018;26(10):1050–1060.

63. Lavretsky H, Reinlieb M, St Cyr N, et al. Citalopram, methylphenidate, or their combination in geriatric depression: a randomized, double-blind, placebo-controlled trial. *Am J Psychiatry.* 2015;172(6):561–569.

64. Zilcha-Mano S, Roose SP, Brown PJ, Rutherford BR. Abrupt symptom improvements in antidepressant clinical trials: transient placebo effects or therapeutic reality? *J Clin Psychiatry.* 2018;80(1). doi:10.4088/JCP.18m12353.

65. Zilcha-Mano S, Brown PJ, Roose SP, et al. Optimizing patient expectancy in the pharmacologic treatment of major depressive disorder. *Psychol Med.* 2018 [Epub before print]. doi:10.1017/S0033291718003343.

66. Arandjelovic K, Eyre HA, Lavretsky H. Clinicians' views on treatment-resistant depression: 2016 survey reports. *Am J Geriatr Psychiatry.* 2016;24(10):913–917.

67. Lenze EJ, Mulsant BH, Blumberger DM, et al. Efficacy, safety, and tolerability of augmentation pharmacotherapy with aripiprazole for treatment-resistant depression in late life: a randomised, double-blind, placebo-controlled trial. *Lancet.* 2015;386(10011):2404–2412.

68. Hsu JH, Mulsant BH, Lenze EJ, et al. Clinical predictors of extrapyramidal symptoms associated with aripiprazole augmentation for the treatment of late-life depression in a randomized controlled trial. *J Clin Psychiatry*. 2018;79(4). doi:10.4088/JCP.17m11764.

69. Kok RM, Vink D, Heeren TJ, Nolen WA. Lithium augmentation compared with phenelzine in treatment-resistant depression in the elderly: an open, randomized, controlled trial. *J Clin Psychiatry*. 2007;68(8):1177–1185.

70. Leach MJ, Pratt NL, Roughead EE. The risk of hip fracture due to mirtazapine exposure when switching antidepressants or using other antidepressants as add-on therapy. *Drugs Real World Outcomes*. 2017;4(4):247–255.

71. Pollock B, Forsyth C, Bies R. The critical role of clinical pharmacology in geriatric psychopharmacology. *Clin Pharmacol Ther*. 2009;85(1):89–93.

72. Unützer J, Park M. Older adults with severe, treatment-resistant depression. *JAMA*. 2012;308(9):909–918.

73. Reynolds CF, Dew MA, Pollock BG, et al. Maintenance treatment of major depression in old age. *N Engl J Med*. 2006;354(11):1130–1138.

74. Lenze EJ, Dew MA, Mazumdar S, et al. Combined pharmacotherapy and psychotherapy as maintenance treatment for late-life depression: effects on social adjustment. *Am J Psychiatry*. 2002;159(3):466–468.

75. Schatzberg AF, Blier P, Culpepper L, et al. An overview of vortioxetine. *J Clin Psychiatry*. 2014;75(12):1411–1418.

76. Katona C, Hansen T, Olsen CK. A randomized, double-blind, placebo-controlled, duloxetine-referenced, fixed-dose study comparing the efficacy and safety of Lu AA21004 in elderly patients with major depressive disorder. *Int Clin Psychopharmacol*. 2012;27(4):215–223.

77. Mørk A, Montezinho LP, Miller S, et al. Vortioxetine (Lu AA21004), a novel multimodal antidepressant, enhances memory in rats. *Pharmacol Biochem Behav*. 2013;105:41–50.

78. Hannestad J, DellaGioia N, Bloch M. The effect of antidepressant medication treatment on serum levels of inflammatory cytokines: a meta-analysis. *Neuropsychopharmacology*. 2011;36(12):2452–2459.

79. Hermida AP, McDonald WM, Steenland K, Levey A. The association between late-life depression, mild cognitive impairment and dementia: is inflammation the missing link? *Expert Rev Neurother*. 2012;12(11):1339–1350.

80. Pierz KA, Thase ME. A review of vilazodone, serotonin, and major depressive disorder. *Prim Care Companion CNS Disord*. 2014;16(1).

81. Eyre H, Siddarth P, Cyr N, et al. Comparing the immune-genomic effects of vilazodone and paroxetine in late-life depression: a pilot study. *Pharmacopsychiatry*. 2017;50(6):256–263.

82. Lenze EJ, Farber NB, Kharasch E, et al. Ninety-six hour ketamine infusion with co-administered clonidine for treatment-resistant depression: a pilot randomised controlled trial. *World J Biol Psychiatry*. 2016;17(3):230–238.

83. Mashour GA, Ben Abdallah A, Pryor KO, et al. Intraoperative ketamine for prevention of depressive symptoms after major surgery in older adults: an international, multicentre, double-blind, randomised clinical trial. *Br J Anaesth*. 2018;121(5):1075–1083.

84. George D, Gálvez V, Martin D, et al. Pilot randomized controlled trial of titrated subcutaneous ketamine in older patients with treatment-resistant depression. *Am J Geriatr Psychiatry*. 2017;25(11):1199–1209.

85. Peciña M, Karp JF, Mathew S, et al. Endogenous opioid system dysregulation in depression: implications for new therapeutic approaches. *Mol Psychiatry*. 2019;24(4):576–587.

86. Karp JF, Butters MA, Begley AE, et al. Safety, tolerability, and clinical effect of low-dose buprenorphine for treatment-resistant depression in midlife and older adults. *J Clin Psychiatry*. 2014;75(8):e785–793.

87. Lin C, Karim HT, Pecina M, et al. Low-dose augmentation with buprenorphine increases emotional reactivity but not reward activity in treatment resistant mid- and late-life depression. *Neuroimage Clin.* 2019;21:101679.

88. Tew JD, Mulsant BH, Haskett RF, et al. Acute efficacy of ECT in the treatment of major depression in the old-old. *Am J Psychiatry.* 1999;156(12):1865–1870.

89. Olfson M, Marcus S, Sackeim HA, et al. Use of ECT for the inpatient treatment of recurrent major depression. *Am J Psychiatry.* 1998;155(1):22–29.

90. Dombrovski AY, Mulsant BH. The evidence for electroconvulsive therapy (ECT) in the treatment of severe late-life depression. ECT: the preferred treatment for severe depression in late life. *Int Psychogeriatr.* 2007;19(1):10–14, 27–35.

91. Dombrovski AY, Mulsant BH, Haskett RF, et al. Predictors of remission after electroconvulsive therapy in unipolar major depression. *J Clin Psychiatry.* 2005;66(8):1043–1049.

92. Kumar S, Mulsant BH, Liu AY, et al. Systematic review of cognitive effects of electroconvulsive therapy in late-life depression. *Am J Geriatr Psychiatry.* 2016;24(7):547–565.

93. Prudic J, Haskett RF, McCall WV, et al. Pharmacological strategies in the prevention of relapse after electroconvulsive therapy. *J ECT.* 2013;29(1):3–12.

94. Kaster TS, Daskalakis ZJ, Noda Y, et al. Efficacy, tolerability, and cognitive effects of deep transcranial magnetic stimulation for late-life depression: a prospective randomized controlled trial. *Neuropsychopharmacology.* 2018;43(11):2231–2238.

95. Duclos M, Gouarne C, Bonnemaison D. Acute and chronic effects of exercise on tissue sensitivity to glucocorticoids. *J Appl Physiol.* 2003;94(3):869–875.

96. Gum AM, Areán PA, Hunkeler E, et al. Depression treatment preferences in older primary care patients. *Gerontologist.* 2006;46(1):14–22.

97. Wetherell JL, Hershey T, Hickman S, et al. Mindfulness-based stress reduction for older adults with stress disorders and neurocognitive difficulties: a randomized controlled trial. *J Clin Psychiatry.* 2017;78(7):e734–e743.

98. Vasudev A, Torres-Platas SG, Kerfoot K, et al. Mind-body interventions in late-life mental illnesses and cognitive disorders: a narrative review. *Am J Geriatr Psychiatry.* 2019;27(5):536–547.

99. Patel K, Abdool PS, Rajji TK, Mulsant BH. Pharmacotherapy of major depression in late life: what is the role of new agents? *Expert Opin Pharmacother.* 2017;18(6):599–609.

/// 26 /// POSTPARTUM DEPRESSION

Identification and Treatment in the Primary Care Setting

NIKITA PATEL, EMILY B. KROSKA,
AND ZACHARY N. STOWE

26.1. OVERVIEW

Postpartum depression (PPD) is a common, and potentially serious, medical illness that affects about 10% to 15% of women after childbirth.[1] The symptoms may interfere with the mother's ability to care for herself, her child, and her family. PPD can be either a continuation or exacerbation of depressive symptoms from pregnancy or new-onset depressive symptoms.[2] Interestingly, approximately 40% of women experience their first depressive episode during the postpartum period,[3] specifically the first two to three months after childbirth.[1] PPD can be confused with other postpartum emotional conditions, the most common being the "baby blues." Nearly 70% of new mothers experience the "baby blues": transient emotional symptoms lasting for a few days during the first two weeks postpartum that typically do not interfere with the mother's functioning. In contrast, postpartum psychosis is an extremely rare and very severe psychiatric illness affecting only 0.1% to 0.5% of new mothers; it occurs within the first month after delivery and requires immediate medical attention. The diagnostic category nomenclature in the fifth edition of the American Psychiatric Association's *Diagnostic and Statistical Manual of Mental Disorders* (DSM-5) does not recognize PPD as a unique diagnosis; instead, PPD is diagnosed as major depressive disorder with the specifier of "with postpartum onset." The symptoms must begin within four weeks of delivery. In practice, however, most clinicians tend to diagnose a woman with PPD if her symptoms arise three to six months postpartum, highlighting the lack of clear consensus regarding the timeline of the postpartum period.[1]

26.1.1. Prevalence

There remain discordant data on the prevalence of PPD. Notably, women from developing countries experience higher rates of PPD than woman from developed countries.[4,5] PPD prevalence rates tend to differ between studies. Woody and colleagues[5] conducted a systematic review of 96 studies and found that discrepancies in the diagnostic methods/instruments employed are likely responsible for differences in rates. Prevalence rates derived using self-report measures (e.g., Edinburgh Postnatal Depression Scale[6]) were generally higher than those derived using diagnostic instruments and structured clinical interviews. Responses on self-report questionnaires may be biased by beliefs and perceptions about depressive symptoms, and self-report measures alone may not always identify women with PPD in need of treatment.

26.1.2. Symptoms

PPD symptoms are often misdiagnosed as the "baby blues," although PPD symptoms are generally more intense and persistent. Symptoms can arise any time during the perinatal period but most commonly occur within the first month of delivery.[7] Common symptoms include severe mood swings, excessive crying, insomnia, withdrawing from activities, fatigue, and overwhelming feelings of anxiety, worthlessness, and guilt. While sleep disruption is a common symptom of PPD, several studies have indicated that quality of sleep also predicts PPD symptom severity, suggesting that clinicians should consider interventions and behavioral suggestions to improve sleep quality in new mothers in order to minimize the development and severity of PPD symptoms.[8,9] A recent report by an international consortium (Postpartum Depression: Action Towards Causes and Treatment) identified significant variations in symptom presentations associated with the timing of symptom onset.[10]

Symptoms of PPD can persist for extended periods and appear to increase the risk for future episodes of major depression. One longitudinal study of PPD symptom trajectory found that depression scores, measured using the Beck Depression Inventory, generally decrease over time.[7] The most significant decrease in depression scores occurred between 4 and 8 weeks and 10 and 14 weeks postpartum; however, depression scores were still elevated above euthymic cutoff scores at two years after delivery for 30.6% of the women. Notably, this cohort had a history of non-postpartum depression and limited social support after delivery.[7]

26.1.3. Risk Factors

Several studies have identified risk factors associated with PPD. Comparison of depression in postpartum women and age-matched women who had not been pregnant found that history of depression and poor partner relationship are associated with depression in both groups of women, but the unique risk factors associated with PPD include not breastfeeding and being a first-time mother.[11] Personal and/or family history of affective disorders has been identified as an important risk factor for PPD. However, data indicate that hormone-related risk factors, such as premenstrual dysphoric disorder (PMDD) and mood sensitivity to iatrogenic alterations in estradiol and progesterone levels, are also associated with PPD symptoms.[12] History of childhood maltreatment can lead to stress response dysregulation across multiple physiological systems over time.[13] While some argue that history of depression is more relevant than history of childhood trauma in predicting PPD,[14] Li and colleagues[13] found that mothers with a childhood maltreatment history were more likely to have higher total depressive symptoms throughout the perinatal period. A prospective investigation of women with a history of depression identified work-related activities, sleep disturbance, and suicidal thoughts during pregnancy as risk factors for later PPD.[15] Interestingly, others argue that high negative affect and low positive affect in the immediate postpartum period (within five days) are better predictors of later depressive symptoms than a history of childhood trauma and depression.[16]

In addition to a history of mental illness and childhood maltreatment, poor partner relationship, negative attitude toward pregnancy, and lack of social support have all been implicated as strong risk factors for PPD among women in both developing and developed countries.[4] Research indicates that women's perception of poor partner support during pregnancy leads to higher Edinburgh Postnatal Depression Scale (EPDS) scores during the postpartum period, suggesting that healthcare professionals should highlight the importance of partner communication during antenatal checkups.[17] Obstetric and pediatric risk factors for women in developed countries remain inconclusive. While some researchers argue that women who undergo cesarean section have a severe acute pain response to childbirth, others argue that women who have infants with medical illnesses have a greater chance of developing PPD.[18,19] Other research indicates that such factors have a minor contribution.[20] Younger maternal age, low education level, and low income have been implicated as playing a small to moderate role in the development of PPD.[21] Screening women, particularly those at increased risk, at both prenatal and postnatal checkups can optimize early identification and treatment planning.

Genetic investigations may eventually provide additional insights or screening options. An initial investigation identified alterations in genes associated with the serotonin transporter in women at high risk for PPD,[22] a finding consistent with studies of other high-risk groups such as trauma victims. Another study identified nine distinct genes that may serve as potential markers for PPD. Five of the nine genes, all related to immune response, were significantly upregulated in PPD women compared to healthy controls, indicating an increase in gene expression in women with PPD.[23] Epigenetics changes, such as methylation and acetylation, are placed throughout the course of an individual's life in response to environmental and natural biological changes.[24] Recent studies have demonstrated an association between oxytocin receptor (OXTR) gene methylation and development of PPD.[25,26] Bell and colleagues[25] found that women with the GG genotype of OXTR had a significantly higher chance of developing PPD compared to "A carriers" despite having similar levels of OXTR methylation, suggesting that certain genotypes are more susceptible to epigenetic variation. In sum, genetic and epigenetic analyses can contribute to the early identification of women at risk for PPD. However, conducting genetic testing as a screening tool and/or adjunct to clinical interviews to identify women at risk for PPD is unlikely to be cost effective in the near future.

26.2. DIAGNOSIS AND SCREENING

To date, the tool most often used by primary care physicians to identify mothers suffering from PPD is the EPDS. The EPDS is a self-report questionnaire that consists of 10 short statements regarding how the mother felt during the past week and has been translated into multiple languages. Each response is rated either 0, 1, 2, or 3, and scores are summed for the total EPDS score. Mothers with scores above 10 are likely to be suffering from PPD, but careful clinical evaluation is needed to confirm the diagnosis.[6] Several studies have demonstrated the validity of the EDPS for identifying women with PPD across different populations from around the world.[27-30] In order to determine the optimal timing of when the EPDS should be administered, one study administered the EPDS to 594 mothers at one, four, and eight weeks postpartum,[31] finding that EPDS scores at one week postpartum were predictive of maternal mood at four and eight weeks postpartum, suggesting that clinicians should administer the EPDS soon after delivery. Furthermore, administration of the EPDS antenatally predicts depressive symptoms in the postpartum period.[32] Although there is no clear consensus regarding the optimal screening time, screening should occur frequently across the perinatal period to ensure that proper preventive measures can be taken.

In addition to the EPDS, three other commonly employed screening instruments for PPD are the Postpartum Depression Screening Scale (PDSS), Beck Depression Inventory (BDI), and Patient Health Questionnaire (PHQ-9). Studies comparing the effectiveness of the screening measures found that the EPDS is the most efficient and accurate tool, followed by the PDSS, BDI, and PHQ-9, in that order.[33,34] Despite its effectiveness in identifying women at risk for PPD, one major limitation of the EPDS is that it uses a one-week timeframe for reporting symptoms, which may result in the extent and magnitude of symptoms being overlooked.[1] Regardless, evidence supports that screening for depressive symptoms reduces both depressive symptoms and prevalence of PPD in a given population.[35]

26.3. ADVERSE CONSEQUENCES

Postpartum maternal depression takes a significant toll on the mother, impacts family stability, and also increases the child's risk for later psychopathology.[36] If PPD is left untreated, it can increase the risk approximately six times for women to develop depression later in life compared to women without PPD.[37]

PPD has significant effects on relationships and may actually increase risks for the mental health of the woman's partner. A study of 128 couples, 60 of which included a woman with PPD, as measured by the EPDS, found that partners of women with PPD had significantly higher levels of depressive symptoms and parenting stress and poorer interactions with their infants.[38] Men whose wives had PPD describe that the absence of a maternal figure, loss of a close adult relationship, and constant preoccupation with their partner's depression prevented them from investing in a father–child relationship.[39]

Mothers with PPD are more likely to demonstrate inadequate levels of maternal sensitivity and attachment that directly impedes the development of infants' social, cognitive, and behavioral skills.[40] For example, mothers with depressive symptoms are more likely to exhibit neutral affect toward their infants during face-to-face interactions and engage in less vocal and visual communication, such as smiling and infant-directed speech.[41,42] This is problematic because face-to-face interactions and infant-directed speech promote social interest and early language learning, respectively.[42,43] Children whose mothers had PPD are four times more likely to have emotional and/or behavioral disorders, which can lead to difficulty interacting with their mothers, behavioral disturbance at home, and social play challenges at school.[36,44] Furthermore, PPD can also affect a child's physical health outcomes, as infants of mothers with PPD show a higher incidence of gastrointestinal symptoms, diarrhea, emergency room visits, and hospitalizations.[45,46] Because PPD mothers are less likely to breastfeed and, instead, formula feed earlier, infants show greater weight gain at six months postpartum and purportedly receive less immune protection.[47]

26.4. TREATMENT OPTIONS

Given the prevalence and consequences of PPD, employing effective treatment options for women suffering from PPD is crucial. While PPD occurs during a unique psychosocial and neuroendocrine window, there are no data suggesting that treatments for non-postpartum depression are less effective. Antidepressant medications, psychological treatments, and the combination of these have all demonstrated clinical efficacy in the treatment of women with PPD. The most widely used antidepressant medications in the treatment of PPD are selective serotonin reuptake inhibitors (SSRIs), such as sertraline, paroxetine, and fluoxetine.[48] Generally,

SSRIs are preferred over the older class of tricyclic medications because they are relatively safer if taken in overdose and have milder side effects, and typically there is more information about use during breastfeeding.[48,49] The small number of randomized, placebo-controlled trials have concluded that SSRIs are more effective than placebos in reducing PPD symptoms. One six-week, randomized, double-blind, placebo-controlled trial of sertraline including 38 women with PPD onset within three months of delivery showed that women in the sertraline group (50 mg) had a more significant decrease in Hamilton Rating Scale for Depression (HAM-D) scores and were twice as likely to be in remission after the trial.[50] Sertraline continues to be one of the more popular SSRIs because of the extant literature in breastfeeding and the relatively low concentrations—if detected—in nursing infants.[51,52] Notably, as a class, antidepressants have more data about use during breastfeeding than all other classes of medication,[53] with sertraline and fluoxetine having the most individually.

A limitation with antidepressant medications is the time it takes to achieve full remission of symptoms; typically two to four weeks elapses before they produce any noticeable effects. A promising new treatment is brexanolone (BRX), a positive allosteric modulator of GABA type A receptors ($GABA_AR$). The results of a phase 3 trial involving BRX indicated that women receiving BRX infusion (60 µg/kg/hour) had greater reductions in HAM-D scores at 60 hours compared to the placebo group. The most prominent adverse effects of BRX are headaches, dizziness, and somnolence.[54] These data indicate that brexanolone treatment has a rapid response rate, warranting additional confirmation and approval from the US Food and Drug Administration (FDA).

The effectiveness of psychological treatments, including counseling, cognitive–behavioral therapy (CBT), interpersonal psychotherapy (IPT), and psychodynamic therapy, has been well supported by the literature.[1] Glavin and colleagues[55] showed that supportive counseling provided by public health nurses significantly reduced EPDS scores at three and six months postpartum. CBT, a form of therapy aimed at changing patterns of thinking and behavior, has demonstrated significant therapeutic effectiveness in treating PPD.[56] A meta-analysis that combined data from 20 randomized controlled trials (RCTs) comparing the effectiveness of CBT versus control found that CBT was associated with lower EPDS scores than controls in both the short and long term, indicating that CBT improves both symptoms and progression of PPD.[57] To increase access to care and minimize barriers to CBT administration, such as lack of trained therapists, long waiting times, and high costs, the success of internet-based CBT (iCBT) in improving stress, anxiety, and depressive symptoms has excited many healthcare providers[58]—though studies in PPD are limited. Studies comparing the efficacy of IPT and psychodynamic therapy versus control show similar efficacy in PPD.[59,60]

Given the effectiveness of pharmacotherapy and psychological treatments, studying the combination of both treatments is of particular interest. Surprisingly, most studies have shown that there are no additional benefits of combining both treatments. The results of one RCT that assigned 45 women with a DSM-IV diagnosis of PPD to receive either CBT, sertraline, or a combination of both for 12 weeks indicated that CBT alone was the superior treatment, and there was no advantage of combining both treatments in the short term.[48] Another study that compared paroxetine, CBT, and the combination found similar results: All three therapies are effective at reducing depression symptoms, but combining the two monotherapies produced no additional benefits.[61]

Despite the availability of effective treatments for PPD, the stigma around mental illness prevents many women, especially minority women, from seeking help.[62] Stigma is associated with lower levels of treatment acceptance for all groups of women, but it does not explain why black women have lower levels of acceptance than white women, suggesting that other factors, such as mistrust in the medical system or limited access to care, may be involved.[63] There is also a significant treatment gap between low/middle-income countries and high-income countries.[64] One major reason for this gap is the lack of experienced treatment providers in developing countries. Prioritization of treatments that are evidence-based, available, cost-effective, and easily delivered may help to ameliorate this gap in service.[64]

26.5. PREVENTION

While there are many effective treatment options for PPD, a focus on prevention is necessary to reduce high prevalence rates and occurrence for at-risk women. A review that synthesized data from 28 RCTs of women at risk for PPD showed that women who received psychosocial and psychological interventions (CBT, IPT, counseling, telephone support, or home visits) antenatally and up to four weeks postpartum were significantly less likely to develop PPD compared to women who received no preventive interventions.[65] The use of pharmacotherapy in the prevention of PPD has also shown some promising results. Treatment with sertraline (50 mg/day) immediately after birth to women with at least one past episode of PPD significantly increased the time of PPD recurrence compared to placebo.[66]

26.6. CONCLUSIONS

PPD is a common and significant mental health problem that has serious potential repercussions for a mother, her child, and her family. It is more common in women with a history of PPD, a history of depression, depressive symptoms during later pregnancy, poor psychosocial support, early adverse life events, and recent stressful life events. Clinicians can identify the majority of women at risk for PPD prior to delivery based on these risk factors; however, many primary care settings may not have the time or expertise to perform in-depth assessments and provide treatment interventions to women at risk for PPD. As a result, the US Preventive Services Task Force recently recommended that clinicians refer pregnant and postpartum women at increased risk for PPD, based on genetic and/or psychosocial factors, to experienced counseling interventions.[67] Such services are not always available, and many women may prefer to receive treatment in the primary care setting. The use of screening tools such as the EPDS during pregnancy and early postpartum visits will increase the likelihood of early identification. Antidepressants have a large reproductive safety database, including use in breastfeeding women, that is well documented, and they are effective in treating women with PPD. Psychotherapy is also efficacious in the treatment of PPD. Antidepressants and psychotherapy are effective in preventing postpartum depressive symptoms in women at high risk. Given the importance of maternal mental health and healthy development of a child, primary care clinicians have a crucial role in screening, recognizing, diagnosing, and treating PPD.

REFERENCES

1. O'Hara MW, McCabe JE. Postpartum depression: current status and future directions. *Annu Rev Clin Psychol*. 2013;9(1):379–407. doi:10.1146/annurev-clinpsy-050212-185612

2. Shakeel N, Sletner L, Falk RS, et al. Prevalence of postpartum depressive symptoms in a multiethnic population and the role of ethnicity and integration. *J Affect Disord*. 2018;241:49–58. doi:10.1016/J.JAD.2018.07.056

3. Wisner KL, Sit DK, McShea MC, et al. Onset timing, thoughts of self-harm, and diagnoses in postpartum women with screen-positive depression findings. *JAMA Psychiatry*. 2013;70(5):490. doi:10.1001/jamapsychiatry.2013.87

4. Norhayati MN, Nik Hazlina NH, Asrenee AR, Wan Emilin WMA. Magnitude and risk factors for postpartum symptoms: a literature review. *J Affect Disord*. 2015;175:34–52. doi:10.1016/J.JAD.2014.12.041

5. Woody CA, Ferrari AJ, Siskind DJ, Whiteford HA, Harris MG. A systematic review and meta-regression of the prevalence and incidence of perinatal depression. *J Affect Disord*. 2017;219:86–92. doi:10.1016/j.jad.2017.05.003

6. Cox JL, Holden JM, Sagovsky R. Detection of postnatal depression: development of the 10-item Edinburgh postnatal depression scale. *Br J Psychiatry*. 1987;150(6):782–786. doi:10.1192/bjp.150.6.782

7. Horowitz JA, Goodman J. A longitudinal study of maternal postpartum depression symptoms. *Res Theory Nurs Pract*. 2004;18(2/3):149–163.

8. Park EM, Meltzer-Brody S, Stickgold R. Poor sleep maintenance and subjective sleep quality are associated with postpartum maternal depression symptom severity. *Arch Womens Ment Health*. 2013;16:539–547. doi:10.1007/s00737-013-0356-9

9. Posmontier B. Sleep quality in women with and without postpartum depression. *J Obstet Gynecol Neonatal Nurs*. 2008;37:722–737. doi:10.1111/j.1552-6909.2008.00298.x

10. Putnam KT, Wilcox M, Robertson-Blackmore E, et al. Clinical phenotypes of perinatal depression and time of symptom onset: analysis of data from an international consortium. *Lancet Psychiatry*. 2017;4(6):477–485. doi:10.1016/S2215-0366(17)30136-0

11. Eberhard-Gran M, Eskild A, Tambs K, et al. Depression in postpartum and non-postpartum women: prevalence and risk factors. *Acta Psychiatr Scand*. 2002;106(6):426–433. doi:10.1034/j.1600-0447.2002.02408.x

12. Bloch M, Rotenberg N, Koren D, Klein E. Risk factors for early postpartum depressive symptoms. *Gen Hosp Psychiatry*. 2006;28(1):3–8. doi:10.1016/J.GENHOSPPSYCH.2005.08.006

13. Li Y, Long Z, Cao D, Cao F. Maternal history of child maltreatment and maternal depression risk in the perinatal period: a longitudinal study. *Child Abuse Negl*. 2017;63:192–201. doi:10.1016/j.chiabu.2016.12.001

14. De Venter M, Smets J, Raes F, et al. Impact of childhood trauma on postpartum depression: a prospective study. *Arch Womens Ment Heal.* 2016;19:337–342. doi:10.1007/s00737-015-0550-z

15. Suri R, Stowe ZN, Cohen LS, et al. Prospective longitudinal study of predictors of postpartum-onset depression in women with a history of major depressive disorder. *J Clin Psychiatry.* 2017;78(8):1110–1116. doi:10.4088/JCP.15m10427

16. Miller ML, Kroska EB, Grekin R. Immediate postpartum mood assessment and postpartum depressive symptoms. *J Affect Disord.* 2017;207:69–75. doi:10.1016/J.JAD.2016.09.023

17. Dennis C-L, Ross L. Women's perceptions of partner support and conflict in the development of postpartum depressive symptoms. *J Adv Nurs.* 2006;56(6):588–599. doi:10.1111/j.1365-2648.2006.04059.x

18. Eisenach JC, Pan PH, Smiley R, et al. Severity of acute pain after childbirth, but not type of delivery, predicts persistent pain and postpartum depression. *Pain.* 2008;140:87–94. doi:10.1016/j.pain.2008.07.011

19. Koutra K, Vassilaki M, Georgiou V, et al. Antenatal maternal mental health as determinant of postpartum depression in a population based mother–child cohort (Rhea Study) in Crete, Greece. *Soc Psychiatry Psychiatr Epidemiol.* 2014;49(5):711–721. doi:10.1007/s00127-013-0758-z

20. Gaillard A, Le Strat Y, Mandelbrot L, et al. Predictors of postpartum depression: Prospective study of 264 women followed during pregnancy and postpartum. *Psychiatry Res.* 2014;215:341–346. doi:10.1016/j.psychres.2013.10.003

21. Kozinszky Z, Dudas RB, Csatordai S, et al. Social dynamics of postpartum depression: a population-based screening in south-eastern Hungary. *Soc Psychiatry Psychiatr Epidemiol.* 2011;46:413–423. doi:10.1007/s00127-010-0206-2

22. Binder EB, Newport DJ, Zach EB, et al. A serotonin transporter gene polymorphism predicts peripartum depressive symptoms in an at-risk psychiatric cohort. *J Psychiatr Res.* 2010;44:640–646. doi:10.1016/j.jpsychires.2009.12.001

23. Landsman A, Aidelman R, Smith Y, et al. Distinctive gene expression profile in women with history of postpartum depression. *Genomics.* 2017;109:1–8. doi:10.1016/j.ygeno.2016.10.005

24. Kumsta R, Hummel E, Chen FS, Heinrichs M. Epigenetic regulation of the oxytocin receptor gene: implications for behavioral neuroscience. *Front Neurosci.* 2013;7:83. doi:10.3389/fnins.2013.00083

25. Bell AF, Carter CS, Steer CD, et al. Interaction between oxytocin receptor DNA methylation and genotype is associated with risk of postpartum depression in women without depression in pregnancy. *Front Genet.* 2015;6:243. doi:10.3389/fgene.2015.00243

26. Kimmel M, Clive M, Gispen F, et al. Oxytocin receptor DNA methylation in postpartum depression. *Psychoneuroendocrinology.* 2016;69:150–160. doi:10.1016/J.PSYNEUEN.2016.04.008

27. Alvarado R, Jadresic E, Guajardo V, Rojas G. First validation of a Spanish-translated version of the Edinburgh Postnatal Depression Scale (EPDS) for use in pregnant women: a Chilean study. *Arch Womens Ment Heal.* 2015;18:607–612. doi:10.1007/s00737-014-0466-z

28. Høivik MS, Burkeland NA, Linaker OM, Berg-Nielsen TS. The Mother and Baby Interaction Scale: a valid broadband instrument for efficient screening of postpartum interaction? A preliminary validation in a Norwegian community sample. *Scand J Caring Sci.* 2013;27(3):733–739. doi:10.1111/j.1471-6712.2012.01060.x

29. Logsdon MC, Usui WM, Nering M. Validation of Edinburgh Postnatal Depression Scale for adolescent mothers. *Arch Womens Ment Heal.* 2009;12:433–440. doi:10.1007/s00737-009-0096-z

30. Wickberg B, Hwang CP. The Edinburgh Postnatal Depression Scale: validation on a Swedish community sample. *Acta Psychiatr Scand.* 1996;94(3):181–184. doi:10.1111/j.1600-0447.1996.tb09845.x

31. Dennis C-L. Can we identify mothers at risk for postpartum depression in the immediate post-partum period using the Edinburgh Postnatal Depression Scale? *J Affect Disord.* 2004;78:163–169. doi:10.1016/S0165-0327(02)00299-9

32. Howard LM, Ryan EG, Trevillion K, et al. Accuracy of the Whooley questions and the Edinburgh Postnatal Depression Scale in identifying depression and other mental disorders in early pregnancy. *Br J Psychiatry.* 2018;212:50–56. doi:10.1192/bjp.2017.9

33. Beck CT, Gable RK. Further validation of the postpartum depression screening scale. *Nurs Res.* 2001;50(3):155–164.

34. Hanusa BH, Scholle SH, Haskett RF, Spadaro K, Wisner KL. Screening for depression in the postpartum period: a comparison of three instruments. *J Women's Heal.* 2008;17(4):585–596. doi:10.1089/jwh.2006.0248

35. O'Connor E, Rossom RC, Henninger M, et al. Primary care screening for and treatment of depression in pregnant and postpartum women. *JAMA.* 2016;315(4):388. doi:10.1001/jama.2015.18948

36. Pawlby S, Sharp D, Hay D, O'Keane V. Postnatal depression and child outcome at 11 years: the importance of accurate diagnosis. *J Affect Disord.* 2008;107(1-3):241–245. doi:10.1016/J.JAD.2007.08.002

37. Josefsson A, Sydsjö G. A follow-up study of postpartum depressed women: recurrent maternal depressive symptoms and child behavior after four years. *Arch Womens Ment Heal.* 2007;10:141–145. doi:10.1007/s00737-007-0185-9

38. Goodman JH. Influences of maternal postpartum depression on fathers and on father-infant interaction. *Infant Ment Health J.* 2008;29(6):624–643. doi:10.1002/imhj.20199

39. Beestin L, Hugh-Jones S, Gough B. The impact of maternal postnatal depression on men and their ways of fathering: an interpretative phenomenological analysis. *Psychol Health.* 2014;29(6):717–735. doi:10.1080/08870446.2014.885523

40. Brummelte S, Galea LAM. Postpartum depression: etiology, treatment and consequences for maternal care. *Horm Behav.* 2016;77:153–166. doi:10.1016/j.yhbeh.2015.08.008

41. Aktar E, Colonnesi C, De Vente W, et al. How do parents' depression and anxiety, and infants' negative temperament relate to parent-infant face-to-face interactions? *Dev Psychopathol.* 2017;29:697–710. doi:10.1017/S0954579416000390

42. Herrera E, Reissland N, Shepherd J. Maternal touch and maternal child-directed speech: effects of depressed mood in the postnatal period. *J Affect Disord.* 2004;81(1):29–39. doi:10.1016/J.JAD.2003.07.001

43. Dettmer AM, Kaburu SSK, Simpson EA, et al. Neonatal face-to-face interactions promote later social behaviour in infant rhesus monkeys. *Nat Commun.* 2016;7(1):11940. doi:10.1038/ncomms11940

44. Murray L, Sinclair D, Cooper P, et al. The socioemotional development of 5-year-old children of postnatally depressed mothers. *J Child Psychol Psychiatry Allied Discip.* 1999;40(8):1259–1271.

45. Darcy JM, Grzywacz JG, Stephens RL, et al. Maternal depressive symptomatology: 16-month follow-up of infant and maternal health-related quality of life. *J Am Board Fam Med.* 2011;24(3):249–257. doi:10.3122/JABFM.2011.03.100201

46. Minkovitz CS, Strobino D, Scharfstein D, et al. Maternal depressive symptoms and children's receipt of health care in the first 3 years of life. *Pediatrics.* 2005;115(2):306–314. doi:10.1542/peds.2004-0341

47. Gaffney KF, Kitsantas P, Brito A, Swamidoss CSS. Postpartum depression, infant feeding practices, and infant weight gain at six months of age. *J Pediatr Heal Care.* 2014;28(1):43–50. doi:10.1016/J.PEDHC.2012.10.005

48. Milgrom J, Gemmill AW, Ericksen J, et al. Treatment of postnatal depression with cognitive behavioural therapy, sertraline and combination therapy: a randomised controlled trial. *Aust New Zeal J Psychiatry.* 2015;49(3):236–245. doi:10.1177/0004867414565474

49. Gjerdingen D. The effectiveness of various postpartum depression treatments and the impact of antidepressant drugs on nursing infants. *J Am Board Fam Pract.* 2003;16:372–382. doi:10.3122/jabfm.16.5.372

50. Hantsoo L, Ward-O'Brien D, Czarkowski KA, et al. A randomized, placebo-controlled, double-blind trial of sertraline for postpartum depression. *Psychopharmacology*. 2014;231(5):939–948. doi:10.1007/s00213-013-3316-1

51. Epperson N, Czarkowski KA, Ward-O'Brien D, et al. Maternal sertraline treatment and serotonin transport in breast-feeding mother-infant pairs. *Am J Psychiatry*. 2001;158(10):1631–1637. doi:10.1176/appi.ajp.158.10.1631

52. Stowe ZN, Hostetter AL, Owens MJ, et al. The pharmacokinetics of sertraline excretion into human breast milk: determinants of infant serum concentrations. *J Clin Psychiatry*. 2003;64(1):73–80.

53. Orsolini L, Bellantuono C. Serotonin reuptake inhibitors and breastfeeding: a systematic review. *Hum Psychopharmacol*. 2015;30:4–20. doi:10.1002/hup.2451

54. Meltzer-Brody S, Colquhoun H, Riesenberg R, et al. Brexanolone injection in post-partum depression: two multicentre, double-blind, randomised, placebo-controlled, phase 3 trials. *Lancet*. 2018;392(1058-1070):1058–1070. doi:10.1016/S0140-6736(18)31551-4

55. Glavin K, Smith L, Sørum R, Ellefsen B. Supportive counselling by public health nurses for women with postpartum depression. *J Adv Nurs*. 2010;66(6):1317–1327. doi:10.1111/j.1365-2648.2010.05263.x

56. Shulman B, Dueck R, Ryan D, et al. Feasibility of a mindfulness-based cognitive therapy group intervention as an adjunctive treatment for postpartum depression and anxiety. *J Affect Disord*. 2018;235:61–67. doi:10.1016/j.jad.2017.12.065

57. Huang L, Zhao Y, Qiang C, Fan BI. Is cognitive behavioral therapy a better choice for women with postnatal depression? A systematic review and meta-analysis. *PLoS One*. 2018;13(10):e0205243. doi:10.1371/journal.pone.0205243

58. Lau Y, Htun TP, Wong SN, et al. Therapist-supported internet-based cognitive behavior therapy for stress, anxiety, and depressive symptoms among postpartum women: a systematic review and meta-analysis. *J Med Internet Res*. 2017;19(4):e138. doi:10.2196/jmir.6712

59. Klier CM, Muzik M, Rosenblum KL, Lenz G. Interpersonal psychotherapy adapted for the group setting in the treatment of postpartum depression. *J Psychother Pract Res*. 2001;10(2):124–131.

60. O'Hara MW, Stuart S, Gorman LL, Wenzel A. Efficacy of interpersonal psychotherapy for postpartum depression. *Arch Gen Psychiatry*. 2000;57(11):1039–1045. doi:10.1001/archpsyc.57.11.1039

61. Misri S, Reebye P, Corral M, Milis L. The use of paroxetine and cognitive-behavioral therapy in postpartum depression and anxiety. *J Clin Psychiatry*. 2004;65(9):1236–1241. doi:10.4088/JCP.v65n0913

62. Corrigan PW, Druss BG, Perlick DA. The impact of mental illness stigma on seeking and participating in mental health care. *Psychol Sci Public Interes*. 2014;15(2):37–70. doi:10.1177/1529100614531398

63. Bodnar-Deren S, Benn EKT, Balbierz A, et al. Stigma and postpartum depression treatment acceptability among black and white women in the first six-months postpartum. *Matern Child Health J*. 2017;21:1457–1468. doi:10.1007/s10995-017-2263-6

64. Nillni YI, Gutner CA. Treatment for perinatal depression: movement towards scalability. *Lancet Psychiatry*. 2019;6(2):83–85. doi:10.1016/S2215-0366(18)30429-2

65. Trivedi D. Cochrane review summary: psychosocial and psychological interventions for preventing postpartum depression. *Prim Health Care Res Dev*. 2017;15:231–233. doi:10.1017/S1463423614000206

66. Wisner KL, Perel JM, Peindl KS, et al. Prevention of postpartum depression: a pilot randomized clinical trial. *Am J Psychiatry*. 2004;161(7):1290–1292. doi:10.1176/appi.ajp.161.7.1290

67. Freeman MP. Perinatal depression: recommendations for prevention and the challenges of implementation. *JAMA*. 2019;321(6):550. doi:10.1001/jama.2018.21247

/// 27 /// DEPRESSION FOLLOWING MILD TRAUMATIC BRAIN INJURY

C. MUNRO CULLUM AND CATHERINE MUNRO

27.1. INTRODUCTION

Depressive symptoms following traumatic brain injury (TBI) are commonly reported and may occur as a result of a multitude of neurobiopsychosocial factors. Estimates of the rates of depression following TBI in general range widely across studies, from approximately 10% to 75% or greater,[1] likely a result of differing methods and sample characteristics. Depressive symptoms have been reported even in mild cases of TBI (mTBI), also referred to as concussions, with reported depression rates ranging from 5% to 40%.[2,3] Major depressive disorder has been reported to occur at higher rates in individuals with mTBI compared with both the general population and to those with orthopedic injuries, with prevalence around 20% when measured three to six months after injury.[4] As many of milder brain injuries often go unreported, these numbers likely reflect an underestimation of actual symptom frequencies. With regard to sports-related concussion, a recent study by Vargas and colleagues[5] found that 23% of collegiate athletes scored in the depressed range on a brief self-report measure following concussion, compared to a pre-injury base rate of depression at 11%. These authors found that depressive symptoms increased at follow-up six to seven weeks later, and, consistent with previously reported data,[6] that higher depressive symptoms at baseline were predictive of greater depressive symptoms at follow-up. Although there appears to be a link between depressive symptoms and mTBI, other data suggest that some of this apparent effect may be explained by more complex neurobiopsychosocial factors associated with injury and response to injury. For example, Mainwaring and colleagues[7] observed elevations in depressive symptoms not only following concussion, but also in their control group of individuals who had

TABLE 27.1. Common Symptom Clusters Following Concussion

Cognitive	Slowed thinking, difficulty concentrating, difficulty remembering new information
Physical	Headache, fatigue, dizziness, light or noise sensitivity, blurry vision, dizziness
Sleep	Sleeping more or less than usual and/or trouble falling asleep
Mood	Irritability, anxiety, depression, emotional lability

suffered anterior cruciate ligament injuries, though both groups showed resolution of depressive symptoms by one week after injury.

Why depressive symptoms may arise following mTBI remains poorly understood but is likely influenced by a host of complex and interrelated neurobiopsychosocial factors that vary across individuals and over the course of recovery. Depression and depression symptoms following mTBI are challenging to study due to the variations in symptom presentation, reporting, preexisting personality factors, past medical history, etiology, co-occurring symptoms (e.g., pain, anxiety), and potential genetic and situational factors, in addition to other intra-individual factors such as socioeconomic status that have also been associated with depressive ideation after mTBI.[8,9] Regardless of etiology, however, changes in mood represent one of the common symptom clusters described in the acute and subacute period following mTBI (Table 27.1). In fact, mood symptoms are such a frequent occurrence following mTBI that a panel of worldwide concussion experts brought together by the National Institute of Neurological Disorders and Stroke and the Department of Defense recommended depression symptom assessment as one of the common data elements that should be included in clinical research studies.[10]

27.2. PREVALENCE

TBI is one of the most common neurologic conditions, affecting millions of people of all ages every year. TBI ranges from mild to severe, with a majority being mild and accounting for approximately 75% of all TBIs. mTBI or concussion has various definitions, but the Concussion in Sport Group defines it simply as "a traumatic brain injury induced by biomechanical forces."[11] The youngest (<5 years) and oldest (>75 years) members of the population are at the greatest risk for TBI, with males being overrepresented at all age levels. Severity of TBI in general is typically characterized in terms of the presence and duration of loss of consciousness (LOC) and post-traumatic amnesia (PTA), with various physical, cognitive, and/or emotional symptoms also reported. The Glasgow Coma Scale (score range = 0–15) is often used to characterize initial TBI severity in emergency department settings, with scores of 13 to 15 reflecting a milder injury and lower scores indicating a more severe injury.

Other indicators that have been used over the years to characterize mTBI include PTA less than 24 hours and LOC under 30 minutes. Despite these general guidelines, however, mTBI is not accompanied by LOC in roughly 90% of cases, and the diagnosis of concussion can be challenging, as most of the common symptoms overlap with other conditions and may have other etiologies. Although the mechanism of TBI varies by age, falls account for the majority of TBIs seen in emergency departments, followed by hitting or being hit by an object, then motor vehicle accidents.[12] TBI is also considered the "signature injury" of recent overseas military conflicts, with many due to blast-related injuries. Regarding sports- and recreation-related concussions, there are an estimated 1.6 million to 3.8 million incidents per year;[13] however, this is no doubt an underestimate, as many concussions go unreported or are treated outside of emergency departments. A meta-analysis and review of the literature on youth sports-related concussions reported that the most common etiologies included rugby, hockey, and American football,[14] although reports vary along these lines depending on samples, setting, age, and gender. A recent review of mechanisms of pediatric concussion in a large hospital system found that while sports-related concussions were the most common, 30% of all injuries were not related to sports, with this percentage being higher in the youngest age group.[15] According to statistics from the Centers for Disease Control and Prevention, the overall number of TBI-related visits to emergency departments has increased steadily in recent years (particularly in young children and in the elderly), perhaps reflecting an increase in frequency of the injury in some groups, but likely also fueled by increased concussion awareness.

27.3. NEUROBIOLOGY OF MTBI

The mechanisms by which neurobehavioral symptoms manifest following mTBI are poorly understood, although several models of injury and recovery have been posited along various neurobiopsychosocial lines of evidence, with particular focus on the acute and post-acute recovery period.

27.3.1. Neuropathologic Cascade

The seminal work on mechanisms of TBI by Hovda and Giza[16] posited a physiologic model of cellular depolarization and influx/efflux of calcium to create a temporary energy-starved state at a point when cells have a maximum need for energy. This model has gained support in numerous nonhuman studies, and the physiologic recovery curves fit with both human and nonhuman animal data.

27.3.2. Axonal Stretching and Tearing

The cerebral white matter makes up the largest percentage of human brain volume, and axonal tracts are responsible for inter- and intra-hemispheric connections across brain regions and neuronal networks. During the process of an acceleration–deceleration injury, the brain endures differential forces on white and gray matter regions based on tissue density. As the physical consistency of the living brain is much like thick Jell-O, neuronal fibers are susceptible to stretching and tearing during trauma. Axons may become temporarily stretched and dysfunctional, or they may become torn, disrupting normal pathways and transmission of nerve impulses. It is currently thought that the main culprit in promoting concussion symptoms is force to the head that results in rotation of the brain and its structures, which may help explain the lack of stronger correlations between concussion symptoms and forces measured by accelerometers and helmet sensors.[17]

27.3.3. Biomarkers and Genetic Factors

Although still an active area of research lacking in definitive associations, a variety of genetic factors have been posited to play a role in short- and/or long-term TBI sequelae, including ApoE, ComT, NFL, BDNF, and S100B,[18] in addition to various indices of inflammation and cytokine dysregulation. Such factors may help explain susceptibility to dysfunction, response to injury, and recovery following mTBI and are the subject of ongoing investigations, as many questions remain in terms of attempts to link genetic factors to neurobehavioral outcomes.[18,19] Similarly, structural neuroimaging of mTBI in routine clinical computed tomography or magnetic resonance imaging scans does not usually show evidence of abnormalities, although as with other biomarkers, promising new neuroimaging techniques and methods are evolving.[18,20] Despite the various posited physiologic mechanisms of mTBI and recovery,[21] however, much less attention has been paid to the potential mechanisms and biomarkers of the emotional symptoms that may arise following mTBI.

27.4. A NEUROBIOPSYCHOSOCIAL MODEL

There is a complex interplay between the various neurobiological, psychological, and psychosocial factors involved in the development and maintenance of postconcussion symptoms; nowhere is this more true than in the case of the psychological symptoms that can arise following mTBI. In addition to the direct or primary potential effects of brain contusion, white matter stretching/shearing, and the metabolic cascade associated with TBI, secondary situational and psychological factors also play a role in symptom presentation and recovery following mTBI.[22] In addition to various mechanistic and physiologic factors, premorbid personality characteristics, response to and recovery from injury in general, resilience, somatization tendencies, expectations for recovery, understanding and attribution of symptoms, and psychosocial environment all may play a role.[23] Figure 27.1 displays some of the general factors that may play a role in symptom expression and recovery from mTBI. As depicted in the figure, various aspects of an individual's life circumstances can play a role in mood and depressive symptoms following mTBI, much like any other injury. In cases where

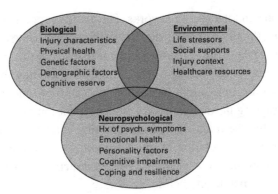

FIGURE 27.1. Biopsychosocial determinants of mTBI outcome.

symptoms arise much later or are prolonged, the role of non-mTBI factors should be given careful consideration.

One saying from healthcare professionals dealing with mTBI is that "no two concussions are alike," referring to the variability in symptoms and recovery patterns across individuals. Whereas certain symptoms are seen with greater frequency than others following mTBI, none are specific to concussion alone. Headache tends to be the most common symptom, but a number of other nonspecific symptoms and symptom clusters are seen with some frequency as well (Box 27.1).

As noted, the specific constellation of symptoms for one patient may be quite different from another, even with a similar injury. This applies similarly to emotional sequelae, including depressive symptoms. Irritability, decreased frustration tolerance, and comorbid factors such as sleep disturbance, pain (headache as well as effects of other physical injuries, if present), light or noise sensitivity, as well as

---

BOX 27.1.
COMMON CONCUSSION SYMPTOMS

- Headache
- Fatigue
- Mental "fogginess"
- Problems with attention and/or working memory
- Irritability
- Depressive symptoms
- Anxiety
- Sleep disturbance
- Tinnitus
- Visual disturbance
- Noise/light sensitivity
- Vestibular/balance disturbance

the disruption in normal daily activities during recovery may all combine to alter an individual's routine and result in an increased awareness of or focus on symptoms. This symptom focus can also result in the misattribution of some "normal" symptoms to the concussion, which can in turn be distressing, thereby resulting in greater stress and emotional symptoms. In a subset of individuals following mTBI, a constellation of symptoms may persist well beyond the typical recovery time course; this has been referred to as "postconcussion syndrome." This condition has been variably defined and remains poorly understood but does appear in the ICD-10. Postconcussion syndrome typically includes a constellation of physical, cognitive, and emotional symptoms that become chronic. Debate continues regarding the biopsychosocial nature of this condition, as some of the symptoms may be related to or perpetuated by non-mTBI factors. Because of its vague and nonspecific nature, the term is of limited utility.

27.5. RECOVERY FROM MTBI

Full recovery from mTBI is the norm, with literature reviews and meta-analyses reflecting prompt and complete resolution of mTBI symptoms in the vast majority of cases. In adults, resolution of acute symptoms within several days or weeks is typical, although a minority of individuals continue to report symptoms weeks or even months later. Estimates of the frequency of this "miserable minority" range from 3% to 20%, with 10% being an oft-cited figure. Factors that may complicate or delay recovery include preexisting psychological factors, the development of depression during the recovery period, concomitant physical injuries requiring treatment, sleep disturbance, and pain. A systematic review of the literature by Iverson and colleagues provides a summary of many variables that have been studied to help predict clinical recovery from mTBI,[24] although this a methodologically challenging endeavor given the complexities of the injury, its identification, assessment, and various comorbid and preexisting factors that can contribute to outcome.[25,26] The extent to which an individual's life routine is upset by the injury also plays a role in the emotional symptoms that can be seen following mTBI (e.g., irritability, anxiety, depression). In general, younger children take longer to recover from mTBI than adolescents (i.e., several weeks), and adolescents take longer to recover than adults, although the elderly also typically have a longer recovery course.

27.6. RISK FACTORS FOR DEPRESSION AFTER MTBI

As we have indicated, the development or recognition of depressive symptoms following mTBI is not rare, although the mechanism(s) and related risk factors are poorly understood. One important distinction to make is that experiencing depressive *symptoms* does not necessarily equate to a formal diagnosis of syndromal *depression*. Self-report checklists are commonly used in screening for depression, with various cutoff scores reflecting an increased *likelihood* of the clinical syndrome of depression. Thus, one can endorse a variety of specific symptoms associated with depressive ideation or symptomatology, but these symptoms may not rise to the level of a clinical diagnosis. When reading the literature related to mTBI, it is important to keep this idea in mind, as some studies make comments or implications about "depression" that may go beyond the data. Since many studies of mTBI do not use standard clinical diagnostic procedures or criteria, this makes a clear interpretation of some findings challenging. A diagnosis of major depression requires that patients meet specific clinical criteria (as per the fifth edition of the American Psychiatric Association's *Diagnostic and Statistical Manual of Mental Disorders*), and brief depression questionnaires alone are inadequate to establish a formal diagnosis. Furthermore, some symptoms of depression overlap significantly with other conditions (e.g., pain, physical disorders, and their related treatments) and thus may be nonspecific; they may not reflect true "depression" per se, but rather may represent isolated physical, cognitive, or emotional aspects and symptoms of the condition. Among athletes, prolonged removal from sport and team activities may contribute to symptoms of depression and anxiety following sport-related concussion as well as other injuries. Thus, depressive symptoms may arise after concussion due to a number of factors and should be assessed and treated as indicated. For recent reviews of psychosocial factors in concussion recovery, see references 27 and 28.

A number of studies have attempted to identify potential indicators of risk of depressive symptoms or depression following mTBI, with mixed results.[2] A review of studies suggests that a variety of potential factors may predispose to or be associated with the development of mood disturbance following mTBI,[29,30] although such predictors are based on group data and may not apply to any individual cases due to the complexity of mTBI mechanisms and individual genotypic, phenotypic, and environmental factors. Regardless, when depression does occur following mTBI, it tends to arise within the first 12 months after injury, although some have suggested that the risk for developing depression may persist.[31] However, few prospective outcome studies specifically focusing on mTBI have been published, and many are lacking in other injury control groups, which may limit conclusions. In a recent review of depressive symptoms and clinical depression in pediatric TBI, Durish, Pereverseff, and Yeates[22] concluded that from the 14 available studies reviewed, depressive symptoms were more common following TBI than in orthopedically injured groups, which they hypothesized might be due to secondary outcomes from brain injury rather than an initial direct effect. A review of mTBI outcomes in military personnel indicated that mTBI was associated with more frequent neuropsychiatric symptoms, including mood, anxiety, and post-traumatic stress.[32] Similarly, retired National Football League players with a history of concussion have been reported to endorse more depressive symptoms than controls,[33] although this remains a complex area of research, as other situational and lifestyle factors may also play a role. Box 27.2 lists some of the more commonly reported risk factors of post-TBI depression, although it is important to keep in mind that depression can arise due to many factors unrelated to TBI per se.

> ### BOX 27.2.
> ## FACTORS ASSOCIATED WITH DEPRESSION FOLLOWING TBI
>
> - Preexisting psychiatric symptoms/disorder
> - More serious injury (as indicated by presence and duration of LOC and PTA)
> - Greater symptoms immediately after injury (especially mood, anxiety, fatigue, sleep disturbance)
> - Female gender
> - Somatization tendencies
> - History of psychosocial problems, family discord, environmental stress
> - Involvement in litigation

27.7. TREATMENT IMPLICATIONS

The primary treatment for mTBI overall is information/education about the injury, expectations for recovery, and initial rest. Early education about mTBI, its common symptoms, and the typical course of recovery is important for patients and their families and may facilitate recovery.[34] Some degree of decreased activity or rest is also useful, although this must be done in moderation and for a limited time. Recent research has demonstrated that being overly restrictive (i.e., "cocooning") or promoting prolonged rest may result in iatrogenic symptoms, including depression and anxiety, which may then be mistakenly ascribed to lingering postconcussion symptoms. A day or two of *relative* physical and cognitive rest is typically advised, followed by a graded return to normal activities over the next several days. As with modern rehabilitation from physical injuries, patients should return to normal activity levels as soon as feasible following mTBI, while monitoring and minimizing symptom exacerbation during the process. Asken and colleagues[35] showed that prompt removal from play was associated with fewer symptoms and more rapid recovery in collegiate athletes following concussion, supporting the notion that some initial rest is beneficial. Working with team neuropsychologists, the National Hockey League and National Football League developed stepwise, graded return-to-play activities that have served as a model for many similar programs in sports. In a graded return-to-play/school/work schema, normal activities are progressively added, and if symptoms worsen or emerge with each step, the physical or cognitive workload/intensity can be decreased accordingly, allowing for a little more time for rest if needed. In addition to treatment for vestibular abnormalities that may be present, other symptoms such as sleep disturbance and headache may require specific interventions; indeed, treatment of symptoms following concussion is key. Recently published data from a rigorous randomized clinical trial suggest that early (i.e., within the first week), graded aerobic exercise may help treat or prevent a variety of persistent postconcussion symptoms,[36] although more clinical trials on concussion recovery interventions are needed.

With respect to mood symptoms in particular, the detailed review of rest following sports concussion by Schneider and colleagues[37] highlights the importance of reasonable return to normal activity, and avoiding over-resting, which may prolong, exacerbate, or result in symptoms. Given the prevalence of mood symptoms following TBI, this merits monitoring, although this can be a complex scenario, particularly in the context of additional physical injuries, disturbed sleep, pain, and disruption of normal social and school/work activities. Removing people from their usual routine and focusing on symptoms after TBI may heighten everyone's attention to even "normal" variations in mood and other symptoms, thereby potentially resulting in symptom misattribution and promoting an over-focus on symptoms and thereby leading to greater or prolonged emotional distress by the patient and/or family.

Along these lines, it is also important to keep in mind an individual's normal base rate of symptoms. For example, a history of migraines is common in individuals who experience lingering post-traumatic headaches, although the frequency and intensity of headaches experienced prior to TBI are important to keep in mind. Not all physical, cognitive, or mood symptoms reported following a TBI are necessarily related to the TBI, and awareness of this fact may facilitate recovery, as the psychological expectation that should be set for all patients following mTBI is recovery. With respect to specific treatments for postconcussion depression, multiple factors must be considered, as depressive symptoms may be related to other factors, including sleep disturbance, pain (e.g., headache), vestibular disturbance, cognitive problems, and/or lifestyle changes. That said, if depressive symptoms rise to the level of a clinical diagnosis of depression, evaluation and treatment should be pursued and targeted to the primary symptoms. Pharmacotherapy, while not specific for post-TBI depression, may be indicated and has been shown to have beneficial results in many cases. Because individuals with TBI may have an elevated sensitivity to psychotropic medications, extra care must be exercised when antidepressant medications are used following mTBI, and selective serotonin reuptake inhibitors (SSRIs) are generally preferred due to their lack of anticholinergic side effects.[31] Psychoeducation, supportive psychotherapy, and cognitive–behavioral therapy can be effective as part of the treatment for post-TBI depression to help patients understand the nature of the injury and the expected course of symptoms, develop coping strategies, and proceed through the recovery process.

27.8. CHRONIC TRAUMATIC ENCEPHALOPATHY AND NEURODEGENERATIVE CONDITIONS LATER IN LIFE

Although not a condition known to arise acutely following mTBI, a brief discussion of chronic traumatic encephalopathy (CTE) and potential later-in-life risks of TBI is in order. The syndrome of traumatic encephalopathy was originally referred to in the early 1900s as "punch drunk syndrome" in boxers and is thought by many to result from repetitive TBIs.[38] CTE is pathologically characterized by the accumulation of the tau protein in characteristic patterns around small blood vessels deep in the cerebral sulci. At this point, the epidemiology of CTE is unknown. It can only be determined neuropathologically, and preliminary criteria for staging the disease have been proposed, based largely on tau appearance and levels in brain.[38] Because tau is seen in other conditions, including normal aging, even postmortem diagnosis can be challenging, particularly when tau is present in small amounts.[39] Additionally, other pathologies commonly coexist with CTE pathology, including characteristic changes associated with Alzheimer's disease, found in more than 50% of CTE cases in some reports. From a clinical perspective, individuals with a postmortem diagnosis of CTE have been retrospectively described as having a number of neurobehavioral changes during life, including cognitive decline, personality change/impulsivity, and depression. Published case descriptions have been largely based on interviews with family members of deceased individuals, and no prospective cohort studies have been completed. Such symptoms obviously overlap with other conditions, including Alzheimer's disease, other neurodegenerative disorders (e.g., frontotemporal dementia), epilepsy, opioid use, and depression. Furthermore, the role of TBI remains unclear in the development of CTE, although repetitive injuries appear to be more common in many but not all cases. To date, the relationship between neuropsychiatric symptoms and the presence of tau in the brain has not been established. Midlife depression and suicidality have been retrospectively reported in some individuals with CTE, although many factors other than a history of mTBI may play a role in the development of depression and/or cognitive decline later in life, particularly when mTBI(s) occurred years or decades earlier. In the case of high-profile retired athletes with CTE, for example, issues surrounding retirement from sport, life circumstances, and behavioral history and other risk factors may all play a role in the evolution of depressive symptoms, whether or not in the context of a history of mTBI.

With respect to other neurodegenerative disorders that arise later in life (e.g., mild cognitive impairment, Alzheimer's disease, frontotemporal dementia), TBI (particularly more serious injuries) and depression have been reported as possible risk factors that may also be associated with an earlier onset of symptoms. However, such studies have been based on analyses of group data and are largely correlational. As such, underlying mechanisms and associated contributing factors remain unclear.[40,41]

27.9. SUMMARY AND FUTURE DIRECTIONS

Concussion or mTBI is a common phenomenon and occurs in relation to a wide range of everyday activities. No two concussions are alike, but certain neurobehavioral sequelae tend to be seen more frequently than others. The development of depressive symptoms or full-blown depression following mTBI is far from rare, and it is crucial to screen for mood disturbance and monitor individuals during the recovery process. Along these lines, identification of risk factors that may be related to the development of postconcussion depression is important, although the emergence of depressive symptoms represents a highly complex neurobiopsychosocial process that merits more multidisciplinary research. In terms of treatment for post-mTBI depression, randomized controlled trials are needed, as is careful consideration and documentation of the nature and length of rest and other adjuvant behavioral and pharmacologic treatments. Also needed are long-term longitudinal studies in order to shed more light on the apparent association between TBI and the later-in-life development of neurodegenerative conditions. Last, it is recommended that more studies of neuropsychiatric disorders, including depression, incorporate information regarding TBI histories as part of routine clinical and research practice so that we may learn more about the potential influence of TBI on the development and course of neuropsychiatric symptoms across the lifespan.

REFERENCES

1. Alderfer BS, Arciniegas DB, Silver JM. Treatment of depression following traumatic brain injury. *J Head Trauma Rehabil.* 2005;20(6):544–562.
2. Busch CR, Alpern HP. Depression after mild traumatic brain injury: a review of current research. *Neuropsychol Rev.* 1998;8(2):95–108.
3. Jorge R, Robinson RG. Mood disorders following traumatic brain injury. *Neurorehabilitation.* 2002;17:311–324.
4. Ponsford J, Always Y, Gould RR. Epidemiology and natural history of psychiatric disorders after TBI. *J Neuropsychiatry Clin Neurosci.* 2018;30(4):262–270. doi:10.1176/appi.neuropsych.18040093.
5. Vargas GA, Rabinowitz AR, Meyer JE, Arnett PA. Predictors and prevalence of postconcussion depression symptoms in collegiate athletes. *J Athl Train.* 2015;50(3):250–255. doi:10.4085/1062-6050-50.3.02.
6. Meier TB, Bellgowan PSF, Singh R, et al. Recovery of cerebral blood flow following sports-related concussion. *JAMA Neurol.* 2015;72(5):530–538. doi:10.1001/jamaneurol.2014.4778.
7. Mainwaring LM, Hutchison M, Bisschop SM, et al. Emotional response to sport concussion compared to ACL injury. *Brain Inj.* 2010;24(4):589–597. doi:10.3109/02699051003610508.
8. Kirkwood M, Janusz J, Yeates KO, et al. Prevalence and correlates of depressive symptoms following traumatic brain injuries in children. *Child Neuropsychol.* 2000;6(3):195–208.
9. Arnett PA, Guty E, Bradson M. Assessment of depression and anxiety in sports concussion evaluations. In: Arnett PA, ed. *Neuropsychology of sports-related concussion.* Washington, DC: American Psychological Association; 2019:71–94.
10. Broglio SP, Kontos AP, Levin H, et al. The National Institute of Neurological Disorders and Stroke and Department of Defense Sport-Related Concussion Common Data Elements version 1.0 recommendations. *J Neurotrauma.* 2018;35(23):2776–2783. doi:10.1089/neu.2018.5643.
11. McCrory P, Meeuwisse W, Dvorak J, et al. Consensus statement on concussion in sport: the 5th International Conference on Concussion in Sport held in Berlin, October 2016. *Br J Sports Med.* 2017;51(11):838–847. doi:10.1136/bjsports-2017-097699.
12. Centers for Disease Control and Prevention. *Report to Congress on Traumatic Brain Injury in the United States: Epidemiology and Rehabilitation. National Center for Injury Prevention and Control; Division of Unintentional Injury Prevention.* Atlanta, GA: Centers for Disease Control and Prevention; 2015.

13. Langlois JA, Rutland-Brown W, Wald MM. The epidemiology and impact of traumatic brain injury: a brief overview. *J Head Trauma Rehabil.* 2006;21(5):375–378.

14. Pfister T, Pfister K, Hagel B, et al. The incidence of concussion in youth sports: a systematic review and meta-analysis. *Br J Sports Med.* 2016;50(5):292–297. doi:10.1136/bjsports-2015-094978.

15. Haarbauer-Krupa J, Arbogast KB, Metzger KB, et al. Variations in mechanisms of injury for children with concussion. *J Pediatr.* 2018;197:241–248. doi:10.1016/jpeds.2018.01.075.

16. Barkhoudarian G, Hovda DA, Giza CC. The molecular pathophysiology of concussive brain injury—an update. *Phys Med Rehabil Clin North Am.* 2016;27(2):373–393. doi:10.1016/j.pmr.2016.01.003.

17. Rowson S, Duma SM, Stemper BD, et al. Correlation of concussion symptom profile with head impact biometrics: a case for individual-specific injury tolerance. *J Neurotrauma.* 2018;35(4):681–690. doi:10.1089/neu.2017.5169.

18. McCrea M, Meier T, Huber D, et al. Role of advanced neuroimaging, fluid biomarkers, and genetic testing in the assessment of sport-related concussion: a systematic review. *Br J Sports Med.* 2017;51(12):919–929. doi:10.1136/bjsports-2016-097447.

19. Zeiler FA, McFadyen C, Newcombe, et al. Genetic influences on patient oriented outcomes in TBI: a living systematic review of non-apolipoprotein e single nucleotide polymorphisms. *J Neurotrauma.* 2018;35:1–17. doi:10.1089/neu.2017.5583.

20. Bigler ED, Abildskov TJ, Goodrich-Hunsaker NJ, et al. Structural neuroimaging findings in mild traumatic brain injury. *Sports Med Arthrosc Rev.* 2016;24(3):e42–52. doi:10.1097/JSA.0000000000000119.

21. Kamins J, Bigler E, Covassin T, et al. What is the physiological time to recovery after concussion? A systematic review. *Br J Sports Med.* 2017;51(12):935–940. doi: 10.1136/bjsports-2016-097464.

22. Durish CL, Pereverseff RS, Yeates KO. Depression and depressive symptoms in pediatric traumatic brain injury: a scoping review. *J Head Trauma Rehabil.* 2018;33(3):E18-E30. doi:10.109/HTR.000000000000343.

23. Kenzie ES, Parks EL, Bigler ED, et al. The dynamics of concussion: mapping pathophysiology, persistence, and recovery with causal-loop diagramming. *Front Neurol.* 2018;9:203. doi:10.3389/fneur.2018.00203.

24. Iverson GL, Gardner AJ, Terry DP, et al. Predictors of clinical recovery from concussion: a systematic review. *Br J Sports Med.* 2017;51(12):941–948. doi:10.1136/bjsports-2017-097729.

25. Covassin T, Elbin RJ, Beidler E, et al. A review of psychological issues that may be associated with a sport-related concussion in youth and collegiate athletes. *Sport Exerc Perform Psychol.* 2017;6(3):220–229. doi:10.1037/spy0000105.

26. Emery CA, Barlow KM, Brooks BL, et al. A systematic review of psychiatric, psychological, and behavioural outcomes following mild traumatic brain injury in children and adolescents. *Can J Psychiatry.* 2016;61(5):259–269. doi:10.1177/0706743716643741.

27. Wilmoth K, Tan A, Hague C, et al. Current state of the literature on psychological and social sequelae of sports-related concussion in school-age children and adolescents. *J Exp Neurosci.* 2019;13:1–9. doi:10.1177/1179069519830421.

28. Brooks BL, Plourde V, Beauchamp MH, et al. Predicting psychological distress after pediatric concussion. *J Neurotrauma.* 2019;36(5):679–685. doi:10.1089/neu.2018.5792.

29. Yrondi A, Brauge D, LeMen J, et al. Depression and sports-related concussion: a systematic review. *Presse Med.* 2017;46(10):890–902. doi:10.1016/j.lpm.2017.08.013.

30. Van der Naalt J, Timmerman ME, de Koning ME, et al. Early predictors of outcome after mild traumatic brain injury (UPFRONT): an observational cohort study. *Lancet Neurol.* 2017;16(7):532–540. doi:10.1016/S1474-4422(17)30117-5.

31. Silver JM, McAllister TW, Arciniegas DB. Depression and cognitive complaints following mild traumatic brain injury. *Am J Psychiatry.* 2009;166(6):653–661. doi:10.1176/appi. ajp.2009.08111676.

32. Scofield DE, Proctor SP, Kardouni JR, et al. Risk factors for mild traumatic brain injury and subsequent post-traumatic stress disorder and mental health disorders among United States Army soldiers. *J Neurotrauma.* 2017;34(23):3249–3255. doi:10.1089/neu.2017.5101.

33. Didehbani N, Cullum CM, Mansinghani S, et al. Depressive symptoms and concussions in aging retired NFL players. *Arch Clin Neuropsychol.* 2013;28(5):418–424. doi:10.1093/arclin/ act028.

34. Kirkwood MW, Peterson RL, Connery AK, et al. A pilot study investigating neuropsychological consultation as an intervention for persistent postconcussive symptoms in a pediatric sample. *J Pediatr.* 2016;169:244–249. doi:10/1016/j.peds.2015.10.014.

35. Asken BM, Bauer RM, Guskiewicz KM, et al. Immediate removal from activity after sport-related concussion is associated with shorter clinical recovery and less severe symptoms in collegiate student-athletes. *Am J Sports Med.* 2018;46(6):1465–1474. doi:10.1177/ 0363546518757984.

36. Leddy JJ, Haider MN, Ellis MJ, et al. Early subthreshold aerobic exercise for sport-related concussion. *JAMA Pediatr.* 2019;173(4):319–325. doi:10.1001/jamapediatrics.2018.4397.

37. Schneider KJ, Iverson GL, Emery CA, et al. The effects of rest and treatment following sport-related concussion: a systematic review of the literature. *Br J Sports Med.* 2013;47(5):304–307. doi:10.1136/bjsports-2013-092190.

38. Iverson GL, Gardner AJ, McCrory P, et al. A critical review of chronic traumatic encephalopathy. *Neurosci Biobehav Rev.* 2015;56:276–293. doi:10.1016/j.neubiorev.2015.05.008.

39. McKee AC, Cairns NJ, Dickson DW, et al. The first NINDS/NIBIB consensus meeting to define neuropathological criteria for the diagnosis of chronic traumatic encephalopathy. *Acta Neuropathol.* 2016;131(1):75–86. doi:10.1007/s00401-015-1515-z.

40. LoBue C, Cullum CM, Didehbani N, et al. Neurodegenerative dementias after traumatic brain injury. *J Neuropsychiatry Clin Neurosci.* 2018;30(1):7–13. doi:10.1176/appi. neuropsych.17070145.

41. Solomon G. Chronic traumatic encephalopathy in sports: a historical and narrative review. *Dev Neuropsychol.* 2018;43(4):279–311. doi:10.1080/87565641.2018.1447575.

PRIMER ON DEPRESSION

Treatment in a Primary Care Setting

ROBERT S. KINNEY AND RADU POP

28.1. VIGNETTES

28.1.1. Scenario 1

Frank is a 34-year-old Caucasian, married father of two, presenting for his annual wellness exam to his primary care physician (Dr. Smith). Frank did not report any concerns during his visit and mentioned scheduling the appointment mainly due to health incentives offered by his workplace. His physical examination was unremarkable, and thus Dr. Smith provided no treatment recommendations prior to Frank leaving the clinic. However, the following week, Dr. Smith saw on the news that Frank had shot and killed himself. Unbeknownst to Dr. Smith was Frank's struggle with untreated depression for the last few years. What, if anything, could Dr. Smith have done differently? What, if any, are Dr. Smith's responsibilities in this case?

28.1.2. Scenario 2

Frank is a 34-year-old Caucasian, married father of two, presenting for his annual wellness exam to his primary care physician. When scheduling his visit, Frank mentioned setting the appointment mainly due to health incentives offered by his workplace. On checking into the clinic, Frank was provided with the initial paperwork and several health questionnaires, which included a depression and suicidality screener. Although Frank denied initial concerns about his mental health, his item responses on the self-report questionnaires suggested clinically significant depressive symptoms and moderate suicidality. Dr. Smith conducted a clinical interview and used Frank's self-report questionnaire to arrive at a depressive diagnosis. This also prompted Dr. Smith to inquire about Frank's safety and to formulate a collaborative safety and treatment plan. Furthermore, Dr. Smith recommended pharmacological treatment and referred Frank to counseling. Dr. Smith further scheduled a follow-up visit with Frank a few weeks later. On his return to the clinic, Frank was given the same questionnaires to assess for depressive symptoms and to evaluate his progress. Frank's responses reflected an improvement in functioning and indicated reduced severity in depressive symptoms, including an absence of suicidality. How does this compare to the previous scenario?

28.2. INTRODUCTION

Optimal approaches for depression screening, diagnosis, and treatment remain debated in the practice of modern medicine. Indeed, many mental health professionals offer differing opinions on the treatment and course of depression, as well as other mental health disorders. A high number of medical providers continue to struggle with the consistent identification and treatment of depression, citing training gaps and time constraints as some of the most significant barriers.[1,2] Despite these and other hurdles to addressing the treatment of depression, antidepressants rank among the most prescribed medications in the United States, with primary care providers dispensing the vast majority of antidepressant prescriptions.[3] However, until recently, psychiatric training was not part of graduate medical education. Even when mental health was included in training curriculum, for many non-psychiatric providers, the treatment of mood disorders has been done by trial and error and has yielded very low remission rates.[4]

This chapter aligns with the recommendations of major accrediting bodies such as the US Preventive Services Task Force (USPSTF) and the American Academy of Pediatrics (AAP), asserting that primary care providers are appropriately poised for screening, diagnosing, and treating most cases of depression. As such, the chapter outlines a theoretical underpinning for the disorder, followed by a description of the major diagnostic categories and most frequently used approaches for identification and treatment. Finally, we describe the most common models of primary care practices that effectively treat depression and result in outcomes that far exceed treatment as usual.

28.3. HISTORY

28.3.1. The Biopsychosocial Model and History of Treatment

Current understandings suggest that biological, psychological, and social factors jointly contribute to the development and maintenance of the disorder. As such, treatments targeting all three of these factors have been the most effective.

28.3.1.1. Biological Factors

While the neurobiological underpinnings of depression are not clearly understood, there is a clear link between genetic predispositions, pre- and perinatal assaults on brain development, and maternal substance abuse/use in utero. In the early 2000s, there was significant focus on the role of cortisol and inflammatory cytokines within the depression literature. Recent evidence has suggested a strong connection between C-reactive protein and a specific subtype of depression.[5,6] In recent years, several commercial genetic tests have also been made available to primary care. These tests have limited empirical support and are marketed at "matching" patients to medications that their body can more easily metabolize.[7] While some studies support the use of genetic panels to better guide psychotropic medication choices for individual patients, the evidence of this pharmacogenomic approach remains inconsistent. Currently, several different classes of medications are prescribed for the treatment of depression, with selective serotonin reuptake inhibitors (SSRIs) often serving as the first line of treatment.[8]

28.3.1.2. Psychological Factors

Emotional wellness directly impacts overall well-being. The integration of psychological components within our conceptualization of patients allows for a better understanding of their functioning and impairment. The burden of stress is an important consideration in development and treatment of depression. It is worth noting that the response to stress greatly varies across patients. It is important to account for patients' coping level and to provide clear avenues to access psychotherapy as a treatment option. Sometimes referred to as counseling, psychotherapy can help patients identify problematic patterns, bolster coping skills, and increase insight into presenting problems. Psychotherapy is an evidence-based depression treatment method with outcomes equal to pharmacotherapy.[9] Psychotherapy gains over time are often more gradual in comparison to medication, yet its impact may be more enduring.[10]

28.3.1.3. Social Factors

Support and structure, living situation, and barriers to care are important factors to evaluate within the primary care setting when addressing depression and initiating treatment. Although it is not always the case, depressed patients may have fewer supports in place than those without. Often patients with depression find themselves isolated and misunderstood by others. Withdrawal and detachment from family and loved ones is a significant symptom of the disease. Patients' social structure, support group, and beliefs are necessary to consider when making treatment recommendations. Group psychotherapy or shared medical education appointments may be a potent treatment in connecting patients with depression to resources and increasing socialization. Conversely, when patients are in depression care, it is important to engage cohabitating family members, social supports, and stakeholders whom patients identify as important. These individuals can help increase adherence and can become valuable adjuncts to treatment. Failing to consider family and friends and even one's faith-based beliefs in the treatment of depression often compounds isolation rather than reducing it.

28.3.2. History of Depression Treatment in the US Medical System and in Primary Care

In the mid-19th century, mental illness became of interest to scientist inquiry and treatment providers. Depression was first identified as a distinct disorder in 1895 by Emil Kraepelin, a contemporary of Sigmund Freud. Initially approached as a purely psychological and social issue, depression was almost entirely treated through psychotherapy and lifestyle change (exercise, sunshine, diet, etc.), with some severe cases treated with a primitive form of electroconvulsive treatment. For the most part, depression was not seen as a disorder that impacted the vast majority of primary care patients.[11] Later, during the 1950s, an early precursor to modern antidepressants, imipramine, a tricyclic antidepressant, was discovered. These medications were initially reserved for severe cases, which were typically seen in hospitalized patient populations of the era.[11] In any event, the accidental discovery of the first antidepressants marked the beginning of a shift to the biological treatment of depression. The 1950s and 1960s also proved to be a time of expansive growth in the theory and practice of psychotherapy and psychopharmacology. By the close of the 1970s psychodynamic psychology shared the field with four other major approaches to the science, and within a few years dozens of other tricyclic antidepressants were marketed for use in the American medical system.[11] In 1963 deinstitutionalization was ushered in by the Community Mental Health Act, designed to give states additional funds to research and treat mental health at a local level. Although the planned agencies were either never built or never funded, most state psychiatric hospitals were closed.

Since that time, there has been a gradual decrease in access to care for patients with mental health disorders. Today, research suggests that within a given year, approximately 37% of adults and 60% of adolescents are untreated for their depressive symptoms.[12] There are significant barriers to care, including shortage of specialty care providers, poor care linkage, a lack of understanding of the physical manifestations of depressive symptoms, low awareness for available treatments, financial limitations, and ongoing stigma.[1,2] Moreover, even with the passage of the Affordable Care Act, many specialty care providers refuse to accept insurance, opting for fee-for-service practices. Primary care remains the de facto choice for many who seek treatment for mood disorders. The evidence also suggests that increasing numbers of primary care providers are prescribing psychotropic medications. For these reasons, primary care has become the primary point of care for many patients and the optimal setting to screen for and begin to address depression.

28.4. CURRENT SYSTEM

28.4.1. Existing Recommendations and Models of Care

The USPSTF and AAP recommend depression screening for ages 12 and up to identify, treat, and provide follow-up for individuals meeting criteria for a depressive disorder.[13–16] Clinical guidelines for these recommendations include the development of a system and set of strategies to address positive screen results. Management of patients with positive screening results includes addressing patient-related risk factors that may include harm to self, harm to others, and risk-taking behavior that may be reported during the screening or subsequent clinical interview. Although a vast body of research has developed on the importance of early identification and treatment of depression, implementation of the recommendation guidelines has yet to become standard practice. Numerous barriers, such as inadequate training and insufficient time, are cited by providers as primary concerns that prevent recommendations from being implemented.[17,18] Even when providers screen for depression and develop a collaborative treatment plan that includes either psychiatry or psychology, the data suggest that the vast majority of patients never make it into care. Practices with a higher rate of success and higher care linkage rates are those that address mental health issues directly or via in-house referrals to a consultant or specialty provider.

A collaborative care model is when specialty providers are integrated within primary care clinics, where they often function as consultants. A patient-centered medical home, which focuses on addressing chronic diseases and on using a multidisciplinary team approach, is another offshoot of integrated care. Other models range from the provision of outside mental health referrals to the direct treatment by primary care providers. While the use of comprehensive and collaborative care has certain advantages and has shown to be effective by improving treatment and patient outcomes[19,20] (see Section 28.4.2 for details), it remains limited by barriers such as implementation costs, care access, and provider availability (Table 28.1 offers more information on barriers). In addition, integrated specialty providers and collaborators will eventually reach a patient limit, rendering many without immediate service availability. The literature has shown that with adequate training, support, and use of measurement-based care (MBC), primary care can be as effective in treating depression as specialty care. Given these results and the above recommendations, the identification, diagnosis, and treatment of depression by primary care providers is a viable and effective solution.

In settings where screening at the primary care level becomes standard of care, the process may comprise the following steps:

1. Patients will complete various self-report questionnaires related to depression, anxiety, and/or other mental health concerns.
2. Providers will conduct a clinical interview and use this information to reach a diagnosis, formulate a treatment plan, and ensure that patients have follow-up.

TABLE 28.1. Barriers to Screening and Treatment of Depression

For Patients:	For Providers:
Discomfort in discussing depression with medical providers	Discomfort in discussing depression with patients
Confidentiality concerns	Lack of training/education in identifying and treating depression
Lack of availability of specialty providers	Lack of available specialty providers for referrals
Stigma	Stigma
Other psychosocial difficulties (e.g., financial constraints/lack of insurance coverage, childcare issues, time off work for treatment)	Time constraints during visits
	Reimbursement difficulties
	Implementation costs for a systemic approach to addressing depression

Data from references 2, 21–23.

    If patient safety issues develop, these would be addressed right away by potentially completing a safety plan, consulting with or referring to a mental health professional, or facilitating triage of patients to the most appropriate level of care based on their current needs.

3. Providers may offer referrals for psychotherapy and/or decide to begin first-line pharmacological treatment (typically SSRIs).
4. Patients who are started on a treatment plan would return for re-evaluation four to six weeks after their initial visit, as per MBC guidelines. Ongoing follow-up while in treatment will continue until sustained remission is achieved, which is typically defined as 10 or more consecutive weeks without symptoms.
5. On reaching remission, patients would be screened at their annual health exams.

    Addressing mental health issues within primary care will likely reduce overall morbidity-associated costs and the number of emergent patient visits. Other associated benefits include increased treatment adherence and improved patient outcomes, as patients would be more functional and productive. This may also break down barriers associated with stigma around mental health, leading to increased comfort in discussing emotional health and well-being.

    The resulting impact on psychiatry is that a large majority of patients with mild or moderate depression may be treated in primary care or in collaboration with available behavioral health personnel. This could subsequently mean that the landscape of specialty care might be geared more to serving severely ill or treatment-resistant patients. In addition, the consulting psychiatry role would be of increased importance to primary care providers, as the reliance on such expertise may likely increase.

28.4.2. Options for Integrating Mental Health Treatment in Primary Care

Table 28.2 reviews three models and lists the benefits and costs of each:

1. *Specialty care outside referral*—In this model, a patient who is identified as having a mental health need is referred to a specialty provider outside of primary care.

2. *Primary care provides mental health service*—Ideally, this model would task providers with screening and treating mental health concerns at the initial point of contact. This model is supported by the USPSTF and AAP[14,16] and stems from recommendations for universal depression screening, treatment, and provision of adequate follow-up care.

3. *Co-location/integrated care*—In this model, primary care providers have direct access to behavioral health providers, and services are often available onsite. This is a multidisciplinary treatment approach that can be applied to various presenting mental health problems. A patient-centered medical home is a specialized integrated care model in which individualized care plans are developed and emerging needs are addressed by the medical team on an ongoing basis.

Several models have been developed to address the implementation of universal screening and treatment of depression in youth within primary care, yet no single solution has been found, and few studies have assessed the feasibility and efficacy of existing models.[14,24] While all three of these models are used in current practice, there is wide variability in adoption and implementation.

The integrated care model may provide various benefits given the availability of behavioral health personnel; however, the use of such a model is likely prohibitive for many primary care and pediatric practices due to significant costs of development and implementation.[14] The initial development of the integrated care framework and emergence of the collaborative care terminology suggested that major depressive disorder can be adequately addressed in primary care setting with available support such as specialty psychiatry consultation.[19] The subsequent initiative of the Texas Medication Algorithm Project yielded evidence that using standardized guidelines and self-rating instruments can result in improved outcomes for depression.[25,26] This paved the way for models such as the Improving Mood-Promoting Access to Collaborative Treatment (IMPACT) model, which consists of depression identification by primary care providers and subsequent treatment by mental health professionals.[27] As a follow-up to IMPACT, the Depression Improvement Across Minnesota-Offering a New Direction (DIAMOND) was created, which included training opportunities and a systemic structure of "evidence-based collaborative care management for depression" to participating clinics and staff.[20] While the IMPACT, DIAMOND, and similar models are more effective than standard care, the major limitation resides in the limited treatment or lack of treatment by

TABLE 28.2. Existing Models for Addressing Mental Health Care Gaps

Model	Description	Benefits	Costs
Specialty care outside referral	• Patients are referred to outside resources; sometimes this model relies on patient self-report, while other times there is a systematic screening procedure.	• Low cost to provider, in terms of effort and finances • Provides greatest patient autonomy	• Poor treatment uptake • Burden for understanding health care system is on patient • Sometimes referrals are not provided • Poor access to providers • Insurance might not cover referrals • Some providers are reticent to treat
Primary care provider initiates mental health treatment	• Providers screen and initiate treatment at the initial point of care.	• Treatment initiated immediately • Supported by USPSTF and AAP	• Requires training • Requires support and consultation from specialty care sources • Requires referral sources be available for more complex cases
Co-location/integrated care	• Care is shared with an embedded behaviorist, usually a social worker or psychologist. • Optimally, scheduling is done in tandem for follow-up visits so that patients receive wraparound care.	• Most comprehensive; Most outpatient cases can be served • Highest likelihood of treatment initiation and follow-up with specialty care • Highest reimbursement	• Most resource intensive • Requires additional space • Requires specialty care providers • Requires complex scheduling procedures for multidisciplinary team visits • Still requires provider to manage medication, unless referred off site • Maximum number of patients who can be treated by a single behavioral health clinician

primary care physicians. This is particularly problematic given the low rate of care linkage when patients are only referred out for mental health concerns.[28] Thus, the task of improving mental health services resides within primary care settings and with providers. Initiating treatment at the initial point of care has been shown to be feasible and efficacious.[29] For more severe and high-risk patients, collaborative treatment through referrals to psychiatric specialty care practice is recommended, so long as continued follow-up in primary care remains ongoing.

28.5. TREATMENTS

28.5.1. Medications

In 2010 more than 250 million prescriptions for antidepressants were filled in the United States (IMS report). Medications are an effective treatment for depression and anxiety. These medications are typically well tolerated and are believed to work by targeting specific neurotransmitters in the brain, effectively changing the way neurons communicate. For approximately half of the depression cases (i.e., mild to moderate) seen in primary care, medication alone is an effective treatment (or psychotherapy alone). For more severe cases, medication and psychotherapy combined is the indicated treatment.

28.5.1.1. SSRIs and Serotonin–Norepinephrine Reuptake Inhibitors

SSRIs were invented in the early 1980s but gained wide popularity when the US Food and Drug Administration approved fluoxetine in 1987. Based on the serotonin hypothesis, these medication classes were developed with the belief that depression was a result of low levels of serotonin in the brain. This concept has been updated to reflect that there are likely additional neurotransmitters implicated in the disorder (e.g., norepinephrine and dopamine). These medications are well tolerated and have low side-effect profiles. Additional information on treatment options is available in other chapters.

28.5.1.2. Sleep Aids

Recent research suggests that treating sleep and correcting drifted sleep cycles can be part of an effective treatment plan for depression. Oversleeping can be a symptom of depression, but more often hyposomnia is the reported symptom, with either difficulty falling asleep or difficulty staying asleep.[30] Additionally, persistent difficulty sleeping has been linked to the development of depressive disorders, and treating insomnia may be effective preventive medicine for depression.[30]

28.5.1.3. Benzodiazepines

Typically thought of as anti-anxiety medications (anxiolytics), this class acts on GABA by increasing its action and creating a sedative effect. While their main function is to reduce anxiety and chances of experiencing an anxiety attack, these medications may occasionally be prescribed for depression in adults. Treatment guidelines suggest that the use of these medications should be sparing and long-term use should be avoided. This medication class has also demonstrated tolerance and a higher propensity for abuse given its potential risks for dependence and withdrawal on discontinuation.[31] Patients with a history of substance or alcohol abuse or post-traumatic stress disorder should not be prescribed this class of medication.[32,33]

28.5.1.4. Non-Benzodiazepine Agents

Several types of medications fall under this category. Sleep-inducing medications called "Z-drugs" and other benzodiazepine receptor agonists are commonly used to treat insomnia, but due to their GABA agonist properties they can lead to anxiety reduction. However, this is often at the cost of a hypnotic effect, among other less desirable side effects. Certain antihistamines and $5\text{-}HT_1$ partial agonists such as buspirone and antidepressants with sedating properties (e.g., sertraline, trazodone, amitriptyline, and mirtazapine) have also proven to be effective for comorbid depression and anxiety symptoms.

28.5.1.5. Other

For more detailed information on additional classes of medications, please refer to the chapters in Section 3 in this volume.

28.5.2. Counseling and Psychotherapy

Traditionally referred to as the "talking cure," counseling usually involves periodic 45- to 60-minute sessions with a mental health professional trained in various modalities and theoretical approaches. The content of these appointments can vary widely. The literature supports that several factors are present in successful treatment. The largest and most significant factors are the therapeutic alliance (including goal consensus and treatment collaboration), empathy, positive regard, therapist factors, and genuineness.[34] Some therapists assign homework, while others may work with the patient to uncover barriers to recovery or engaging in social relationships. Psychologists do not usually have prescriptive authority, but they do have extensive knowledge of the biological underpinnings of depression, anxiety, and other mental health disorders. Therapy is an effective standalone treatment and may also be initiated in conjunction with pharmacotherapy. The majority of the current literature suggests that counseling and medication are equally efficacious for mild to moderate depression, while combination treatment should be reserved for treatment-resistant or severe cases in adults. With the increased focus on treatment of mental health within primary care, there is a need for therapeutic interventions to be provided within that setting by clinicians and other professionals.

28.5.2.1 Cognitive–Behavioral Therapy

Cognitive–behavioral therapy (CBT) is an umbrella term for many approaches to psychotherapy treatment. Although these approaches vary, many of them represent standardized, evidence-based psychotherapy treatments that are time limited and goal oriented. Focused on understanding the relationship among one's thoughts, feelings, and actions and how this can result in mental health difficulties, many patients prefer this treatment because of the easy-to-understand approach. Traditional CBT models follow an 8- to 12-week, 50-minute session course. CBT and various components (e.g., motivational interviewing, problem-solving techniques) are widely used in medical and outpatient psychotherapy settings. CBT has been shown to be an effective treatment for depression, mood disorders, and other mental health disorders.

28.5.2.2. Interpersonal Psychotherapy

Interpersonal psychotherapy is an evidence-based, time-limited treatment, focused primarily on interpersonal difficulties. The number of sessions can range from 6 to 20, depending on the level of emotional distress and the presenting concerns.

28.5.2.3. Problem-Solving Therapy in Primary Care

Originally adapted in the early 1990s, problem-solving therapy in primary care is a brief treatment intervention for depression and anxiety, requiring some training for primary care providers. This modality uses 6 to 10 30-minute sessions with a non-mental health professional (physician, nurse, etc.) to help patients focus on positive action. The focus of these session is "here and now" problems, with a focus on solutions.[35] The underlying theory of this approach is that symptoms of depression and anxiety are likely a consequence of poor problem solving, and that identifying and implementing positive coping strategies will lead to symptom cessation.[36]

28.5.2.4. Other Treatments

There are many other evidence-based psychotherapies that may benefit patients presenting to primary care. Examples include group psychotherapy, dialectical behavioral therapy, psychodynamic psychotherapy, acceptance and commitment therapy, and couple and family therapy. The types of professionals who offer these services also vary. Psychologists, licensed counselors, social workers, and marriage and family therapists may all provide some or all of these services. It is important to develop a relationship with referral resources so that patients are more likely to follow through with your clinical recommendations.

28.5.2.5. Patient Education

Providing information directly to patients and families helps them understand the presenting problem, as well as potential solutions and treatments, in an effort to increase motivation for patients to commit to the therapeutic process.

28.5.2.6. Lifestyle Adjustments

Exercise, fish intake, sleep, the use of melatonin, stress management techniques, healthy eating habits, and meditation/mindfulness exercises are shown to be beneficial for patients with depression.

28.5.3. Special Treatment Considerations

28.5.3.1. Children

Depression in children and adolescents may often manifest as irritability in lieu of or sometimes accompanying sad or down mood. Parents, teachers, and peers may notice increased anger, a higher frequency of arguments, outbursts, and difficulties with social interactions. The appetite symptoms may also present as increased cravings for carbohydrate-rich foods.[37] The rate of teen depression has increased over the last few years to nearly 13%,[12] with some studies citing the onset of a mood disorder in as many as one in seven youth.[38]

28.5.3.2. Older Adults

Older adults may be at a higher risk for the development of depression as a result of various life changes and adjustments. New roles, different responsibilities, potential health concerns, and other stressors could result in a higher incidence of the disorder. In the 65-and-older age group, depression prevalence rates are approximately 1% to 5%.[39,40] Within the general geriatric community, up to 15% of individuals could meet criteria for depression.[41]

28.5.3.3. Gender Differences

Women are at elevated risk for developing depression. The existing literature indicates that the female-to-male ratio for depression is approximately 2:1, which begins to differentiate during adolescence. During preadolescence, depression rates for females and males are nearly identical (1:1 ratio).

28.5.4. Risk Assessment

State and local agencies, as well as certifying and licensing boards, have varying requirements regarding safety assessment, and duty to warn, when a client reports imminent risk. This section will provide a general overview of suicidality and risk assessment. Homicidality and psychotic symptoms can be part of a depressive presentation, although the base rates of this clinical presentation are quite low; specialty care or a call to emergency services is needed.

Because thoughts of death can be a symptom of depression, all patients presenting with symptoms should be screened for risk of harm to self. These thoughts usually present as vague or fleeting ideas about escape (e.g., "I just don't want to deal with this"), a wish for the depressive symptoms to end (e.g., "I want the pain to stop"), or guilt about one's perceived burden on family or friends. Some patients with depression might present with suicidal ideation or a history of suicide attempts. Suicidal thoughts represent a more severe depressive presentation and require additional action by the provider. When you become aware of this information during screening procedures and the clinical interview, it is necessary to ask follow-up questions and formulate a collaborative safety plan. Obtaining additional information about frequency, intensity, planning, and intent will clarify whether immediate action is necessary. Emergent steps include triaging patients to a higher level of care, such as an emergency center or a mental health facility, and providing resources for mental health, the national suicide lifeline, or other local resources. If your client is reporting suicidality, it is important to assess safety and not leave the client alone until you have been able to (1) determine that the client's risk level is appropriate for self-management or (2) secure a more thorough assessment by a qualified mental health professional. If you feel that a patient is not safe to function on an outpatient basis, in many regions it is your duty to notify authorities and maintain chain of custody. It is important to check with your local licensing board to clearly understand your clinical responsibility.

28.6. CONCLUSION

With adequate training and use of MBC principles, primary care providers can appropriately identify and treat depression in various medical settings. The responsibility of implementation ultimately falls on providers and their clinic/facility, as a standardized plan of action and follow-up is necessary from both a clinical standpoint and an ethical perspective. Accrediting bodies such as the AAP and USPSTF have taken various steps toward promoting depression and mental health screening in recent years, yet in order to make this a regular occurrence, barriers related to training, time, cost, and stigma have to be overcome.

A step-by-step process for employing a standardized depression identification, treatment, and follow-up system is as follows:

1. Obtain training on depression, treatment, and the use of MBC principles—many low- or no-cost opportunities are available through accrediting bodies or offered as continuing medical education units.
2. Develop a standardized screening, treatment, and follow-up system within your clinic/facility.
   a. Engage all necessary personnel such as nurses, front desk staff, and other providers.
   b. Implement either paper or electronic screening tools such as the Patient Health Questionnaire (PHQ-9) and Generalized Anxiety Questionnaire (GAD-7). Most questionnaires are available at little or no charge and can be obtained electronically.
   c. Develop a workflow for your clinic that accounts for time taken for patients to complete measures and for you to review the results and to document and counsel accordingly.

    d. Establish a plan for triage when acute issues arise and/or how to manage suicidality concerns.

3. Actively discuss mental health concerns with patients and families. You have already established a working relationship with your patients and developed rapport. Patients are more likely to follow up on your recommendations once trust is created.

4. Collaborate with mental health providers when necessary so that you can refer to or consult with these resources for cases that are more severe.

REFERENCES

1. Sanchez K. Collaborative care in real-world settings: barriers and opportunities for sustainability. *Patient Prefer Adherence*. 2017;11:71–74.

2. Whitebird RR, Solberg LI, Margolis KL, et al. Barriers to improving primary care of depression: perspectives of medical group leaders. *Qual Health Res*. 2013;23(6):805–814.

3. Mark TL, Levit KR, Buck JA. Datapoints: psychotropic drug prescriptions by medical specialty. *Psychiatr Serv*. 2009;60(9):1167.

4. Pence BW, O'Donnell JK, Gaynes BN. The depression treatment cascade in primary care: a public health perspective. *Curr Psychiatry Rep*. 2012;14(4):328–335.

5. Kohler-Forsberg O, Buttenschon HN, Tansey KE, et al. Association between C-reactive protein (CRP) with depression symptom severity and specific depressive symptoms in major depression. *Brain Behav Immun*. 2017;62:344–350.

6. Jha MK, Minhajuddin A, Gadad BS, et al. Can C-reactive protein inform antidepressant medication selection in depressed outpatients? Findings from the CO-MED trial. *Psychoneuroendocrinology*. 2017;78:105–113.

7. Bousman CA, Forbes M, Jayaram M, et al. Antidepressant prescribing in the precision medicine era: a prescriber's primer on pharmacogenetic tools. *BMC Psychiatry*. 2017;17(1):60.

8. Ng CW, How CH, Ng YP. Managing depression in primary care. *Singapore Med J*. 2017;58(8):459–466.

9. Cuijpers P, Sijbrandij M, Koole SL, et al. The efficacy of psychotherapy and pharmacotherapy in treating depressive and anxiety disorders: a meta-analysis of direct comparisons. *World Psychiatry*. 2013;12(2):137–148.

10. DeRubeis RJ, Siegle GJ, Hollon SD. Cognitive therapy versus medication for depression: treatment outcomes and neural mechanisms. *Nat Rev Neurosci*. 2008;9(10):788–796.

11. Horwitz AV. How an age of anxiety became an age of depression. *Milbank Q*. 2010;88(1):112–138.

12. Mental Health Services Administration. *Results from the 2016 National Survey on Drug Use and Health: detailed tables*. Rockville, MD: Center for Behavioral Health Statistics and Quality; 2017.

13. Cheung AH, Zuckerbrot RA, Jensen PS, et al. Guidelines for Adolescent Depression in Primary Care (GLAD-PC): Part II. Treatment and ongoing management. *Pediatrics*. 2018;141(3). doi:10.1542/peds.2017-4082.

14. Zuckerbrot RA, Cheung A, Jensen PS, et al. Guidelines for Adolescent Depression in Primary Care (GLAD-PC): Part I. Practice preparation, identification, assessment, and initial management. *Pediatrics*. 2018;141(3). doi:10.1542/peds.2017-4081.

15. Siu AL, Force USPST, Bibbins-Domingo K, et al. Screening for depression in adults: US Preventive Services Task Force Recommendation Statement. *JAMA*. 2016;315(4):380–387.

16. O'Connor EA, Whitlock EP, Gaynes B, Beil TL. *Screening for depression in adults and older adults in primary care: an updated systematic review*. Rockville, MD: Agency for Healthcare Research and Quality; 2009.

17. Barkil-Oteo A. Collaborative care for depression in primary care: how psychiatry could "troubleshoot" current treatments and practices. *Yale J Biol Med.* 2013;86(2):139–146.

18. Grazier KL, Smith JE, Song J, Smiley ML. Integration of depression and primary care: barriers to adoption. *J Prim Care Community Health.* 2014;5(1):67–73.

19. Katon W, Von Korff M, Lin E, et al. Collaborative management to achieve treatment guidelines. Impact on depression in primary care. *JAMA.* 1995;273(13):1026–1031.

20. Solberg LI, Crain AL, Jaeckels N, et al. The DIAMOND initiative: implementing collaborative care for depression in 75 primary care clinics. *Implement Sci.* 2013;8:135.

21. Richardson LP, Lewis CW, Casey-Goldstein M, et al. Pediatric primary care providers and adolescent depression: a qualitative study of barriers to treatment and the effect of the black box warning. *J Adolesc Health.* 2007;40(5):433–439.

22. Asarnow JR, Jaycox LH, Duan N, et al. Effectiveness of a quality improvement intervention for adolescent depression in primary care clinics: a randomized controlled trial. *JAMA.* 2005;293(3):311–319.

23. Olson AL, Kelleher KJ, Kemper KJ, et al. Primary care pediatricians' roles and perceived responsibilities in the identification and management of depression in children and adolescents. *Ambul Pediatr.* 2001;1(2):91–98.

24. Asarnow JR, Rozenman M, Wiblin J, Zeltzer L. Integrated medical-behavioral care compared with usual primary care for child and adolescent behavioral health: a meta-analysis. *JAMA Pediatr.* 2015;169(10):929–937.

25. Crismon ML, Trivedi M, Pigott TA, et al. The Texas Medication Algorithm Project: report of the Texas Consensus Conference Panel on Medication Treatment of Major Depressive Disorder. *J Clin Psychiatry.* 1999;60(3):142–156.

26. Kobak KA, Greist JH, Jefferson JW, Katzelnick DJ. Computer-administered clinical rating scales: a review. *Psychopharmacology.* 1996;127(4):291–301.

27. Unutzer J, Katon W, Callahan CM, et al. Collaborative care management of late-life depression in the primary care setting: a randomized controlled trial. *JAMA.* 2002;288(22): 2836–2845.

28. Trivedi MH, Daly EJ. Measurement-based care for refractory depression: a clinical decision support model for clinical research and practice. *Drug Alcohol Depend.* 2007;88(Suppl 2):S61–S71.

29. Trivedi MH, Rush AJ, Wisniewski SR, et al. Evaluation of outcomes with citalopram for depression using measurement-based care in STAR*D: implications for clinical practice. *Am J Psychiatry.* 2006;163(1):28–40.

30. Nutt D, Wilson S, Paterson L. Sleep disorders as core symptoms of depression. *Dialogues Clin Neurosci.* 2008;10(3):329–336.

31. Olfson M, King M, Schoenbaum M. Benzodiazepine use in the United States. *JAMA Psychiatry.* 2015;72(2):136–142.

32. DuPont RL. Should patients with substance use disorders be prescribed benzodiazepines? No. *J Addict Med.* 2017;11(2):84–86.

33. Guina J, Rossetter SR, De RB, et al. Benzodiazepines for PTSD: a systematic review and meta-analysis. *J Psychiatr Pract.* 2015;21(4):281–303.

34. Wampold BE. How important are the common factors in psychotherapy? An update. *World Psychiatry.* 2015;14(3):270–277.

35. Oxman TE, Hegel MT, Hull JG, Dietrich AJ. Problem-solving treatment and coping styles in primary care for minor depression. *J Consult Clin Psychol.* 2008;76(6):933–943.

36. Barrett JE, Williams JW, Jr., Oxman TE, et al. Treatment of dysthymia and minor depression in primary care: a randomized trial in patients aged 18 to 59 years. *J Fam Pract.* 2001;50(5):405–412.

37. American Psychiatric Association. *Diagnostic and statistical manual of mental disorders, 5th ed.* Washington, DC: American Psychiatric Association; 2013.

38. Merikangas KR, He JP, Burstein M, et al. Lifetime prevalence of mental disorders in U.S. adolescents: results from the National Comorbidity Survey Replication—Adolescent Supplement (NCS-A). *J Am Acad Child Adolesc Psychiatry.* 2010;49(10):980–989.

39. Hasin DS, Goodwin RD, Stinson FS, Grant BF. Epidemiology of major depressive disorder: results from the National Epidemiologic Survey on Alcoholism and Related Conditions. *Arch Gen Psychiatry.* 2005;62(10):1097–1106.

40. Fiske A, Wetherell JL, Gatz M. Depression in older adults. *Annu Rev Clin Psychol.* 2009;5:363–389.

41. Blazer DG. Depression in late life: review and commentary. *J Gerontol A Biol Sci Med Sci.* 2003;58(3):249–265.

42. IMS Institute for Healthcare Informatics. "The use of medicines in the United States: Review of 2010." 2011.

/// 29 /// PRECISION MEDICINE FOR THE TREATMENT OF DEPRESSION

MADHUKAR H. TRIVEDI, FARRA KAHALNIK, AND TRACY L. GREER

29.1. INTRODUCTION

Major depressive disorder (MDD) is characterized by biological heterogeneity and variable symptom presentation that is not sufficiently captured by clinical assessment alone. As such, diagnosis and treatment selection often follow a trial-and-error paradigm without reference to individual variability in genes, brain structure, function, and/or psychological factors [1]. This likely accounts for the poor prognosis in effectively treating patients with depression. For example, MDD patients typically stay on ineffective medications for too long, switch treatments too early, or simply drop out of care [2–4]. While most individuals show some improvement with initial treatment strategies, remission rates with currently available treatments are low, the duration to attain therapeutic benefit is long, and the treatment-emergent side-effect burden is significant [5–7]. Treatments are selected based on patient or provider preferences as opposed to linking specific treatments to the individual patient [8]. Unlike in other fields of medicine, such as breast cancer [9], asthma [10], macular degeneration [11], and multiple sclerosis [12], there are no available and/or valid biomarkers that enable the field of mental health to move toward precise, targeted treatment for this devastating, lifelong illness. Personalized treatment for patients with MDD will maximize the likelihood of treatment response and continuation and is urgently needed to reduce the suffering and burden experienced by people with this disorder [13, 14].

Clinical, demographic, and lifestyle factors have failed to provide subtypes of depression or moderate treatment outcomes. However, recent advances in technology

475

allow us to examine biological data to potentially clarify the heterogeneity of the disease thus far. Targeted progress has been made regarding the search for biomarkers that are correlated not only with subtypes of the illness but also with treatment response. However, a comprehensive biomarker profile that guides treatment decisions and informs rapid antidepressant response is still lacking. To this end, the National Institute of Mental Health (NIMH)'s Research Domain Criteria (RDoC) initiative was designed to facilitate and encourage a novel approach for this search. RDoC, along with other exciting innovations that explore novel biological pathways or integrate known shared pathways, have the potential to significantly advance the search for breakthrough biomarker discovery.

29.2. FACTORS THUS FAR

A multitude of variables contribute to the clinical heterogeneity of MDD, and each one may hold important modulatory factors that improve treatment outcomes. Examination of broad features, such as demographic characteristics, has provided some signal that could guide future understanding to optimize and personalize treatment decisions. Sex-specific responses to the selective serotonin reuptake inhibitor (SSRI) citalopram have indicated better responses in women than men [15]; racial and socioeconomic factors impact treatment response [16], as do social support [17] or social status [18].

Lifetime severity, chronicity, and complexity of illness also differentially impact treatment response. Remission is more difficult to achieve in patients with greater baseline severity of depression, chronic index episodes [20], longer length of illness [17], family history of mood disorders [17], presence of anxious features [21], and comorbid psychiatric disorders including posttraumatic stress disorder, drug abuse, and hypochondriasis [16].

Despite these significant observations and findings, this literature as a whole has proven to be of limited utility [22–27] when it comes to accurately predicting differential treatment response to antidepressant medications or other treatment strategies.

The limitations of current diagnostic criteria for psychiatric illnesses have led to the RDoC initiative by the NIMH [28]. This institution-wide initiative was designed to guide new ways of designing research questions and studies using known neuroscientific paradigms to inform psychiatric study. In the field of depression, where clinical syndrome-based subtyping has failed to identify personalized treatment, the framework postulated in RDoC offers an exciting and promising way forward. A few constructs, which may drive findings forward, are under current study. For example, aberrant neuroplasticity related to a genetic predisposition and early life trauma appears to be a promising subtype. Further, chronic inflammation may define a subgroup of patients, as suggested by the mouse models and elevated cytokine levels in depressed patients. The comorbidity of metabolic syndrome and depression is another promising avenue to identify subtypes of depression. However, a report by Toups et al. failed to identify obesity as a predictor of differential outcomes with combinations of antidepressant medications [29]. Thus, the continued search for biomarkers will likely require a thorough theoretical rationale to guide the research study followed by appropriately rigorous clinical testing.

There is strong evidence based on the literature that dysregulation in selective cytokines and interleukins reliably produces depression-like symptoms with strong homology to idiopathic MDD. This may provide continued momentum to the previously discussed case study of immune markers as biomarkers to guide antidepressant selection and push it toward a further understanding of the underlying role that inappropriate immune signaling plays in the development of depression. This may eventually support the creation of a new subtype of depression, for example the "immuno-type." Current large-scale studies have already started toward subtyping [30] and may in the near future provide the clear evidence to assign these subtypes before antidepressant treatment. Overall, diagnosis based on a more specific depression subtype will open up new avenues to understanding the pathophysiology of MDD and find the associations of related biomarkers to truly personalize treatment. Thus, biological markers may provide objective measurement to help assess treatment response or suitability [31, 32] and have the potential to bridge the knowledge gap to achieve personalized treatment for MDD.

29.3. INVESTIGATED BIOMARKERS OF ANTIDEPRESSANT RESPONSE

Several biomarkers have been studied in order to improve our understanding of antidepressant treatment response. These biomarkers typically are characterized as blood-based biomarkers (e.g., markers of genetic activity, expression, or transcription; protein changes; or changes in functionality of known regulators) or brain-based biomarkers (e.g., neuroimaging to map changes in neural structure or function).

29.3.1. Blood-Based Biomarkers

It is understood that antidepressant treatment response is likely influenced by an individual's genetic makeup; however, the process of discovering exactly which genes may be most meaningful is ongoing. Chapter 5 provides an excellent overview of our current evidence base for blood-based biomarkers. A few markers do hold some promise to achieve more targeted antidepressant response for the near future, including polymorphisms in the multidrug-resistance gene (MDR1), polymorphisms in serotonin regulation (SLC6A4, HTR2A, among others), messenger ribonucleic acid (mRNA) transcripts, and certain inflammatory markers (e.g., C-reactive protein and several cytokines). However, not all studies can confirm these relationships. In general, most genetic association studies indicate the heritability aspect of antidepressant response and likely also highlight aspects of the known heritability of depression risk. Clinical data indicating the true clinical utility of these biomarkers remain to be discovered.

29.3.2. Brain-Based Biomarkers

Brain-based biomarkers are primarily gathered through neuroimaging techniques to either directly or indirectly image the structure, function, and processes important for pharmacology of the nervous system. Neuroimaging modalities under investigation for biomarkers of antidepressant response include positron emission tomography, magnetic resonance imaging (MRI) of brain structure (structural MRI), functional metabolic activity (functional MRI), diffusion tensor imaging, and electroencephalography. Like much of the blood-based biomarker work, some of the brain-based biomarkers still require additional evidence to push them toward clinical utility. However, some indications of reasonable candidates are appearing. Phillips et al. recently published a detailed review of neuroimaging predictors of antidepressant response [33] and found that baseline predictors of better response to antidepressant medications include hypermetabolism in anterior cingulate cortex (ACC) and increased activity in ACC and amygdala in response to emotional stimuli. Additionally, Mayberg et al. [34] have identified metabolic activity of anterior insula to predict antidepressant response [35]. They found that hypometabolism in anterior insula was associated with a greater likelihood of remission with cognitive–behavioral therapy and poor response to escitalopram [36].

Investigations using electroencephalography have reported greater response to SSRI treatment in patients with a strong response to the loudness dependency of auditory evoked potentials (LDAEP) assessment at baseline, while patients with flat LDAEP respond better to non-serotonergic antidepressant treatment [37–40]. In a recently published report, higher baseline theta activity in rostral ACC was not associated with increased response to antidepressant medication, and this was attributed to previous treatment failures [41]. Cordance, a quantitative electroencephalographic measure related to underlying brain tissue functioning and perfusion [42–44], has been shown to predict antidepressant treatment outcomes in multiple studies [45–49]. The antidepressant treatment response index is calculated from alpha and theta waves measured with five electrodes placed over frontal brain regions at baseline and one week after treatment initiation. The probability of antidepressant response is scored from 0 (low) to 100 (high) [50]. Several studies have reported use of this index to predict response to SSRIs [8, 51] as well as non-serotonergic antidepressants [51, 52]. However, determining the best candidate or candidates for biomarkers still requires further exploration and evaluation.

29.4. COGNITIVE PROCESSES

With the launch of the RDoC framework, increased attention to cognitive processes has led researchers to begin examining the vast elements of cognitive disturbances associated with depression. While the primary symptoms of MDD include depressed mood and diminished interest or pleasure in activities once pleasurable to the person, the diminished ability to concentrate, or being indecisive, is one of the diagnostic criteria for a major depressive episode per the fifth edition of the American Psychiatric Association's *Diagnostic and Statistical Manual of Mental Disorders*. Yet, this symptom definition does not capture the variability of cognitive disturbances that individuals with depression often report. Cognitive dysfunction presents early in the course of disease and is possibly premorbid [53]. Moreover, the presence of cognitive dysfunction in MDD is associated with greater illness severity and poorer functioning than MDD severity alone. Prior research has found no consistent relationship between mood and cognitive impairment, with unresolved cognitive impairment occurring frequently despite improvement in overall depressive symptoms [54]. However, increasing evidence has associated impaired cognition with impaired function, accounting for the link between psychosocial dysfunction (e.g., workplace performance) and MDD [55]. Moving toward defining functional recovery, including cognition, may assist in defining targeted, novel approaches to treating MDD and increasing remission.

Cognitive function is impaired across a wide range of cognitive domains. Part of the movement in the field is to differentiate between cognitive processes that are emotionally dependent ("hot") from those that are independent of emotion ("cold") to aid both diagnostic (subgrouping) and treatment prediction (decision making) in MDD. Treating hot and cold top-down cognition in depression considerations include (1) cognitive–behavioral therapy can train patients to challenge their top-down hot biases (negative expectations) and thereby resolve dysfunctional negative schemata and (2) transcranial magnetic stimulation directly activates the dorsolateral prefrontal cortex and interconnected structures, improving cold top-down cognitive control and emotional regulation. However, dysfunctional monoamine transmission and bottom-up negative biases (negative perceptions) are not treated directly by cognitive–behavioral therapy or transcranial magnetic stimulation and may thus persist. Treating hot bottom-up cognition in depression considerations include (1) antidepressant medications target the monoamine systems (5-HT, NE, and DA), which may be disrupted in some depressed patients, thereby resolving bottom-up hot biases (negative perceptions) and (2) deep brain stimulation in the subgenual ACC may influence circuits instantiating bottom-up negative biases directly, via connections with other regions in limbic circuits. However, top-down negative biases (negative expectations) are not treated directly by antidepressant medications or deep brain stimulation and may thus persist. RDoC has been helpful in aligning constructs with relevant sub-constructs and associated tasks probing systems such as positive and negative valence (similar to hot aspects of cognitions).

Incorporation of biological, neurochemical, and other related biomarkers will more likely lead to better characterization of cognitive function and appropriate treatments, particularly those translational approaches that focus on early resolution of cognitive symptoms to increase function and remission rates.

29.5. DATA-DRIVEN BIOMARKER DISCOVERY

29.5.1. Informatics

Bioinformatics, the study of information processing in biological systems, gained widespread prominence with the large volume of data arising out of the Human Genome Project [56]. Bioinformatics computer programming tools are now widely used to analyze the biological systems in the fields of genomics, transcriptomics, epigenomics, proteomics, and metabolomics. One example is the ongoing Human Connectome Project, which is scanning 1,200 healthy adults and using robust informatics tool to analyze this large volume of data to map the neural network and understand the functional connections in the human brain [57]. Furthermore, the directive from National Institutes of Health to share data for studies that they sponsor [58] has brought these large datasets into the public domain, raising the possibility of crowdsourcing biomarker discovery.

29.5.2. Health Information Technology

The last decade has seen a significant push toward the incorporation of health information technology tools into clinical practice [59, 60]. Most hospitals in the United States now use some form of an electronic health record (EHR) [61]. Patients also contribute data on a regular basis through patient health records [62], allowing for assessments in between clinic or hospital visits. Health information exchanges are being developed to allow information sharing between different EHR systems [63]. Computational tools of natural language processing allow extraction of meaningful information from narrative texts of EHR [64]. Recent initiatives by the Centers for Medicare and Medicaid Services will lead to greater adoption of structured instruments like the Patient Health Questionnaire in routine clinical care. These advances are being used to improve not only the care of patients with chronic medical conditions [65], but also the feasibility of conducting large-scale biomarker discovery studies. For example, Perlis et al. used billing codes and natural language processing from EHR data to develop a scheme of classifying patients with treatment-resistant depression [66]. Using DNA extracted from discarded blood, O'Dushlaine et al. conducted analyses of rare copy number variants in these patients and then used previously collected publicly shared data from the STAR*D cohort to replicate their findings [67]. As we continue to expand research by combining large samples and collecting a variety of clinical and biological variables, bioinformatics and novel statistical methods will become increasingly important.

29.6. AN INTEGRATED APPROACH

Precision medicine takes into account the complex interplay between individual variability in genes, biological function, brain activity, and clinical phenotypes to predict differential treatment response [68]. The individual biomarkers investigated thus far have substantially contributed to our knowledge base. However, to maximize the chances of success, we may need to go beyond individual biomarkers and venture toward generating biosignatures by systematically evaluating combinations of both clinical and biological markers.

Decades ago, the hallmark Framingham Heart Study was initiated to assess the epidemiology of cardiovascular disease (CVD). In 1948, over 5,000 participants were enrolled in the first of three cohorts, which were comprehensively assessed and followed longitudinally for decades. As a result, several individual CVD risk factors—including hypertension, obesity, cigarette smoking, and high cholesterol— were been identified [69, 70] and now serve as gold-standard metrics for heart disease. Importantly, a multivariate "risk score" was also developed and is now the premise for identifying an individual's 10-year risk of developing CVD [71, 72]. The Framingham Risk Score is derived from the integration of data collected across several modalities, including demographics (e.g., age), lifestyle (e.g., cigarette smoking), and biology (e.g., cholesterol). Today, both patients and the general public are much more aware of the contributors to CVD risk, and it is standard clinical practice for physicians to routinely assess this risk, which can provide guidance for both lifestyle changes and preventive treatments. With the Framingham approach in mind, we must strive for the same integrated, comprehensive examination of data that will lead us to a more thorough understanding and awareness of depression.

While informative, these studies largely focused on characterizing individual biomarkers rather than undertaking an integrated biomarker approach that takes into account features that span multiple modalities. Recent studies, such as the Establishing Moderators and Biosignatures of Antidepressant Response for Clinical Care (EMBARC) and the international Study to Predict Optimized Treatment for Depression (iSPOT), are first steps toward this endeavor. Only by *integrating* predictors or moderators across modalities and assessing clinical or biological features *over time* will we develop a better understanding of how these factors affect disease burden and/or treatment outcome, which is what is ultimately needed to significantly move the field forward.

REFERENCES

1. Gelenberg, A., et al., Practice Guideline for the Treatment of Patients with Major Depressive Disorder, 3rd ed. Arlington, VA: American Psychiatric Association; 2010.
2. Burton, C., A.J. Cochran, and I.M. Cameron, Restarting antidepressant treatment following early discontinuation: a primary care database study. Fam Pract, 2015. 43(5): pp. 520–524.
3. Rush, A.J., et al., Selecting among second-step antidepressant medication monotherapies: predictive value of clinical, demographic, or first-step treatment features. Arch Gen Psychiatry, 2008. 65(8): pp. 870–880.
4. Warden, D., et al., Predictors of attrition during initial (citalopram) treatment for depression: a STAR*D report. Am J Psychiatry, 2007. 164(8): pp. 1189–1197.

5. Warden, D., et al., The STAR*D Project results: a comprehensive review of findings. Curr Psychiatry Rep, 2007. **9**(6): pp. 449–459.

6. Trivedi, M.H., et al., Evaluation of outcomes with citalopram for depression using measurement-based care in STAR*D: implications for clinical practice. Am J Psychiatry, 2006. **163**(1): pp. 28–40.

7. Rush, A.J., et al., Combining medications to enhance depression outcomes (CO-MED): acute and long-term outcomes of a single-blind randomized study. Am J Psychiatry, 2011. **168**(7): pp. 689–701.

8. Cook, I.A., et al., Quantitative electroencephalogram biomarkers for predicting likelihood and speed of achieving sustained remission in major depression: a report from the Biomarkers for Rapid Identification of Treatment Effectiveness in Major Depression (BRITE-MD) trial. J Clin Psychiatry, 2013. **74**(1): pp. 51–56.

9. Dowsett, M., and A.K. Dunbier, Emerging biomarkers and new understanding of traditional markers in personalized therapy for breast cancer. Clin Cancer Res, 2008. **14**(24): pp. 8019–8026.

10. Lima, J.J., et al., Pharmacogenetics of asthma. Curr Opin Pulm Med, 2009. **15**(1): pp. 57–62.

11. Lee, A.Y., et al., Pharmacogenetics of complement factor H (Y402H) and treatment of exudative age-related macular degeneration with ranibizumab. Br J Ophthalmol, 2009. **93**(5): pp. 610–613.

12. Vosslamber, S., L.G. van Baarsen, and C.L. Verweij, Pharmacogenomics of IFN-beta in multiple sclerosis: towards a personalized medicine approach. Pharmacogenomics, 2009. **10**(1): pp. 97–108.

13. Kessler, R.C., et al., The epidemiology of major depressive disorder. JAMA, 2003. **289**(23): pp. 3095–3105.

14. Murray, C.J., et al., The state of US health, 1990–2010: burden of diseases, injuries, and risk factors. JAMA, 2013. **310**(6): pp. 591–608.

15. Young, E.A., et al., Sex differences in response to citalopram: a STAR*D report. J Psychiatr Res, 2009. **43**(5): pp. 503–511.

16. Friedman, E.S., et al., Sociodemographic, clinical, and treatment characteristics associated with worsened depression during treatment with citalopram: results of the NIMH STAR(*)D trial. Depress Anxiety, 2009. **26**(7): pp. 612–621.

17. Trivedi, M.H., et al., What moderator characteristics are associated with better prognosis for depression? Neuropsychiatr Dis Treat, 2005. **1**(1): pp. 51–57.

18. Lesser, I., et al., Depression outcomes of Spanish- and English-speaking Hispanic outpatients in STAR*D. Psychiatr Serv, 2008. **59**(11): pp. 1273–1284.

19. Friedman, E.S., et al., Baseline depression severity as a predictor of single and combination antidepressant treatment outcome: results from the CO-MED trial. Eur Neuropsychopharmacol, 2012. **22**(3): pp. 183–199.

20. Rush, A.J., et al., Is prior course of illness relevant to acute or longer-term outcomes in depressed out-patients? A STAR*D report. Psychol Med, 2012. **42**(6): pp. 1131–1149.

21. Fava, M., et al., Difference in treatment outcome in outpatients with anxious versus nonanxious depression: a STAR*D report. Am J Psychiatry, 2008. **165**(3): pp. 342–351.

22. Arnow, B.A., et al., Depression subtypes in predicting antidepressant response: a report from the iSPOT-D trial. Am J Psychiatry, 2015. **172**(8): pp. 743–750.

23. Bobo, W.V., et al., Randomized comparison of selective serotonin reuptake inhibitor (escitalopram) monotherapy and antidepressant combination pharmacotherapy for major depressive disorder with melancholic features: a CO-MED report. J Affect Disord, 2011. **133**(3): pp. 467–476.

24. Chan, H.N., et al., Correlates and outcomes of depressed out-patients with greater and fewer anxious symptoms: a CO-MED report. Int J Neuropsychopharmacol, 2012. **15**(10): pp. 1387–1399.

25. Sung, S.C., et al., The impact of chronic depression on acute and long-term outcomes in a randomized trial comparing selective serotonin reuptake inhibitor monotherapy versus each of 2 different antidepressant medication combinations. J Clin Psychiatry, 2012. **73**(7): pp. 967–976.

26. Sung, S.C., et al., Does early-onset chronic or recurrent major depression impact outcomes with antidepressant medications? A CO-MED trial report. Psychol Med, 2013. **43**(5): pp. 945–960.

27. Sung, S.C., et al., Pre-treatment insomnia as a predictor of single and combination antidepressant outcomes: a CO-MED report. J Affect Disord, 2015. **174**: pp. 157–164.

28. Insel, T., et al., Research domain criteria (RDoC): toward a new classification framework for research on mental disorders. Am J Psychiatry, 2010. **167**(7): pp. 748–751.

29. Toups, M.S.P., et al., Relationship between obesity and depression: characteristics and treatment outcomes with antidepressant medication. Psychosom Med, 2013. **75**(9): pp. 863–872.

30. Lamers, F., et al., Metabolic and inflammatory markers: associations with individual depressive symptoms. Psychol Med, 2018. **48**(7): pp. 1102–1110.

31. Biomarkers Definitions Working Group. Biomarkers and surrogate endpoints: preferred definitions and conceptual framework. Clin Pharmacol Ther, 2001. **69**(3): pp. 89–95.

32. Strimbu, K., and J.A. Tavel, What are biomarkers? Curr Opin HIV AIDS, 2010. **5**(6): pp. 463–466.

33. Phillips, M.L., et al., Identifying predictors, moderators, and mediators of antidepressant response in major depressive disorder: neuroimaging approaches. Am J Psychiatry, 2015. **172**(2): pp. 124–138.

34. Dunlop, B.W., and H.S. Mayberg, Neuroimaging-based biomarkers for treatment selection in major depressive disorder. Dialogues Clin Neurosci, 2014. **16**(4): pp. 479–490.

35. Dunlop, B.W., et al., Preliminary findings supporting insula metabolic activity as a predictor of outcome to psychotherapy and medication treatments for depression. J Neuropsychiatry Clin Neurosci, 2015. **27**(3): pp. 237–239.

36. McGrath, C.L., et al., Toward a neuroimaging treatment selection biomarker for major depressive disorder. JAMA Psychiatry, 2013. **70**(8): pp. 821–829.

37. Gallinat, J., et al., The loudness dependency of the auditory evoked N1/P2-component as a predictor of the acute SSRI response in depression. Psychopharmacology, 2000. **148**(4): pp. 404–411.

38. Juckel, G., et al., Differential prediction of first clinical response to serotonergic and noradrenergic antidepressants using the loudness dependence of auditory evoked potentials in patients with major depressive disorder. J Clin Psychiatry, 2007. **68**(8): pp. 1206–1212.

39. Linka, T., et al., The intensity dependence of auditory evoked ERP components predicts responsiveness to reboxetine treatment in major depression. Pharmacopsychiatry, 2005. **38**(3): pp. 139–143.

40. Lee, T.W., et al., Loudness dependence of the auditory evoked potential and response to antidepressants in Chinese patients with major depression. J Psychiatry Neurosci, 2005. **30**(3): pp. 202–205.

41. Arns, M., et al., Frontal and rostral anterior cingulate (rACC) theta EEG in depression: implications for treatment outcome? Eur Neuropsychopharmacol, 2015. **25**(8): pp. 1190–1200.

42. Leuchter, A.F., et al., Cordance: a new method for assessment of cerebral perfusion and metabolism using quantitative electroencephalography. Neuroimage, 1994. **1**(3): pp. 208–219.

43. Leuchter, A.F., et al., Assessment of cerebral perfusion using quantitative EEG cordance. Psychiatry Res, 1994. **55**(3): pp. 141–152.

44. Leuchter, A.F., et al., Relationship between brain electrical activity and cortical perfusion in normal subjects. Psychiatry Res, 1999. **90**(2): pp. 125–140.

45. Adamczyk, M., et al., Cordance derived from REM sleep EEG as a biomarker for treatment response in depression—a naturalistic study after antidepressant medication. J Psychiatr Res, 2015. **63**: pp. 97–104.

46. Bares, M., et al., The change of prefrontal QEEG theta cordance as a predictor of response to bupropion treatment in patients who had failed to respond to previous antidepressant treatments. Eur Neuropsychopharmacol, 2010. **20**(7): pp. 459–466.

47. Bares, M., et al., Early reduction in prefrontal theta QEEG cordance value predicts response to venlafaxine treatment in patients with resistant depressive disorder. Eur Psychiatry, 2008. **23**(5): pp. 350–355.

48. Bares, M., et al., Changes in QEEG prefrontal cordance as a predictor of response to antidepressants in patients with treatment resistant depressive disorder: a pilot study. J Psychiatr Res, 2007. **41**(3–4): pp. 319–325.

49. Cook, I.A., et al., Early changes in prefrontal activity characterize clinical responders to antidepressants. Neuropsychopharmacology, 2002. **27**(1): pp. 120–131.

50. Leuchter, A.F., et al., Comparative effectiveness of biomarkers and clinical indicators for predicting outcomes of SSRI treatment in major depressive disorder: results of the BRITE-MD study. Psychiatry Res, 2009. **169**(2): pp. 124–131.

51. Leuchter, A.F., et al., Effectiveness of a quantitative electroencephalographic biomarker for predicting differential response or remission with escitalopram and bupropion in major depressive disorder. Psychiatry Res, 2009. **169**(2): pp. 132–138.

52. Caudill, M.M., et al., The antidepressant treatment response index as a predictor of reboxetine treatment outcome in major depressive disorder. Clin EEG Neurosci, 2014. **46**(4): pp. 277–284.

53. Trivedi, M.H., and T.L. Greer., Cognitive dysfunction in unipolar depression: implications for treatment. J Affect Disord, 2014. 152–154: pp. 19–27.

54. Fava, M., et al., A cross-sectional study of the prevalence of cognitive and physical symptoms during long-term antidepressant treatment. J Clin Psychiatry, 2006. **67**(11): pp. 1754–1759.

55. McIntyre, R., et al., Cognitive deficits and functional outcomes in major depressive disorder: determinants, substrates, and treatment interventions. Depress Anxiety, 2013. **30**: pp. 515–527.

56. Hogeweg, P., The roots of bioinformatics in theoretical biology. PLoS Comput Biol, 2011. **7**(3): p. e1002021.

57. Toga, A.W., et al., Mapping the human connectome. Neurosurgery, 2012. **71**(1): pp. 1–5.

58. http://grants.nih.gov/grants/guide/notice-files/NOT-OD-03–032.html Accessed August 17, 2015.

59. Stark, P., Congressional intent for the HITECH Act. Am J Manag Care, 2010. **16**(12 Suppl HIT): p. Sp24–Sp28.

60. Brailer, D.J., Presidential leadership and health information technology. Health Aff, 2009. **28**(2): pp. w392–w398.

61. Adler-Milstein, J., et al., More than half of US hospitals have at least a basic EHR, but stage 2 criteria remain challenging for most. Health Aff, 2014. **33**(9): pp. 1664–1671.

62. Halamka, J.D., K.D. Mandl, and P.C. Tang, Early experiences with personal health records. J Am Med Inform Assoc, 2008. **15**(1): pp. 1–7.

63. Hripcsak, G., et al., The United Hospital Fund meeting on evaluating health information exchange. J Biomed Inform, 2007. **40**(6 Suppl): pp. S3–S10.

64. Ohno-Machado, L., P. Nadkarni, and K. Johnson, Natural language processing: algorithms and tools to extract computable information from EHRs and from the biomedical literature. J Am Med Informatics Assoc, 2013. **20**(5): pp. 805.

65. Young, A.S., et al., Information technology to support improved care for chronic illness. J Gen Intern Med, 2007. **22**(Suppl 3): pp. 425–430.

66. Perlis, R.H., et al., Using electronic medical records to enable large-scale studies in psychiatry: treatment-resistant depression as a model. Psychol Med, 2012. **42**(01): pp. 41–50.

67. O'Dushlaine, C., et al., Rare copy number variation in treatment-resistant major depressive disorder. Biol Psychiatry, 2014. **76**(7): pp. 536–541.

68. Committee on a Framework for Development a New Taxonomy of Disease; National Research Council, Toward Precision Medicine: Building a Knowledge Network for Biomedical Research and a New Taxonomy of Disease. Washington, DC: National Academies Press; 2011.

69. Wilson, P.W., et al., Prediction of coronary heart disease using risk factor categories. Circulation, 1998. **97**(18): pp. 1837–1847.

70. Gordon, T., et al., Diabetes, blood lipids, and the role of obesity in coronary heart disease risk for women: the Framingham study. Ann Intern Med, 1977. **87**(4): pp. 393–397.

71. Kannel, W.B., D. McGee, and T. Gordon, A general cardiovascular risk profile: the Framingham study. Am J Cardiol, 1976. **38**(1): pp. 46–51.

72. Gordon, T., and W.B. Kannel, Multiple risk functions for predicting coronary heart disease: the concept, accuracy, and application. Am Heart J, 1982. **103**(6): pp. 1031–1039.

INDEX

Figures, tables, and boxes are indicated by *f*, *t*, and *b*, respectively, following the page number.

For the benefit of digital users, indexed terms that span two pages (e.g., 52–53) may, on occasion, appear on only one of those pages.